DNA Repair and Genetic Instability

DNA Repair and Genetic Instability

Edited by Adrian Bradley

hayle
medical

New York

Hayle Medical,
750 Third Avenue, 9th Floor,
New York, NY 10017, USA

Visit us on the World Wide Web at:
www.haylemedical.com

ISBN: 978-1-63241-491-5

Trademark Notice: Registered trademark of products or corporate names are used only for explanation and identification without intent to infringe.

Cataloging-in-Publication Data

DNA repair and genetic instability / edited by Adrian Bradley.
    p. cm.
Includes bibliographical references and index.
ISBN 978-1-63241-491-5
1. DNA repair. 2. Genetic disorders. I. Bradley, Adrian.
QH467 .D53 2018
572.864 59--dc23

Table of Contents

Preface

Every book is initially just a concept it takes months of research and hard work to give it the final shape in which the readers receive it. In its early stages, this book also went through rigorous reviewing. The notable contributions made by experts from across the globe were first molded into patterned chapters and then arranged in a sensibly sequential manner to bring out the best results.

DNA molecules undergo chemical reactions which may alter their structure and DNA repair is the process by which such damages are repaired. Significant damage may hinder the RNA transcription process as well as cause mutations in the DNA molecule. Cell aging, apoptosis and cancerous tumors are common outcomes of long-term damage to DNA. Cellular processes such as the stress to reactive oxygen species as well as exposure to ionizing radiation and large amounts of ultraviolet light are sources of DNA damage. This book explores all the important aspects of DNA repair in the present day scenario. Scientists and students actively engaged in this field will find this book full of crucial and unexplored concepts.

It has been my immense pleasure to be a part of this project and to contribute my years of learning in such a meaningful form. I would like to take this opportunity to thank all the people who have been associated with the completion of this book at any step.

Editor

Association between the XRCC1 Polymorphisms and Thyroid Cancer Risk: A Meta-Analysis from Case-Control Studies

Fei-Fei Wu[1], Xiao-Feng He[2], Hu-Wei Shen[3], Gui-Jun Qin[1]*

1 Department of Endocrinology, First Affiliated Hospital of Zhengzhou University, Zhengzhou, China, 2 Department of Research, Peace Hospital of Changzhi Medical College, Changzhi, China, 3 Department of Endocrinology, Peace Hospital of Changzhi Medical College, Changzhi, China

Abstract

Background: The previous published data on the association between the X-ray repair cross-conplementation group 1 (XRCC1) polymorphisms and thyroid cancer risk remained controversial. Hence, we performed a meta-analysis on all available studies that provided 1729 cases and 3774 controls (from 11 studies) for XRCC1 Arg399Gln, 1040 cases and 2487 controls for Arg194Trp (from 7 studies), and 1432 cases and 3356 controls for Arg280His (from 8 studies).

Methodology/Principal Findings: PubMed, CNKI, and EMBASE database were searched to identify relevant studies. Overall, no significant association was found between XRCC1 Arg399Gln (recessive model: OR = 0.95, 95% CI = 0.77–1.15; dominant model: OR = 0.89, 95% CI = 0.75–1.05; homozygote model: OR = 0.92, 95% CI = 0.69–1.23; Heterozygote model: OR = 0.91, 95% CI = 0.80–1.03; additive model: OR = 0.93, 95% CI = 0.81–1.07), Arg194Trp (recessive model: OR = 1.41, 95% CI = 0.62–3.23; dominant model: OR = 1.01, 95% CI = 0.77–1.34; homozygote model: OR = 1.42, 95% CI = 0.55–3.67; Heterozygote model: OR = 1.03, 95% CI = 0.85–1.26; additive model: OR = 1.08, 95% CI = 0.81–1.42), and Arg280His (recessive model: OR = 1.08, 95% CI = 0.56–2.10; dominant model: OR = 1.01, 95% CI = 0.84–1.22; homozygote model: OR = 1.00, 95% CI = 0.51–1.96; Heterozygote model: OR = 1.04, 95% CI = 0.75–1.42; additive model: OR = 1.03, 95% CI = 0.86–1.23) and thyroid cancer risk when all the eligible studies were pooled into the meta-analysis. In the further stratified and sensitivity analyses, significant association was still not found in these three genetic polymorphisms.

Conclusions/Significance: In summary, this meta-analysis indicates that XRCC1 Arg399Gln, Arg280His, and Arg194Trp are not associated with thyroid cancer.

Editor: Jacques Emile Dumont, Universite Libre de Bruxelles (ULB), Belgium

Funding: The authors have no funding or support to report.

Competing Interests: The authors have declared that no competing interests exist.

* Email: qinguijun123@163.com

Introduction

Thyroid carcinomas are the most frequent endocrine malignancies which among these thyroid carcinomas, more than 90 percent are differentiated thyroid carcinomas (DTC). Pathologically, DTC include papillary, follicular, and Hürthle cell carcinoma [1]. To date, exposure to ionizing radiation is the only known risk factor for thyroid cancer [2]. However, there are evidences that some gene variants including DNA repair genes influence on DTC susceptibility. XRCC1 is one of the candidate genes which its variant relationship with thyroid cancer has not been extensively studied [3].

The *XRCC* (X-Ray cross-complementing) genes were initially discovered through their role in DNA damage response caused by ionizing radiation. They are important components of various DNA repair pathways contributing to DNA-damage processing and genetic stability [4]. X-ray cross-complementing gene 1 (*XRCC1*) is involved in the repair of DNA base damage and singlestrand DNA breaks by binding DNA ligase III at its carboxyl and DNA polymerase β and poly (ADP-ribose) polymerase at the

site of damaged DNA [5] and is known to participate in base excision repair (BER) of small lesions such as oxidized or reduced bases, fragmented or nonbulky adducts, and lesions caused by methylating agents [6]. Three common polymorphisms within the *XRCC1* have been identified at codon 194, 280, and 399 (Arg194Trp, Arg280His, and Arg399Gln) [7].

Many studies have reported the association of *XRCC1* polymorphisms at 194, 280, and 399 (Arg194Trp, Arg280His, and Arg399Gln) with thyroid cancer risk [16–25], but the results were inconclusive, some original studies thought that these polymorphisms were associated with thyroid cancer risk, but others had different opinions. In addition, attention has been mainly drawn at a meta-analytical level upon the association of *XRCC1* polymorphisms at 194, 280, and 399 with thyroid cancer risk [8,9]. However, the previous meta-analyses on *XRCC1* Arg194Trp, Arg280His, and Arg399Gln with thyroid cancer risk have shown conflicting conclusions. In order to explore the association between Arg399Gln, Arg194Trp, and Arg280His polymorphisms with thyroid cancer risk, an updated meta-analysis was conducted to summarize the data. Meta-analysis is a good method for summarizing the different studies. It can not only overcome the problem of small size and inadequate statistical power of genetic studies of complex traits, but also provide more reliable results than a single case–control study.

Materials and Methods

Identification and eligibility of relevant studies

A bibliographical search was performed in PubMed, CNKI, and EMBASE database to identify studies that evaluated XRCC1 polymorphisms and thyroid cancer up to April 10, 2014. The search terms used were: (polymorphism or mutation or variant) and (XRCC1 or "X-ray repair cross-conplementation group 1") and thyroid. The search was not limited to language. Additional studies were identified by hand searching references in original articles and review articles. Authors were contacted directly regarding crucial data not reported in original articles. In addition, studies were identified by a manual search of the reference lists of reviews and retrieved studies. We included all the case–control studies and cohort studies that investigated the association between XRCC1 Arg399Gln, Arg194Trp, and Arg280His polymorphisms and thyroid cancer risk with genotyping data. All eligible studies were retrieved, and their bibliographies were checked for other relevant publications. When the same sample was used in several publications, only the most complete information was included following careful examination.

Inclusion criteria

The included studies needed to have met the following criteria: (1) only the case–control studies or cohort studies were considered, (2) evaluated the XRCC1 Arg399Gln, Arg194Trp, and Arg280His polymorphisms and thyroid cancer risk, and (3) the genotype distribution of the polymorphisms in cases and controls were described in details and the results were expressed as odds ratio (OR) and corresponding 95% confidence interval (95% CI). Major reasons for exclusion of studies were as follows: (1) not for cancer research, (2) only case population, and (3) duplicate of previous publication.

Data extraction

Information was carefully extracted from all eligible studies independently by two investigators according to the inclusion criteria listed above. The following data were collected from each study: first author's name, year of publication, country of origin, ethnicity, source of controls, genotyping method, and numbers of cases and controls in the XRCC1 Arg399Gln, Arg194Trp, and Arg280His genotypes whenever possible. Ethnicity was categorized as "Caucasian," "African," (including African Americans) and "Asian." We considered the samples of studies from India and Pakistan as of "Indian'" ethnicity, and samples from Middle Eastern countries as "Middle Eastern" ethnicity. When one study did not state which ethnic groups was included or if it was impossible to separate participants according to phenotype, the sample was termed as "mixed population." We did not define any minimum number of patients to include in this meta-analysis. Articles that reported different ethnic groups and different countries or locations, we considered them different study samples for each category cited above.

Statistical analysis

Crude odds ratios (ORs) together with their corresponding 95% CIs were used to assess the strength of association between the XRCC1 Arg399Gln, Arg194Trp, and Arg280His polymorphisms and thyroid cancer risk. The pooled ORs were performed for dominant model (Arg399Gln: Arg/Gln+Gln/Gln *versus* Arg/Arg, Arg194Trp: Arg/Trp+Trp/Trp *versus* Arg/Arg, and Arg280His: Arg/Gln+His/His *versus* Arg/Arg); recessive model (Arg399Gln: Gln/Gln *versus* Arg/Gln+Arg/Arg, Arg194Trp: Trp/Trp *versus* Arg/Trp+Arg/Arg, and Arg280His: His/His *versus* Arg/His+ Arg/Arg); Homozygote model (Arg399Gln: Gln/Gln *versus* Arg/ Arg, Arg194Trp: Trp/Trp *versus* Arg/Arg, and Arg280His: His/ His *versus* Arg/Arg), Heterozygote model (Arg399Gln: Arg/Gln *versus* Arg/Arg, Arg194Trp: Arg/Trp *versus* Arg/Arg, and Arg280His: Arg/Gln *versus* Arg/Arg), and additive model (Arg399Gln: Gln *versus* Arg, Arg194Trp: Trp *versus* Arg, and Arg280His: His *versus* Arg), respectively. Heterogeneity assumption was checked by a chi-square-based Q test (Heterogeneity was considered statistically significant if $P<0.10$) [26] and quantified using the I^2 value, a value that describes the percentage of variation across studies that are due to heterogeneity rather than chance, where $I^2 = 0\%$ indicates no observed heterogeneity, with 25% regarded as low, 50% as moderate, and 75% as high [27]. If results were not heterogeneous, the pooled ORs were calculated by the fixed-effect model (we used the Q-statistic, which represents the magnitude of heterogeneity between-studies) [28]. Otherwise, a random-effect model was used (when the heterogeneity between-studies were significant) [29]. In addition to the comparison among all subjects, we also performed stratification analyses by ethnicity and histological subtype (papillary thyroid cancer and follicular thyroid cancer). Moreover, the extent to which the combined risk estimate might be affected by individual studies was assessed by consecutively omitting every study from the meta-analysis (leave-one-out sensitivity analysis). This approach would also capture the effect of the oldest or first positive study (first study effect). In addition, sensitivity analysis was also performed, excluding studies whose allele frequencies in controls exhibited significant deviation from the Hardy–Weinberg equilibrium (HWE), given that the deviation may denote bias. Deviation of HWE may reflect methodological problems such as genotyping errors, population stratification or selection bias. HWE was calculated by using the goodness-of-fit test, and deviation was considered when $P<0.05$. Begg's funnel plots [30] and Egger's linear regression test [31] were used to assess publication bias. A meta-regression analysis was carried out to identify the major sources of between-studies variation in the results, using the log of the ORs from each study as dependent variables, and ethnicity and source of controls as the possible sources of heterogeneity. All of the calculations were performed using STATA version 10.0 (STATA Corporation, College Station, TX).

Results

Literature Search and Meta-analysis Databases

Relevant publications were retrieved and preliminarily screened. As shown in **Fig. 1**, 45 publications were identified, among which 17 irrelevant papers were excluded. Thus, 28 publications were eligible. Among these publications, 17 articles were excluded because they were review articles, case reports, and other polymorphisms of *XRCC1*. In addition, one was excluded because the data of genotyping distribution was missing [32]. As summarized in Table 1, 10 articles with 25 case–control studies publications were selected in the final meta-analysis, including 1729 cases and 3774 controls for *XRCC1* Arg399Gln (from 11 studies), 1,040 cases and 2,487 controls for Arg194Trp (from 7 studies), 1,432 cases and 3,356 controls for Arg280His (from 8 studies). **Tables 1** list all essential information such as the publication year, first author, Country, ethnicity, source of controls, and Genotyping method for XRCC1 Arg399Gln,

Arg194Trp, and Arg280His, respectively. Genotype frequencies for thyroid cancer cases and controls were listed in **Table 2–4**. Among these, two separated case-control studies were included from Akulevich et al. [19] and were considered separately. And one publication was analyzed only in dominant model because Sigurdson et al. [25] provide the limited genotyping information for two XRCC1 polymorphisms (Arg194Trp and Arg280His). Among them, six studies focused on PTC (18, 20, 22, 24, 25) and only Santos et al. [16] on both PTC and FTC. All of the cases were pathologically confirmed.

Quantitative synthesis

Table 5 listed the main results of the meta-analysis of *XRCC1* polymorphisms and thyroid cancer risk. For Arg399Gln, there was no significant association between this polymorphism and thyroid cancer risk in any genetic model when all the eligible studies were pooled together. Similarly, the combined results did not showed any association between Arg194Trp/Arg280His polymorphisms and thyroid cancer risk for all genetic models. However, in the subgroup analysis by ethnicity, the results showed that Arg/His genotype was associated with an increased risk of thyroid cancer among Caucasians (dominant model: $OR = 1.43$, 95% $CI = 1.08$–1.89, P value of heterogeneity test $[F_h] = 0.513$, $I^2 = 0.0\%$; additive model: $OR = 1.38$, 95% $CI = 1.05$–1.80, $P_h = 0.551$, $I^2 = 0.0\%$; Heterozygote model: $OR = 1.45$, 95% $CI = 1.09$–1.93, $P_h = 0.495$, $I^2 = 0.0\%$). And carriers of the 399Gln variant allele have a decreased thyroid cancer risk in mixed population (dominant model: $OR = 0.73$, 95% $CI = 0.55$–0.97, $P_h = 0.326$, $I^2 = 0.0\%$; additive model: $OR = 0.73$, 95% $CI = 0.59$–0.92, $P_h = 0.308$, $I^2 = 3.6\%$; recessive model: $OR = 0.56$, 95% $CI = 0.34$–0.93, $P_h = 0.588$, $I^2 = 0.0\%$; homozygote model: $OR = 0.50$, 95% $CI = 0.30$–0.85, $P_h = 0.460$, $I^2 = 0.0\%$). We also detected that the Trp allele of Arg194Trp polymorphism was significantly increased thyroid cancer risk in mixed population (additive model: $OR = 1.49$, 95% $CI = 1.02$–2.17). When subgroup analysis by histological subtype, the results showed that Arg194Trp polymorphism was associated with decreased papillary

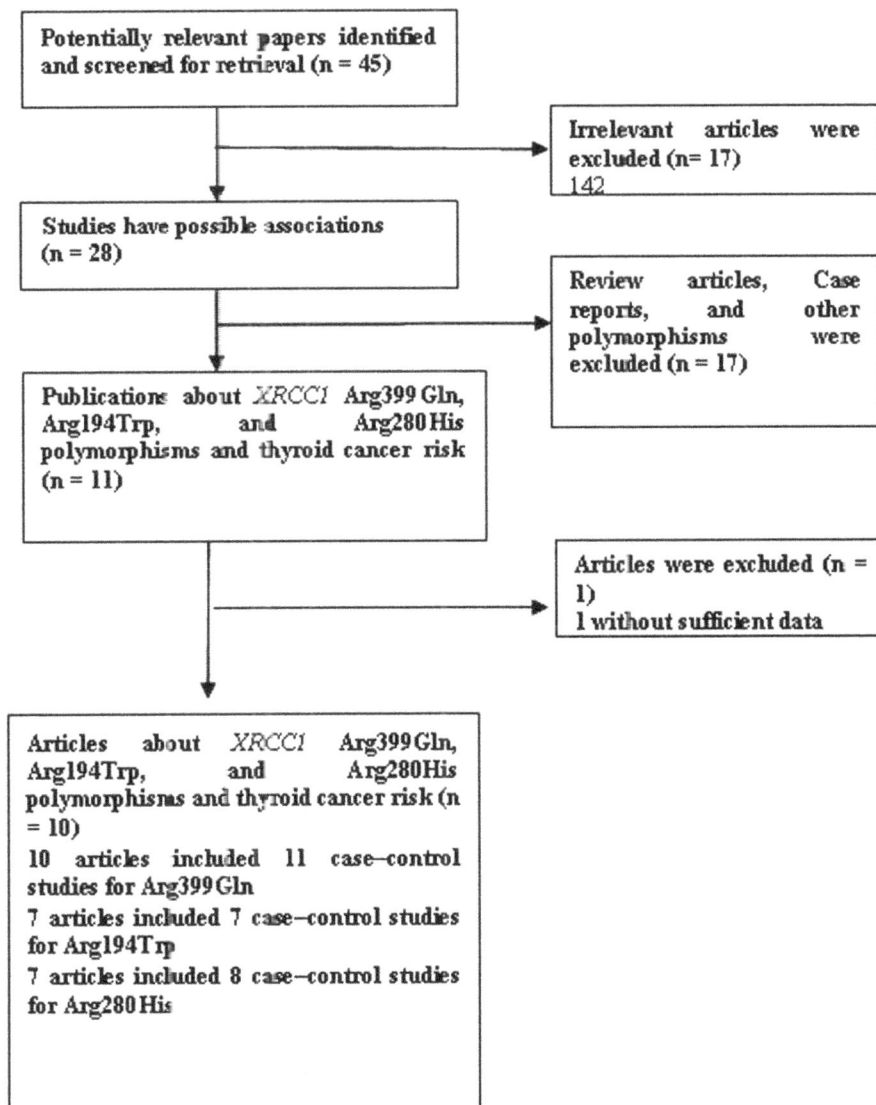

Figure 1. Study flow chart explaining the selection of the 10 eligible articles included in the meta-analysis.

Table 1. Characteristics of studies included in the meta-analysis.

First author	Year	Country	Ethnicity	SC	SNP	Genotyping method
Santos [16]	2012	Portugal	Caucasian	HB	Arg399Gln	PCR-RFLP
Santos [16]	2012	Portugal	Caucasian	HB	Arg194Trp	PCR-RFLP
Fard-Esfahani [17]	2011	Iran	Caucasian	HB	Arg399Gln	PCR-RFLP
Fard-Esfahani [17]	2011	Iran	Caucasian	HB	Arg194Trp	PCR-RFLP
Fard-Esfahani [17]	2011	Iran	Caucasian	HB	Arg280His	PCR-RFLP
Ryu [18]	2011	Korea	Asian	HB	Arg399Gln	PCR-RFLP
Ryu [18]	2011	Korea	Asian	HB	Arg194Trp	PCR-RFLP
García-Quispes [19]	2011	Spain	Caucasian	HB	Arg399Gln	iPLEX
García-Quispes [19]	2011	Spain	Caucasian	HB	Arg280His	iPLEX
Akulevich [20]	2009	RB	Caucasian	HB	Arg399Gln	PCR-RFLP
Akulevich [20]	2009	RB	Caucasian	PB	Arg399Gln	PCR-RFLP
Akulevich [20]	2009	RB	Caucasian	HB	Arg280His	PCR-RFLP
Akulevich [20]	2009	RB	Caucasian	PB	Arg280His	PCR-RFLP
Ho [21]	2009	USA	Mixed	HB	Arg399Gln	PCR-RFLP
Ho [21]	2009	USA	Mixed	HB	Arg194Trp	PCR-RFLP
Ho [21]	2009	USA	Mixed	HB	Arg280His	PCR-RFLP
Siraj [22]	2009	Saudi	ME	HB	Arg399Gln	PCR-RFLP
Siraj [22]	2009	Saudi	ME	HB	Arg280His	PCR-RFLP
Chiang [23]	2008	China	Asian	HB	Arg399Gln	Taqman
Chiang [23]	2008	China	Asian	HB	Arg194Trp	Taqman
Chiang [23]	2008	China	Asian	HB	Arg280His	Taqman
Zhu [24]	2004	China	Asian	HB	Arg399Gln	PCR-RFLP
Zhu [24]	2004	China	Asian	HB	Arg194Trp	PCR-RFLP
Sigurdson [25]	2009	Kazakhstan	Mixed	N	Arg399Gln	Taqman
Sigurdson [25]	2009	Kazakhstan	Mixed	N	Arg194Trp	Taqman
Sigurdson [25]	2009	Kazakhstan	Mixed	N	Arg280His	Taqman

HT, Histological type; RB Russia and Belarus, HB hospital-based studies, N nested case-control studies, PB population-based studies, SC source of controls,

thyroid cancer (PTC) risk in dominant model (OR = 0.71, 95% CI = 0.50–0.99, $P_h = 0.525$, $I^2 = 0.0\%$).

Test of heterogeneity and sensitivity

There was significant heterogeneity among these studies for dominant model comparison (Arg399Gln: $P_h = 0.089$, Arg194Trp: $P_h = 0.088$, and Arg280His: $P_h = 0.061$), recessive model (Arg194Trp: $P_h = 0.041$), homozygote model comparison (Arg399Gln: $P_h = 0.090$, Arg194Trp: $P_h = 0.014$), heterozygote model (Arg280His: $P_h = 0.035$), and additive model comparison (Arg399Gln: $P_h = 0.031$, Arg194Trp: $P_h = 0.019$). Then, we assessed the source of heterogeneity by ethnicity and source of controls. The results of meta-regression indicated that ethnicity (dominant model: $P = 0.039$ for Arg399Gln and $P = 0.001$ for Arg280His; additive model: $P = 0.001$ for Arg399Gln; homozygote model: $P = 0.002$ for Arg399Gln; heterozygote model: $P < 0.001$ for Arg280His) but not source of controls (dominant model: $P = 0.799$ for Arg399Gln and $P = 0.086$ for Arg280His; additive model: $P = 0.500$ for Arg399Gln; homozygote model: $P = 0.388$ for Arg399Gln; heterozygote model: $P = 0.159$ for Arg280His) contributed to substantial heterogeneity among the meta-analysis. Although there were two studies [18,25] deviated from HWE for Arg399Gln polymorphism, the corresponding pooled ORs were not materially altered by excluding these studies in overall and subgroup analyses. However, when the study of Ho et al. [21] was

excluded, the results were changed in mixed population for Arg399Gln (dominant model: OR = 1.06, 95% CI = 0.47–2.40; additive model: OR = 1.00, 95% CI = 0.53–1.88; recessive model: OR = 0.82, 95% CI = 0.19–3.55; homozygote model: OR = 0.86, 95% CI = 0.19–3.92).

For Arg194Trp polymorphism, when one study was excluded, the results were also changed in mixed population (data not shown) and PTC (dominant model: OR = 0.85, 95% CI = 0.55–1.29). For Arg280His polymorphism, when one study was excluded, the results were also changed in Caucasians (dominant model: OR = 1.25, 95% CI = 0.84–1.85; additive model: OR = 1.21, 95% CI = 0.83–1.76; Heterozygote model: OR = 1.28, 95% CI = 0.86–1.90).

Publication bias

Both Begg's funnel plot and Egger's test were performed to access the publication bias of this meta-analysis. Begg's funnel plots did not reveal any evidence of obvious asymmetry in any genetic model in the overall meta-analysis (**Figure 2–4**). The Egger's test results also suggested no evidence of publication bias in the meta-analysis of Arg399Gln ($P = 0.523$ for dominant model, $P = 0.466$ for recessive model, $P = 0.796$ for additive model, $P = 0.598$ for homozygote model, and $P = 0.329$ for heterozygote model), Arg194Trp ($P = 0.224$ for dominant model, $P = 0.758$ for recessive model, $P = 0.618$ for additive model, $P = 0.822$ for

Table 2. Genotype distribution of XRCC1 Arg399Gln polymorphism used in the meta-analysis.

First author	Year	Case			Control			HWE	MAF
		Arg/Arg	Arg/Gln	Gln/Gln	Arg/Arg	Arg/Gln	Gln/Gln		
Santos [16]	2012	46	50	13	87	105	25	0.43	0.36
Fard-Esfahani [17]	2011	78	60	17	83	87	20	0.69	0.33
Ryu [18]	2011	87	17	7	72	19	9	<0.01	0.19
Garcia-Quispes [19]	2011	153	186	47	196	212	66	0.48	0.36
Akulevich [20]	2009	65	53	14	158	193	47	0.30	0.36
Akulevich [20]	2009	55	50	18	75	100	22	0.18	0.37
Ho [21]	2009	133	99	19	220	216	67	0.23	0.35
Siraj [22]	2008	35	13	2	142	72	15	0.16	0.22
Chiang [23]	2008	150	110	23	777	165	27	0.71	0.23
Zhu [24]	2004	49	44	12	57	45	3	0.09	0.24
Sigurdson [25]	2009	12	10	2	460	343	89	0.036	0.29

HWE, Hardy-Weinberg equilibrium; MAF minor aller freqyency; Arg, the major allele, Gln, the minor allele.

Table 3. Genotype distribution of XRCC1 Arg280His polymorphism used in the meta-analysis.

First author	Year	Case			Control			HWE	MAF
		Arg/Arg	Arg/His	His/His	Arg/Arg	Arg/His	His/His		
Fard-Esfahani [17]	2011	146	23	1	173	18	2	0.07	0.06
Garcia-Quispes [19]	2011	337	58	3	426	44	3	0.12	0.05
Akulevich [20]	2009	117	15	0	366	32	0	0.40	0.04
Akulevich [20]	2009	113	10	0	176	19	0	0.47	0.05
Ho [21]	2009	229	22	0	453	50	0	0.24	0.05
Siraj [22]	2009	33	12	5	129	79	21	0.09	0.26
Chiang [23]	2008	224	54	5	349	113	7	0.53	0.14
Sigurdson [25]	2009	24	1		800	96		-	-

HWE, Hardy-Weinberg equilibrium; MAF minor aller freqyency; Arg, the major allele, His, the minor allele.

Table 4. Genotype distribution of XRCC1 Arg194Trp polymorphism used in the meta-analysis.

First author	Year	Case			Control			HWE	MAF
		Arg/Arg	Arg/Trp	Trp/Trp	Arg/Arg	Arg/Trp	Trp/Trp		
Santos [16]	2012	98	8	2	196	21	0	0.45	0.05
Fard-Esfahani [17]	2011	136	18	3	166	20	1	0.64	0.06
Ryu [18]	2011	59	43	9	37	49	14	0.73	0.39
Ho [21]	2009	203	45	3	433	69	1	0.31	0.07
Zhu [24]	2004	50	52	3	48	51	6	0.11	0.30
Sigurdson [25]	2009	20	5		665	241			-
Chiang [23]	2008	127	119	37	234	199	36	0.48	0.29

HWE, Hardy-Weinberg equilibrium; MAF minor aller freqency; Arg, the major allele; Trp, the minor allele.

homozygote model, and $P = 0.293$ for heterozygote model), and Arg280His ($P = 0.656$ for dominant model, $P = 0.236$ for recessive model, $P = 0.821$ for additive model, $P = 0.588$ for homozygote model, and $P = 0.992$ for heterozygote model), respectively.

Discussion

DNA is continuously damaged by endogenous and exogenous mutagens and carcinogens. The damages are fixed by multiple DNA repair pathways including base excision repair, nucleotide excision repair, mismatch repair, and double-strand break repair [15]. Cells with unrepaired DNA damage undergo either apoptosis or unregulated growth to malignancy. A defect or reduced efficiency in repairing DNA damage therefore plays a pivotal role in the development of cancer. One of the DNA repair genes exhibiting polymorphic variation is XRCC1, which is located on chromosome 19q13.2 and encodes a M_r 70,000 protein [10]. XRCC1 (X-ray cross-complementing group 1 protein) is involved in the repair of DNA base damage and single-strand DNA breaks by binding DNA ligase III at its carboxyl and DNA polymerase β and poly (ADP-ribose) polymerase at the site of damaged DNA [11]. Deletion of the XRCC1 gene in mice results in an embryonic lethal phenotype [12]. Chinese hamster ovary cell lines with mutations in the XRCC1 have shown a reduced ability to repair single-strand breaks in DNA and concomitant cellular hypersensitivity to ionizing radiation and alkylating agents [13]. These suggest that XRCC1 plays an essential role in the removal of endogenous and exogenous DNA damage. Three polymorphisms in coding regions of the XRCC1 gene at codons 194 (Arg to Trp), 280 (Arg to His), and 399 (Arg to Gln) have been recently identified [14]. A number of epidemiological studies have evaluated the association between XRCC1 Arg399Gln, Arg194Trp, and Arg280His polymorphisms and thyroid cancer risk, but the results remain inconclusive. In order to resolve this conflict, a meta-analysis was performed to examine the association between *XRCC1* polymorphisms and thyroid cancer risk, by critically reviewing 11 studies on *XRCC1* Arg399Gln (a total of 1729 cases and 3774 controls), 7 studies on Arg194Trp (1040 cases and 2487 controls), and 8 studies on Arg280His (1432 cases and 3356 controls).

Overall, no significant association was found between *XRCC1* Arg399Gln, Arg280His, and Arg194Trp when all the eligible studies were pooled into the meta-analysis. And In the further stratified and sensitivity analyses, significant association was still not found in these three genetic polymorphisms. Zhu et al. [24] in 2004, Santos et al. [16], Sigurdson et al. [25], and Ho et al. [21] reported that the XRCC1 Arg194Trp was not associated with the risk of thyroid cancer. Ryu et al. [18] in 2011, Santos et al. [16], Sigurdson et al. [25], García-Quispes et al. [19], Fard-Esfahani et al. [17], Chiang et al. [23] and Akulevich et al. [20] reported that the XRCC1 Arg399Gln polymorphism was not associated with the risk of thyroid cancer. Sigurdson et al. [25], Fard-Esfahani et al. [17] Akulevich et al. [20], and Chiang [23] et al. reported that the XRCC1 Arg280His polymorphism was not associated with the risk of thyroid cancer. The results of our meta-analysis supported the negative association between XRCC1 Arg399Gln, Arg194Trp, and Arg280His polymorphisms and thyroid cancer risk. However, a careful matching should be considered in future larger genetic association studies including multiple ethnic groups. In the present meta-analysis, between-studies heterogeneity was observed for XRCC1 Arg399Gln, Arg280His, and Arg194Trp. The results of meta-regression indicated that ethnicity but not source of controls contributed to substantial heterogeneity among the meta-analysis of Arg280His and Arg399Gln. Hence, the same

Table 5. Results of meta-analysis for Arg399Gln, Arg194Trp, and Arg280His polymorphisms and the risk of thyroid cancer.

Generic model	n	Recessive model OR (95%CI)	P_h	I^2 (%)	Dominant model OR (95%CI)	P_h	I^2 (%)	Homozygote OR (95%CI)	P_h	I^2 (%)	Heterozygote OR (95%CI)	P_h	I^2 (%)	Additive model OR (95%CI)	P_h	I^2 (%)
Arg399Gln		**Gln/Gln vs. Arg/Gln+Arg/Arg**			**Arg/Gln+Gln/Gln vs. Arg/Arg**			**Gln/Gln vs. Arg/Arg**			**Arg/Gln vs. Arg/Arg**			**Gln vs. Arg**		
Overall	11 (1729/3774)	0.95 (0.77–1.15)	0.160	30.0	0.89 (0.75–1.05)	0.089	39.1	0.92 (0.69–1.23)*	0.090	38.9	0.91 (0.80–1.03)	0.240	21.4	0.93 (0.81–1.07)*	0.031	49.5
Ethnicity																
Caucasian	5 (905/1476)	0.97 (0.75–1.26)	0.822	0.0	0.87 (0.74–1.03)	0.342	11.2	0.91 (0.69–1.19)	0.937	0.0%	0.87 (0.72–1.04)	0.193	34.2	0.92 (0.82–1.05)	0.744	0.0
Asian	3 (499/674)	1.50 (0.64–3.50)	0.086	59.2	1.19 (0.93–1.51)	0.217	34.6	1.56 (0.63–3.86)*	0.067	63.1	1.14 (0.88–1.47)	0.451	0.0	1.15 (0.81–1.63)*	0.086	59.2
Mixed	2 (275/1395)	0.56 (0.34–0.93)	0.588	0.0	0.73 (0.55–0.97)	0.376	0.0	0.50 (0.30–0.85)	0.460	0.0%	0.80 (0.59–1.07)	0.403	0.0	0.72 (0.59–0.92)	0.308	3.6
Histological subtype																
PTC	7 (623/2138)	1.13 (0.82–1.57)	0.323	14.1	0.85 (0.70–1.04)	0.382	5.9	1.02 (0.73–1.43)	0.238	25.1	0.82 (0.66–1.01)	0.620	0.0	0.94 (0.80–1.09)	0.188	31.4
Arg194Trp		**Trp/Trp vs. Arg/Trp+Arg/Arg**			**Arg/Trp+Trp/Trp vs. Arg/Arg**			**Trp/Trp vs. Arg/Arg**			**Arg/Trp vs. Arg/Arg**			**Trp vs. Arg**		
Overall	7 (1040/2487)	1.41 (0.62–3.23)	0.041	56.8	1.01 (0.77–1.34)	0.088	45.6	1.42 (0.55–3.67)*	0.014	65.1	1.03 (0.85–1.26)	0.202	31.2	1.08 (0.81–1.42)*	0.019	63.1
Ethnicity																
Caucasian	2 (265/404)	5.38 (0.89–32.5)	0.591	0.0	1.10 (0.67–1.82)	0.634	0.0	5.37 (0.89–32.5)	0.605	0.0	0.95 (0.56–1.60)	0.509	0.0	1.25 (0.79–1.99)	0.779	0.0
Asian	3 (499/674)	0.88 (0.33–2.32)	0.025	72.9	0.87 (0.52–1.44)*	0.026	72.7	0.78 (0.24–2.52)*	0.007	79.8	0.95 (0.74–1.21)	0.118	53.2	0.90 (0.57–1.43)*	0.006	80.7%
Mixed	2 (276/1409)	6.07 (0.63–58.7)	–	–	1.30 (0.90–1.87)	0.168	47.4	6.40 (0.66–61.9)	–	–	1.39 (0.92–2.10)	–	–	1.49 (1.02–2.17)	–	–
Histological subtype																
PTC	4 (318/1328)	0.71 (0.35–1.40)	0.112	54.3	0.71 (0.50–0.99)	0.525	0.0	0.75 (0.18–3.12)*	0.088	58.8	0.71 (0.49–1.03)	0.314	13.8	0.76 (0.58–1.01)	0.302	16.5
Arg280His		**His/His vs. Arg/His+Arg/Arg**			**Arg/His+His/His vs. Arg/Arg**			**His/His vs. Arg/Arg**			**Arg/His vs. Arg/Arg**			**His vs. Arg**		
Overall	8 (1432/3356)	1.08 (0.56–2.10)	0.957	0.0	1.01 (0.84–1.22)*	0.061	48.2	1.00 (0.51–1.96)	0.958	0.0	1.04 (0.75–1.42)*	0.035	55.9	1.03 (0.86–1.23)	0.118	40.9
Ethnicity																
Caucasian	4 (823/3356)	0.94 (0.25–3.50)	0.614	0.0	1.43 (1.08–1.89)	0.513	0.0	0.99 (0.26–3.70)	0.608	0.0	1.45 (1.09–1.93)	0.495	0.0	1.38 (1.05–1.80)	0.551	0.0
Mixed	2 (276/1399)	–	–	–	0.80 (0.48–1.32)	0.382	0.0	–	–	–	0.87 (0.51–1.47)	–	–	0.88 (0.52–1.46)	–	–
Histological subtype																
PTC	4 (330/1718)	1.10 (0.39–3.07)	–	–	0.87 (0.59–1.29)	0.263	24.7	0.93 (0.33–2.65)	–	–	0.91 (0.61–1.38)	0.173	43.0	0.95 (0.67–1.36)	0.316	13.2

[1] All summary ORs were calculated using fixed-effects models. In the case of significant heterogeneity (indicated by *), ORs were calculated using random-effects models.

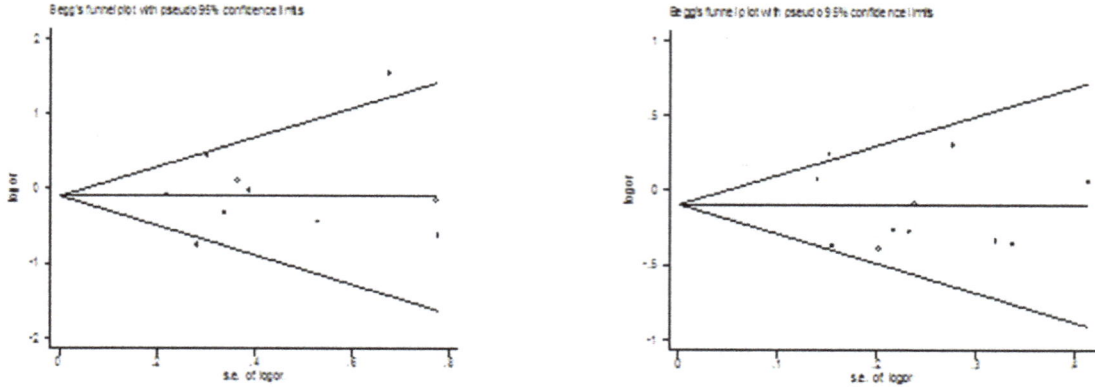

Figure 2. Begg's funnel plot of the meta-analysis of thyroid cancer risk and XRCC1 Arg399Gln polymorphism. (Homozygote model and dominant model).

polymorphisms may play different roles in different ethnicity, because cancer is a complicated multi-genetic disease, and different genetic backgrounds may contribute to the discrepancy. And even more importantly, the low penetrance genetic effects of single polymorphism may largely depend on interaction with other polymorphisms and/or a particular environmental exposure.

Previous meta-analyses on *XRCC1* Arg399Gln, Arg194Trp, and Arg280His polymorphisms with thyroid cancer risk showed conflicting results. The study of Hu et al. [33] suggested that XRCC1 Arg399Gln polymorphism is not associated with differentiated thyroid carcinoma risk, while a decreased risk is observed among Caucasian population. The study of Qian et al. [8] suggested that XRCC1 Arg399Gln polymorphism might be associated with decreased thyroid cancer risk among Caucasians and XRCC1 Arg194Trp may be associated with a tendency for increased thyroid cancer risk in the two larger sample size trials. The study of Bao et al. [9] suggested that Arg280His might contribute to the susceptibility of Differentiated Thyroid Carcinoma (DTC) among Caucasians, whereas it might provide protective effects in Asians against the risk of DTC. Additionally, their results supported the protective role of Arg194Trp polymorphism in developing PTC, and showed evidence of an association between Arg399Gln polymorphism and decreased risk of DTC in mixed population. The study of Du et al. [34] suggested that XRCC1 Arg194Trp may be a risk factor for DTC development.

The study of Wang et al. [35] demonstrated that the XRCC1 Arg399Gln, Arg194Trp, and Arg280His may be associated with developing of thyroid cancer. However, the results of the present meta-analysis are not in accordance with those reported by the previous meta-analysis [8,9,33–35]. Our meta-analysis indicates that XRCC1 Arg399Gln, Arg280His, and Arg194Trp are not associated with thyroid cancer. Our results seem to confirm and establish the trend in the meta-analysis of the XRCC1 Arg399Gln, Arg280His, and Arg194Trp polymorphisms because this meta-analysis performed a more complete sensitivity analysis than the previous meta-analysis [8,9,33–35]. We found that previous meta-analysis [8,9,33–35] did not seriously perform the sensitivity analysis. hence, their meta-analysis results may be inaccurate.

There are several limitations in this meta-analysis. First, the controls were not uniformly defined. Although most of them were common populations, some controls were population-based; other controls were hospital-based. Hence, non–differential misclassification bias is possible. Second, in the subgroup analysis may have had insufficient statistical power to check an association, Third, we were also unable to examine the interactions among gene-environment, lacking of the original data of the included studies limited our further evaluation of potential interactions, which may be an important component of the association between XRCC1 Arg399Gln, Arg280His, and Arg194Trp polymorphisms and environment and thyroid cancer risk. Four, it was much difficult

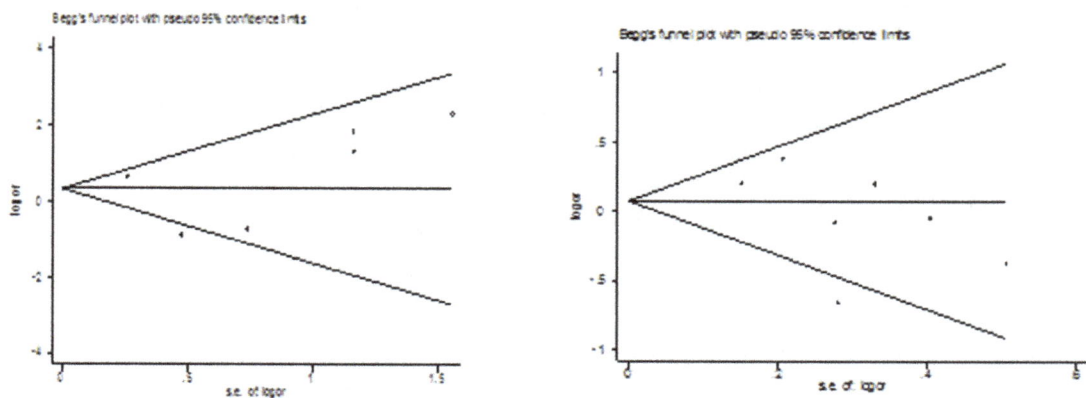

Figure 3. Begg's funnel plot of the meta-analysis of thyroid cancer risk and XRCC1 Arg194Trp polymorphism. (Homozygote model and dominant model).

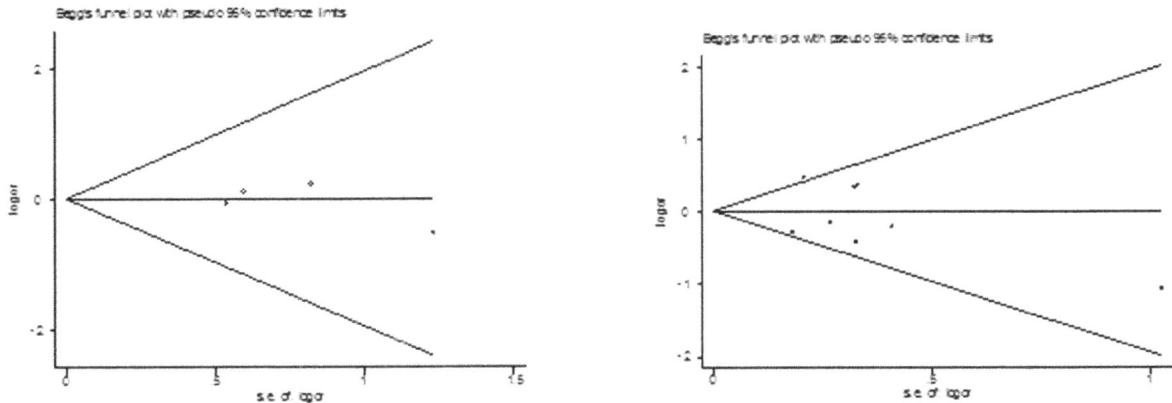

Figure 4. Begg's funnel plot of the meta-analysis of thyroid cancer risk and XRCC1 Arg194Trp polymorphism. (Homozygote model and dominant model).

to get the all articles published in various language. Last, our results were based on unadjusted published estimates. Because of data limitations, we were unable to adjust them such as age and alcohol consumption et al. Our meta-analysis also has several strengths. First, a meta-analysis of the association of XRCC1 Arg399Gln, Arg280His, and Arg194Trp polymorphisms with thyroid cancer risk is statistically more powerful than any single study. Second, the quality of eligible studies included in current meta-analysis was satisfactory and met our inclusion criterion.

In summary, this meta-analysis indicates that XRCC1 Arg399Gln, Arg280His, and Arg194Trp are not associated with thyroid cancer. However, it is necessary to conduct large sample studies using standardized unbiased genotyping methods, homogeneous cancer patients and well-matched controls. Moreover, further studies estimating the effect of gene–gene and gene–

environment interactions may eventually lead to our better, comprehensive understanding of the association between the XRCC1 Arg399Gln, Arg280His, and Arg194Trp polymorphisms and thyroid cancer risk.

Supporting Information

Checklist S1　PRISMA Checklist.

Author Contributions

Conceived and designed the experiments: FFW EWS GJQ. Performed the experiments: FFW HWS. Analyzed the data: XFH FFW. Contributed reagents/materials/analysis tools: FFW XFH GJQ. Wrote the paper: FFW XFH.

References

1. Wein RO, Weber RS (2005) Contemporary management of differentiated thyroid carcinoma. Otolaryngol Clin North Am 38:161–178.
2. Prestor-Martin S, Franceschi S, Ron E, Negri E (2003) Thyroid cancer pooled analysis from 14 case–control studies: what have we learned? Cancer Causes Control 14:787–789.
3. Akulevich NM, Saenko VA, Rogounovitch TI, Drozd VM, Lushnikov EF, et al. (2009) Polymorphisms of DNA damage response genes in radiation-related and sporadic papillary thyroid carcinoma. Endocr Relat Cancer 16:491–503.
4. Thacker J, Zdzienicka MZ (2003) The mammalian XRCC genes: their roles in DNA repair and genetic stability. DNA Repair (Amst) 2:655–672.
5. Caldecott KW, Aoufouchi S, Johnson P, Shall S (1996) XRCC1 polypeptide interacts with DNA polymerase beta and possibly poly (ADP-ribose) polymerase, and DNA ligase III is a novel molecular nick-sensor in vitro. Nucleic Acids Res 24:4387–4397.
6. Caldecott KW (2003) XRCC1 and DNA strand break repair. DNA Repair (Amst) 2:955–969.
7. Shen MR, Jone IM, Mohrenweiser H (1998) Nonconservative amino acid substitution variants exist at polymorphic frequency in DNA repair genes in healthy humans. Cancer Res 58:604–608.
8. Qian K, Liu KJ, Xu F, Chen XY, Chen GN, et al. (2012) X-Ray Repair Cross-Complementing Group 1(XRCC1) Genetic Polymorphisms and Thyroid Carcinoma Risk: a Meta-Analysis. Asian Pac J Cancer Prev 13:6385–6390.
9. Bao Y, Jiang L, Zhou JY, Zou JJ, Zheng JY, et al. (2013) XRCC1 Gene Polymorphisms and the Risk of Differentiated Thyroid Carcinoma (DTC): A Meta-Analysis of Case–Control Studies. PLoS One 2013;8:e64851.
10. Lamerdin J, Montgomery M, Stilwagen S, Scheidecker L, Tebbs R, et al. (1995) Genomic sequence comparison of the human and mouse XRCC1 DNA repair gene regions. Genomics 25:547–554.
11. Caldecott KW, Aoufouchi S, Johnson P, Shall S (1996) XRCC1 polypeptide interacts with DNA polymerase? and possibly poly(ADP-ribose) polymerase, and DNA ligase III is a novel molecular "nick sensor" in vitro. Nucleic Acids Res 24:4387–4397.
12. Tebbs RS, Flannery ML, Meneses JJ, Hartmann A, Tucker JD, et al. (1999) Requirement for the Xrcc1 DNA base excision repair gene during early mouse development. Dev Biol 208:513–529.
13. Shen MR, Zdzienicka MZ, Mohrenweiser H, Thompson LH, Thelen MP (1998) Mutations in hamster single-strand break repair gene XRCC1 causing defective DNA. Nucleic Acids Res 26:1032–1037.
14. Shen MR, Jones IM, Mohrenweiser H (1998) Nonconservative amino acid substitution variants exist at polymorphic frequency in DNA repair genes in healthy humans. Cancer 58:604–608.
15. Goode EL, Ulrich CM, Potter JD (2002) Polymorphisms in DNA repair genes and associations with cancer risk. Cancer Epidemiol Biomark Prev 11:1513–1530.
16. Santos LS, Branco SC, Silva SN, Azevedo AP, Gil OM, et al. (2012) Polymorphisms in base excision repair genes and thyroid cancer risk. Oncol Rep 28:1859–1868.
17. Fard-Esfahani P, Fard-Esfahani A, Fayaz S, Gharbarzadeh B, Saidi P, et al. (2011) Association of Arg194Trp, Arg280His and Arg399Gln polymorphisms in X-ray repair cross-complementing group gene and risk of differentiated thyroid carcinoma in Iran. Iran Biomed J 15:73–78.
18. Ryu RA, Tae K, Min HJ, Jeong JH, Cho SH, et al. (2011) XRCC1 polymorphisms and risk of papillary thyroid carcinoma in a Korean sample. J Korean Med Sci 26:991–995.
19. García-Quispes WA, Pérez-Machado G, Akdi A, Pastor S, Galofré P, et al. (2011) Association studies of OGG1, XRCC, XRCC2 and XRCC3 polymorphisms with differentiated thyroid cancer. Mutat Res 709–710:67–72.
20. Akulevich NM, Saenko VA, Rogounovitch TI, Drozd VM, Lushnikov EF, et al. (2009) Polymorphisms of DNA damage response genes in radiation-related and sporadic papillary thyroid carcinoma. Endocr Relat Cancer 16:491–503.
21. Ho T, Li G, Lu J, Zhao C, Wei Q, et al. (2009) Association of XRCC1 polymorphisms and risk of differentiated thyroid carcinoma: a case–control analysis. Thyroid 19:129–135.
22. Siraj AK, Al-Rasheed M, Ibrahim M, Siddiqui K, Al-Dayel F, et al. (2008) RAD52 polymorphisms contribute to the development of papillary thyroid cancer susceptibility in Middle Eastern population. J Endocrinol Invest 31:893–899.
23. Chiang FY, Wu CW, Hsiao PJ, Kuo WR, Lee KW, et al. (2008) Association between polymorphisms in DNA base excision repair genes XRCC1, APE1, and ADPRT and differentiated thyroid carcinoma. Clin Cancer Res 14:5919–5924.

24. Zhu QX, Bian JC, Shen Q, Jiang F, Tang HW, et al. (2004) Genetic polymorphisms in X-ray repair cross-complementing gene 1 and susceptibility to papillary thyroid carcinoma. Zhonghua Liu Xing Bing Xue Za Zhi 25:702–705.
25. Sigurdson AJ, Land CE, Bhatti P, Pineda M, Brenner A, et al. (2009) Thyroid nodules, polymorphic variants in DNA repair and RET-related genes, and interaction with ionizing radiation exposure from nuclear tests in Kazakhstan. Radiat Res 171:77–88.
26. Davey SG, Egger M (1997) Meta-analyses of randomized controlled trials. Lancet 350:1182.
27. Higgins JP, Thompson SG, Deeks JJ, Altman DG (2003) Measuring inconsistency in meta-analysis. Br Med J 327:557–560.
28. Mantel N, Haenszel W (1959) Statistical aspects of the analysis of data from retrospective studies of disease. Natl Cancer Inst 22:719–748.
29. DerSimonian R, Laird N (1986) Meta-analysis in clinical trials. Control Clin Trials 7:177–188.
30. Begg CB, Mazumdar M (1994) Operating characteristics of a rank correlation test for publication bias. Biometrics 50:1088–1101.
31. Egger M, Smith DG, Schneider M, Minder C (1997) Bias in meta-analysis detected by a simple, graphical test. Br Med J 315:629–634.
32. Neta G, Brenner AV, Sturgis EM, Pfeiffer RM, Hutchinson AA, et al. (2011) Common genetic variants related to genomic integrity and risk of papillary thyroid cancer. Carcinogenesis 32: 1231–1237.
33. Hu Z, Hu X, Long J, Su L, Wei B (2013) XRCC1 polymorphisms and differentiated thyroid carcinoma risk: a meta-analysis. Gene 528:67–73.
34. Du Y, Han LY, Li DD, Liu H, Gao YH, et al. (2013) Associations between XRCC1 Arg399Gln, Arg194Trp, and Arg280His polymorphisms and risk of differentiated thyroid carcinoma: a meta-analysis. Asian Pac J Cancer Prev 14:5483–5487.
35. Wang C, Ai Z (2014) Association of XRCC1 polymorphisms with thyroid cancer risk. Tumour Biol 35:4791–4797.

2

Impact of α-Targeted Radiation Therapy on Gene Expression in a Pre-Clinical Model for Disseminated Peritoneal Disease when Combined with Paclitaxel

Kwon Joong Yong, Diane E. Milenic, Kwamena E. Baidoo, Martin W. Brechbiel*

Radioimmune & Inorganic Chemistry Section, Radiation Oncology Branch, National Cancer Institute, National Institutes of Health, Bethesda, Maryland, United States of America

Abstract

To better understand the molecular basis of the enhanced cell killing effected by the combined modality of paclitaxel and ^{212}Pb-trastuzumab (Pac/^{212}Pb-trastuzumab), gene expression in LS-174T i.p. xenografts was investigated 24 h after treatment. Employing a real time quantitative PCR array (qRT-PCR array), 84 DNA damage response genes were quantified. Differentially expressed genes following therapy with Pac/^{212}Pb-trastuzumab included those involved in apoptosis (*BRCA1, CIDEA, GADD45α, GADD45γ, GML, IP6K3, PCBP4, PPP1R15A, RAD21,* and *p73*), cell cycle (*BRCA1, CHK1, CHK2, GADD45α, GML, GTSE1, NBN, PCBP4, PPP1R15A, RAD9A,* and *SESN1*), and damaged DNA repair (*ATRX, BTG2, EXO1, FEN1, IGHMBP2, OGG1, MSH2, MUTYH, NBN, PRKDC, RAD21,* and *p73*). This report demonstrates that the increased stressful growth arrest conditions induced by the Pac/^{212}Pb-trastuzumab treatment suppresses cell proliferation through the regulation of genes which are involved in apoptosis and damaged DNA repair including single and double strand DNA breaks. Furthermore, the study demonstrates that ^{212}Pb-trastuzumab potentiation of cell killing efficacy results from the perturbation of genes related to the mitotic spindle checkpoint and BASC (BRCA1-associated genome surveillance complex), suggesting cross-talk between DNA damage repair and the spindle damage response.

Editor: Subhra Mohapatra, University of South Florida, United States of America

Funding: This research was supported by the Intramural Research Program of the National Institutes of Health, National Cancer Institute, Center for Cancer Research, and AREVA Med LLC. The funders had no role in study design, data collection and analysis, decision to publish, or preparation of the manuscript.

* Email: martinwb@mail.nih.gov

Introduction

Microtubule-targeting cancer therapies, such as paclitaxel (Pac), perturb the dynamics of the mitotic spindle, blocking cells in mitosis from progressing through the cell cycle by activating the mitotic checkpoint. Paclitaxel is an FDA approved chemotherapeutic treatment for ovarian, breast, and lung carcinomas [1,2]. This chemotherapeutic has been combined with low LET photon radiation for the treatment of cancer. High LET radiation such as α-particles, however, is more effective in cell killing than low LET radiation [3–5]. To take advantage of the cell killing efficiency of α-radiation, α-emitting radionuclides have been successfully carried on vector antibodies in radioimmunotherapy (RIT) to effect targeted therapy of cancer [6–9]. In combination with chemotherapeutics, such as gemcitabine and paclitaxel, highly enhanced therapeutic efficacy has been demonstrated by the α-particle targeted radioimmunotherapeutic ^{212}Pb-trastuzumab [10,11]. Application of α-emitter immunoconjugates, such as ^{212}Pb-trastuzumab either as monotherapy or in combination with chemotherapeutics, are promising therapeutic options for treatment of carcinomas that are characterized by dissemination of single tumor cells in the peritoneum like ovarian or gastric cancer. This success has translated to an ongoing Phase I human clinical

trial at the University of Alabama with 16 patients treated to date [12].

Exposure of cells to ionizing radiation activates multiple signal transduction pathways resulting in complex alterations in gene expression. Despite a long history of studies regarding the mechanisms of action of paclitaxel and photon radiation used individually, little is understood about how paclitaxel and radiation together promote *in vivo* tumor cell death. In particular, gene modulations associated with the cytocidal response have not been clearly defined following exposure of cells to α-particle RIT combined with paclitaxel [13,14]. A recent report from this laboratory showed that paclitaxel potentiates ^{212}Pb-trastuzumab cytotoxicity, in part, by perturbing the mitotic spindle checkpoint [15]. Gene expression profiling provides a potentially powerful approach towards understanding the molecular basis of the cellular response to therapeutic agents. The use of high LET radiation such as α-particles originating from radionuclides such as ^{211}At and ^{213}Bi on different biological systems has identified gene expression profiles [16,17]. Irradiation results in major damage to DNA while paclitaxel affects microtubules. Modifications in gene expression invoked by Pac/^{212}Pb-trastuzumab may thus derive mainly from perturbation of the microtubule network and DNA damage signaling pathways. In order to better understand the molecular basis of the therapeutic efficacy of targeted α-radiation in combination with paclitaxel, changes in gene expression induced by Pac/^{212}Pb-trastuzumab therapy were investigated. For this purpose, mice bearing human colon cancer LS-174T i.p. xenografts were pre-treated with paclitaxel, followed 24 h later by treatment with ^{212}Pb-trastuzumab. The gene expression of LS-174T i.p. tumor xenografts from mice that received paclitaxel plus specifically targeted α-RIT (^{212}Pb-trastuzumab) was compared to paclitaxel plus a non-specifically labeled control (^{212}Pb-HuIgG), paclitaxel alone, and untreated control tumors. Gene expression was quantified using a real time quantitative PCR (qRT-PCR) array covering 84 genes in the DNA damage signaling pathway.

Materials and Methods

Cell line

The human colon carcinoma cell line (LS-174T) was used for all *in vivo* studies. LS-174T was grown in supplemented Dubelcco's Modified Eagle's Medium (DMEM) as previously described in the published reference [18]. All media and supplements were obtained from Lonza (Walkersville, MD). The cell line has been screened for mycoplasma and other pathogens before *in vivo* use according to National Cancer Institute (NCI) Laboratory Animal Sciences Program policy. No authentication of the cell line was conducted by the authors.

Chelate synthesis, mAb conjugation, and radiolabeling

The synthesis, characterization, and purification of the bifunctional ligand TCMC has been previously described [19]. Trastuzumab (Genentech, South San Francisco, CA) was conjugated with TCMC by established methods using a 10-fold molar excess of ligand to mAb. A 10 mCi (0.37 GBq) ^{224}Ra/^{212}Pb generator was purchased from AlphaMed (Lakewood, NJ). HuIgG was also conjugated with the TCMC ligand and radiolabeled, providing a non-specific control antibody for the experiments.

Tumor model, treatment, and tumor harvesting

Studies were performed with 19–21 g female athymic mice (NCI-Frederick) bearing intraperitoneal (i.p.) LS-174T xenografts as previously reported [19]. The viability of the LS-174T cells (> 95%) was determined using trypan-blue. Athymic mice were injected i.p. with 1×10^8 LS-174T cells in 1 mL of DMEM. The inoculum size for this cell line represents the minimum amount of cells required for tumor growth in 100% of the mice. Two days after tumor cell inoculation, the mice (n = 10–15) were given i.p. injections of paclitaxel (600 μg; Hospira, Inc, Lake Forest, IL). ^{212}Pb-trastuzumab ((10 μCi (0.37 MBq) in 0.5 mL PBS)) was administered i.p. to the mice 24 h later. Mice were euthanized in their home cages with the specialized euthanasia lid attached to the CO$_2$ line. The flow rate of CO$_2$ was 2 L/min. When breathing ceases for all mice, the mice were removed from the CO$_2$-filled cage. After euthanasia, the tumor tissues from the 24 h time point were pooled together, macroscopically inspected, and adherent tissues were removed. The tumor tissues were then thoroughly rinsed in ice-cold PBS 3 times, divided, and processed accordingly for each assay. This treatment group was compared with sets of tumor bearing mice (n = 10–15) that received paclitaxel or Pac/^{212}Pb-HuIgG. All animal protocols were approved by the NCI Animal Care and Use Committee.

RNA purification

Total RNA was isolated from harvested tumor tissues using the RNeasy Mini Kit (Qiagen, Santa Clarita, CA) according to the manufacturer's instruction and stored at −80°C until assayed.

Purity of isolated total RNA was measured using a NanoDrop spectrophotometer (Thermo Scientific, Wilmington, DE) and PCR with β-actin primers. Only total RNA with A260/A280 ratio >1.9 and without detectable contamination of DNA (PCR) were employed for gene expression array (qRT-PCR array).

Human DNA damage PCR array

The cDNA were reverse transcribed from RNA using the First Strand cDNA Synthesis Kit (SABiosciences, Frederick, MD). Comparison of the relative expression of the 84 DNA damage related genes was characterized by human DNA Damage PCR array (SABiosciences) and the RT^2 real-time SYBR Green/Rox PCR master mix (SABiosciences) on a 7500 real time PCR system (Applied Biosystems, Rockville, MD). The array includes genes involved in apoptosis, cell cycle and damaged DNA binding and repair (Table S1). Data was analyzed using the RT^2 Profiler PCR Array Data Analysis v3.5 software (Qiagen). The fold change in gene expression was calculated using the equation $2(-\Delta\Delta C_T)$. In cases in which a gene was down-regulated (less than 1 fold change), the value was reported as the negative inverse.

Chromatin immunoprecipitation

The chromatin immunoprecipitation (ChIP) assay kit (Upstate Biotechnology, Billerica, MA) was utilized according to the manufacturer's instructions with minor adjustments. The lysates were prepared and aliquoted. Ten μL of antibody (1:100) for E2F1 (Upstate Biotechnology) was added to a lysate aliquot; the resulting DNA-protein complexes were isolated by protein G agarose beads. The samples were subjected to 65°C for 5 h, the DNA extracted, and dissolved in elution reagent. The immunoprecipitated DNA was amplified by PCR using *BRCA1* and *p73* promoter specific primers (Applied Biosystems) and analyzed by electrophoresis using 2% agarose gels.

Immunblot analysis

Immunoblot analysis following standard procedures was performed with total protein isolates using tissue protein extraction reagent (Thermo Scientific, Asheville, NC) containing protease inhibitors (Roche, Indianapolis, IN). Fifty μg of total protein per lane was separated on a 4–20% tris-glycine gel and transferred to a nitrocellulose membrane. Antibodies against MAD2 (Cell Signaling, Beverly, MA), CYCLIN B1, EMI1, and GEMININ (SantaCruz, Santa Cruze, CA) were used at a dilution of 1:1000 in PBS containing 5% BSA and 0.05% Tween-20. Horseradish peroxidase conjugated rabbit secondary antibodies were used at 1:5000 in 3% non-fat dry milk. The blots were developed using the ECL plus chemoluminescent detection kit (GE Healthcare, Pascataway, NJ and images were acquired using a Fuji LAS 4000 imager (GE Healthcare, Pascataway, NJ).

Statistics

A minimum of at least three independent experiments were conducted for each treatment described. Student *t* test was used for paired data and multiple comparisons were performed with the ANOVA. A *p*-value <0.05 was considered statistically significant.

Results

To explore the molecular basis of α-particle RIT in combination with paclitaxel therapy in LS-174T i.p. xenografts, qRT-PCR array was employed for gene expression analysis of 84 genes of the DNA damage signaling pathway in three independent experiments. The qRT-PCR array identified the genes significantly up- or down-regulated at 24 h after radioactivity injection. Each treatment group was separately compared with the untreated group using a 2-fold change cut-off.

Pac/²¹²Pb-trastuzumab-induced cell killing is associated with an increased expression of genes involved in apoptosis

Of the 84 genes examined (Table S1), 13 genes are involved in regulation of the apoptotic process and eight of those genes (*CIDEA, GADD45α, GADD45γ, GML, IP6K3, PCBP4, PPP1R15A,* and *p73*) were up-regulated in tumors collected from mice treated with Pac/²¹²Pb-trastuzumab (Table 1). Of these up-regulated genes, the greatest impact was on the expression of *CIDEA* (14.0-fold increase, $p<0.0067$), *GML* (26.4-fold increase, $p<0.0004$), and *IP6K3* (18.1-fold increase, $p<0.0001$) in the LS-174T tumor xenografts. There was also a clear difference between this group and the groups that received the Pac/²¹²Pb-HuIgG or only Pac (Pac/²¹²Pb-trastuzumab *vs* paclitaxel, $p<0.01$; Pac/²¹²Pb-trastuzumab *vs* Pac/²¹²Pb-HuIgG, $p<0.01$). Among the other genes for which an up-regulation of expression was noted, the differences between the Pac/²¹²Pb-trastuzumab and Pac/²¹²Pb-HuIgG were either modest (GADD45α), or negligible (GADD45γ and PCBP4). Treatment with either Pac/²¹²Pb-trastuzumab or Pac/²¹²Pb-HuIgG resulted in an increase in the expression of *p73*, however, a greater fold increase was observed in the latter group. The expression of two genes, *BRCA1* and *Rad21*, were down-regulated by Pac/²¹²Pb-trastuzumab, albeit their expression was also found to be down-regulated to a lesser degree by Pac/²¹²Pb-HuIgG.

Pac/²¹²Pb-trastuzumab-induced cell killing may be associated with differential expression of genes involved in the regulation of cell cycle arrest and cell cycle check point

Genes involved in regulation of cell cycle arrest (15 genes) and cell cycle checkpoint (8 genes) were another component of the array used in this gene profiling study. Expression of six genes was found to be up-regulated while five genes were down-regulated 24 h after the sequential exposure to Pac and ²¹²Pb-trastuzumab (Table 2). The genes associated with cell cycle arrest that demonstrated an increase in expression were *GADD45α, GML, PCBP4, PP1R15A, RAD9A,* and *SESN1*. In contrast, the *CHK1, CHK2* and *GTSE1* genes were down-regulated. When compared to the group treated with Pac/²¹²Pb-HuIgG, the Pac/²¹²Pb-trastuzumab treatment elicited a modestly greater response of *CHK1, RAD9A,* and *SENS1*. The Pac/²¹²Pb-trastuzumab treatment had the greatest effect on the expression of *GML* (26.4-fold increase, $p<0.0004$), compared to the set of tumors treated with Pac and the non-specifically targeted ²¹²Pb-HuIgG (Pac/²¹²Pb-trastuzumab *vs* paclitaxel, $p<0.01$; Pac/²¹²Pb-trastuzumab *vs* Pac/²¹²Pb-HuIgG, $p<0.01$). *GML* has been suggested to have a possible role in arresting cell cycle in the G2/M phase [20]. Of the eight genes involved in the cell cycle checkpoint, an alteration in only *BRCA1* and *NBN* gene expression was noted. For *NBN* genes, the difference between the Pac/²¹²Pb-trastuzumab and Pac/²¹²Pb-HuIgG treated tumor tissue was negligible. There was approximately a four-fold reduction in *BRCA1* expression for Pac/²¹²Pb-trastuzumab versus a three-fold reduction of expression for Pac/²¹²Pb-HuIgG treatment as compared to a two-fold reduction for paclitaxel treatment alone (Pac/²¹²Pb-trastuzumab *vs* paclitaxel, $p<0.05$).

Table 1. Expression of genes involved in apoptosis in LS-174T i.p. xenografts following treatment with Paclitaxel and ²¹²Pb-trastuzumab.

Symbol	Gene name	GeneBank ID	Fold change					
			Paclitaxel-²¹²Pb-trastuzumab	p	Paclitaxel-²¹²Pb-HuIgG	p	Paclitaxel	p
BRCA1	Breast Cancer 1, early onset	NM_007294	-3.8	0.0005	-3.0	0.0022	-2.1	0.0061
CIDEA	Cell death-inducing DEFA-like effector a	NM_001279	14.0	0.0067	3.8	0.0654	1.1	0.4741
GADD45α	Growth arrest and DNA-damage-inducible, alpha	NM_001924	5.9	0.0001	3.8	0.0002	1.9	0.0962
GADD45γ	Growth arrest and DNA-damage-inducible, gamma	NM_006705	10.9	0.0001	9.4	0.0002	2.4	0.0067
GML	Glycosylphosphatidylinositol anchored molecule like protein	NM_002066	26.4	0.0004	2.7	0.0023	-1.4	0.4430
IP6K3	Inositol hexakisphosphate kinase 3	NM_054111	18.1	0.0001	8.7	0.0843	-1.1	0.6288
PCBP4	Poly(rC)binding protein 2	NM_020418	3.1	0.0116	2.8	0.0012	1.6	0.0205
PPP1R15A	Protein phosphatase 1, regulatory subunit 15A	NM_014330	2.6	0.0115	1.4	0.0399	-1.1	0.4490
RAD21	RAd21 homolog	NM_006265	-3.1	0.0001	-2.5	0.0002	-1.7	0.0184
p73	Tumor protein p73	NM_005427	2.6	0.0009	5.6	0.0021	2.9	0.0628

Mice bearing i.p. LS-174T xenografts were treated by Pac/²¹²Pb-trastuzumab for 24 h. qRT-PCR array was used for gene expression analysis in three independent experiments. The numbers indicate fold change compared to untreated control (2-fold change cut-off). Additional groups included paclitaxel alone and Pac/²¹²Pb-HuIgG as a nonspecific control antibody. Results represent the average of a minimum of three replicates. A p-value <0.05 was considered significantly significant.

Table 2. Expression of genes involved in cell cycle in LS-174T i.p. xenografts following treatment with Paclitaxel and ^{212}Pb-trastuzumab.

Symbol	Gene name	GeneBank ID	Fold change					
			Paclitaxel-^{212}Pb-trastuzumab	p	Paclitaxel-^{212}Pb-HuIgG	p	Paclitaxel	p
BRCA1	Breast Cancer 1, early onset	NM_007294	−3.8	0.0005	−3.0	0.0022	−2.1	0.0061
CHK1	CHK1 checkpoint homolog	NM_001274	−4.0	0.0001	−3.2	0.0002	−2.4	0.0018
CHK2	CHK2 checkpoint homolog	NM_007194	−2.0	0.0016	−1.9	0.0025	−2.4	0.0032
GADD45α	Growth arrest and DNA-damage-inducible, alpha	NM_001924	5.9	0.0001	3.8	0.0002	1.9	0.0962
GML	Glycosylphosphatidylinositol anchored molecule like protein	NM_002066	26.4	0.0004	2.7	0.0023	−1.4	0.4430
GTSE1	G-2 and S-phase expressed 1	NM_016426	−9.3	0.0014	−4.3	0.0025	−3.1	0.0043
NBN	Nibrin	NM_002485	−2.0	0.0303	−2.1	0.0065	−1.4	0.0999
PCBP4	Poly(rC)binding protein 2	NM_020418	3.1	0.0116	2.8	0.0012	1.6	0.0205
PPP1R15A	Protein phosphatase 1, regulatory subunit 15A	NM_014330	2.6	0.0115	1.4	0.0399	−1.1	0.4490
RAD9A	RAD9 homolog A	NM_004584	2.4	0.0016	1.6	0.0006	−1.3	0.0132
SESN1	Sestrin1	NM_014454	4.6	0.0001	3.8	0.0006	2.8	0.0004

Impact of Pac/^{212}Pb-trastuzumab on expression of genes involved in damaged DNA repair

The LS-174T tumor xenografts were also probed to identify those genes involved in DNA repair that were affected by the combined treatment modality. These genes fall into several categories (Table S1) which include damaged DNA binding (DDBR; 26 genes) as well as those that comprise single strand break repair, nucleotide excision repair (NER; 12 genes), base-excision (BER; 7 genes) and mismatch repair (MMR; 14 genes). Nine genes pivotal in double-strand break repair (DSB) were also screened using the same qRT-PCR array. The array includes 15 other uncategorized genes that are related to DNA repair. Again, using the criteria of a 2-fold difference, several genes presented with a difference in expression at 24 h subsequent to the administration of Pac/^{212}Pb-trastuzumab (Table 3). Among these genes, however, only six demonstrated a clear difference between the tumors harvested from mice that had been treated with Pac/^{212}Pb-trastuzumab and those that had received the Pac/^{212}Pb-HuIgG. These genes were *ATRX, BTG2, IGHMBP2, FEN1* and *p73*, and *XPC*. The first three, *ATRX, BTG2,* and *IGHMBP2*, fall into the category of other genes related to DNA repair. *FEN1* and *XPC* are involved in repair of DDBR while *p73* is involved in MMR. One caveat to observations related to the latter gene is that the tumors from the Pac/^{212}Pb-HuIgG group demonstrated a greater increase (Pac/^{212}Pb-trastuzumab *vs* Pac/^{212}Pb-HuIgG, $p<0.05$) than the tumors treated with Pac/^{212}Pb-trastuzumab (a 2.7- fold increase, $p<0.0009$ *vs* a 5.6-fold increase, $p<0.0021$). *FEN1* was the only gene demonstrating a decrease (a 4.5-fold decrease, $p<0.0024$) in expression (Pac/^{212}Pb-trastuzumab *vs* paclitaxel, $p<0.05$; Pac/^{212}Pb-trastuzumab *vs* Pac/^{212}Pb-HuIgG, $p<0.05$).

Of the remaining genes for which differential expression was observed, nine were down-regulated (*BRCA1, EXO1, MSH2, NBN, OGG1, PRKDC, RAD18, RAD21* and *XRCC2*), while only 3 were up-regulated (*MUTYH, PNKP* and *SEM4A*). Eight of these genes play a role in DDBR, three in MMR, two each in NER and DSB repair, and finally one in BER. There were only modest to negligible differences between Pac/^{212}Pb-trastuzumab and Pac/^{212}Pb-HuIgG treated tumors amongst these genes.

Pac/^{212}Pb-trastuzumab down-regulates gene expression related to BASC

BASC (BRCA1-associated genome surveillance complex) is a multi-subunit complex, which includes BRCA1 and other DNA damage proteins such as MSH2-MSH6 and MLH1, as well as ATM, NBS1 (NBN), MRE11 and BLM [21]. BRCA1 may function as a coordinator of multiple activities required for maintenance of genomic integrity during the process of DNA replication. Genetic instability caused by BRCA1 deficiency triggers cellular responses to DNA damage that blocks cell proliferation and induces apoptosis [22]. Among genes identified in the profile, *BRCA1, MSH2,* and *NBN*, which are associated with BASC, were found to be down-regulated after the Pac/^{212}Pb-trastuzumab treatment. To investigate the effect on BASC by Pac/^{212}Pb-trastuzumab, the expression of *MSH2* and *BRCA1* were determined at the transcriptional level. Indeed, Pac/^{212}Pb-trastuzumab reduced expression of *MSH2* and *BRCA1* at the transcriptional level (Untreated *vs* Pac/^{212}Pb-trastuzumab, $p< 0.01$; Pac/^{212}Pb-trastuzumab *vs* Pac/^{212}Pb-HuIgG, $p<0.05$), suggesting that transcription-coupled repair (Mismatch repair; *MSH2* and DNA double stand repair; *BRCA1*) might be defective (Figure 1A).

Table 3. Expression of gene expression involved in DNA repair in LS-174T i.p. xenografts following treatment with Paclitaxel and ^{212}Pb-trastuzumab.

Symbol	Gene name	GeneBank ID	Fold change					
			Paclitaxel-^{212}Pb-trastuzumab	p	Paclitaxel-^{212}Pb-HuIgG	p	Paclitaxel	p
ATRX	Alpha thalassemia/mental retardation	NM_000489	2.8	0.0018	1.4	0.1413	1.1	0.4611
BRCA1	Breast Cancer 1, early onset	NM_007294	−3.8	0.0005	−3.0	0.0022	−2.1	0.0061
BTG2	BTG family, member 2	NM_006763	7.5	0.0006	5.4	0.0003	2.7	0.0001
EXO1	Exonuclease 1	NM_130398	−4.5	0.0004	−4.0	0.0003	−2.1	0.0030
FEN1	Flap structure-specific endonuclease 1	NM_004111	−4.5	0.0024	−5.8	0.0017	−2.4	0.0072
IGHMBP2	Immunoglobulin mu binding protein 2	NM_002180	2.4	0.0013	1.8	0.0307	−1.4	0.0430
MSH2	MutS homolog 2	NM_000251	−2.9	0.0080	−2.7	0.0085	−1.9	0.0249
MUTYH	MutY homolog	NM_012222	2.8	0.0002	2.0	0.0019	−1.4	0.0837
NBN	Nibrin	NM_002485	−2.0	0.0303	−2.1	0.0065	−1.4	0.0999
OGG1	8-oxoguanine DNA glycosylase	NM_002542	−2.2	0.1217	−2.2	0.1214	−1.9	0.2046
PNKP	Polynucleotide kinase 3'-phosphatase	NM_007254	2.4	0.0063	2.1	0.0014	−1.5	0.0084
PPP1R15A	Protein phosphatase 1, regulatory unit 15A	NM_014330	2.6	0.0115	1.4	0.0399	−1.1	0.4490
PRKDC	Protein kinase, DNA-activated, catalytic polypeptide	NM_006904	−2.7	0.0187	−2.5	0.0126	−1.9	0.0306
RAD18	RAD18 homolog	NM_020165	−2.3	0.0030	−1.9	0.0003	−1.6	0.0001
RAD21	RAD21 homolog	NM_006265	−3.1	0.0001	−2.5	0.0002	−1.7	0.0184
SEMA4A	Semadomain, immunoglobulin domain, cycloplastic domain 4A	NM_022367	2.8	0.0350	2.7	0.0031	1.3	0.3131
p73	Tumor protein p73	NM_005427	2.7	0.0009	5.6	0.0021	2.9	0.0628
XPC	Xeroderma pigmentosum, complementation group C	NM_004628	5.1	0.0001	3.7	0.0001	1.9	0.0141
XRCC2	X-ray repair complementing defective repair in Chinese hamster cells 2	NM_005431	−3.5	0.0020	−3.0	0.0003	−2.2	0.0025

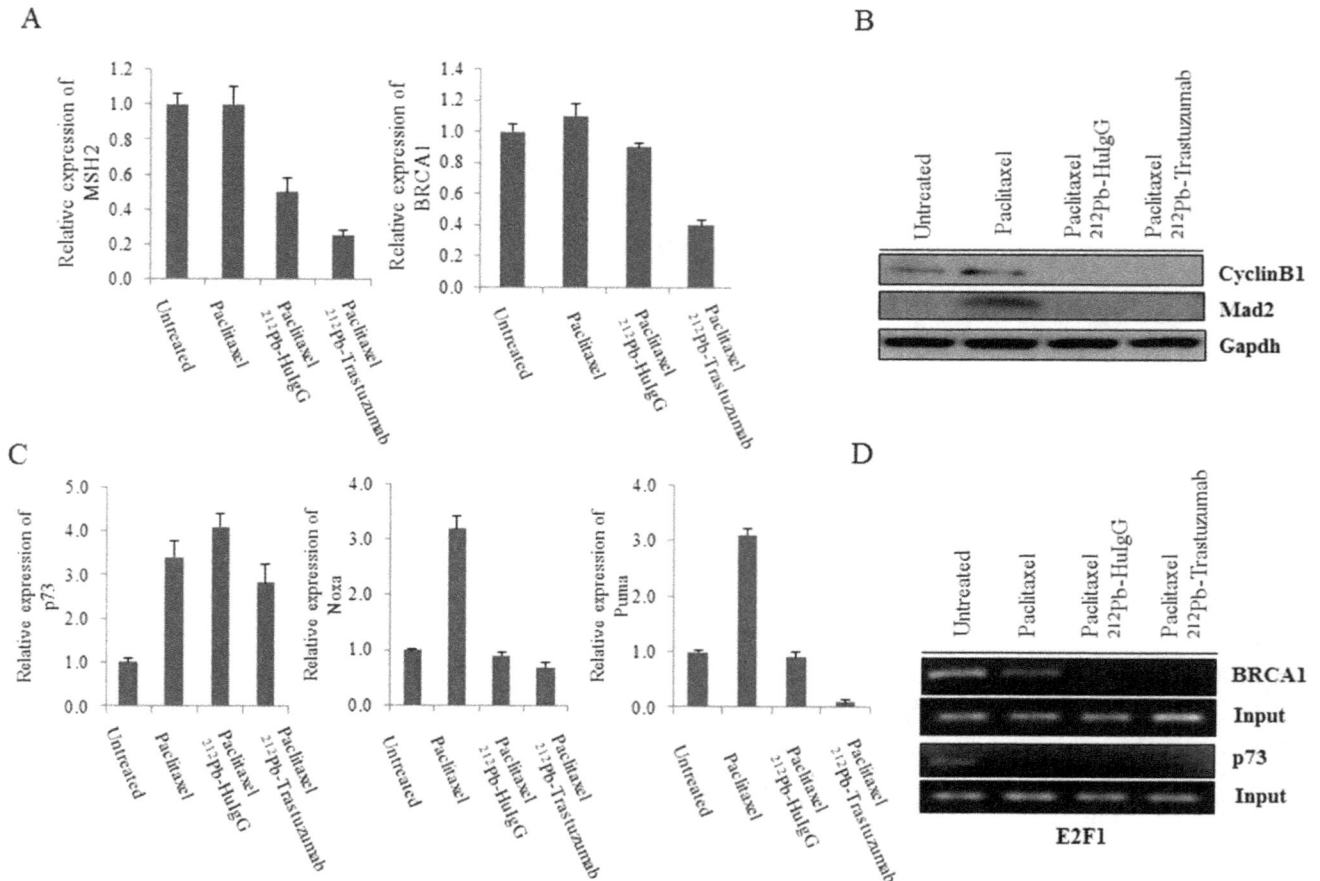

Figure 1. Expression of BASC (BRCA1-associated genome surveillance complex) related genes and *p73* expression in response to Pac/^{212}Pb-trastuzumab. Mice bearing i.p. LS-174T xenografts were treated by Pac/^{212}Pb- trastuzumab for 24 h. A. Expression of *MSH2* and *BRCA1* was determined by RT-PCR. Results represent the average of a minimum of three replications. B. Immunoblot analysis for MAD2 and CYCLIN B1 was performed with tumor collected 24 h after Pac/^{212}Pb-trastuzumab treatment. MAD2 and CYCLIN B1 were detected 22 kDa and 48 kDa, respectively. Equal protein loading control was GAPDH. C. Expression of *p73*, *NOXA*, and *PUMA* was determined by RT-PCR. Results represent the average of a minimum of three replications. D. Binding abundance to E2F1 was determined by ChIP using specific primers for *p73 and BRCA1*.

CHK-mediated phosphorylation of *BRCA1* is required for proper and timely assembly of mitotic spindles. Down-regulation of *BRCA1* reduces the mitotic index and triggers premature CYCLIN B1 degradation and decreases expression of genes that are involved in the spindle checkpoint including MAD2 [23]. To examine the role of BRCA1 in mitosis, the expression of DNA damage response genes such as CYCLIN B1 and MAD2 were determined using immunoblot analysis (Figure 1B). Pac/^{212}Pb-trastuzumab revoked the expression of CYCLIN B1 and MAD2, induced by the administration of paclitaxel alone suggesting that down-regulation in BASC by Pac/^{212}Pb-trastuzumab may result in genomic instability. The decrease in the level of these two proteins was also observed in the tumors that had been treated with Pac/^{212}Pb-HuIgG.

Pac/^{212}Pb-trastuzumab may induce chromosomal instability as a result of interfere with E2F1/p73 signaling

Reports have indicated that p73 interacts with spindle assembly checkpoint (SAC) proteins and that loss of p73 causes mislocalization at the kinetochore and reduced kinase activity of BubR1, leading to chromosome instability [24]. The expression of *p73* at the transcriptional level appeared to be up-regulated, as the *p73* gene expression was increased for paclitaxel alone, but there is a

reduction in *p73* expression with Pac/^{212}Pb-trastuzumab (Table 3). To examine the effect on genome instability induced by Pac/^{212}Pb-trastuzumab, the expression of *p73* and *NOXA/PUMA*, down-stream effectors of p73, was determined at the transcriptional level. Pac/^{212}Pb-trastuzumab treatment seemed to marginally increase the expression of *p73* at the gene level (Figure 1C). However, the expression of *p73* downstream effectors that was apparent after the initial Pac treatment was reduced (Untreated *vs* Pac/^{212}Pb-trastuzumab, $p<0.05$). p73 is a transcriptional target of E2F1 and therefore p73 regulation may be mediated by E2F1 [25]. BRCA1 promoter also has E2F binding sites to bring about transcriptional regulation [26]. With these in mind, the abundances of E2F1 association with *BRCA1* and *p73* promoters in tumors exposed to Pac/^{212}Pb-trastuzumab were evaluated using the ChIP assay. Pac/^{212}Pb-trastuzumab and Pac/^{212}Pb-HuIgG (Figure 1D) attenuated the binding capacity at *BRCA1* and *p73* promoters, implicating a disturbance in activation of E2F1/p73 signaling.

Pac/^{212}Pb-trastuzumab may induce chromosomal instability by the regulating mitotic spindle checkpoint

Reduced BUBR1 activity results in the premature activation of the anaphase promoting complex/cyclosome (APC/C), which negatively regulates its substrates such as GEMININ [27]. To further investigate the effect on genome instability induced by Pac/^{212}Pb-trastuzumab, the expression of *BUBR1*, one of the spindle assembly checkpoint (SAC) proteins, was determined at the transcriptional level (Figure 2A). Upon incubation with paclitaxel alone, *BUBR1* expression was found to be elevated. The increase in expression of *BUBR1* was reversed at the transcription level upon subsequent treatment with ^{212}Pb-trastuzumab consistent with an earlier study from this laboratory [15]. Topoisomerase II helps to bring about a high order of compaction of chromatin to form condensed mitotic chromosomes [28]. Topoisomerase II expression was also reduced by Pac/^{212}Pb-trastuzumab (Untreated *vs* Pac/^{212}Pb-trastuzumab, $p<0.01$; Pac/^{212}Pb-trastuzumab *vs* Pac/^{212}Pb-HuIgG, $p<0.01$), suggesting possible chromosome instability through perturbation of SAC proteins. Pac/^{212}Pb-HuIgG elicited similar effects in the tumors, but, in this case, the levels of *BUBR1* and *TOPOISOMERASE II* were comparable to the untreated controls and much higher than that of the Pac/^{212}Pb-trastuzumab treatment.

EMI1 (early mitotic inhibitor) suppresses APC/C activity during the cell cycle, and is believed to be required for proper mitotic entry. EMI1 depletion induces re-replication due to premature activation of APC/C that results in destabilization of GEMININ [29,30]. The effect on EMI1 and GEMININ in tumors exposed to Pac/^{212}Pb-trastuzumab was examined using immunoblot analysis. Pac/^{212}Pb-trastuzumab reduced the expression level of EMI1 and GEMININ to a greater extent than paclitaxel alone (Figure 2B), implicating aberrant DNA re-replication which may result in DNA replication fork collision and double strand breaks.

Discussion

The therapeutic potential of ^{212}Pb-trastuzumab, α-emitting radioimmunotherapeutic, has been successfully demonstrated for the treatment of disseminated peritoneal disease in murine models [31]. Studies investigating the molecular basis of this efficacy have revealed that ^{212}Pb-trastuzumab results in the induction of apoptosis, G2/M cell cycle arrest and blocks double strand DNA damage repair [32]. The molecular basis of this action is thought to be mediated through the p73/GADD45 signaling pathway via p38 kinase signaling [33]. Addition of paclitaxel to the treatment protocol resulted in greater therapeutic efficacy in the LS-174T i.p. tumor xenograft model [15]. The inclusion of paclitaxel in the regimen was found to increase mitotic catastrophe and apoptosis. Concomitantly, a redistribution of DNA content into the G2/M phase of the cell cycle, a decrease in the phosphorylation of histone H3, an increase in multi-micronuclei, and an increase in positively stained γH2AX foci, suggested possible effects on the mitotic spindle assembly checkpoint (SAC) by this combined modality therapy. Paclitaxel induces the arrest of spindle assembly checkpoint (SAC) through suppression of the spindle microtubule dynamics by binding to the β-subunit of tubulin and stabilizing microtubules. The resultant mitotic arrest rapidly triggers onset of the p53-independent apoptotic pathway [34]. To better understand the interplay between ^{212}Pb-trastuzumab and paclitaxel that produces enhancement of the α-radiation cytotoxicity, gene expression profiling was performed with LS-147T i.p. tumor xenografts treated *in vivo* to identify affected genes.

A

B

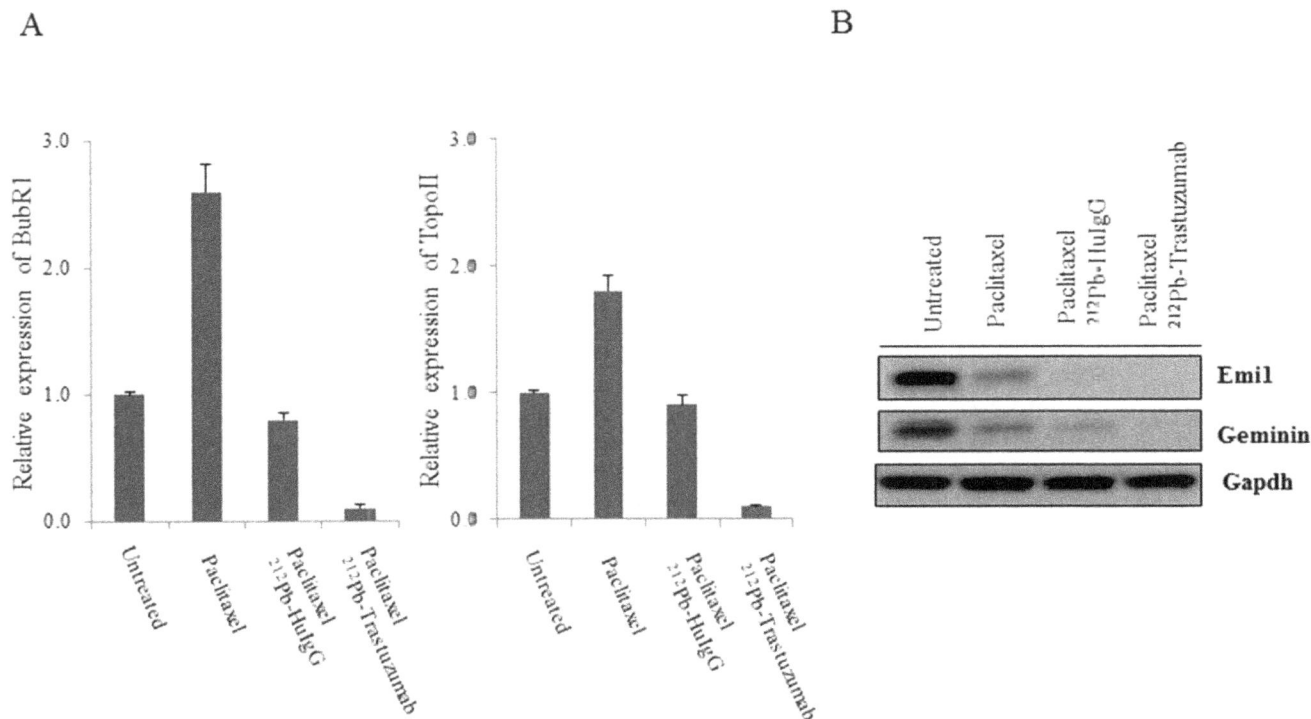

Figure 2. Pac/^{212}Pb-trastuzumab may induce chromosomal instability as a result of suppression of BUBR1 and EMI1 expression.
Mice bearing i.p. LS-174T xenografts were treated by Pac/^{212}Pb-trastuzumab for 24 h. A. Expression of *BUBR1* and *TOPOII* was determined by RT-PCR using specific primers for *BUBR1* and *TOPOISOMERASE II*. Results represent the average of a minimum of three replications. B. Immunoblot analysis for EMI1 and GEMININ was performed with tumor tissue collected 24 h after Pac/^{212}Pb- trastuzumab treatment. The EMI1 and GEMININ were detected at 56 kDa and 35 kDa, respectively. Equal protein loading control was GAPDH.

Eighty-four genes were assessed using a real-time quantitative PCR (qRT-PCR) array. Thirty genes were identified (Tables 1-3) in the LS-174T tumors that were differentially expressed 24 h following the administration of paclitaxel followed the next day by [212]Pb-trastuzumab treatment. Differential expression of eight genes had been previously identified following treatment with [212]Pb-trastuzumab alone [33]. In each of the categories that were evaluated, apoptosis, cell cycle regulation and damaged DNA repair, more genes were affected by the combination of paclitaxel with [212]Pb-trastuzumab. This is perhaps not surprising considering that paclitaxel was added to the treatment regimen to introduce other mechanisms of effecting or enhancing tumor cell killing. What is more striking when comparing the two studies is that more genes were down-regulated in their expression by the Pac/[212]Pb-trastuzumab, nine of which are involved in DNA repair. This suggests a more compromised cancer tissue in its effort to overcome the stress induced by the combined modality.

Eleven genes in the apoptosis panel demonstrated altered expression in the LS-174T tumors following treatment with Pac/[212]Pb-trastuzumab. Six (CIDEA, GADD45α, GADD45γ, IP6K3, PCBP4 and p73) were found previously to be affected by [212]Pb-trastuzumab [33]. More important, however, is that paclitaxel enhanced the expression of five of the genes, with two (CIDEA and IP6K3) having a 2.9- and 3.9-fold increase over the [212]Pb-trastuzumab alone. Interestingly, even though the expression of p73 was increased, the expression was lower in this study as compared to its expression following [212]Pb-trastuzumab alone. Overall, the combined modality appears to have had the greatest effect on the expression of CIDEA, GML and IP6K3. These three are involved in apoptosis with GML also having a role in cell cycle regulation. In the presence of paclitaxel, GML is hypothesized to monitor the status of microtubules and transduces a signal to activate apoptosis, cooperating with or enhancing the effect of paclitaxel [35]. GML has also been implicated in the enhancement of G2/M arrest and apoptosis following α-irradiation [20]. However, an increase in the expression of this gene was not detectable following the exposure to α-radiation alone, and differential expression by paclitaxel treatment alone was not significant. Thus the 26.4-fold ($p<0.0004$) increased expression of GML by the combined Pac/[212]Pb-trastuzumab treatment may be a special response of the cells to the prior paclitaxel treatment. Interestingly, Pac/[212]Pb-HuIgG, the non-specific control also increased GML expression by 2.7-fold ($p<0.0023$) indicating that the α-radiation and paclitaxel together are important for GML expression. Paclitaxel can also result in stress-reaction-induced apoptosis through the up-regulation of the GADD gene family [36,37]. GADD45α and PPP1R15A were both up-regulated following the Pac/[212]Pb-trastuzumab treatment. Again, the higher level of GADD45 expression noted in the present study and the addition of PPP1R15A to the list of responsive genes attests to the increased stress on the LS-174T tumors by the combined modality. RAD21 (Rad21 homolog) is a central component of the cohesin complex which consists of RAD21, SMC1, SMC3, and SCC3. RAD21 expression confers poor prognosis and resistance to chemotherapy and knockdown of RAD21 results in enhanced sensitivity to chemotherapeutic drugs [38]. In this study, RAD21 expression was reduced to a greater extent by Pac/[212]Pb-trastuzumab treatment than Pac/[212]Pb-HuIgG or paclitaxel alone. These results suggest that [212]Pb-trastuzumab and to a lesser extent, also [212]Pb-HuIgG might increase cell sensitivity to therapy by up-regulating genes involved in apoptosis and down-regulating genes involved in desensitizing cells to chemotherapeutics. For α-particle irradiation, micronucleus induction has a biphasic phenomenon containing a low-dose hypersensitivity

characteristic and its dose response could be well stimulated with a state vector model where radiation-induced bystander effects are involved. The increase in the micronucleus frequency in bystander cells provides evidence for indirect DNA damage signal or a bystander phenomenon released by irradiated cells. The non-specific effect in α-particle and bystander effects have been recognized in the past and occur as with β⁻-emitter therapy. Therefore, consideration toward greater studies of these specific responses must be given to these effects of radiation.

A total of eleven genes in the cell cycle category were found to be differentially regulated in the Pac/[212]Pb-trastuzumab treated xenografts, five of which were cross-overs into the apoptosis category. Four genes (GADD45α, GTSE1, PCBP4 and SESN1) had been found to have an altered expression following treatment with [212]Pb-trastuzumab alone [33]. The effect of paclitaxel alone was less pronounced. BRCA1 was one of the genes down-regulated by Pac/[212]Pb-trastuzumab. A deficiency in BRCA1 causes abnormalities in the S-phase checkpoint, G2/M check-point, spindle checkpoint and centrosome duplication [22]. CHK1 is required to delay entry of cells with damaged or unreplicated DNA into mitosis. CHK1 protects cells against spontaneous chromosome missegregation and is required to sustain anaphase delay when spindle function is disrupted by paclitaxel. The requirement of CHK1 for spindle checkpoints has been elucidated [39]. Spindle checkpoint failure in CHK1-deficient cells correlates with decreased AuroraB kinase activity, and impaired phosphorylation and kinetochore localization of BUBR1 [40].

DNA damage corrupts the integrity and translation of essential information in the genome. Two major strategies for repair are single strand break repair and double strand break repair (DSBR). The former includes nucleotide excision repair (NER), base excision repair (BER), mismatch repair (MMR), while the latter encompasses non-homologous end joining (NHEJ) and homologous recombination [41]. Eighteen genes involved in DNA repair were affected in the LS-174T tumor xenografts following the Pac/[212]Pb-trastuzumab treatment. These genes represented those involved in damaged DNA binding (DDB, 5 genes), NER (2 genes), BER (3 genes), MMR (2 genes), DSBR (3 genes) as well as 3 others related to DNA repair. In comparison to [212]Pb-trastuzumab alone [33], the addition of paclitaxel to the treatment regimen not only resulted in an alteration in more genes involved in DNA repair, but also affected each of the major repair pathways. Interestingly, most of the genes involved in DNA single and double break repair, were differentially down-regulated, suggesting that Pac/[212]Pb-trastuzumab impairs both single and double strand break repair. Expression of several genes involved in DNA repair may be determinant of tumor sensitivity to the anti-mitotic chemotherapy. Severe DNA double-strand breaks are known to be caused by α-emitters that are also inefficiently repaired, leading to cell death [6,32,42]. A lack of specificity in this category of genes is worth noting. A comparison of the tumor response between the Pac/[212]Pb-trastuzumab and the Pac/[212]Pb-HuIgG groups gives the impression that there is little difference in the differential expression of most of the responding genes. However, there are differences between the two groups in the expression levels of the ATRX, BTG2 and XPC genes. Loss of ATRX (alpha thalassemia/mental retardation syndrome X-linked) protein and mutations in the ATRX gene are associated with genome instability, defects in the G2/M checkpoint, and altered double strand break (DSB) repair in alternative lengthening of telomeres pathway. Recent developments suggest that ATRX plays a variety of key roles at tandem repeat sequences within the genome, including the deposition of a histone variant, prevention of replication fork stalling, and the suppression of a homologous

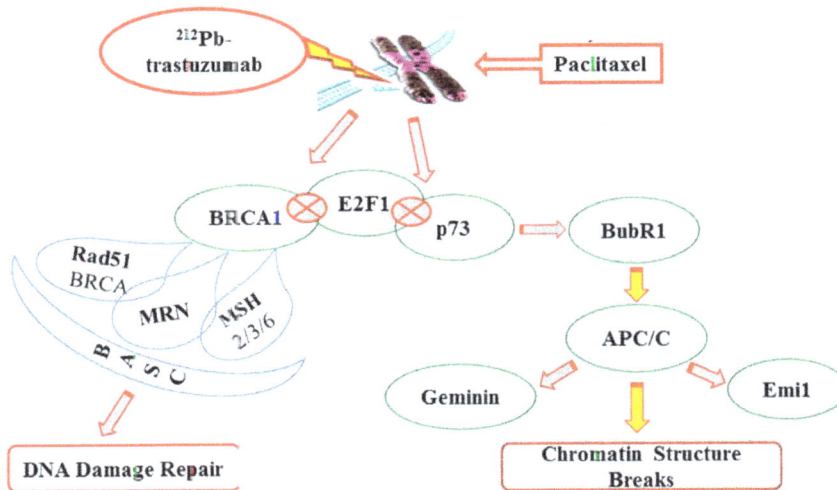

Figure 3. Proposed mode of action in the induction of chromosomal instability by Pac/²¹²Pb-trastuzumab treatment. See text for details.

recombination-based pathway of telomere maintenance [43]. *BTG2* (BTG family member 2) is induced through a p53 dependent mechanism and that expression of BTG2 promotes the repair of DSBs and reduces apoptosis by blocking the damage signal from p-ATM(S1981) to Chk2(T68)-p53(S20) via the activation of Mre11 and PRMT1 [44].

BRCA1 associates with tumor suppressor and DNA damage proteins to form a large complex, BRCA1-associated genome surveillance complex (BASC), which recognizes and repairs aberrant DNA structures. BASC contains BRCA1, ATM and BLM as well as four subprotein complexes; 1) RAD50-MRE11-NBN, 2) MSH2-MSH6, 3) MLH1-PMS2 and 4) RFCA. All of the BASC proteins can also form complexes independent of BRCA1. BASC is a dynamic structure in which multiple complexes assemble and disassemble at various sites of BRCA1 functions, DSB being one example [21]. The proteins all share the potential to act either as sensors of abnormal DNA structure or as effectors of repair. These properties of BASC lend a great deal of flexibility to the structure and allows for a rapid response for repair of DNA aberrations [21]. *MSH2* and *NBN* were two of the genes in the profile that were found to be differentially down-regulated by Pac/²¹²Pb-trastuzumab along with *BRCA1*. Not only is the ability to bind damaged DNA hindered with the loss of *BRCA1* and *NBN*, but there is also the loss of one of the DNA repair mechanisms with lowered expression level of *MSH2*. Additionally, down-regulation of BRCA1 reduces the mitotic index and triggers premature CYCLIN B1 degradation and decrease in genes that are involved in the spindle checkpoint, including MAD2, which are key components that inhibit the anaphase-promoting complex [23]. Consistent with this notion, expressions of CYCLIN B1 and MAD2 that increased upon paclitaxel treatment alone were abrogated upon subsequent treatment with ²¹²Pb-trastuzumab or ²¹²Pb-HuIgG, suggesting the role of BRCA1 as a sensor of abnormal DNA structure or as effector of repair failed, resulting in chromosome instability following the α-radiation treatment. The effects of the decrease in BRCA1 is expected to be more pronounced for the Pac/²¹²Pb-trastuzumab treatment compared with the Pac/²¹²Pb-HuIgG treatment because of the greater reduction in BRCA1 expression for Pac/²¹²Pb-trastuzumab than ²¹²Pb-HuIgG.

p73 is a member of the *p53* tumor suppressor gene family and induces cell cycle arrest and cell death in response to DNA damage. Loss of p73 can lead to mitotic arrest defects and p73 regulates the spindle checkpoint by modulating BUBR1 activity [24]. In this study, Pac/²¹²Pb-trastuzumab treatment seemed to marginally increase the expression of *p73* at the gene level. However, expression of its downstream effectors, *NOXA* and *PUMA* at the transcriptional level was reduced. *p73* and *BRCA1* have also been shown to be transcriptional targets of E2F1. ChIP analysis revealed that the abundances of E2F1 on *p73* and *BRCA1* promoters were also down-regulated. These results were discordant. It would have been expected that increased expression of *p73* would result in an increased expression of its downstream effectors as well as an increase in the interaction with E2F1. These effects are most likely a result of the aberrant regulation, or lack thereof, of the BRCA1-associated target genes such as CHK1, E2F1, and p73 in response to Pac/²¹²Pb-trastuzumab. It must be emphasized that the *in vivo* mechanisms invoked after the massive damage to DNA by the α-radiation are complex. Thus, we may not be able to explain all the results because of the myriad responses to the injury. However, the results obtained with the downstream effectors of *p73* indicate that the E2F1/p73 signaling pathway becomes defective after the combined paclitaxel and α-radiation treatment. p73 interacts with spindle assembly checkpoint (SAC) proteins and that loss of p73 causes mislocalization at the kinetochore and reduced kinase activity of BUBR1, leading to chromosome instability [24]. Studies from this laboratory recently demonstrated that paclitaxel potentiates ²¹²Pb-trastuzumab induced cell killing by perturbing the mitotic spindle checkpoint, including BUBR1 [15]. Reduced BUBR1 activity results in the premature activation of the anaphase promoting complex/cyclosome (APC/C), which negatively regulates its substrates such as GEMININ [27]. In this study, α-radiation also suppressed EMI1 (early mitotic inhibitor), leading to unscheduled anaphase promoting complex/cyclosome (APC/C) activity as evidenced by down-regulation of GEMININ, an APC/C substrate, which plays redundant roles in preventing re-replication. The resulting aberrant DNA re-replication may result in DNA replication fork collision and double strand breaks. The presence of premature sister chromatid separation and chromosome breaks will compromise cell division and survival of the cells.

Clearly, the addition of paclitaxel resulted in a greater number of genes responding to the therapy especially those involved in DNA repair compared to [212]Pb-trastuzumab treatment alone. The [212]Pb-trastuzumab treatment is either potentiating the effect of paclitaxel, or, the paclitaxel is enhancing the effect of the [212]Pb-trastuzumab. The findings suggest that perturbation of DNA damage repair and the mitotic checkpoint in tumors exposed to paclitaxel and [212]Pb-trastuzumab may be responsible for the cell death. A fine cross-talk between DNA damage and the spindle damage response is evident (Figure 3). It must be noted that non-apoptotic death during mitotic catastrophe cannot be excluded as typically there is a mixture of apoptotic and non-apoptotic cell death during mitosis and after multinucleation. These studies represent a starting point for future investigations that will focus on the refinement of the identification of genes pivotal to the therapeutic response evoked by the combination of paclitaxel and targeted α-radiation using monoclonal antibodies such as trastuzumab. Analysis of later time points may reveal greater differences between specific and non-specifically delivered α-radiation.

The impact of the xenograft study results on understanding findings pertaining to the ongoing clinical trial at this time is limited since this is a Phase 1 trial that evaluates safety of [212]Pb-labeled trastuzumab. The real impact is more directed towards future trials wherein our understanding of the results of these pre-clinical studies on targeted α-particle RIT might be applied to improve integration of this modality with standards of care chemotherapy, particularly so with respect to normal tissues toxicity as doses increase. Further elucidation of these mechanisms could aid in the development of more precise diagnostic and prognostic tools to promote clinical transition in the treatment of cancer.

Supporting Information

Table S1 Functional gene grouping. Comparison of the relative expression of 84 DNA damage related genes involved in apoptosis (Figure 1), cell cycle (Figure 2), and DNA damage repair (Figure 3) was characterized with the human DNA damage signaling pathway PCR array.

Author Contributions

Conceived and designed the experiments: KJY DEM KEB MWB. Performed the experiments: KJY DEM KEB. Analyzed the data: KJY. Contributed reagents/materials/analysis tools: KJY DEM KEB. Wrote the paper: KJY.

References

1. Matson DR, Stukenberg PT (2011) Spindle poisons and cell fate: a tale of two pathways. Mol Interv 11: 141–150.
2. Dalton WB, Yang VW (2009) Role of prolonged mitotic checkpoint activation in the formation and treatment of cancer. Future Oncol 5: 1363–1370.
3. Barbet J, Bardies M, Bourgeois M, Chatal JF, Cherel M, et al. (2012) Radiolabeled antibodies for cancer imaging and therapy. Methods Mol Biol 907: 681–697.
4. Navarro-Teulon I, Lozza C, Pelegrin A, Vives E, Pouget JP (2013) General overview of radioimmunotherapy of solid tumors. Immunotherapy 5: 467–487.
5. Jurcic JG (2013) Radioimmunotherapy for hematopoietic cell transplantation. Immunotherapy 5: 383–394.
6. Yong KJ, Brechbiel MW (2011) Towards translation of [212]Pb as a clinical therapeutic; getting the lead in! Dalton Trans 40: 6068–6076.
7. Dahle J, Abbas N, Bruland OS, Larsen RH (2011) Toxicity and relative biological effectiveness of alpha emitting radioimmunoconjugates. Curr Radiopharm 4: 321–328.
8. Kim YS, Brechbiel MW (2012) An overview of targeted alpha therapy. Tumour Biol 33: 573–590.
9. Seidl C (2014) Radioimmunotherapy with α-particle-emitting radionuclides. Immunotherapy 6: 431–458.
10. Milenic DE, Garmestani K, Brady ED, Albert PS, Adulla A, et al. (2007) Potentiation of high-LET radiation by gemcitabine: targeting HER2 with trastuzumab to treat disseminated peritoneal disease. Clin Cancer Res 13: 1926–1935.
11. Milenic DE, Garmestani K, Brady ED, Baidoo KE, Albert PS, et al. (2008) Multimodality therapy: potentiation of high linear energy transfer radiation with paclitaxel for the treatment of disseminated peritoneal disease. Clin Cancer Res 14: 5108–5115.
12. Meredith RF, Torgue J, Azure MT, Shen S, Saddekni S, et al. (2014) Pharmacokinetics and imaging of [212]Pb-TCMC-trastuzumab after intraperitoneal administration in ovarian cancer patients. Cancer Biother Radiopharm 29: 12–17.
13. Chauhan V, Howland M, Chen J, Kutzner B, Wilkins RC (2011) Differential effects of α-particle radiation and X-irradiation on genes associated with apoptosis. Radiol Res Pract doi:10.1155/2011/679806.
14. Chen JG, Yang CP, Cammer M, Horwtz SB (2003) Gene expression and mitotic exit induced by microtubule-stabilizing drugs. Cancer Res 63: 7891–7899.
15. Yong KJ, Milenic DE, Baidoo KE, Brechbiel MW (2013) Paclitaxel potentiates [212]Pb-radioimmunotherapy-induced cell killing efficacy by perturbing mitotic spindle checkpoint. Br J Cancer 108: 2013–2020.
16. Danielsson A, Caesson K, Parris TZ, Helou K, Nemes S, et al. (2013) Differential gene expression in human fibroblasts after alpha-particle emitter [211]At compared with ^{60}Co irradiation. Int J Radiat Biol 89: 250–258.
17. Seidl C, Port M, Apostolidis C, Bruchertseifer F, Schwaiger M, et al. (2010) Differential gene expression triggered by highly cytotoxic α-emitter-immunoconjugates in gastric cancer cells. Invest New Drugs 28: 49–60.
18. Tom BH, Rutzky LP, Jakstys MM, Oyasu R, Kahan BD (1976) Human colonic adenocarcinoma cells. I. Establishment and description of a new cell line. In Vitro 12: 180–191.
19. Chappell LL, Dadachova E, Milenic DE, Garmestani K, Wu C, et al. (2000) Synthesis, characterization, and evaluation of a novel bifunctional chelating agent for the lead isotopes [203]Pb and [212]Pb. Nucl Med Biol 27: 93–100.
20. Kagawa K, Inoue T, Tokino T, Nakamura Y, Akiyama T (1997) Overexpression of GML promotes radiation-induced cell cycle arrest and apoptosis. Biochem Biophys Res Commun 241: 481–485.
21. Wang Y, Cortez D, Yazdi P, Neff N, Elledge SJ, et al. (2000) BASC, a super complex of BRCA1-associated proteins involved in the recognition and repair of aberrant DNA structures. Genes & Dev 14: 927–939.
22. Deng CX (2006) BRCA1: cell cycle checkpoint, genetic instability, DNA damage response and cancer evolution. Nucleic Acids Res 34: 1416–1426.
23. Wang RH, Yu H, Deng CX (2004) A requirement for breast cancer associated gene1 (BRCA1) in spindle checkpoint. Proc Natl Acad Sci USA 101: 17108–17113.
24. Tomasini R, Tsuchihara K, Tsuda C, Lau SK, Wilhelm M, et al. (2009) Tap73 regulates the spindle assembly checkpoint by modulating BubR1 activity. Proc Natl Acad Sci USA 106: 797–702.
25. Tophkhane C, Yang SH, Jiang Y, Ma Z, Subramaniam D, et al. (2012) p53 inactivation up-regulates p73 expression through E2F1 mediated transcription. PLoS One 7: e43564. doi:10.1371
26. Bindra RS, Gibson SL, Meng A, Westermark U, Jasin M, et al. (2005) Hypoxia-induced down-regulation of BRCA1 expression by E2Fs. Cancer Res 65: 11597–11604.
27. Taylor WR, Stark GR (2001) Regulation of the G2/M transition by p53. Oncogene 20: 1803–1815.
28. Dai W, Wang Q, Liu T, Swamy M, Fang Y, et al. (2004) Slippage of mitotic arrest and enhanced tumor development in mice with BubR1 haploin sufficiency. Cancer Res 64: 440–445.
29. Sivaprasad U, Machida YJ, Dutta A (2007) APC/C-master controller of origin licensing? Cell Div 2: 8.
30. Machida Y, Dutta A (2007) The APC/C inhibitor, Emil, is essential for prevention of replication. Cell Div 2: 184–194.
31. Milenic DE, Garmestani K, Brady ED, Albert PS, Ma D, et al. (2005) Alpha-particle radioimmunotherapy of disseminated peritoneal disease using a [212]Pb-labeled radioimmunoconjugate targeting HER2. Cancer Biother Radiopharm 5: 557–568.
32. Yong KJ, Milenic DE, Baidoo KE, Brechbiel MW (2012) [212]Pb-Radioimmunotherapy induces G2 cell cycle arrest and delays DNA damage repair in tumor xenografts in a model for disseminated intraperitoneal disease. Mol Cancer Ther 11: 639–648.
33. Yong KJ, Milenic DE, Baidoo KE, Kim YS, Brechbiel MW (2013) Gene expression profiling upon [212]Pb-TCMC-trastuzumab treatment in the LS-174T i.p. xenograft model. Cancer Med 2: 646–653.
34. Abal M, Andreu JM, Barasoain I (2003) Taxane: microtubule and centrosome targets and cell cycle dependent mechanisms of action. Curr Cancer Drug Targets 3: 193–203.
35. Kimura Y, Furuhata T, Shiratsuchi T, Nishimori H, Hirata K, et al. (1997) GML sensitizes cancer cells to Taxol by induction of apoptosis. Oncogene 15: 1369–1374.

36. Sugimura M, Sagae S, Ishioka S, Nishioka Y, Tsukada K, et al. (2004) Mechanisms of paclitaxel-induced apoptosis in an ovarian cancer cell line and its paclitaxel-resistant clone. Oncology 66: 53–61.

37. Hollander MC, Poola-Kella S, Fornace AJ (2003) Gad44 functional domains involved in growth suppression and apoptosis. Oncogene 22: 3827–3832.

38. Xu H, Yan M, Patra J, Natrajan R, Yan Y, et al. (2012) Enhanced RAD21 cohesion expression confers poor prognosis and resistance to chemotherapy in high grade luminal, basal and HER2 breast cancers. Breast Cancer Res 13:R69.

39. Carrassa L, Sanchez Y, Erba E, Damia G (2009) U2OS cells lacking Chk1 undergo aberrant mitosis and fail to activate the spindle checkpoint. J Cell Mol Med 13: 1565–1576.

40. Zachos G, Black EJ, Walker M, Scott MT, Vagnarelli F, et al. (2007) Chk1 is required for spindle checkpoint function. Dev Cell 12: 247–260.

41. Olive PL (1998) The role of DNA single- and double-strand breaks in cell killing by ionization radiation. Radiat Res 150: 42–51.

42. Sgouros G, Roeske JC, McDevitt MR, Palm S, Allen BJ, et al. (2010) MIRD Pamphlet No. 22 (abridged): radiobiology and dosimetry of alpha-particle emitters for targeted radionuclide therapy. J Nucl Med 51: 311–328.

43. Lovejoy CA, Li W, Reisenweber S, Thongthip S, Bruno J, et al. (2012) Loss of ATRX, Genome Instability, and an altered DNA damage response are hallmarks of the alternative lengthening of telomeres pathway. PloS Genet 8:e1002772.

44. Choi KS, Kim JY, Lim SK, Choi YW, Kim YH, et al. (2012) TIS21(BTG2/PC3) accelerates the repair of DNA double strand breaks by enhancing Mre11 methylation and blocking damage signaling transfer to Chk2(T68)-p53(S20) pathway. DNA Repair 11: 965–975.

3

A PCNA-Derived Cell Permeable Peptide Selectively Inhibits Neuroblastoma Cell Growth

Long Gu[1]*, Shanna Smith[1], Caroline Li[1], Robert J. Hickey[2], Jeremy M. Stark[3], Gregg B. Fields[4], Walter H. Lang[5], John A. Sandoval[5], Linda H. Malkas[1]

1 Department of Molecular & Cellular Biology, Beckman Research Institute of City of Hope, Duarte, California, United States of America, 2 Department of Molecular Pharmacology, Beckman Research Institute of City of Hope, Duarte, California, United States of America, 3 Department of Radiation Biology, Beckman Research Institute of City of Hope, Duarte, California, United States of America, 4 Torrey Pines Institute for Molecular Studies, Port St. Lucie, Florida, United States of America, 5 Department of Surgery, St. Jude Children's Research Hospital, Memphis, Tennessee, United States of America

Abstract

Proliferating cell nuclear antigen (PCNA), through its interaction with various proteins involved in DNA synthesis, cell cycle regulation, and DNA repair, plays a central role in maintaining genome stability. We previously reported a novel cancer associated PCNA isoform (dubbed caPCNA), which was significantly expressed in a broad range of cancer cells and tumor tissues, but not in non-malignant cells. We found that the caPCNA-specific antigenic site lies between L126 and Y133, a region within the interconnector domain of PCNA that is known to be a major binding site for many of PCNA's interacting proteins. We hypothesized that therapeutic agents targeting protein-protein interactions mediated through this region may confer differential toxicity to normal and malignant cells. To test this hypothesis, we designed a cell permeable peptide containing the PCNA L126-Y133 sequence. Here, we report that this peptide selectively kills human neuroblastoma cells, especially those with *MYCN* gene amplification, with much less toxicity to non-malignant human cells. Mechanistically, the peptide is able to block PCNA interactions in cancer cells. It interferes with DNA synthesis and homologous recombination-mediated double-stranded DNA break repair, resulting in S-phase arrest, accumulation of DNA damage, and enhanced sensitivity to cisplatin. These results demonstrate conceptually the utility of this peptide for treating neuroblastomas, particularly, the unfavorable *MYCN*-amplified tumors.

Editor: Anja-Katrin Bielinsky, University of Minnesota, United States of America

Funding: This work was supported in part by research awards to LHM from the Department of Defense (W81XWH-11-1-0786), National Institutes of Health/ National Cancer Institute (R01 CA121289), St Baldrick' Foundation (www.stbaldricks.org), and the ANNA Fund (www.annafund.com) and by the National Institutes of Health/National Cancer Institute grant RO1CA120954 to JMS. In addition, research reported in this publication was supported by National Cancer Institute of the National Institutes of Health under grant number P30CA033572. The content is solely the responsibility of the authors and does not necessarily represent the official views of the National Institutes of Health. The funders had no role in study design, data collection and analysis, decision to publish, or preparation of the manuscript.

Competing Interests: The authors have declared that no competing interests exist.

* E-mail: lgu@coh.org

Introduction

Neuroblastoma (NB) is one of the most common childhood neoplasms which originates from neural crest progenitor cells of the sympathetic nervous system and accounts for about 15% of all pediatric cancer deaths [1]. The prognosis of NB patients depends on the risk stratification. Survival is excellent in low and intermediate risk groups and localized perinatal adrenal tumors often spontaneously regress [2]. In contrast, patients in the high-risk group have very aggressive disease and represents a significant clinical hurdle [3]. Modern treatment for high-risk NB consists of induction treatment (conventional chemotherapy and surgery with or without radiotherapy), high-dose chemotherapy and autologous stem cell transplantation (HDCT/autoSCT) as a consolidation treatment, and 13-*cis*-retinoid acid to reduce relapse from minimal residual disease. Despite aggressive therapy, approximately 50% of patients with advanced disease are refractory to treatment or relapse and the survival rate for high-risk NB patients is dismal [4,5]. Thus, there is a significant unmet medical need for new

therapies to improve the treatment outcomes of this aggressive tumor phenotype.

Proliferating cell nuclear antigen (PCNA) is an evolutionally conserved protein found in all eukaryotic cells. It is an extensively used tumor progression marker, due to its function in DNA replication and its peak expression during S and G2 phases [6–8]. PCNA forms a homotrimeric ring structure encircling DNA [9,10] and acts as a sliding clamp that provides anchorage for many proteins [11]. A major interaction site in PCNA is the interdomain connecting loop that spans from amino acid M121 to Y133 [9]. This loop is recognized by proteins including p21 (CDKN1A) [12], DNA polymerase ä (Pol ä) [13], flap endonuclease 1 (FEN1) [14], DNA methyltransferase MeCTr [15], and DNA ligase 1 (LIGI) [16], which interact with PCNA through their PIP-box domains [11,17]. By recruiting these proteins to chromatin, PCNA plays a critical role in regulating DNA replication, cell cycle progression, and DNA damage responses [18]. Given the essential role of PCNA in coordinating these cellular processes that are fundamental to the proliferation and survival of cancer cells, inhibition of PCNA is viewed as an effective way to suppress tumor growth [19]. Extensive structural studies have enabled blockade of PCNA interaction by rational designs [20–22]. Several attempts have been made in recent years to block various aspects of PCNA function with promising results [12,23–27], demonstrating the potential of PCNA as a target for anti-cancer therapies.

We previously reported a novel cancer associated PCNA isoform (caPCNA) [28], which is present in a broad range of cancer cells and tumor tissues, but not highly expressed in non-malignant cells. We determined that caPCNA arises not because of a genetic mutation but as a result of posttranslational modification [29]. caPCNA actively participates in DNA replication and interacts with cellular DNA polymerases [28]. Epitope analysis using monoclonal antibodies raised against caPCNA reveals that the caPCNA-specific antigenic site lies between L126 and Y133 within the interconnector domain of PCNA ([28] and to be reported elsewhere). Using an *in vitro* Biacore assay, we observed that the peptide corresponding to L126-Y133 (caPep) can block the PCNA interaction with the PIP-box sequence of FEN1. Interestingly, the L126-Y133 region is only accessible to immunohistochemistry staining by a monoclonal antibody specific to this region in tumor cells, suggesting that this region is structurally altered and becomes more accessible for protein-protein interaction in tumor cells. We hypothesized that therapeutic agents targeting protein-protein interaction mediated through this peptide region may confer differential toxicity to normal and malignant cells. To test this hypothesis, we designed a cell permeable peptide containing the L126-Y133 sequence of PCNA (R9-caPep, see Materials and Methods). Here, we report that this peptide selectively kills NB cells with much less toxicity to human peripheral blood mononuclear cells (PBMC) or neural crest stem cells. R9-caPep also suppressed NB cell growth in a mouse xenograft model. Interestingly, *MYCN*-amplified NB cell lines are more sensitive to R9-caPep treatment than non-*MYCN*-amplified lines. Mechanistically, R9-caPep is able to selectively block PCNA interactions in cancer cells. It interferes with DNA synthesis and homologous recombination (HR) mediated double-stranded DNA break (DSB) repair, resulting in S-phase arrest, accumulation of DNA damage, and enhanced sensitivity to cisplatin. These results demonstrate that targeting protein-protein interactions involving the L126-Y133 region of PCNA may prove to be an effective approach to treating high-risk *MYCN*-amplified NB patients with reduced side effects.

Materials and Methods

Peptides

The eight amino acid caPeptide (caPep) corresponds to the L126-Y133 sequence of human PCNA. The cell permeable peptide, R9-caPep ($R_DR_DR_DR_DR_DR_DR_DR_DR_D$CCLGIPEQEY) was created by fusing the caPep to the C-terminus of a nine D-arginine sequence (R9) through a spacer of two cysteines (CC). Peptides containing nine D-arginines and two cysteines only (R9-CC) or the R9-CC sequence fused to the same amino acid residues as in the PCNA L126-Y133 region, but in a scrambled order (R9-srbPep: $R_DR_DR_DR_DR_DR_DR_DR_DR_D$CCEPGLIYEQ) were synthesized as controls. 5/6-Fluorescein (5-FAM) labeled R9-caPep and R9-srbPep were utilized for fluorescence microscopy and FACS analysis. All peptides were synthesized by AnaSpec (Fremont, CA).

Kinetic analysis of PCNA interaction by surface plasmon resonance (SPR)

All experiments were conducted on the Biacore T100 (GE Healthcare Life Sciences, Piscataway, NJ) in the running buffer

HBS-EP+ (10 mM HEPES pH 7.4, 0.15 M NaCl, 3 mM EDTA, 0.05% v/v Surfactant P20). FEN1 peptide containing the PIP-box (SKSRQGSTQGRLDDFF) was immobilized on a carboxymethylated dextran modified CM5 chip using carbodiimide covalent linkage procedures outlined by the manufacturer (GE Healthcare Life Sciences). Recombinant PCNA (rPCNA), purchased from Surmodics, Inc. (Edina, MN), were serially diluted in the HBS-EP+ buffer and flowed over the FEN1-coated sensor chip in the presence of 0, 500, or 1000 nM of caPep at a 5 il/min flow rate with a contact time of 3 minutes, followed by dissociation under the same buffer condition and regeneration of the chip surface in 10 mM glycine-HCl (pH 2.0). Binding curves were recorded for rPCNA concentrations ranging from 250 to 1000 nM in the presence of 0, 500, or 1000 nM of caPep. Kinetic parameters from Biacore binding data were determined using Biacore T100 Evaluation Software Version 2.0.3.

Cell permeability analysis

Cells were treated by various concentrations of 5-FAM labeled R9-caPep or R9-srbPep for 6 h. After being washed twice by PBS and detached by trypsin treatment, cells were further washed twice by the cell culture medium. The uptake of the fluorescent peptides was measured by a FACS analysis. The median fluorescent intensity was determined by the FlowJo program for each cell population under different treatment conditions. In addition, cells treated by 10 μM 5-FAM labeled R9-caPep or R9-srbPep were examined by confocal microscopy to determined the subcellular localization of the peptides.

Plasmids and Cell Lines

The human NB cell lines, SK-N-DZ, SK-N-BE(2)c, SK-N-AS, SK-N-SH, and SK-N-FI were obtained from the American Type Culture Collection (Rockville, MD). Cells were maintained in DMEM with 10% fetal bovine serum (FBS), 100 units/ml penicillin, and 100 μg/ml streptomycin in the presence of 5% CO_2 at 37°C. Human PBMCs from a healthy donor were purchased from Sanguine BioSciences (Valencia, CA) and grown in RPMI1640 with10% FBS, 100 units/ml penicillin, 100 μg/ml streptomycin, and 10 ng/ml IL-2 in the presence of 5% CO_2 at 37°C. Human embryonic progenitor cell line 7SM0032 was acquired from Millipore (Billerica, MA) and grown in the hEPM-1 Media Kit purchased from the same company.

The plasmid pCBASce expresses the rare cutting I-SceI meganuclease [30]. The U2OS-derived cell lines, DR-GFP, EJ5-GFP, and SA-GFP contain a stably transfected reporter gene for DSB repair mediated by HR, end joining (EJ), and single-strand annealing (SSA), respectively [31]. These cell lines were cultured in DMEM medium with 10% FBS at 37°C in the presence of 5% CO_2.

Cell growth and terminal deoxynucleotidyl transferase–mediated dUTP nick end labeling (TUNEL) assays

To measure cell growth, cells were seeded at 3×10^4/ml. After being allowed to attach overnight, cells were treated with various concentrations of the peptides for 72 h. Cell growth was measured by the CellTitor-Glo assay (Promega, Madison, WI) according to manufacturer's instruction. To measure apoptosis, cells were seeded at 1×10^5/ml onto a chamber slide. Once attached, cells were treated with the peptides for 48 h. Cells were fixed and analyzed by a TUNEL assay using the TMR red *in situ* cell death detection kit (Roche Diagnostics, Indianapolis, IN).

Cell Cycle Analysis

Cells were seeded at 1×10^5/ml. Once attached, cells were treated with or without R9-caPep for 48 hours. Cells were fixed in 60% ethanol and stained with propidium iodide (PI). The cellular PI fluorescence intensity was determined by flow cytometry. The flow cytometry data were analyzed by the FlowJo program to model various cell populations.

Immunofluorescence

Cells were seeded at 1×10^5/ml onto a chamber slide and were allowed to attach overnight. To analyze the interaction of PCNA with FEN1, LIGI, or Pol ä, we first synchronize cells at the G1/S boundary. The synchronization is achieved by starving cells in medium containing 0.25% FBS for 24 h. Cells were further cultured in the complete medium containing 400 μM of mimosine for 24 h. To release cells into S phase, cells were washed and incubated in mimosine-free medium containing 30 μM R9-caPep or R9-srbPep for 6 h. We pre-determined that the majority of cells were in the S-phase 6 h after mimosine was removed (data not shown). Cells were fixed in ice-cold methanol:acetone (50%:50%) for 10 min or in 4% paraformaldehyde for 20 min at room temperature. Cells were incubated with a goat polyclonal anti-PCNA antibody (Santa Cruz) and a mouse monoclonal anti-FEN1 antibody (Santa Cruz), a mouse anti-POLD3 antibody (Sigma, St. Louis, MO), or a mouse anti-LIGI antibody (Abcam, Cambridge, MA) for 1 h at room temperature. After being washed with PBS, cells were incubated with Alexa Fluor 488 conjugated anti-mouse IgG and Alexa Fluor 555 conjugated anti-goat IgG antibodies (Invitrogen, Grand Island, NY) for 1 h. Cells were mounted in Vectashield with DAPI (Vector Labs, Burlingame, CA) and visualized by a confocal microscope.

To study DNA damage and repair, attached cells were pretreated with the peptides for 2 h and were then ä-irradiated (5 Gy). After irradiation, cells were cultured in the presence of the peptides for the indicated time. For analyzing äH2A.X foci formation, cells were fixed in a solution of methanol and acetone (70%:30% v/v) for 15 min at $-20°C$. The slides were air-dried for storage and rehydrated in PBS prior to immunostaining. Cells were stained by a mouse monoclonal antibody specific to äH2A.X (Millipore, Billerica, MA) followed by an Alexa Fluor 488 conjugated anti-mouse IgG antibody. For analyzing Rad51 foci formation, cells were fixed in PBS buffered 4% paraformaldehyde at room temperature for 15 min. After being washed twice by PBS, cells were permeabilized in PBS containing 0.5% triton for 15 min on ice. The fixed and permeabilized cells were stained with a rabbit polyclonal antibody raised against the human Rad51 (Santa Cruz) followed by an Alexa Fluor 488 conjugated anti-rabbit IgG antibody. Stained cells were visualized and imaged by a confocal microscope.

BrdU incorporation assay

SK-N-BE(2)c cells were treated with the peptides for 7.5 h and then incubated in 10 imol/L BrdU for an additional 30 min in the continuous presence of the peptides. Cells were detached with trypsin and fixed in Cytofix/Cytoperm buffer according to the manufacturer's instructions (BD Bioscience, San Jose, CA). Fixed cells were treated with DNase to expose incorporated BrdU and stained with FITC-conjugated anti-BrdU antibody (BD Bioscience) for 1 h at room temperature. Samples were analyzed by flow cytometry to quantify the amount of BrdU incorporation. Percentages of FITC-positive cells were determined by analysis with the FlowJo software. Statistical analysis was conducted using a two-tailed t-test.

SV40 DNA replication assay

The assay was performed essentially as described [32], except that nuclear extracts from SK-N-BE(2)c cells were used in the assay.

DSB repair assays

DR-GFP, EJ5-GFP, and SA-GFP cell lines were seeded at 2.5×10^4 cells/cm^2 in a 12-well plate. Once attached overnight, cells were transfected with 1.2 μg of the pCBASce I-SceI expression plasmid mixed with 3.6 μl of Lipofectamine 2000 (Invitrogen) in 200 μl of Optimem media (Invitrogen). After incubation for 3 h, the media containing transfection complexes was aspirated and replaced with fresh media containing 30 μM of the peptides. The HR, EJ, and SSA-mediated DSB repair, indicated by the restoration of a functional GFP gene in the respective cell lines, were quantified by measuring the relative abundance of GFP-positive cells by flow cytometry 3 d after transfection.

Clonogenic Assay

Three hundred fifty SK-N-BE(2)c cells were seeded onto a 60-mm tissue culture dish. Once attached overnight, cells were treated with or without cisplatin for 2 h. Cells were washed twice with growth medium and were cultured in fresh medium with or without R9-caPep for 3 weeks to allow colony formation. The medium was changed every 3 d. The colonies formed under each treatment conditions were counted after being stained with 0.5% crystal violet.

Western blot

Cell extracts were prepared by dissolving cell pellets directly into the Laemmli sample buffer and resolved in a 4–12% SDS polyacrylamide gel. Resolved proteins were blotted onto a nitrocellulose membrane. The membrane was blocked with 5% nonfat dry milk and incubated with an antibody specific to äH2A.X (Millipore), total H2A.X (Cell Signaling Technology, Danvers, MA), MYCN (Cell Signaling Technology), or actin (Sigma) in the blocking buffer. After incubation with peroxidase-conjugated secondary antibodies, the protein of interest was detected using an ECL kit purchased from GE Healthcare.

In vivo tumor model

All experiments involving live animals were carried out in strict accordance with the recommendations in the Guide for the Care and Use of Laboratory Animals of the National Institutes of Health. The protocol (#11034) was reviewed and approved by the City of Hope Institutional Animal Care and Use Committee. Nude mice 6 weeks of age were purchased from the Jackson Laboratory (Bar Harbor, ME). SK-N-BE(2)c cells were harvested and washed twice in PBS. Cells were suspended in Matrigel (BD Biosciences) at 5×10^7/ml. 0.1 ml of suspended cells was subcutaneously injected into the right flank of each of 30 nude mice. Seven days after tumor inoculation, mice were randomly grouped into three groups with 10 mice in each group. The mice were treated with PBS, R9-srbPep, or R9-caPep 3 times a week by intratumoral injection. Tumor growth was measured weekly as well as at the end of the experiment by a dial caliper. Tumor volumes were estimated based on the length (L) and width (W) of the tumors ($V = L \times W^2 \times 0.5$). At the end of the experiment, tumors were isolated from sacrificed mice and their masses were measured.

Results

Cell permeable R9-caPep selectively inhibits the growth of NB cells

To determine the cytotoxic potential of blocking protein-protein interaction involving the L126-Y133 region of PCNA in cancer cells, we generated the R9-caPep by fusing the L126-Y133 sequence of PCNA to the C-terminus of a nine D-arginine sequence (R9) through a spacer of two cysteines. We also generated peptides R9-CC and R9-srbPep as controls (see Materials and Methods). To determine cell permeability of the peptides, we treated SK-N-DZ NB cells with various concentrations of 5-FAM labeled R9-caPep and R9-srbPep and measured their fluorescence intensity by flow cytometry. Quantification of the median fluorescence intensity of each cell population under various treatment conditions revealed that both peptides are cell permeable and are taken by cells with similar efficiencies in a dose dependent manner (Fig 1a). By fluorescence microscopy, we observed that R9-caPep and R9-srbPep localized to the cytosol, throughout the nucleoplasma, and likely in nucleoli (Fig 1b). They both formed small spots in the nucleoplasma with slightly different patterns presumably caused by their different affinities to nucleoproteins. R9-caPep inhibited the growth of a panel of NB cell lines with IC_{50} ranging from 10 to 32 μM (Fig 1c & d). In contrast, control peptides R9-srbPep and R9-CC did not significantly affect cell growth up to 50 μM (data not shown). In addition, R9-caPep was well tolerated by non-malignant cells including human peripheral blood mononuclear cells (PBMC) and human neural crest stem cells (Fig 1c) with IC_{50} of 98 μM and more than 100 μM on these cells respectively, indicating that the R9-caPep selectively inhibits the growth of NB cancer cells. Interestingly, NB cell lines with *MYCN* amplification were uniformly more sensitive to R9-caPep than NB cell lines without *MYCN* amplification (Fig 1c, d, & e). These observations demonstrate the potential utility of R9-caPep or R9-caPep derived agents for treating NB, especially the subset containing *MYCN* amplification associated with a particularly poor prognosis.

The R9-caPep blocks PCNA interactions

One essential function of PCNA is coordinating DNA replication by recruiting many interacting proteins, including FEN1, LIGI, and Pol ä, to replication foci. Binding of these proteins to PCNA not only brings them to the site of DNA replication, but also is often essential to their functional activity or processivity. To explore the mechanism by which R9-caPep kills cancer cells, we first examined whether the caPeptide (caPep) interferes with PCNA interaction *in vitro* by SPR (see Materials and Method for details). Given the fact that caPep is derived from the interdomain connecting loop of PCNA that usually contacts the PIP-box sequence in PCNA-binding proteins [11,17], we tested whether caPep can block interaction between PCNA and the PIP-box sequence of FEN1. Shown in Fig 2a are the real-time response curves recorded for 1000 nM recombinant PCNA (rPCNA) flowing over the PIP-box sequence of FEN1 immobilized to the surface of a CM5 chip in the presence of 0, 500, or 1000 nM caPep. The presence of caPep significantly reduced rPCNA interaction with the immobilized FEN1 PIP-box sequence (Fig 2a). We also recorded binding curves under other rPCNA concentrations ranging between 250 and 1000 nM in the presence of 0, 500, or 1000 nM of caPep and observed that rPCNA binds to the immobilized FEN1 PIP-box sequence in a dose-dependent manner (data not shown). The dose-dependent PCNA binding to the immobilized FEN1 PIP-box sequence recorded under each caPep concentration was used for calculating dissociation constant

(K_D). As shown by the K_D in the inserted table in Fig 2a, caPep decrease the affinity of PCNA-FEN1 PIP-box interaction in a dose-dependent manner, indicating its antagonistic effect on PCNA interaction.

We sought to determine whether R9-caPep treatment interferes with the interaction of PCNA with these proteins during DNA replication. Cells were synchronized by serum starvation followed by mimosine treatment (see Methods for details). We pre-determined that more than 60% of the cells were in the S-phase 6 h after mimosine was removed (data not shown). We treated synchronized cells with R9-caPep or R9-srbPep for 6 h as they were entering S-phase after being released from mimosine-induced growth arrest. Cell cycle analyses indicated that neither peptide significantly affected cell cycle progress within 6 h (data not shown) and a longer treatment increased the relative abundance of cells in S-phase (Fig. 3c). We determined the subcellular localization of PCNA, FEN1, LIGI, and POLD3 (the subunit of Pol ä that directly interacts with PCNA) by immunofluorescence microscopy. In cells treated with R9-srbPep, PCNA co-localized with FEN1 and LIGI at discrete foci (Fig 2b and c). The PCNA foci were also visible in cells treated with R9-caPep. However, LIGI co-localization to PCNA-positive foci was largely blocked by the R9-caPep (Fig 2c). In addition, the few remaining FEN1 foci in cells treated by the R9-caPep didn't appear to overlap the PCNA foci (Fig 2b). Since R9-caPep treatment didn't affect intracellular LIGI or FEN1 level in a western blot assay (data not shown), the lack of FEN1 or LIGI foci co-localized with PCNA indicated that R9-caPep interfered with the recruitment of FEN1 and LIGI to PCNA without dissociating PCNA from replication foci. Interestingly, R9-caPep did not seem to affect the recruitment of POLD3 to PCNA (Fig 2d), indicating a degree of selectivity in the R9-caPep effect on PNCA interactions.

R9-caPep inhibits DNA replication and induces cancer cell cycle arrest and apoptosis

Because R9-caPep affects the PCNA interaction with FEN1 and LIGI, both of which are involved in the maturation of the lagging chain during DNA replication, we determined whether the peptide interferes with DNA replication in NB cells by determining the effect of R9-caPep on DNA synthesis using a BrdU incorporation assay. R9-caPep treatment induced a significant reduction in the percentage of BrdU-positive cells in comparison to the treatment by R9-srbPep (Fig 3a), indicating stalled DNA replication in cells treated with R9-caPep.

We further examined the effect of R9-caPep on SV40 T-antigen-dependent DNA replication *in vitro*. The SV40 viral system is a widely used model for studying eukaryotic DNA replication, partly because SV40 encodes only a single replication protein, the T antigen, and extensively utilizes cellular replication machinery [33]. As a result, the viral and eukaryotic DNA replications share remarkable resemblance. R9-caPep inhibited SV40 T-antigen-dependent DNA replication *in vitro* (Fig 3b), confirming the effect of R9-caPep on DNA replication observed in the BrdU incorporation assay. Consistent with these observations, R9-caPep treatment caused S-phase arrest in NB cells (Fig 3c). After 48 h of treatment by 40 μM of R9-caPep, NB cells start to die through apoptosis as indicated by the rise of a sub-G1 cell population (Fig 3c) and by increased TUNEL positivity (Fig 3d & e). In contrast, significantly less effect on cell cycle progression and cell survival were seen in non-malignant 7SM0032 cells under the same R9-caPep treatment (Fig 3c, d, & e). Collectively, these observations support the hypothesis that the R9-caPep exerts its effect on cancer cells at least partly by interfering with DNA

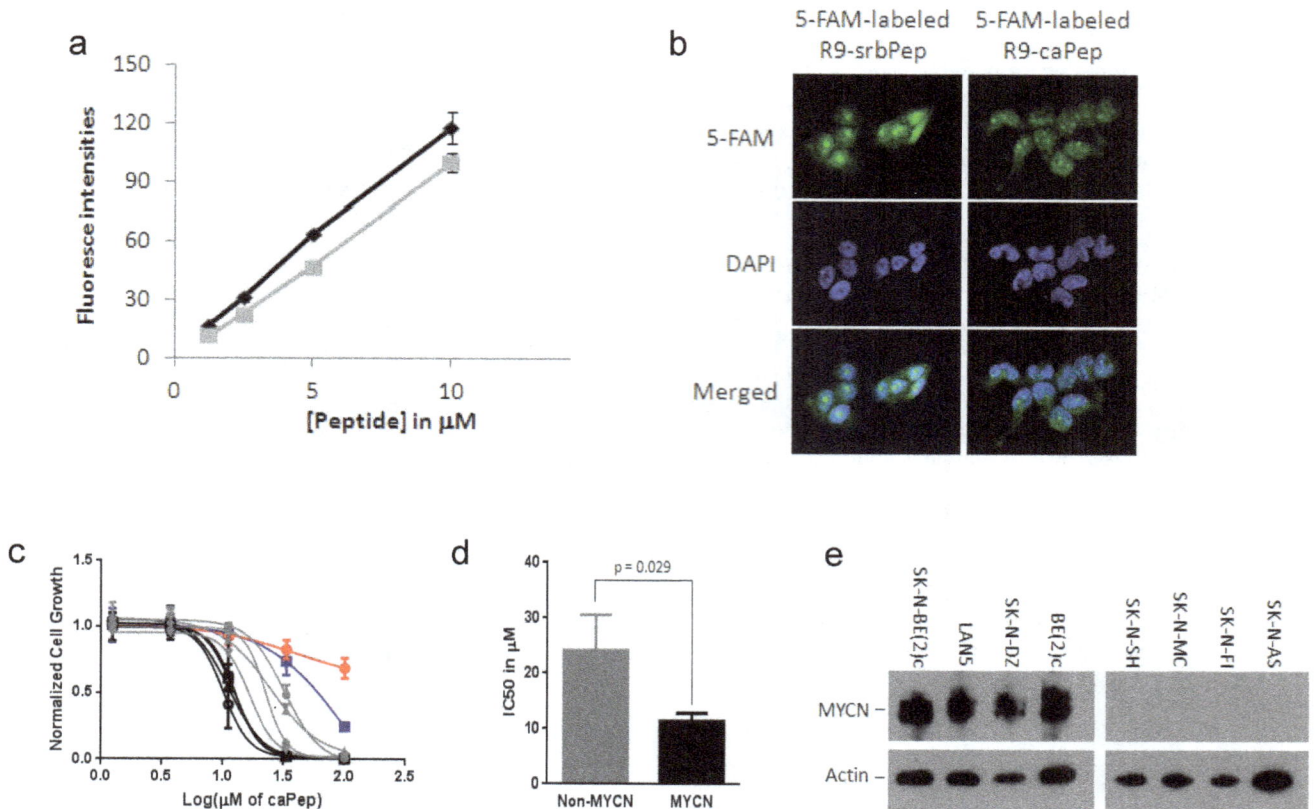

Figure 1. Permeability and selective cytotoxicity of R9-caPep in NB cells. a) SK-N-DZ NB cells were treated in triplicates by various concentrations of 5-FAM labeled R9-caPep (gray) or R9-srbPep (dark). After cells were treated by trypsin and washed, their fluorescence intensities were determined by flow cytometry. The median fluorescence intensities for triplicate cell populations under each treatment condition were averaged and graphed plus/minus standard deviations. b) Cells treated by 10 μM 5-FAM labeled R9-caPep or R9-srbPep were examined by confocal microscopy. The nuclear areas were indicated by DAPI staining. c) Four NB cell lines with *MYCN* amplification (in black), four NB cell lines without *MYCN* amplification (in grey), human PBMCs (red cycles), and human neural crest stem cell line 7SM0032 (blue squares) were cultured in the presence of various concentrations of the R9-caPep for 72 h. Cell growth was determined by a CellTiter-Glo luminescence assay (Promega). Cells cultured in the absence of the R9-caPep were used as control. Luminescent signals in triplicates normalized to the control for each cell line were averaged and graphed plus/minus standard deviations. Black filled squares: LAN5, black triangles: SK-N-DZ, black circles: SK-N-BE(2)c, black empty squares: BE(2)c, grey diamond: SK-N-AS, grey circle: SK-N-SH, grey triangle: SK-N-MC, and grey square: SK-N-FI. d) The IC_{50}s of the peptide on cell lines with or without *MYCN* amplification, determined by non-linear fit of Prism 6 (GraphPad Software, La Jolla, CA), were averaged and graphed plus/minus standard deviations. e) Total cell lysates were extracted from the indicated cell lines. The expression of MYCN and actin in these cell lines were determined by western blot.

replication through blocking PCNA interactions with its binding proteins.

R9-caPep interferes with HR-mediated DSB repair

In addition to its role as the processivity clamp for the DNA replication machinery, PCNA also plays a broad role in repairing DNA damage including the lethal DSB [18]. To investigate whether R9-caPep treatment affects DNA DSB repair, we induced DSB by ã-irradiation of cells pre-treated with R9-caPep or R9-srbPep. Western blot analysis showed that the levels of ãH2A.X, a marker of double-stranded DNA damage, increased within 30 min following ã-irradiation in cells treated with either peptide (Fig 4a). In cells treated by the control R9-srbPep, the ãH2A.X level went down to a basal level by 48 h after ã-irradiation, suggesting the completion of DSB repair. In contrast, the ãH2A.X level remained elevated in cells treated by the R9-caPep, indicating the continued presence of unresolved DSB after 48 h. This result was further confirmed by immunofluorescence studies showing that R9-caPep treatment delayed the resolution of ãH2A.X foci induced by ã-

irradiation (Fig 4b & c), indicating an impaired capacity for DSB repair in cells treated with R9-caPep.

Double-stranded DNA breaks, if not resolved in time, are lethal to cells. Cells deal with double-stranded DNA breaks through several DNA repair pathways, including HR, EJ, and SSA mediated DNA repair [34,35]. Reporter cell lines have been established to monitor each of these DNA repair pathways [31]. These cells lines each contain a reporter with a GFP expression cassette disrupted by recognition site(s) for the endonuclease I-SceI. Introduction of exogenous I-SceI creates DSB(s) within the reporters. Each reporter is designed such that repair of the I-SceI-induced DSB(s) by a specific pathway can result in restoration of the GFP cassette: HR for DR-GFP, EJ for EJ5-GFP, and SSA for SA-GFP. The relative abundance of GFP-positive cells determined by flow cytometry, therefore, reflects the efficiency of the respective DSB repair pathway in these reporter cell lines. Using these characterized reporter cell lines, we observed that R9-caPep treatment significantly inhibited HR-mediated DNA repair, while causing only small effects on EJ or SSA (Fig 4d). The DSB repair event measured by DR-GFP (HR), but not EJ or SSA, is promoted

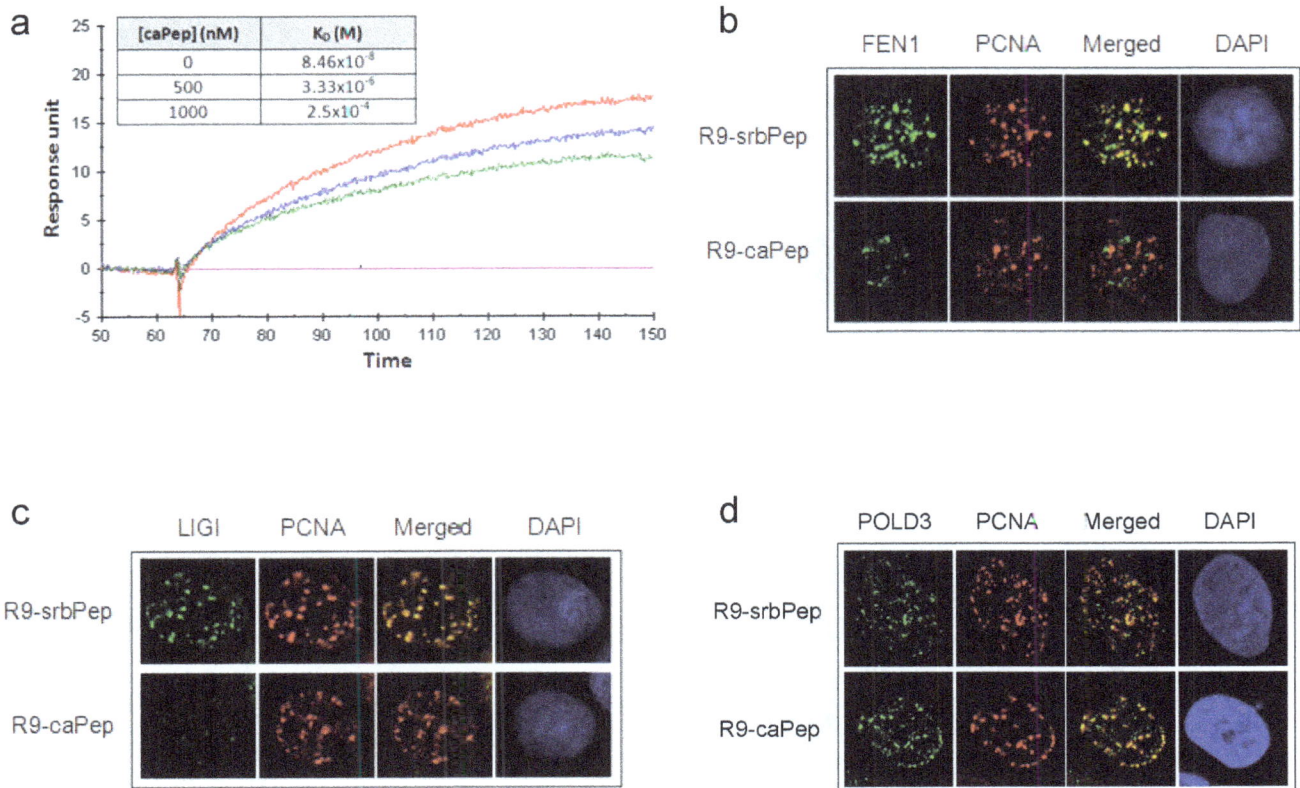

Figure 2. Inhibition of PCNA interactions by caPep and R9-caPep. a) The real-time SPR response curves were recorded for 1000 nM recombinant PCNA (rPCNA) flowing over the PIP-box sequence of FEN1 immobilized to the surface of a CM5 chip in the presence of 0 (red), 500 (blue), or 1000 (green) nM caPep. The dose-dependent binding of rPCNA to the immobilized FEN1 PIP-box sequence were also recorded under other rPCNA concentrations ranging between 250 and 1000 nM in the presence of 0, 500, or 1000 nM caPep (response curve not shown) and were used to calculate K_D of PCNA-FEN1 PIP-box interaction, as shown in the inserted table. SK-N-AS NB cells were treated with R9-caPep or R9-srbPep. Cells were fixed and immunostained with: b) mouse anti-FEN1 and goat anti-PCNA antibodies; c) mouse anti-LIGI and goat anti-PCNA antibodies; d) mouse anti-POLD3 and goat anti-PCNA antibodies. After DAPI counterstaining, nuclear co-localization of PCNA with FEN1, LIGI, or POLD3 was visualized by fluorescence confocal microscopy.

by the recombinase Rad51 [30], which mediates strand exchange between sister chromatids. Accordingly, HR requires the recruitment of Rad51 to DNA damage, often measured as its accumulation into nuclear foci, which is dependent on BRCA1 and BRCA2 [36]. The formation of the Rad51-DNA recombination complex is known to be regulated by PCNA and its interacting proteins [37,38]. We measured the effect of R9-caPep on the formation and/or resolution of Rad51 foci in response to ã-irradiation in SK-N-BE(2)c cells. Immunofluorescence microscopy indicated that R9-caPep treatment reduced the number of Rad51-positive cells at 4 h after ã-irradiation (Fig 4e and f). By 48 h after ã-irradiation, cells treated with the control R9-srbPep were able to almost completely resolve the Rad51 foci. In contrast, nearly all the cells treated with R9-caPep showed a strong and diffused background staining of Rad51, indicating an enhanced expression of Rad51. Over this strong background staining, Rad51 foci remain visible, suggesting that DNA repair following Rad51-DNA complex formation was blocked in R9-caPep treated cells.

R9-caPep enhances the sensitivity of cancer cells to cisplatin

HR-mediated DNA repair plays an important role in repairing cross-linked DNA [39,40] caused by common chemotherapeutic drugs, such as cisplatin. We performed a clonogenic assay to investigate whether the peptide would increase NB cells' sensitivity to cisplatin. We treated SK-N-BE(2)c cells with or without 1 µM cisplatin for 2 h to induce DNA cross-linking. After being washed twice with growth medium, cells were cultured in fresh medium with or without 20 µM of R9-caPep in the absence of cisplatin for 3 weeks to allow colony formation. Whereas R9-caPep or cisplatin alone reduced the number of colonies formed by less than 30%, sequential treatment of cells with cisplatin and R9-caPep was able to reduce the number of colonies by about 80% (Fig 5), demonstrating the potential of combining R9-caPep-derived therapies with conventional chemotherapeutic drugs in treating NB patients.

R9-caPep inhibits tumor growth in mice

Given the favorable potential therapeutic properties of R9-caPep seen in cell-based assays, we asked whether we could recapitulate its anti-cancer activity in vivo. We tested R9-caPep in nude mice bearing xenograft tumors derived from the SK-N-BE2(c) cells and found that R9-caPep significantly and nearly completely inhibited tumor growth in terms of tumor volume and mass (Fig 6a & b) in comparison to the control groups that were treated with PBS or R9-srbPep. These in vivo results corroborate with our in vitro results and further suggest the potential of the PCNA L126-Y133 region in conceptualizing NB therapeutics.

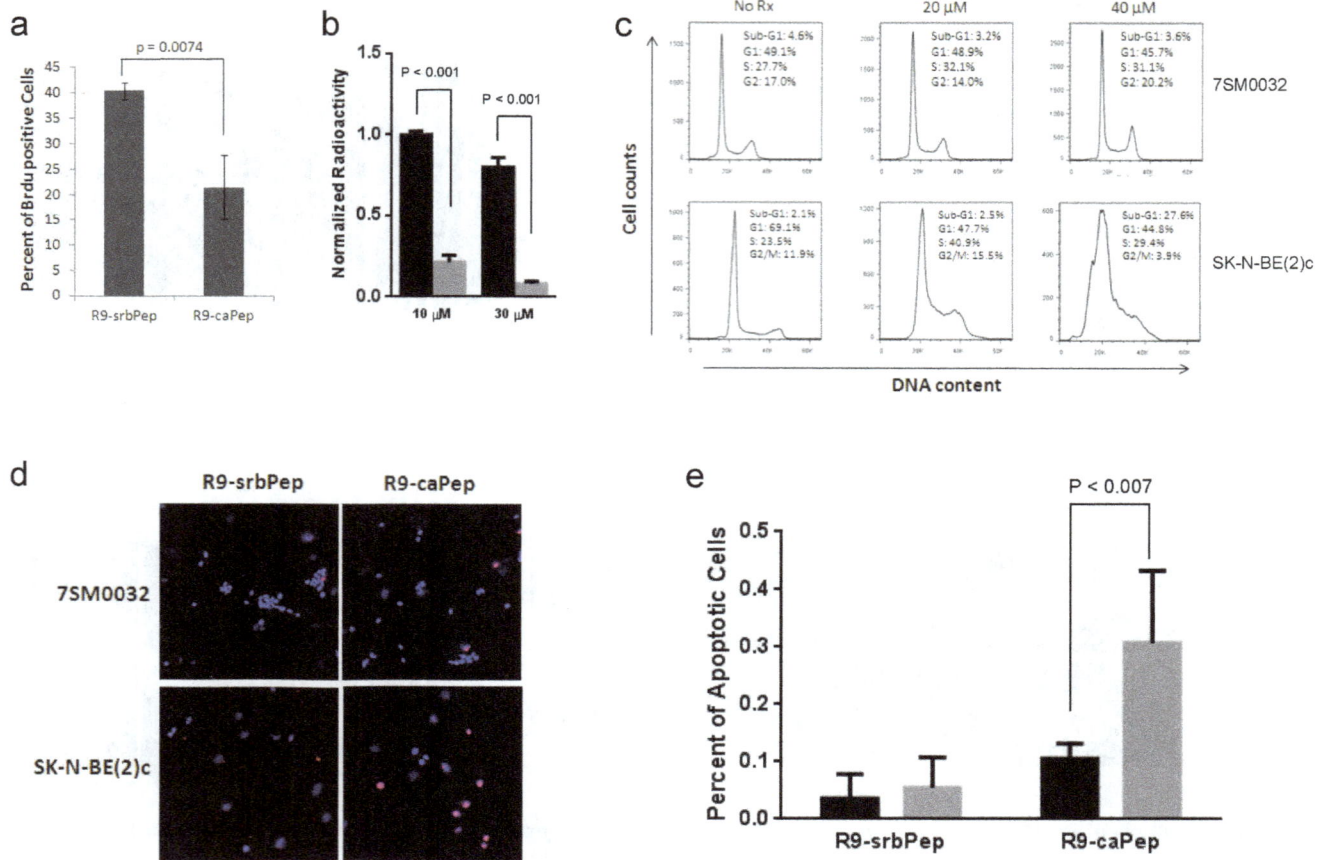

Figure 3. Inhibition of DNA replication and induction of S-phase arrest and apoptosis by R9-caPep. a) SK-N-BE(2)c cells were pulsed in 10 µM of BrdU for 30 min after being pre-treated with R9-caPep or R9-srbPep for 7.5 h. The relative abundances of BrdU-positive cells in triplicates were averaged and graphed plus/minus standard deviations. b) Nuclear extracts from SK-N-BE(2)c cells were incubated with the indicated concentrations of R9-caPep (grey bars) or R9-srbPep (black bars) for 20 min. SV40 T-antigen was then added to the nuclear extracts along with premixed reaction buffer containing ^{32}P dCTP. A complete reaction mixture except for SV40 T-antigen was used as control for T-antigen-independent nucleotide incorporation. The polymerized radioactivity was measured by a scintillation counter. The T-antigen-dependent incorporation of ^{32}P dCTP was calculated by subtracting T-antigen-independent radioactivity from the total radioactivity and was normalized to the T-antigen-dependent radioactivity in PBS-treated samples. Triplicates of normalized T-antigen-dependent radioactivity for each treatment condition were averaged and graphed plus/minus standard deviations. c) SK-N-BE(2)c and non-malignant 7SM0032 cells were fixed and stained with propidium iodide (PI) after being treated with the indicated concentrations of R9-caPeptide for 48 h. The cellular PI fluorescence intensity determined by flow cytometry was analyzed by the FlowJo to model various cell populations. d) Cells grown on chamber slides were treated by R9-caPep or R9-srbPep at 40 µM for 48 h. Cells were fixed and analyzed by a TUNEL assay. Cells were imaged by a confocal microscope. TMR-red is the fluorophore that was attached to the free DNA ends. DAPI (blue) indicates the location of nuclei. The pink dots derived from the merged TMR-red and DAPI staining indicate apoptosis. e) The abundance of apoptotic cells relative to the total number of cells in six randomly selected fields were averaged and graphed plus/minus standard deviations (right). The dark and gray bars represent results from 7SM0032 and SK-N-BE(2)c cells respectively.

Discussion

Cancer cells depend on DNA replication as well as multiple DNA repair pathways to proliferate and survive. It is no coincidence that many chemotherapeutic agents act by damaging DNA or interfering with DNA replication or repair. These traditional chemotherapeutic drugs are widely used as first line therapies for treating a broad range of cancers, including NB. However, they are also toxic to normal cells, causing severe, debilitating side effects. In addition, there is a high risk of developing resistance to these drugs through mutations, resulting from the genetic instability characteristic of many cancers and redundancy in DNA synthesis and repair pathways. There is currently a considerable interest in the development of PCNA inhibitors as broad spectrum anti-cancer agents, because of the indispensible role of PCNA in regulating DNA replication and

most DNA repair pathways. Proteins and peptides in general exhibit greater specificities to their targets than small molecules and are increasingly recognized as structural leads for the development of novel therapeutic small molecules. With the recent advancement in protein and peptide delivery technology, a number of protein and peptide based drugs have successfully reached markets or are currently working their way through different stages of clinical trials [41]. To target cancer cells selectively, we developed the therapeutic peptide, R9-caPep, which contains the L126-Y133 octapeptide region of PCNA and demonstrated that this peptide selectively kills NB cells and is especially toxic to *MYCN*-amplified NB cell lines, demonstrating its potential utility in treating patients with high-risk *MYCN*-amplified tumors.

Our work demonstrates that R9-caPep interfered with DNA replication and HR-mediated DNA repair presumably by binding

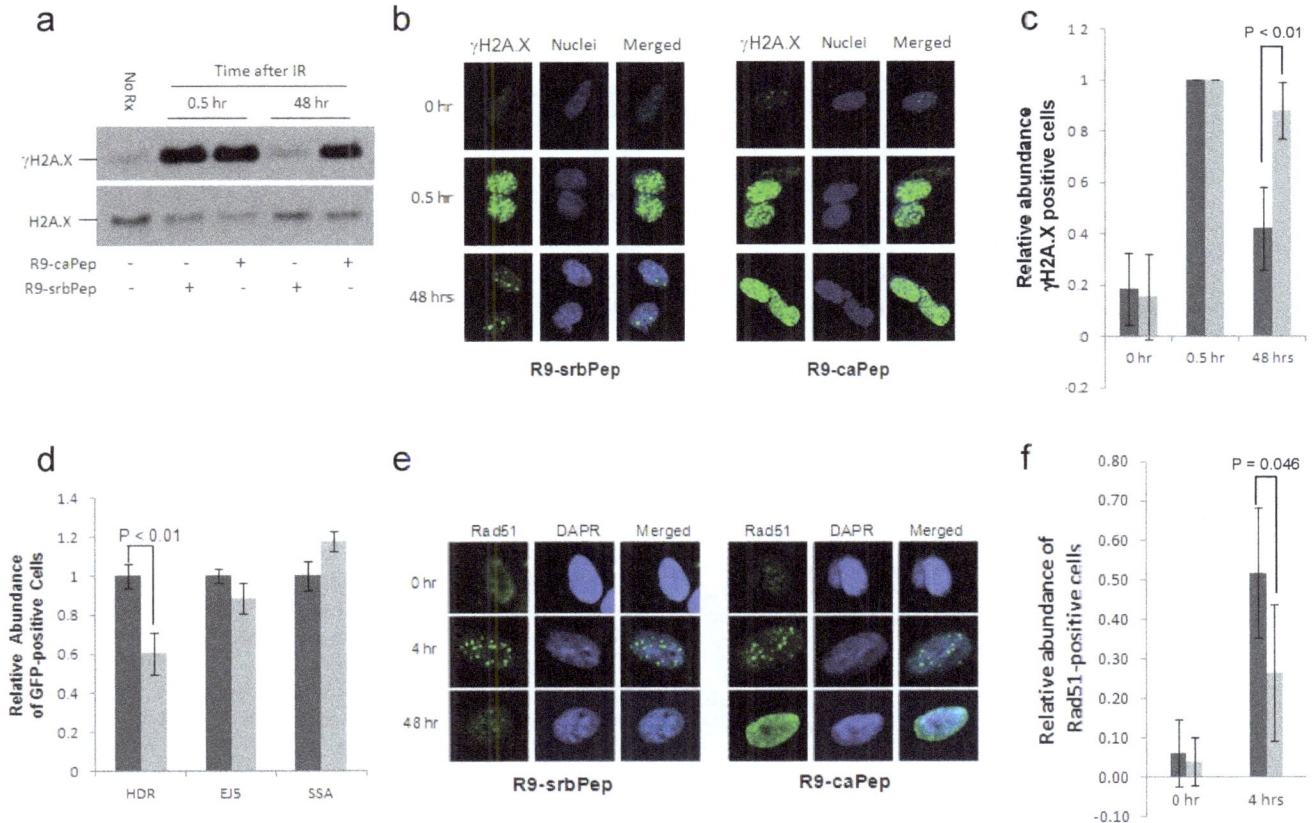

Figure 4. Inhibition of DSB repair by R9-caPep. Cells pretreated with 30 μM R9-caPep or R9-srbPep for 2 h were irradiated by a ã-irradiator (5 Gy). After irradiation, cells were cultured in the presence of R9-caPep or R9-srbPep for the indicated time. a) Intracellular ãH2A.X and total H2A.X levels were determined by western blot. b) The formation of intra-nuclear ãH2A.X foci was analyzed by immunofluorescence microscopy. c) Cells containing at least 5 ãH2A.X foci were counted as ãH2A.X positive cells. The relative abundance of ãH2A.X positive cells in five randomly selected fields were averaged and graphed plus/minus standard deviation. Dark bars represent results from cells treated with the scrambled R9-srbPep; Light bars represent results from cells treated with R9-caPep. d) The DR-GFP, EJ5-GFP, and SA-GFP cell lines were transiently transfected by the pCBASce plasmid that expresses the I-SceI meganuclease. The HR, EJ, and SSA-mediated DSB repair events, indicated by the restoration of a functional GFP gene in the respective cell lines, were quantified by measuring the relative abundance of GFP-positive cells by flow cytometry. The relative abundance of GFP-positive cells in R9-caPep treated samples (light bars) were normalized to those treated with R9-srbPep (dark bars). Results from triplets for each cell line and treatment condition were averaged and graphed plus/minus standard deviations. e) Cells pretreated with R9-caPep or R9-srbPep for 2 h were ã-irradiated (5 Gy). The formation of intra-nuclear Rad51 foci was analyzed at the indicated time after ã-irradiation by immunofluorescence microscopy. f) The relative abundance of Rad51-positive cells (containing at least 5 foci) as a percent of the total number of cells in five randomly selected fields were averaged and graphed plus/minus standard deviations. The dark and gray bars represent results from cells treated by R9-srbPep or R9-caPep respectively.

to proteins that interact with PCNA through the L126-Y133 region, thereby preventing them from functionally being recruited to PCNA. Indeed, the caPep interfered with PCNA interaction with the PIP-box sequence of FEN1 *in vitro* and the R9-caPep blocked the co-localization of fen-1 and LIGI to the PCNA foci in cells undergoing DNA replication. Given the essential role these two proteins play in the processing of Okazaki fragments, the R9-caPep may stall replication of lagging strands by blocking Okazaki fragment maturation. The R9-caPep was also observed to block the repair of ã-irradiation-induced DSB. The effect of the R9-caPep on DSB repair appears to be specific to the HR-mediated pathway, since the peptide has little effect on the EJ pathway and slightly enhances DNA repair through SSA. The HR-mediated DNA repair is a major DSB repair mechanism in S and G2 phases and plays a vital role in resolving stalled replication forks [42]. When faced with DNA replication stress, cells attempt to overcome the stalled replication forks by transiently introducing DSB, which, if not resolved, is lethal to cells. By causing DNA

replication stress and inhibiting HR-mediated DNA repair, the R9-caPep delivers a lethal one-two punch to cancer cells.

The most intriguing finding of this study is that NB cells with *MYCN* amplification are more sensitive to R9-caPep treatment than NB cells without *MYCN* amplification, as *MYCN*-amplified NB cancers are characteristically aggressive and resistant to therapy. We speculate that this phenomenon might be related to the dysregulated cell cycle control and DNA damage response in *MYCN*-amplified cells. *MYCN* is a member of the MYC proto-oncogene family that also comprises *MYC* and *MYCL*. It has been shown that MYC proteins promote the entry of S phase [43,44] and inhibit G1 arrest after DNA damage [44–46]. Consequently, cells overexpressing MYC proteins are more likely to enter S-phase with unrepaired DNA damage. In the *MYCN*-amplified NB cell line, SK-N-BE(2)c, knockdown of MYCN expression by siRNA can restore DNA damage induced G1 arrest [44], indicating a causal relationship between MYCN overexpression and dysregulation of the G1 check point. In addition, both MYCN

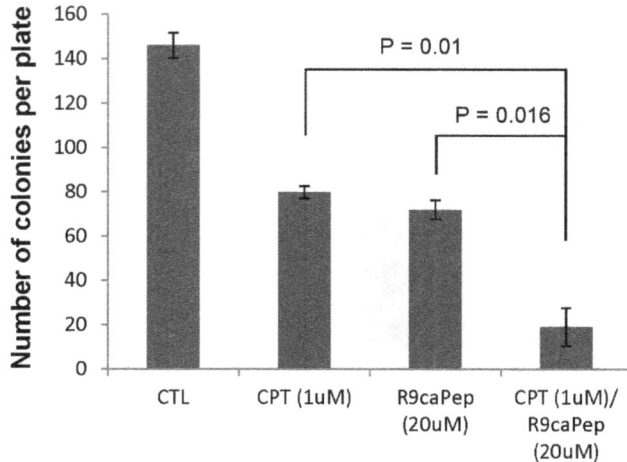

Figure 5. Enhanced sensitivity to cisplatin by R9-caPep. Human SK-N-BE2c NB cells were treated with or without 1 μM cisplatin for 2 h. Cells were washed twice with growth medium and were cultured in fresh medium with or without 20 μM R9-caPep for 3 weeks to allow colony formation. The colony counts in 3 dishes under each treatment condition were averaged and graphed plus/minus standard deviations.

[47] and MYC [48] have been shown to directly induce DNA replication stress. Taken together, overexpression of MYC proteins likely makes cancer cells more dependent on HR-mediated DNA repair to resolve stalled DNA replication and, consequently, more sensitive to the blockade of DNA repair by R9-caPep. Consistent with this hypothesis, cancer cells overexpressing MYC proteins are addicted to DNA helicase, WRN, which plays an important role in resolving replication stress [43,49]. The expression of a number of genes involved in the HR-mediated DSB repair pathway is also enhanced in NB tumors and cell lines containing *MYCN* amplification ([50] and data not shown). Given the structural similarity [51] and functional redundancy [52,53] between MYCN and MYC, R9-caPep might be effective in treating cancers that overexpress MYC as well.

In addition to NB cells, the peptide is selectively toxic to breast, lung, and pancreatic cancer cell lines in comparison with non-malignant cell lines of their respective tissue origins (data not shown). The exact mechanism for such a specificity against a broad spectrum of malignancy remains to be elucidated. The interconnector domain of PCNA that contains the L126-Y133 sequence is a major binding site for many PCNA interacting proteins. Interestingly, whereas the R9-caPep blocked the co-localization of fen-1 and LIG1 to the PCNA, it did not block PCNA and p21 interaction *in vitro* (data not shown) or the recruitment of POLD3 to PCNA foci in cells (Fig 2c). The differences in the ability of R9-caPep to block the recruitment of different PCNA interacting proteins may reflect the different affinities of these proteins to PCNA. It might also result from different binding affinities between the R9-caPep and these PCNA interacting proteins. We believe that the anti-cancer specificity of the R9-caPep is likely related to the unique profile of R9-caPep affinities towards various potential targets and their structural responses to R9-caPep binding. Identification of R9-caPep binding proteins by proteomic studies will be an important step toward understanding and further improving R9-caPep-type therapeutics. It has been shown that single amino acid substitutions in the L126-Y133 region can cause significant changes in the affinity profiles of PCNA for its interacting proteins in yeast [54]. Mutagenesis studies of the R9-caPep are ongoing to identify peptides with improved potency and therapeutic window. The structural and mechanistic insight gained from such studies will provide valuable information for the design of non-peptide mimetics of the R9-caPep. The fact that R9-caPep confers higher sensitivity to the DNA damaging agent cisplatin indicates its potential for combination therapy.

Acknowledgments

We thank the City of Hope Analytical Cytometry Core for help with flow cytometry work and the Microscopy Core for help with fluorescence imaging. The authors dedicate the work in memory of Anna Olivia Healey.

Author Contributions

Conceived and designed the experiments: LG SS CL RJH JMS GBF JAS LHM. Performed the experiments: LG SS CL WHL. Analyzed the data:

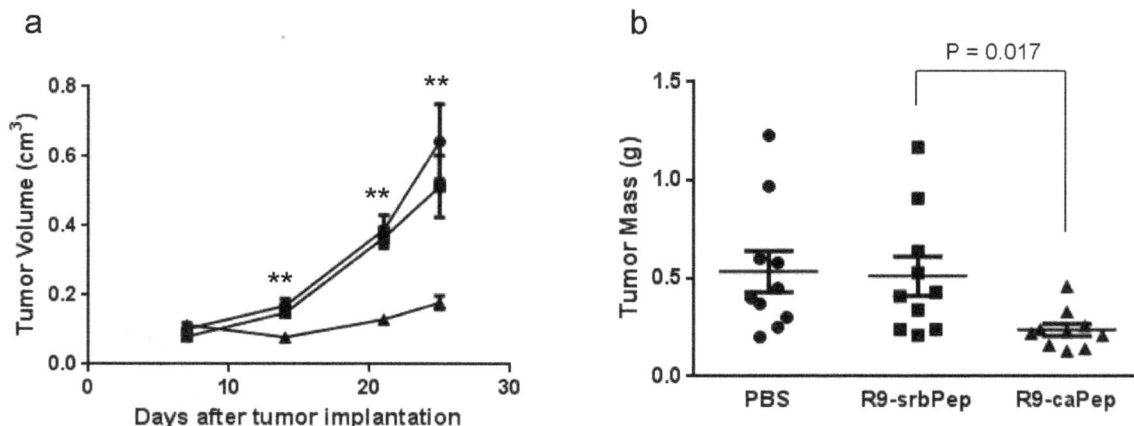

Figure 6. Inhibition of tumor growth by R9-caPep *in vivo*. a) Nude mice were randomly divided into 3 groups of 10 mice after each being injected with 5×10^6 SK-N-BE(2)c cells in Matrigel. Each group was treated with PBS (circle), R9-srbPep (square), or R9-caPep (triangle) by intratumoral injection. Tumor sizes were measured at the indicated time points and tumor volumes were estimated based on the length and width of the tumors ($V = L \times W2 \times 0.5$). The mean tumor volume for each treatment group was graphed plus/minus standard errors. ** indicates p<0.01. b) Tumor masses were measured at the end of the experiment and graphed in a scatter plot with mean plus/minus standard errors.

LG SS CL RJH JMS GBF JAS LHM. Contributed reagents/materials/ analysis tools: LG CL RJH JMS GBF WHL JAS LHM. Wrote the paper: LG SS CL RJH JMS GBF WHL JAS LHM.

References

1. Brodeur GM (2003) Neuroblastoma: biological insights into a clinical enigma. Nat Rev Cancer 3: 203–216.
2. De Bernardi B, Gerrard M, Boni L, Rubie H, Canete A, et al. (2009) Excellent outcome with reduced treatment for infants with disseminated neuroblastoma without MYCN gene amplification. J Clin Oncol 27: 1034–1040.
3. Bhatnagar SN, Sarin YK (2012) Neuroblastoma: a review of management and outcome. Indian J Pediatr 79: 787–792.
4. Maris JM, Hogarty MD, Bagatell R, Cohn SL (2007) Neuroblastoma. Lancet 369: 2106–2120.
5. Park JR, Eggert A and Caron H (2010) Neuroblastoma: biology, prognosis, and treatment. Hematol Oncol Clin North Am 24: 65–86
6. Aaltomaa S, Lipponen P, Syrjanen K (1993) Proliferating cell nuclear antigen (PCNA) immunolabeling as a prognostic factor in axillary lymph node negative breast cancer. Anticancer Res 13: 533–538.
7. Chu JS, Huang CS, Chang KJ (1998) Proliferating cell nuclear antigen (PCNA) immunolabeling as a prognostic factor in invasive ductal carcinoma of the breast in Taiwan. Cancer Lett 131: 145–152.
8. Tahan SR, Neuberg DS, Dieffenbach A, Yacoub L (1993) Prediction of early relapse and shortened survival in patients with breast cancer by proliferating cell nuclear antigen score. Cancer 71: 3552–3559.
9. Krishna TS, Kong XP, Gary S, Burgers PM, Kuriyan J (1994) Crystal structure of the eukaryotic DNA polymerase processivity factor PCNA. Cell 79: 1233–1243.
10. Schurtenberger P, Egelhaaf SU, Hindges R, Maga G, Jonsson ZO, et al. (1998) The solution structure of functionally active human proliferating cell nuclear antigen determined by small-angle neutron scattering. J Mol Biol 275: 123–132.
11. Warbrick E (2000) The puzzle of PCNA's many partners. Bioessays 22: 997–1006.
12. Waga S, Hannon GJ, Beach D, Stillman B (1994) The p21 inhibitor of cyclin-dependent kinases controls DNA replication by interaction with PCNA. Nature 369: 574–578.
13. Ducoux M, Urbach S, Baldacci G, Hubscher U, Koundrioukoff S, et al. (2001) Mediation of proliferating cell nuclear antigen (PCNA)-dependent DNA replication through a conserved p21(Cip1)-like PCNA-binding motif present in the third subunit of human DNA polymerase delta. J Biol Chem 276: 49258–49266.
14. Warbrick E, Lane DP, Glover DM, Cox LS (1997) Homologous regions of Fen1 and p21Cip1 compete for binding to the same site on PCNA: a potential mechanism to co-ordinate DNA replication and repair. Oncogene 14: 2313–2321.
15. Chuang LS, Ian HI, Koh TW, Ng HH, Xu G, et al. (1997) Human DNA-(cytosine-5) methyltransferase-PCNA complex as a target for p21WAF1. Science 277: 1996–2000.
16. Levin DS, McKenna AE, Motycka TA, Matsumoto Y, Tomkinson AE (2000) Interaction between PCNA and DNA ligase I is critical for joining of Okazaki fragments and long-patch base-excision repair. Curr Biol 10: 919–922.
17. Jonsson ZO, Hindges R, Hubscher U (1998) Regulation of DNA replication and repair proteins through interaction with the front side of proliferating cell nuclear antigen. EMBO J 17: 2412–2425.
18. Strzalka W, Ziemienowicz A (2011) Proliferating cell nuclear antigen (PCNA): a key factor in DNA replication and cell cycle regulation. Ann Bot 107: 1127–1140.
19. Stoimenov I, Helleday T (2009) PCNA on the crossroad of cancer. Biochem Soc Trans 37: 605–613.
20. Bozza WP, Yang K, Wang J, Zhuang Z (2012) Developing peptide-based multivalent antagonists of proliferating cell nuclear antigen and a fluorescence-based PCNA binding assay. Analytical biochemistry 427: 69–78.
21. Xu H, Zhang P, Liu L, Lee MY (2001) A novel PCNA-binding motif identified by the panning of a random peptide display library. Biochemistry 40: 4512–4520.
22. Zheleva DI, Zhelev NZ, Fischer PM, Duff SV, Warbrick E, et al. (2000) A quantitative study of the in vitro binding of the C-terminal domain of p21 to PCNA: affinity, stoichiometry, and thermodynamics. Biochemistry 39: 7388–7397.
23. Muller R, Misund K, Holien T, Bachke S, Gilljam KM, et al. (2013) Targeting proliferating cell nuclear antigen and its protein interactions induces apoptosis in multiple myeloma cells. PLoS One 8: e70430.
24. Punchihewa C, Inoue A, Hishiki A, Fujikawa Y, Connelly M, et al. (2012) Identification of small molecule proliferating cell nuclear antigen (PCNA) inhibitor that disrupts interactions with PIP-box proteins and inhibits DNA replication. J Biol Chem 287: 14289–14300.
25. Tan Z, Wortman M, Dillehay KL, Seibel WL, Evelyn CR, et al. (2012) Small-molecule targeting of proliferating cell nuclear antigen chromatin association inhibits tumor cell growth. Mol Pharmacol 81: 311–319.
26. Yu YL, Chou RH, Liang JH, Chang WJ, Su KJ, et al. (2013) Targeting the EGFR/PCNA signaling suppresses tumor growth of triple-negative breast cancer cells with cell-penetrating PCNA peptides. PLoS One 8: e61362.
27. Zhao H, Lo YH, Ma L, Waltz SE, Gray JK, et al. (2011) Targeting tyrosine phosphorylation of PCNA inhibits prostate cancer growth. Mol Cancer Ther 10: 29–36.
28. Malkas LH, Herbert BS, Abdel-Aziz W, Dobrolecki LE, Liu Y, et al. (2006) A cancer-associated PCNA expressed in breast cancer has implications as a potential biomarker. Proc Natl Acad Sci U S A 103: 19472–19477.
29. Hoelz DJ, Arnold RJ, Dobrolecki LE, Abdel-Aziz W, Loehrer AP, et al. (2006) The discovery of labile methyl esters on proliferating cell nuclear antigen by MS/MS. Proteomics 6: 4808–4816.
30. Bennardo N, Cheng A, Huang N, Stark JM (2008) Alternative-NHEJ is a mechanistically distinct pathway of mammalian chromosome break repair. PLoS Genet 4: e1000110.
31. Gunn A, Bennardo N, Cheng A, Stark JM (2011) Correct end use during end joining of multiple chromosomal double strand breaks is influenced by repair protein RAD50, DNA-dependent protein kinase DNA-PKcs, and transcription context. J Biol Chem 286: 42470–42482.
32. Malkas LH, Hickey RJ, Li C, Pedersen N, Baril EF (1990) A 21S enzyme complex from HeLa cells that functions in simian virus 40 DNA replication in vitro. Biochemistry 29: 6362–6374.
33. Challberg MD, Kelly TJ (1982) Eukaryotic DNA replication: viral and plasmid model systems. Annu Rev Biochem 51: 901–934.
34. Kasparek TR, Humphrey TC (2011) DNA double-strand break repair pathways, chromosomal rearrangements and cancer. Semin Cell Dev Biol 22: 886–897.
35. Symington LS, Gautier J (2011) Double-strand break end resection and repair pathway choice. Annu Rev Genet 45: 247–271.
36. Kass EM, Jasin M (2010) Collaboration and competition between DNA double-strand break repair pathways. FEBS letters 584: 3703–3708.
37. Hashimoto Y, Puddu F, Costanzo V (2012) RAD51- and MRE11-dependent reassembly of uncoupled CMG helicase complex at collapsed replication forks. Nat Struct Mol Biol 19: 17–24.
38. Branzei D, Vanoli F, Foiani M (2008) SUMOylation regulates Rad18-mediated template switch. Nature 456: 915–920.
39. Al-Minawi AZ, Lee YF, Hakansson D, Johansson F, Lundin C, et al. (2009) The ERCC1/XPF endonuclease is required for completion of homologous recombination at DNA replication forks stalled by inter-strand cross-links. Nucleic Acids Res 37: 6400–6413.
40. Raschle M, Knipscheer P, Enoiu M, Angelov T, Sun J, et al. (2008) Mechanism of replication-coupled DNA interstrand crosslink repair. Cell 134: 969–980.
41. Stevenson CL (2009) Advances in peptide pharmaceuticals. Curr Pharm Biotechnol 10: 122–137.
42. Shibata A, Conrad S, Birraux J, Geuting V, Barton O, et al. (2011) Factors determining DNA double-strand break repair pathway choice in G2 phase. EMBO J 30: 1079–1092.
43. Robinson K, Asawachaicharn N, Galloway DA, Grandori C (2009) c-Myc accelerates S-phase and requires WRN to avoid replication stress. PLoS One 4: e5951.
44. Yu UY, Cha JE, Ju SY, Cho KA, Yoo ES, et al. (2008) Effect on cell cycle progression by N-Myc knockdown in SK-N-BE(2) neuroblastoma cell line and cytotoxicity with STI-571 compound. Cancer Res Treat 40: 27–32.
45. Sheen JH, Dickson RB (2002) Overexpression of c-Myc alters G(1)/S arrest following ionizing radiation. Mol Cell Biol 22: 1819–1833.
46. Bell E, Premkumar R, Carr J, Lu X, Lovat PE, et al. (2006) The role of MYCN in the failure of MYCN amplified neuroblastoma cell lines to G1 arrest after DNA damage. Cell Cycle 5: 2639–2647.
47. Petroni M, Veschi V, Prodosmo A, Rinaldo C, Massimi I, et al. (2011) MYCN sensitizes human neuroblastoma to apoptosis by HIPK2 activation through a DNA damage response. Mol Cancer Res 9: 67–77.
48. Dominguez-Sola D, Ying CY, Grandori C, Ruggiero L, Chen B, et al. (2007) Non-transcriptional control of DNA replication by c-Myc. Nature 448: 445–451.
49. Moser R, Toyoshima M, Robinson K, Gurley KE, Howie HL, et al. (2012) MYC-driven tumorigenesis is inhibited by WRN syndrome gene deficiency. Mol Cancer Res 10: 535–545.
50. Valentijn LJ, Koster J, Haneveld F, Aissa RA, van Sluis P, et al. (2012) Functional MYCN signature predicts outcome of neuroblastoma irrespective of MYCN amplification. Proc Natl Acad Sci U S A 109: 19190–19195.
51. Henriksson M, Luscher B (1996) Proteins of the Myc network: essential regulators of cell growth and differentiation. Adv Cancer Res 68: 109–182.
52. Mukherjee B, Morgenbesser SD, DePinho RA (1992) Myc family oncoproteins function through a common pathway to transform normal cells in culture: cross-interference by Max and trans-acting dominant mutants. Genes Dev 6: 1480–1492.
53. Malynn BA, de Alboran IM, O'Hagan RC, Bronson R, Davidson L, et al. (2000) N-myc can functionally replace c-myc in murine development, cellular growth, and differentiation. Genes Dev 14: 1390–1399.
54. Fridman Y, Palgi N, Dovrat D, Ben-Aroya S, Hieter P, et al. (2010) Subtle alterations in PCNA-partner interactions severely impair DNA replication and repair. PLoS Biol 8: e1000507.

4

The Effect of *XPD* Polymorphisms on Digestive Tract Cancers Risk

Haina Du[1,9], Nannan Guo[1,9], Bin Shi[3,9], Qian Zhang[1], Zhipeng Chen[2], Kai Lu[3], Yongqian Shu[1], Tao Chen[3*], Lingjun Zhu[1*]

1 Department of Oncology, The First Affiliated Hospital of Nanjing Medical University, Nanjing, China, 2 Department of Oncology, The first people's Hospital of Zhangjiagang City, Suzhou, China, 3 Department of Gastrointestinal Surgery, The First Affiliated Hospital of Nanjing Medical University, Nanjing, China

Abstract

Background: The Xeroderma pigmento-sum group D gene (*XPD*) plays a key role in nucleotide excision repair. Single nucleotide polymorphisms (SNP) located in its functional region may alter DNA repair capacity phenotype and cancer risk. Many studies have demonstrated that *XPD* polymorphisms are significantly associated with digestive tract cancers risk, but the results are inconsistent. We conducted a comprehensive meta-analysis to assess the association between *XPD* Lys751Gln polymorphism and digestive tract cancers risk. The digestive tract cancers that our study referred to, includes oral cancer, esophageal cancer, gastric cancer and colorectal cancer.

Methods: We searched PubMed and EmBase up to December 31, 2012 to identify eligible studies. A total of 37 case-control studies including 9027 cases and 16072 controls were involved in this meta-analysis. Statistical analyses were performed with Stata software (version 11.0, USA). Odds ratios (ORs) with 95% confidence intervals (CIs) were used to assess the strength of the association.

Results: The results showed that *XPD* Lys751Gln polymorphism was associated with the increased risk of digestive tract cancers (homozygote comparison (GlnGln *vs.* LysLys): OR = 1.12, 95% CI = 1.01–1.24, $P = 0.029$, $P_{heterogeneity} = 0.133$). We found no statistical evidence for a significantly increased digestive tract cancers risk in the other genetic models. In the subgroup analysis, we also found the homozygote comparison increased the susceptibility of Asian population (OR = 1.28, 95% CI = 1.01–1.63, $P = 0.045$, $P_{heterogeneity} = 0.287$). Stratified by cancer type and source of control, no significantly increased cancer risk was found in these subgroups. Additionally, risk estimates from hospital-based studies and esophageal studies were heterogeneous.

Conclusions: Our meta-analysis suggested that the *XPD* 751Gln/Gln genotype was a low-penetrate risk factor for developing digestive tract cancers, especially in Asian populations.

Editor: Robert W. Sobol, University of Pittsburgh, United States of America

Funding: This study was partially supported by the Postdoctoral Science Foundation of Jiangsu Province (528), the Health Department guidance project of Jiangsu Province (Z201201), the Program for Development of Innovative Research Team in the First Affiliated Hospital of NJMU and the Project Funded by the Priority Academic Program Development of Jiangsu Higher Education Institutions (JX10231801), the Jiangsu Province Clinical science and technology projects (Clinical Research Center, BL2012008) and the Summit of the Six Top Talents Program of Jiangsu Province (2013-WSN-034). The funders had no role in study design, data collection and analysis, decision to publish, or preparation of the manuscript.

Competing Interests: The authors have declared that no competing interests exist.

* E-mail: ct55979@163.com (TC); zhulingjun@njmu.edu.cn (LZ)

9 These authors contributed equally to this work.

Introduction

Digestive tract cancers, especially gastric, esophageal and colorectal cancers, are a major global health problem. Globocan data in 2008 showed [1] that the standardized incidence of colorectal cancer, gastric cancer and esophageal cancer were located in 4th, 6th and 9th in all tumors, respectively. The standardized mortality rate of gastric cancer, coming after lung cancer and breast cancer, ranked the third place. Moreover, colorectal cancer and esophageal cancer also ranked top ten in cancer mortality rankings. The incidence of different cancer varies widely among different racial and ethnic groups which may be partly attributed to lifestyle and genetic background [2]. Exposure to environmental carcinogens can cause different types of DNA damage that subsequently lead to carcinogenesis of different tissues, if left unrepaired [3].

DNA repair mechanisms, such as the nucleotide excision repair (NER), base excision repair pathway (BER) and double-strand break pathway, are essential for maintaining genome integrity and preventing carcinogenesis. NER, the most versatile, well studied DNA repair mechanism in humans, is mainly responsible for repairing bulky DNA damage, such as DNA adducts caused by UV radiation, mutagenic chemicals, or chemotherapeutic drugs [4]. The major component of NER, xeroderma pigmentosum group D (*XPD* or *ERCC2*), mapped in chromosome 19q13.3, spans over 20 kb, contains 23exons and encodes the 761-amino acid

Table 1. Characteristics of XPD polymorphisms Included in the Meta-analysis.

study	Year	Ethnicity	Source of controls	Cases				Controls				P for HWE
				N	Genotypes			N	Genotypes			
					Lys/Lys	Lys/Gln	Gln/Gln		Lys/Lys	Lys/Gln	Gln/Gln	
Oral cancer												
Surya	2005	Asian	PB	110	49	46	15	110	71	31	8	0.09
Da-Tian	2007	Asian	HB	154	134	18	2	105	89	15	1	0.68
Mousumi	2007	Asian	HB	388	190	158	40	309	158	125	26	0.85
Suparp	2005	Asian	PB	105	83	21	1	164	126	36	2	0.74
Esophageal cancer												
Xing	2002	Asian	HB	433	367	63	3	524	451	70	3	0.87
Xing	2003	Asian	HB	325	278	44	3	383	331	49	3	0.43
Yu	2004	Asian	HB	135	108	16	11	152	133	17	2	0.10
Alan	2005	European	HB	56	31	21	4	95	34	46	15	0.93
Ye	2006	European	PB	303	99	156	48	472	198	203	71	0.11
Geoffrey	2007	European	HB	182	61	98	23	336	143	161	32	0.16
Ranbir	2007	Asian	HB	120	52	61	7	160	63	77	20	0.63
Darren	2008	European	HB	312	104	159	49	453	193	208	52	0.72
Heather	2008	European	PB	208	80	94	34	247	91	121	35	0.60
James	2008	European	PB	263	108	123	32	1337	575	588	174	0.22
Jennifer	2009	European	HB	346	137	153	56	456	187	216	53	0.43
Zhai	2009	Asian	HB	200	167	31	2	200	148	51	1	0.12
Huang	2012	Asian	HB	213	150	55	8	358	274	79	5	0.79
Gastric cancer												
Huang[a]	2005	European	PB	279	381	107	126	46	145	163	73	0.03
Lou	2006	Asians	HB	238	205	30	3	200	164	33	3	0.38
Ye	2006	European	PB	126	49	61	16	472	198	203	71	0.11
Ruzzo	2007	European	PB	89	29	44	16	94	25	53	16	0.18
Zhou	2006	Asians	PB	253	224	26	3	612	522	86	4	0.82
Gabriel	2000	European	HB	245	99	105	41	1172	447	555	170	0.91
Doecke	2008	European	PB	303	127	140	36	1337	575	588	174	0.22
Zhang	2009	Asians	PB	207	166	39	2	212	172	39	1	0.43
Domenico	2010	European	PB	295	90	157	48	546	177	284	85	0.09
EMEL	2010	European	PB	40	14	18	8	247	102	114	31	0.92
Long[a]	2010	Asians	HB	361	616	139	151	71	400	164	52	0.00
Ayse[a]	2011	European	HB	106	116	30	56	20	40	43	33	0.01
Colorectal cancer												

Table 1. Cont.

study	Year	Ethnicity	Source of controls	Cases N	Genotypes Lys/Lys	Lys/Gln	Gln/Gln	Controls N	Genotypes Lys/Lys	Lys/Gln	Gln/Gln	P for HWE
Camilla	2006	Asians	PB	105	43	47	15	331	148	142	41	0.44
Mariana	2006	European	PB	740	387	298	55	789	392	317	80	0.18
Skjelbred	2006	European	PB	156	58	76	22	398	175	173	50	0.48
Victor	2006	European	HB	357	158	150	49	318	135	145	38	0.92
Mariana	2007	Asians	PB	303	251	48	4	1163	998	159	6	0.90
Chih-Ching	2007	Asians	HB	717	602	112	3	731	631	96	4	0.86
Rikke	2007	European	PB	396	160	178	58	798	311	382	105	0.47
Tomasz	2009	European	HB	100	56	33	11	100	42	41	17	0.21
Wang	2010	Asians	HB	302	138	130	34	291	137	117	37	0.13
Jelonek	2010	European	PB	123	54	47	22	153	66	68	19	0.81
Canbay	2011	European	PB	79	31	37	11	247	102	114	31	0.92

HB: hospital based.
PB: population based.
a: Hardy-Weinberg Equilibrium (HWE) in controls: $P < 0.05$. Overall analysis and subgroup analysis does not include these studies' data.

protein. It has two functions: nucleotide excision repair and basal transcription as part of the transcription factor complex (TFIIH) [5]. Mutations on different sites in *XPD* gene can give rise to repair and transcription defects, and altered DNA repair capacity can render a higher risk of developing different types of cancer [5–11]. Several polymorphisms of *XPD* were identified, like Asp312Asn, Lys751Gln, Arg194Trp and Arg399Gln. The XPD polymorphic loci that has been of particular interest in molecular epidemiology studies is the Lys751Gln polymorphism (rs13181) in exon 23 [12]. The lysine to glutamine transition at position 751 in exon 23 may affect different protein interactions, diminish the activity of TFIIH complexes, and alter the genetic susceptibility to cancer [13].

Genetic variant in *XPD* Lys751Gln had been demonstrated to be associated with some cancers risk in different meta-analysis, such as esophageal cancer, gastric cancer, colorectal cancer, breast cancer, prostate cancer, lung cancer and bladder cancer [14–23]. However, due to an insufficient number of publications, they did not calculate pooled odds ratios (ORs) of digestive tract cancers comprehensively. In consideration of the extensive role of *XPD* in digestive tract cancers, we performed a meta-analysis of all 37 eligible case–control studies: oral cancer, esophageal cancer, gastric cancer http://www.sciencedirect.com/science/article/pii/S0188440911000853 - bib10and colorectal cancer, to derive a more precise association of *XPD* Lys751Gln polymorphism and different types of digestive tract cancers risk.

Materials and Methods

Identification of eligible studies

Using PubMed, we identified all published case–control studies which investigated the association between the *XPD* Lys751Gln polymorphism and digestive tract cancers risk using a retrieving query formulation "(*XPD* or ERCC2) polymorphisms AND (colorectal cancer OR gastric cancer OR esophageal cancer OR oral cancer)". The digestive tract cancers in this article refer to oral cancer, esophageal cancer, gastric cancer and colorectal cancer. We also searched references in published articles and reviews on this topic in PubMed. Eligible studies had to meet the following criteria: (a) only case-control designs were considered, (b) The study explored the correlation between different types of digestive tract cancers and *XPD* Lys751Gln polymorphism. Major exclusion criteria were (a) no control population, (b) no available genotype frequency. (c) Genotypic distribution of the controls was not in agreement with Hardy-Weinberg equilibrium (HWE). (d) Duplication of the previous publications, the largest or most recent publication was selected.

Data Extraction

Information was carefully extracted from all eligible publications independently by two authors according to the inclusion criteria listed above. If the two pieces of typed data were different, a third investigator would be asked to check and to make sure all data were right. The following information was extracted from each study: first author, year of publication, country of study population, ethnicity, source of controls, number of cases and controls with different genotypes and HWE (Table 1).

Statistical Analysis

We assessed the departure from the Hardy–Weinberg equilibrium for the control group in each study using Pearson's goodness-of-fit χ^2 test with 1 degree of freedom. Heterogeneity among studies was checked by the random-effects model (the Der Simonian and Laird method) if there was significant heterogeneity [24]. A *P* value of more than the nominal level of 0.05 for the Q

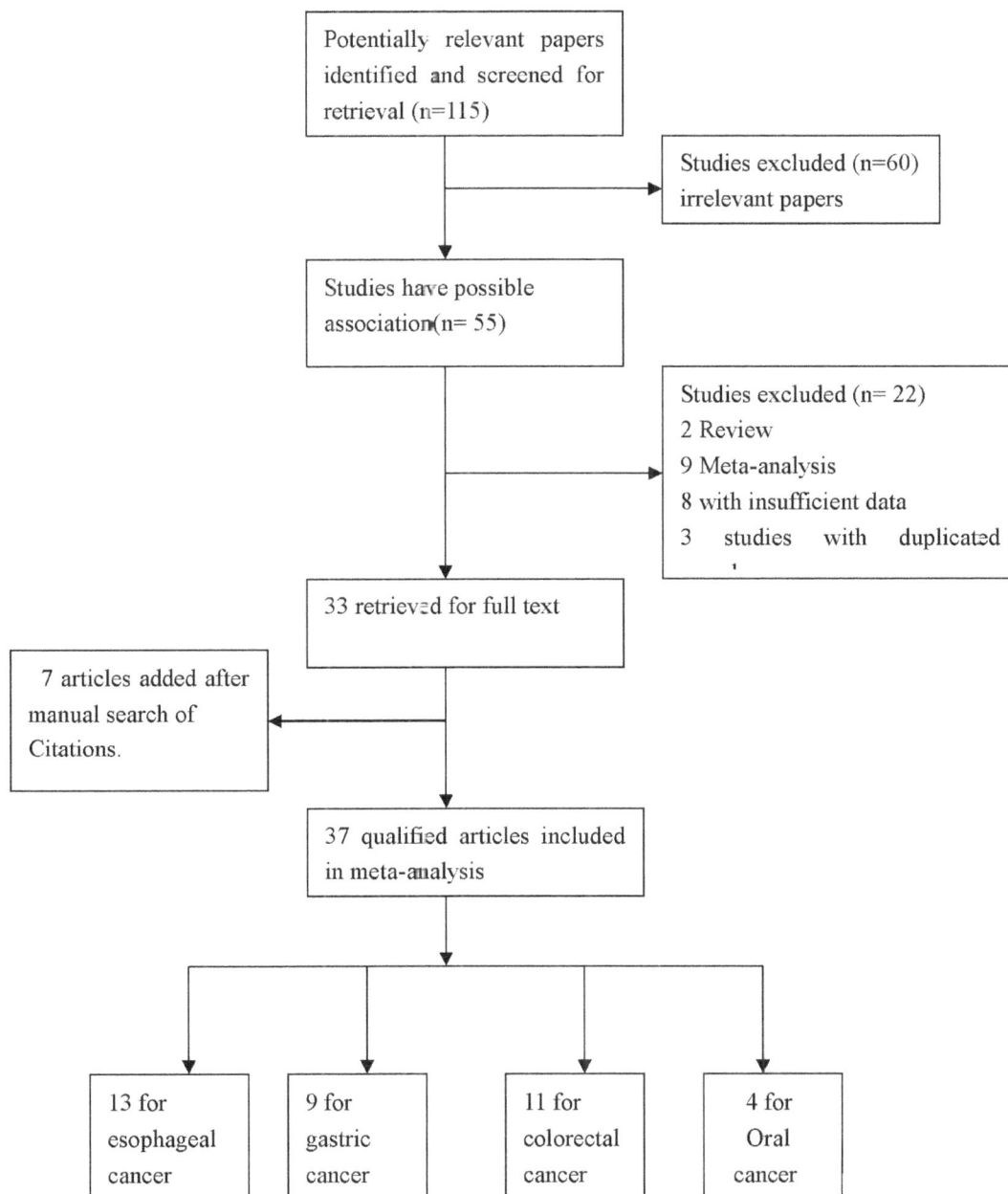

Figure 1. Flow diagram of studies identification.

statistic indicated a lack of heterogeneity across studies, allowing for the use of the fixed -effects model (the Mantel–Haenszel method) [25]. If *P* value less than 0.05 was considered as having heterogeneity, the results can not be pooled together and discussed. The risks ORs of digestive tract cancers associated with the *XPD* Lys751Gln polymorphism were estimated for each study. The pooled ORs were evaluated on co-dominant model (Lys/Gln *vs.*Lys/Lys, Gln/Gln *vs.* Lys/Lys), dominant model (Gln/Gln + Lys/Gln *vs.* Lys/Lys), recessive model (Gln/Gln *vs.* Lys/Gln+Lys/ Lys), respectively. Subgroup analyses were performed by cancer types, ethnicity and source of controls. The publication bias was diagnosed by the funnel plot, in which the standard error of log (OR) of each study was plotted against its log (OR). Funnel plot asymmetry was assessed by Egger's linear regression test. The

significance of the intercept was determined by the t test suggested by Egger (*P*<0.05 was considered representative of statistically significant publication bias) [26]. All the statistical tests were performed with STATA version11.0 (Stata Corporation, College Station, TX, USA).

Results

Study characteristic

A total of 107 potential relevant studies were retrieved through PubMed (Figure 1). After carefully reviewing, 40 eligible case-control studies (3 studies not consistent with HWE were also

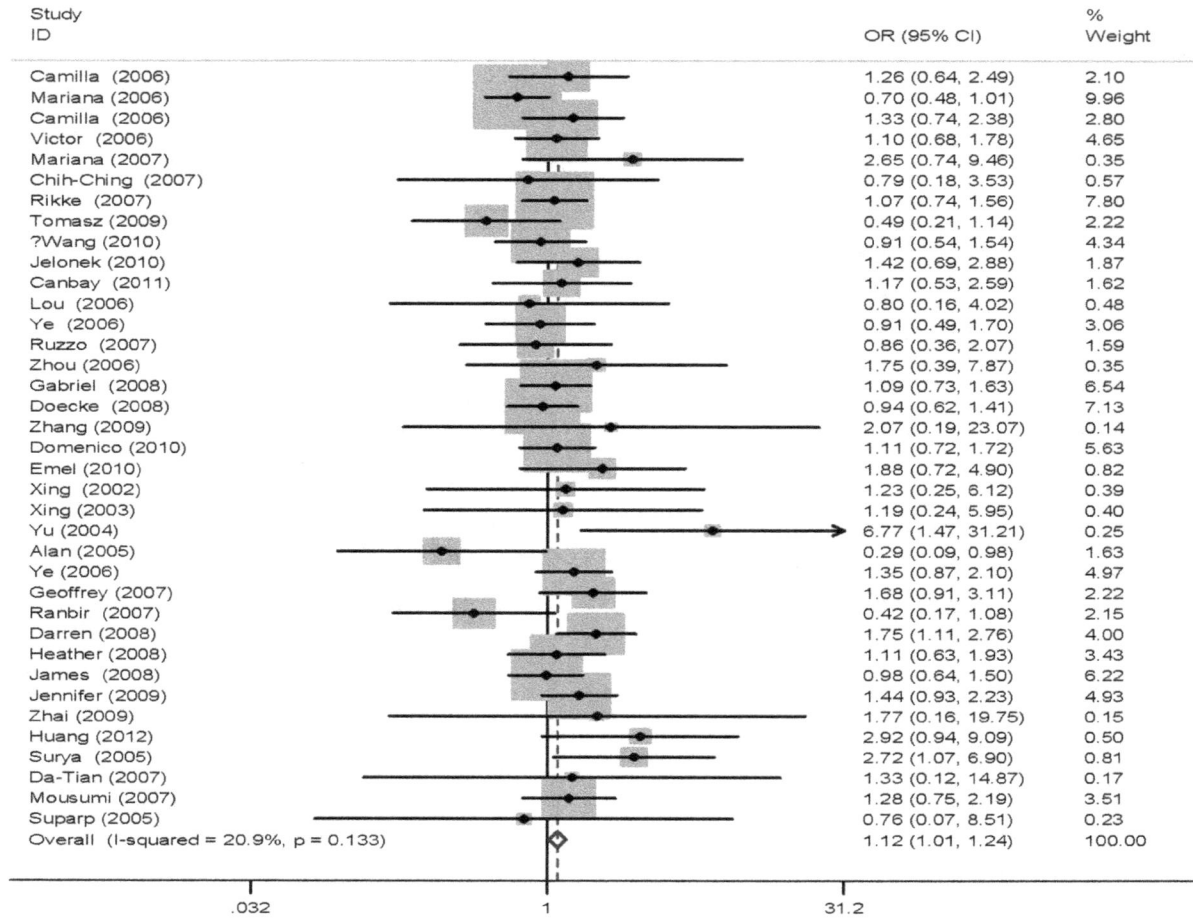

Figure 2. Forest plot of digestive cancer risk associated with the XPD Lys751Gln polymorphisms. Homozygote comparison.

shown) on the relationship between *XPD* Lys715Gln polymorphism and digestive cancers risk were involved in this meta-analysis, including 4 oral cancer studies [62–65], 13 esophageal cancer studies [27–39], 12 gastric cancer studies [36,40–50] and 11 colorectal cancer studies [51–61]. As shown in Table 1, 17 studies were conducted in Asians, 20 studies in Europeans. In addition, there were 18 hospital-based studies, 19 population-based studies. Diverse genotyping methods were used, including PCR-RFLP, PCR-SSCP, Taqman, Real-time PCR and SEB PCR. All studies indicated that the genotypic distribution of the controls were consistent with HWE.

Meta-analysis

Table2 lists the main results of the meta-analysis for *XPD* Lys751Gln: having the Gln/Gln genotype is a risk factor for digestive tract cancers: GlnGln *vs.* LysLys: OR = 1.12, 95% CI = 1.01–1.24, $P = 0.029$, $P_{heterogeneity} = 0.133$. $I^2 = 20.9\%$ (Figure 2). We did not find any significant association between the other genetic models and digestive tract cancers. The results of stratified analysis by cancer type, source of controls and ethnicity were shown in table 2. The Gln/Gln vs. Lys/Lys genotype had an elevated risk in Asian population (OR = 1.28, 95% CI = 1.01–1.63, $P = 0.045$, $P_{heterogeneity} = 0.287$, $I^2 = 14.2\%$; Figure 3). High heterogeneity was found in esophageal cancer and hospital-based studies, so the results can not be pooled together. In addition, the results did not suggest any association between *XPD* Lys751Gln

polymorphism and digestive cancers susceptibility for all genetic models in European individuals or in population-based studies overall.

Sensitivity analysis

In the sensitivity analysis, when each particular study had been removed meta-analyses were conducted repeatedly. The corresponding pooled ORs were not qualitatively altered with or without this study. As shown in Figure 4, the most influencing single study on the overall pooled OR estimates seemed to be the one conducted by Mariana et al, which had a relatively large sample size. However, after the removal of the study, the result of the meta-analysis did not been influenced significantly: Gln/Gln vs. Lys/Lys: OR = 1.17, 95% CI: 1.05–1.30, indicating high stability of our results.

Heterogeneity analysis

There was moderate heterogeneity among these studies in GlnGln+GlnLys *vs.*LysLys comparisons and Gln/Gln *vs.* Lys/Lys comparisons, but not in the other genetic models. We explored the source of heterogeneity for dominant model by cancer type, ethnicity, source of control, and found that esophageal cancer and hospital-based studies contributed to substantial heterogeneity (Table3). One reason may be that hospital-based studies had relatively small samples and were more prone to random error and false positive or negative results. Furthermore, it is very likely that

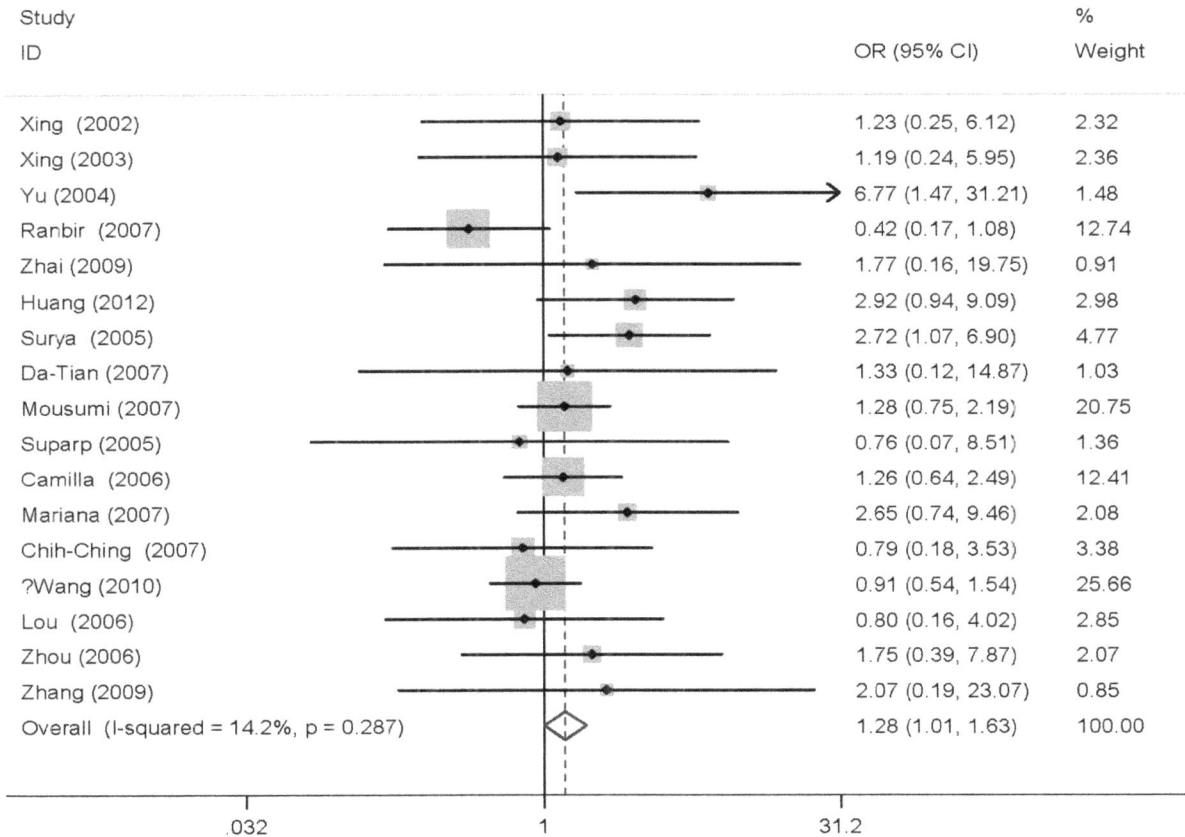

Figure 3. Forest plot of digestive cancer risk associated with the XPD Lys751Gln polymorphisms in Asian subgroups **(based on homozygote comparison).** A fixed-effects model was used. The squares and horizontal lines correspond to the study-specific OR and 95% CI. The area of the squares reflects the weight (inverse of the variance). The diamond represents the summary OR and 95% CI.

the heterogeneity in esophageal studies and hospital-based studies are related since hospital-based studies predominate among the esophageal studies.

Publication Bias

Begg's rank correlation method and Egger's weighted regression method were used to assess publication bias. There was no evidence of publication bias in XPD Lys751Gln (Begg's test $P = 0.284$, Egger's test $P = 0.324$, t = 1.00, 95% CI = 0.41–1.21). We present funnel plot for ORs of Gln/Gln versus Lys/Lys (Figure 5).

Discussion

XPD plays a crucial role in NER, which is significant in the elimination of certain DNA cross-links, ultraviolet (UV) photolesions, and bulky chemical adducts. The XPD protein possesses both single-strand DNA-dependant ATP ase and 5'-3' DNA helicase activities, which is essential for NER pathway and transcription [66]. Genetic variation in XPD may contribute to impaired DNA repair capacity and increased cancer risk. The Lys to Gln change at position 751 of XPD results in complete changes about the charge configuration of the amino acid, which affects the interactions of XPD protein and its helicase activator [67]. To date, a number of epidemiological studies have been conducted to evaluate the role of Lys751Gln polymorphism on several cancer risks, but the results remain controversial. As far as we know,

several previous meta-analyses on XPD Lys751Gln polymorphism and cancers risk have been performed, such as gastric cancer, colorectal cancer, esophageal cancer, breast cancer and bladder cancer [14–23]. But to date, there is no meta-analysis on the association between digestive tract cancers risk and XPD Lys751Gln polymorphism. In order to derive a more precise estimation of relationship, we performed this meta-analysis of 37 studies, including 9027 cases and 16072 controls.

Through analyzing genotypes from the 37 eligible studies, we found the Gln/Gln genotype carries might be at potential risk to digestive tract cancers. The Lys to Gln variation on position 751 of XPD resulted in complete changes about the electronic configuration of the amino acid, which affected the interactions of XPD protein and its helicase activator [68]. Digestive tract cancers represent a homogenous group of malignancies in some ways. Different primary sites of digestive tract cancers have some shared risk factors. For example, except for smoking and alcohol consumption, eating rough, spicy, hot and non-digestible food is likely to damage the digestive tract tissue. In addition, H.Pylori infection is a major cause of gastric cancer, while nitrites derived from red meat and processed meat is a key risk factor for esophageal cancer and colorectal cancer. Such risk factors and their tissue specificity raise the possibility that the XPD polymorphism may be associated with digestive tract cancers risk. The functional XPD Lys751Gln polymorphism resulting in decreased activity of XPD protein may increase risk of digestive tract cancers on the basis of damage tissue.

Table 2. Pooled ORs and 95%CIs of stratified meta-analysis.

Stratification	No.case/control	GlnGln vs.LysLys OR (95%CI)	P	GlnLys vs.LysLys OR (95%CI)	P	GlnGln+GlnLys vs.LysLys OR (95%CI)	P	GlnGln vs.GlnLys+LysLys OR (95%CI)	P
Total	40(9773/17185)	1.12(1.01,1.24)	0.029	1.04(0.98–1.11)	0.194	1.06(1.00,1.12)[b]	0.064	1.09(0.99,1.20)	0.072
Cancer type									
Colorectal cancer	11(3378/5319)	0.99(0.3,1.17)	0.870	0.99(0.89,1.09)	0.776	0.99(0.90,1.09)	0.790	1.00(0.85,1.17)	0.954
Gastric cancer	12(2542/5905)	1.05(0.85,1.29)	0.639	0.97(0.85,1.10)	0.612	0.98(0.86,1.11)	0.744	1.05(0.87,1.28)	0.630
Esophageal cancer	13(3096/5173)	1.29(1.08,1.54)[b]	0.005	0.90(0.81,1.00)[b]	0.056	0.91(0.77,1.07)[b]	0.235	0.84(0.66,1.07)	0.159
Oral cancer	4(757/688)	1.50(0.96,2.35)	0.078	0.88(0.60,1.30)	0.518	0.85(0.56,1.28)	0.430	0.72(0.47,1.12)	0.147
Ethnicity									
Asian	18(4669/6521)	1.28(1.01,1.63)	0.045	1.05(0.95,1.17)	0.340	1.08(0.98,1.19)	0.133	1.21(0.96,1.53)	0.110
European	22(5104/10564)	1.09(0.97,1.22)	0.144	1.04(0.96,1.12)	0.363	1.05(0.97,1.13)	0.232	1.07(0.96,1.19)	0.210
Source of control									
HB	20(5290/7075)	1.19(1.01,1.40)[b]	0.038	1.02(0.93,1.12)	0.703	1.02(0.89, 1.16)[b]	0.787	1.16(0.95,1.41)	0.140
PB	20(4483/10010)	1.08(0.94,1.23)	0.267	1.06(0.98,1.16)	0.157	1.07(0.98,1.15)	0.122	1.04(0.92,1.18)	0.715

NO: involved studies' number; *Gln Lys VS.Lys*Lys: Heterozygote comparison; GlnGln vs.LysLys: Homozygote comparison; GlnGln+GlnLys vs. LysLys: Dominant model; GlnGln vs. GlnLys+LysLys: Recessive model; Random model was chosen for data pooling when $P<0.10$ and/or $I^2>50\%$; otherwise fixed model was used.
[b]the results were excluded due to potential heterogeneity.

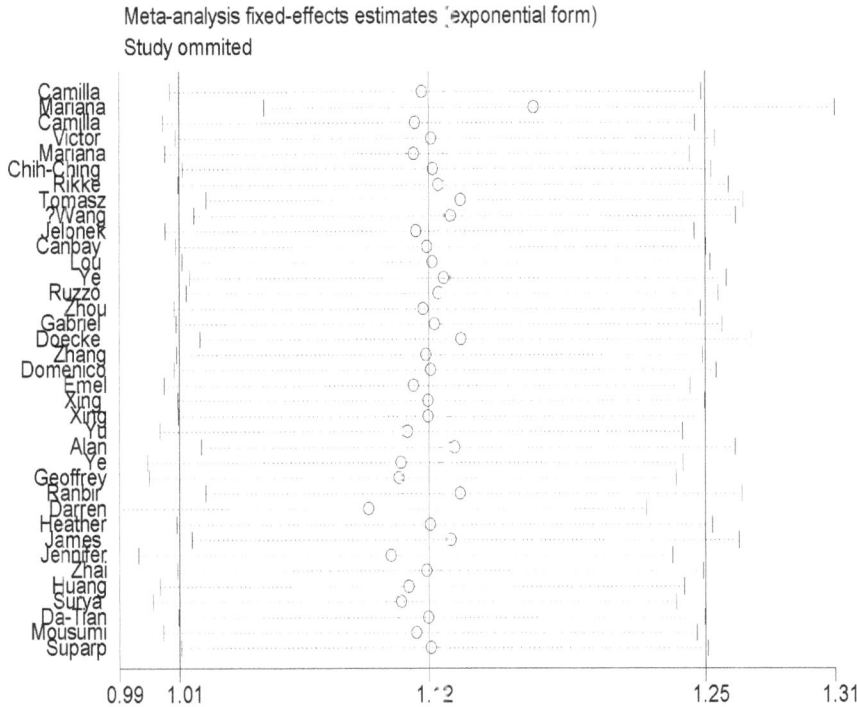

Figure 4. Influence analysis of the summary odds ratio coefficients on the association between XPD Lys751Gln homozygote comparison with digestive tract cancers risk. Results were computed by omitting each study (left column) in turn. Bars, 95% CI.

In stratified analysis by cancer type, we found that all genetic models did not appear to have an effect on the risks of esophageal, gastric, colorectal and oral cancers. This was different from Ling Yuan's and Wu XB's studies [69,70]. However Bo Chen et al. [71] detected that Gln/Gln genotype carriers might have an increased risk of gastric cancer in the Helico-bacter pylori (H.pylori)-positive population, but not in the Helico-bacter pylori (H. pylori)-negative population. One possible explanation is that the modulation of digestive tract cancers risk may depend not only on a single gene/single nucleotide polymorphism, but also on a joint effect of multiple polymorphisms within different genes or pathways, or on close interaction between polymorphisms and environmental factor. The other is that Helicobacter pylori infection is one of the clear etiologies of gastric cancer and maybe there is some relationship between helicobacter pylori and the polymorphic loci. In the subgroup of ethnicity, we found significant association

Table 3. Heterogeneity test.

Stratification	Gln Gln vs.LysLys	Gln Lys vs.LysLys	GlnGln+GlnLys vs.LysLys	GlnGln vs. GlnLys+LysLys
	Ph, I^2 (%)	Ph, I^2 (%)	Ph, I^2 (%)	Ph, I^2 (%)
Digestive cancers	0.133, 20.9	0.064,27.6	0.011, 38.3	0.385, 4.9
Cancer type				
Esophageal cancer	0.033, 46.6	0.022, 49.3	0.004,58.2	0.084,37.4
Gastric cancer	0.930,0	0.554,0	0.698,0	0.664,0
Colorectal cancer	0.310,13	0.470,0	0.328,12.2	0.387,5.9
Oral cancer	0.529, 0	0.095, 52.5	0.052,61.1	0.795, 0
Source of control				
Hospital-based	0.043,39.6	0.051,38.2	0.006,51.6	0.180,23.2
Population-based	0.550,0	0.243,17.3	0.184,22.3	0.715,0
Ethnicity				
Asian	0.287,14.2	0.174,24.2	0.057,38.0	0.353,8.6
European	0.137, 26.3	0.074,334	0.029,41.2	0.414,3.4

Ph: P-value of Q-test for heterogeneity identification; I^2 index: a quantitative measurement which indicates the proportion of total variation in study estimates that is due to between-study heterogeneity.

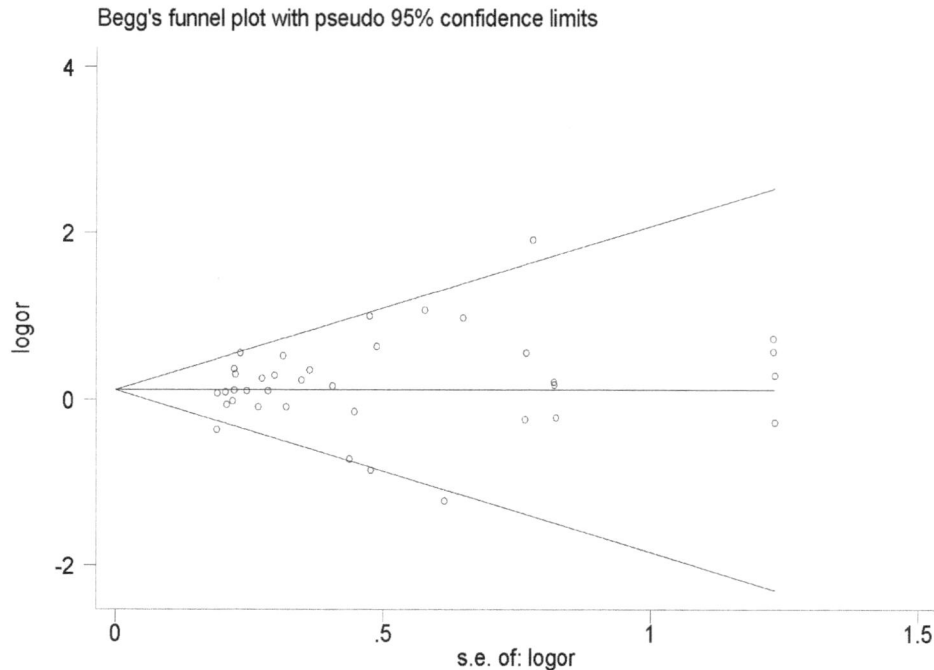

Figure 5. Begg's funnel plot for publication bias test (Homozygote comparison). Each point represents a separate study for the indicated association.

between *XPD* Gln/Gln polymorphism and increased risks of digestive tract cancers in Asians but not in European. We think ethnic differences and diverse live environment may partly explain the phenomenon. Furthermore, we believed differences in diet, such as food structure and cooking way, were the main cause of this result. In addition, it was also likely that the observed ethnic differences may be due to chance because studies with small sample size may have insufficient statistical power to detect a slight effect or may have generated a fluctuated risk estimate [72].

In summary, this meta-analysis indicated that *XPD* Lys751Gln polymorphism, individuals carrying the variant homozygote Gln/Gln may increase the susceptibility of digestive tract cancers. And, significant associations were detected among Asians population. It should be noted explicitly: first, the effective sample size is much smaller for the Gln/Gln vs. Lys/Lys analyses than the other genetic models and therefore it is more prone to random error and false positive results; second, the results for GlnGln vs. GlyLys+ LysLys, while not statistically significant (OR 1.09, 95% CI = 0.99–1.20, $P = 0.072$, $P_{heterogeneity} = 0.385$), strengthen our

conclusion about which genetic model is most appropriate. Large-scale case-control and population-based association studies are warranted to validate the risk identified in the current meta-analysis and investigate the potential gene-gene and gene-environment interactions on digestive tract cancers risk.

Supporting Information

Checklist S1

Author Contributions

Conceived and designed the experiments: HND NNG YQS TC LJZ. Performed the experiments: HND BS QZ ZPC KL TC LJZ. Analyzed the data: HND ZPC LJZ QZ. Contributed reagents/materials/analysis tools: HND ZPC LJZ QZ. Wrote the paper: HND ZPC NNG. Designed the software used in analysis: HND NNG ZPC QZ.

References

1. Ferlay J, Shin HR, Bray F, Forman D, Mathers C, et al. (2010) Estimates of worldwide burden of cancer in 2008: GLOBOCAN 2008. Int J Cancer 127: 2893–2917.
2. Iscovich J, Howe GR (1998) Cancer incidence patterns (1972–91) among migrants from the Soviet Union to Israel. Cancer Causes Control 9: 29–36.
3. Zhu ML, Wang M, Cao ZG, He J, Shi TY, et al. (2012) Association between the ERCC5 Asp1104His polymorphism and cancer risk: a meta-analysis. PLoS One 7: e36293.
4. Shi TY, He J, Qiu LX, Zhu ML, Wang MY, et al. (2012) Association between XPF polymorphisms and cancer risk: a meta-analysis. PLoS One 7: e38606.
5. Spitz MR, Wu X, Wang Y, Wang LE, Shete S, et al. (2001) Modulation of nucleotide excision repair capacity by XPD polymorphisms in lung cancer patients. Cancer Res 61: 1354–1357.
6. Shen H, Spitz MR, Qiao Y, Guo Z, Wang LE, et al. (2003) Smoking, DNA repair capacity and risk of nonsmall cell lung cancer. Int J Cancer 107: 84–88.
7. Shi Q, Wang LE, Bondy ML, Brewster A, Singletary SE, et al. (2004) Reduced DNA repair of benzo[a]pyrene diol epoxide-induced adducts and common XPD polymorphisms in breast cancer patients. Carcinogenesis 25: 1695–1700.
8. Ramos JM, Ruiz A, Colen R, Lopez ID, Grossman L, et al. (2004) DNA repair and breast carcinoma susceptibility in women. Cancer 100: 1352–1357.
9. Wei Q, Lee JE, Gershenwald JE, Ross MI, Mansfield PF, et al. (2003) Repair of UV light-induced DNA damage and risk of cutaneous malignant melanoma. J Natl Cancer Inst 95: 308–315.
10. Hu JJ, Hall MC, Grossman L, Hedayati M, McCullough DL, et al. (2004) Deficient nucleotide excision repair capacity enhances human prostate cancer risk. Cancer Res 64: 1197–1201.
11. Hemminki K, Xu G, Angelini S, Snellman E, Jansen CT, et al. (2001) XPD exon 10 and 23 polymorphisms and DNA repair in human skin in situ. Carcinogenesis 22: 1185–1188.
12. Shen MR, Jones IM, Mohrenweiser H (1998) Nonconservative amino acid substitution variants exist at polymorphic frequency in DNA repair genes in healthy humans. Cancer Res 58: 604–608.

13. Shen MR, Jones IM, Mohrenweiser H (1998) Nonconservative amino acid substitution variants exist at polymorphic frequency in DNA repair genes in healthy humans. Cancer Res 58: 604–608.
14. Xue H, Lu Y, Lin B, Chen J, Tang F, et al. (2012) The effect of XPD/ERCC2 polymorphisms on gastric cancer risk among different ethnicities: a systematic review and meta-analysis. PLoS One 7: e43431.
15. Zhu S, Zhang H, Tang Y, Wang J (2012) Polymorphisms in XPD and hOGG1 and prostate cancer risk: a meta-analysis. Urol Int 89: 233–240.
16. Yuan H, Niu YM, Wang RX, Li HZ, Chen N (2011) Association between XPD Lys751Gln polymorphism and risk of head and neck cancer: a meta-analysis. Genet Mol Res 10: 3356–3364.
17. Ding DP, Ma WL, He XF, Zhang Y (2012) XPD Lys751Gln polymorphism and esophageal cancer susceptibility: a meta-analysis of case-control studies. Mol Biol Rep 39: 2533–2540.
18. Yuan L, Cui D, Zhao EJ, Jia CZ, Wang LD, et al. (2011) XPD Lys751Gln polymorphism and esophageal cancer risk: a meta-analysis involving 2288 cases and 4096 controls. World J Gastroenterol 17: 2343–2348.
19. Zhang Y, Ding D, Wang X, Zhu Z, Huang M, et al (2011) Lack of association between XPD Lys751Gln and Asp312Asn polymorphisms and colorectal cancer risk: a meta-analysis of case-control studies. Int J Colorectal Dis 26: 1257–1264.
20. Zhan P, Wang Q, Wei SZ, Wang J, Qian Q, et al. (2010) ERCC2/XPD Lys751Gln and Asp312Asn gene polymorphism and lung cancer risk: a meta-analysis involving 22 case-control studies. J Thorac Oncol 5: 1337–1345.
21. Pabalan N, Francisco-Pabalan O, Sung L, Jarjanazi H, Ozcelik H (2010) Meta-analysis of two ERCC2 (XPD) polymorphisms, Asp312Asn and Lys751Gln, in breast cancer. Breast Cancer Res Treat 124: 531–541.
22. Qiu LX, Yao L, Zhang J, Zhu XD, Zhao XM, et al. (2010) XPD Lys751Gln polymorphism and breast cancer susceptibility: a meta-analysis involving 28,709 subjects. Breast Cancer Res Treat 124: 229–235.
23. Wang M, Gu D, Zhang Z, Zhou J (2009) XPD polymorphisms, cigarette smoking, and bladder cancer risk: a meta-analysis. J Toxicol Environ Health A 72: 698–705.
24. DerSimonian R, Laird N (1986) Meta-analysis in clinical trials. Control Clin Trials 7: 177–188.
25. Mantel N, Haenszel W (1959) Statistical aspects of the analysis of data from retrospective studies of disease. J Natl Cancer Inst 22: 719–748.
26. Egger M, Davey Smith G, Schneider M, Minder C (1997) Bias in meta-analysis detected by a simple, graphical test. BMJ 315: 629–634.
27. Huang CG, Liu T, Lv GD, Liu Q, Feng JG, et al. (2012) Analysis of XPD genetic polymorphisms of esophageal squamous cell carcinoma in a population of Yili Prefecture, in Xinjiang, China. Mol Biol Rep 39: 709–714.
28. Liu G, Zhou W, Yeap BY, Su L, Wain JC, et al. (2007) XRCC1 and XPD polymorphisms and esophageal adenocarcinoma risk. Carcinogenesis 28: 1254–1258.
29. Xing DY, Qi J, Tan W, Miao XP, Liang G, et al. (2003) Association of genetic polymorphisms in the DNA repair gene XPD with risk of lung and esophageal cancer in a Chinese population in Beijing. Zhonghua Yi Xue Yi Chuan Xue Za Zhi 20: 35–38.
30. Xing D, Qi J, Miao X, Lu W, Tan W, et al. (2002) Polymorphisms of DNA repair genes XRCC1 and XPD and their associations with risk of esophageal squamous cell carcinoma in a Chinese population. Int J Cancer 100: 600–605.
31. Xing D, Tan W, Lin D (2003) Genetic polymorphisms and susceptibility to esophageal cancer among Chinese population (review). Oncol Rep 10: 1615–1623.
32. Yu HP, Wang XL, Sun X, Su YH, Wang YJ, et al. (2004) Polymorphisms in the DNA repair gene XPD and susceptibility to esophageal squamous cell carcinoma. Cancer Genet Cytogenet 154: 10–15.
33. Casson AG, Zheng Z, Evans SC, Veugelers PJ, Porter GA, et al. (2005) Polymorphisms in DNA repair genes in the molecular pathogenesis of esophageal (Barrett) adenocarcinoma. Carcinogenesis 26: 1536–1541.
34. Ye W, Kumar R, Bacova G, Lagergren J, Hemminki K, et al. (2006) The XPD 751Gln allele is associated with an increased risk for esophageal adenocarcinoma: a population-based case-control study in Sweden. Carcinogenesis 27: 1835–1841.
35. Tse D, Zhai R, Zhou W, Heist RS, Asomaning K, et al. (2008) Polymorphisms of the NER pathway genes, ERCC1 and XPD are associated with esophageal adenocarcinoma risk. Cancer Causes Control 19: 1077–1083.
36. Doecke J, Zhao ZZ, Pandeya N, Sadeghi S, Stark M, et al. (2008) Polymorphisms in MGMT and DNA repair genes and the risk of esophageal adenocarcinoma. Int J Cancer 123: 174–180.
37. Ferguson HR, Wild CP, Anderson LA, Murphy SJ, Johnston BT, et al. (2008) No association between hOGG1, XRCC1, and XPD polymorphisms and risk of reflux esophagitis, Barrett's esophagus, or esophageal adenocarcinoma: results from the factors influencing the Barrett's adenocarcinoma relationship case-control study. Cancer Epidemiol Biomarkers Prev 17: 736–739.
38. Pan J, Lin J, Izzo JG, Liu Y, Xing J, et al. (2009) Genetic susceptibility to esophageal cancer: the role of the nucleotide excision repair pathway. Carcinogenesis 30: 785–792.
39. Xing DY, Qi J, Tan W, Miao XP, Liang G, et al. 2003) Association of genetic polymorphisms in the DNA repair gene XPD with risk of lung and esophageal cancer in a Chinese population in Beijing. Zhonghua Yi Xue Yi Chuan Xue Za Zhi 20: 35–38.
40. Lou Y, Song Q, He XM(2006) Association of single nucleotide polymorphism in DNA repair gene XPD with gastric cancer in Han population from northeast region of China. World Chinese Journal of Digestology 14: 3143–3146.
41. Canbay E, Agachan B, Gulluoglu M, Isbir T, Balik E, et al. (2010) Possible associations of APE1 polymorphism with susceptibility and HOGG1 polymorphism with prognosis in gastric cancer. Anticancer Res 30: 1359–1364.
42. Palli D, Polidoro S, D'Errico M, Saieva C, Guarrera S, et al. (2010) Polymorphic DNA repair and metabolic genes: a multigenic study on gastric cancer. Mutagenesis 25: 569–575.
43. Zhang CZ, Chen ZP, Xu CQ, Ning T, Li DP, et al. (2009) Correlation of XPD gene with susceptibility to gastric cancer. Ai Zheng 28: 1163–1167.
44. Ruzzo A, Canestrari E, Maltese P, Fizzagalli F, Graziano F, et al. (2007) Polymorphisms in genes involved in DNA repair and metabolism of xenobiotics in individual susceptibility to sporadic diffuse gastric cancer. Clin Chem Lab Med 45: 822–828.
45. Capella G, Pera G, Sala N, Agudo A, Rico F, et al. (2008) DNA repair polymorphisms and the risk of stomach adenocarcinoma and severe chronic gastritis in the EPIC-EURGAST study. Int J Epidemiol 37: 1316–1325.
46. Ye W, Kumar R, Bacova G, Lagergren J, Hemminki K, et al. (2006) The XPD 751Gln allele is associated with an increased risk for esophageal adenocarcinoma: a population-based case-control study in Sweden. Carcinogenesis 27: 1835–1841.
47. Zhou RM, Li Y, Wang N, Zhang XJ, Dong XJ, et al. (2006) [Correlation of XPC Ala499Val and Lys939Gln polymorphisms to risks of esophageal squamous cell carcinoma and gastric cardiac adenocarcinoma]. Ai Zheng 25: 1113–1119.
48. Engin AB, Karahalil B, Engin A, Karakaya AE (2011) DNA repair enzyme polymorphisms and oxidative stress in a Turkish population with gastric carcinoma. Mol Biol Rep 38: 5379–5336.
49. Long XD, Ma Y, Huang YZ, Yi Y, Liang QX, et al. (2010) Genetic polymorphisms in DNA repair genes XPC, XPD, and XRCC4, and susceptibility to Helicobacter pylori infection-related gastric antrum adenocarcinoma in Guangxi population, China. Mol Carcinog 49: 611–618.
50. Huang WY, Chow WH, Rothman N, Lissowska J, Llaca V, et al. (2005) Selected DNA repair polymorphisms and gastric cancer in Poland. Carcinogenesis 26: 1354–1359.
51. Canbay E, Cakmakoglu B, Zeybek U, Sozen S, Cacina C, et al. (2011) Association of APE1 and hOGG1 polymorphisms with colorectal cancer risk in a Turkish population. Curr Med Res Opin 27: 1295–1302.
52. Jelonek K, Gdowicz-Klosok A, Pietrowska M, Borkowska M, Korfanty J, et al. (2010) Association between single-nucleotide polymorphisms of selected genes involved in the response to DNA damage and risk of colon, head and neck, and breast cancers in a Polish population. J Appl Genet 51: 343–352.
53. Wang J, Zhao Y, Jiang J, Gajalakshmi V, Kuriki K, et al. (2010) Polymorphisms in DNA repair genes XRCC1, XRCC3 and XPD, and colorectal cancer risk: a case-control study in an Indian population. J Cancer Res Clin Oncol 136: 1517–1525.
54. Sliwinski T, Krupa R, Wisniewska-Jarosinska M, Pawlowska E, Lech J, et al. (2009) Common polymorphisms in the XPD and hOGG1 genes are not associated with the risk of colorectal cancer in a Polish population. Tohoku J Exp Med 218: 185–191.
55. Skjelbred CF, Saebo M, Wallin H, Nexo BA, Hagen PC, et al. (2006) Polymorphisms of the XRCC1, XRCC3 and XPD genes and risk of colorectal adenoma and carcinoma, in a Norwegian cohort: a case control study. BMC Cancer 6: 67.
56. Hansen RD, Sorensen M, Tjonneland A, Overvad K, Wallin H, et al. (2007) XPA A23G, XPC Lys939Gln, XPD Lys751Gln and XPD Asp312Asn polymorphisms, interactions with smoking, alcohol and dietary factors, and risk of colorectal cancer. Mutat Res 619: 68–80.
57. Stern MC, Conti DV, Siegmund KD, Corral R, Yuan JM, et al. (2007) DNA repair single-nucleotide polymorphisms in colorectal cancer and their role as modifiers of the effect of cigarette smoking and alcohol in the Singapore Chinese Health Study. Cancer Epidemiol Biomarkers Prev 16: 2363–2372.
58. Moreno V, Gemignani F, Landi S, Gioia-Patricola L, Chabrier A, et al. (2006) Polymorphisms in genes of nucleotide and base excision repair: risk and prognosis of colorectal cancer. Clin Cancer Res 12: 2101–2108.
59. Yeh CC, Sung FC, Tang R, Chang-Chieh CR, Hsieh LL (2007) Association between polymorphisms of biotransformation and DNA-repair genes and risk of colorectal cancer in Taiwan. J Biomed Sci 14: 183–193.
60. Stern MC, Siegmund KD, Conti DV, Corral R, Haile RW (2006) XRCC1, XRCC3, and XPD polymorphisms as modifiers of the effect of smoking and alcohol on colorectal adenoma risk. Cancer Epidemiol Biomarkers Prev 15: 2384–2390.
61. Skjelbred CF, Saebo M, Wallin H, Nexo BA, Hagen PC, et al. (2006) Polymorphisms of the XRCC1, XRCC3 and XPD genes and risk of colorectal adenoma and carcinoma, in a Norwegian cohort: a case control study. BMC Cancer 6: 67.
62. Bau DT, Tsai MH, Huang CY, Lee CC, Tseng HC, et al. (2007) Relationship between polymorphisms of nucleotide excision repair genes and oral cancer risk in Taiwan: evidence for modification of smoking habit. Chin J Physiol 50: 294–300.
63. Majumder M, Sikdar N, Ghosh S, Roy B (2007) Polymorphisms at XPD and XRCC1 DNA repair loci and increased risk of oral leukoplakia and cancer among NAT2 slow acetylators. Int J Cancer 120: 2148–2156.

64. Ramachandran S, Ramadas K, Hariharan R, Rejnish Kumar R, Radhakrishna Pillai M (2006) Single nucleotide polymorphisms of DNA repair genes XRCC1 and XPD and its molecular mapping in Indian oral cancer. Oral Oncol 42: 350–362.

65. Kietthubthew S, Sriplung H, Au WW, Ishida T (2006) Polymorphism in DNA repair genes and oral squamous cell carcinoma in Thailand. Int J Hyg Environ Health 209: 21–29.

66. Lunn RM, Helzlsouer KJ, Parshad R, Umbach DM, Harris EL, et al. (2000) XPD polymorphisms: effects on DNA repair proficiency. Carcinogenesis 21: 551–555.

67. Pavanello S, Pulliero A, Siwinska E, Mielzynska D, Clonfero E (2005) Reduced nucleotide excision repair and GSTM1-null genotypes influence anti-B[a]PDE-DNA adduct levels in mononuclear white blood cells of highly PAH-exposed coke oven workers. Carcinogenesis 26: 169–175.

68. Coin F, Marinoni JC, Rodolfo C, Fribourg S, Pedrini AM, et al. (1998) Mutations in the XPD helicase gene result in XP and TTD phenotypes, preventing interaction between XPD and the p44 subunit of TFIIH. Nat Genet 20: 184–188.

69. Yuan L, Cui D, Zhao EJ, Jia CZ, Wang LD, et al. (2011) XPD Lys751Gln polymorphism and esophageal cancer risk: a meta-analysis involving 2288 cases and 4096 controls. World J Gastroenterol 17: 2343–2348.

70. Wu XB, Dai LP, Wang YP, Wang KJ, Zhang JY (2009) [DNA repair gene xeroderma pigmentosum group D 751 polymorphism and the risk on esophageal cancer: a meta-analysis]. Zhonghua Liu Xing Bing Xue Za Zhi 30: 281–285.

71. Chen B, Zhou Y, Yang P, Wu XT (2011) ERCC2 Lys751Gln and Asp312Asn polymorphisms and gastric cancer risk: a meta-analysis. J Cancer Res Clin Oncol 137: 939–946.

72. Wacholder S, Chanock S, Garcia-Closas M, El Ghormli L, Rothman N (2004) Assessing the probability that a positive report is false: an approach for molecular epidemiology studies. J Natl Cancer Inst 96: 434–442.

5

Association of BLM and BRCA1 during Telomere Maintenance in ALT Cells

Samir Acharya, Zeenia Kaul, April Sandy Gocha, Alaina R. Martinez, Julia Harris, Jeffrey D. Parvin, Joanna Groden*

Department of Molecular Virology, Immunology and Medical Genetics, College of Medicine, The Ohio State University, Columbus Ohio, United States of America

Abstract

Fifteen percent of tumors utilize recombination-based alternative lengthening of telomeres (ALT) to maintain telomeres. The mechanisms underlying ALT are unclear but involve several proteins involved in homologous recombination including the BLM helicase, mutated in Bloom's syndrome, and the BRCA1 tumor suppressor. Cells deficient in either BLM or BRCA1 have phenotypes consistent with telomere dysfunction. Although BLM associates with numerous DNA damage repair proteins including BRCA1 during DNA repair, the functional consequences of BLM-BRCA1 association in telomere maintenance are not completely understood. Our earlier work showed the involvement of BRCA1 in different mechanisms of ALT, and telomere shortening upon loss of BLM in ALT cells. In order to delineate their roles in telomere maintenance, we studied their association in telomere metabolism in cells using ALT. This work shows that BLM and BRCA1 co-localize with RAD50 at telomeres during S- and G2-phases of the cell cycle in immortalized human cells using ALT but not in cells using telomerase to maintain telomeres. Co-immunoprecipitation of BRCA1 and BLM is enhanced in ALT cells at G2. Furthermore, BRCA1 and BLM interact with RAD50 predominantly in S- and G2-phases, respectively. Biochemical assays demonstrate that full-length BRCA1 increases the unwinding rate of BLM three-fold in assays using a DNA substrate that models a forked structure composed of telomeric repeats. Our results suggest that BRCA1 participates in ALT through its interactions with RAD50 and BLM.

Editor: Michael Shing-Yan Huen, The University of Hong Kong, Hong Kong

Funding: This work was supported by funding from the National Institutes of Health [CA117898 to J.G.]; National Cancer Institute-T32 [Z.K.]; National Science Foundation Award GRFP DGE-0822215 [J.L.H.]; The Ohio State University Pelotonia Fellowship Program [A.S.G; Z.K.]; The project described was supported by Award Number 8UL1TR000090-05, 8KL2TR000112-05, and 8TL1TR000091-05 from the National Center For Advancing Translational Sciences. The funders had no role in study design, data collection and analysis, decision to publish, or preparation of the manuscript.

Competing Interests: The authors have declared that no competing interests exist.

* Email: joanna.groden@osumc.edu

Introduction

Telomeres are DNA-protein complexes comprised of repetitive non-coding DNA sequences at the ends of eukaryotic chromosomes and the proteins that bind these sequences. In mammals, telomeres consist primarily of TTAGGG sequences [1–5]. Telomeres prevent chromosome erosion and loss of coding sequences due to the end-replication problem. Loss of telomeric DNA is linked with cellular senescence and aging, and likely resembles double-strand breaks that activate DNA damage response pathways [6–9]. While cell growth continuously reduces telomere length, cancer cells become immortalized by activating mechanisms of telomere maintenance. The most common mechanism is expression of the enzyme telomerase, which catalyzes the addition of repeats to maintain telomere length. Approximately 15% of human tumors maintain telomeres independently of telomerase and use a recombination-based mechanism known as alternative lengthening of telomeres (ALT) to maintain telomere lengths [10–17]. ALT cells are typified by the presence of ALT-associated PML bodies (APBs) that include telomeric DNA and telomeric proteins [15,18]. Although the functions of APBs are unclear, they are considered primary sites of telomere metabolism. Aberrant telomere metabolism results in telomere dysfunction, yield chromosomal abnormalities, such as chromosome end-to-end fusions, telomeric translocations, tri- and quadri-radial chromosomes, and limit growth potential [8,19–22].

The mechanisms of ALT remain unclear. However, several DNA damage response proteins are implicated in ALT due to their association with telomeres or APBs, including the recQ-like helicases BLM (defective in Bloom's syndrome) and WRN (defective in Werner's syndrome), and the tumor suppressor BRCA1 [23–30]. BLM inhibits recombination by facilitating the resolution of recombination and replication intermediates. Through its structure-specific unwinding activity, BLM helps to resolve DNA damage-induced replication blocks that if left unresolved will result in aberrant recombination and chromosomal breakage. BLM associates with numerous proteins involved in DNA repair including BRCA1, DNA topoisomerases, DNA mismatch repair proteins and Fanconi anemia proteins, and is a component of the BRCA1-associated genome surveillance complex (BASC) [31–33]. BLM also associates with several telomere-specific proteins, such as POT1, TRF1 and TRF2 [34–37]. Biochemically, POT1 stimulates BLM unwinding of telomeric DNA end structures including D-loops and G-quadruplexes during DNA replication and/or recombination. TRF1 and TRF2 also modulate BLM function using telomeric substrates. The role of BLM in telomere metabolism is emphasized by telomere dysfunction in cells from those with Bloom's syndrome or cells lacking BLM, including increased telomeric associations and increased frequency of anaphase bridges involving telomeres [25,28,38–40]. While BLM plays a major role in regulating genomic sister chromatid exchange, studies investigating telomeric sister chromatid exchange (T-SCE) in cells lacking BLM have yielded inconsistent results but do not support a major role for BLM in regulating T-SCEs in ALT cells [38–40].

The tumor suppressor BRCA1 performs a key role in the cellular DNA-damage response and recombination repair by promoting both homologous recombination and non-homologous end-joining [41–48]. Its recruitment to DNA double strand breaks (DSB) is facilitated by the damage sensor MRN (MRE11-RAD50-NBS1 complex) and is critical for further assembly and employment of other recombination proteins to the site. BRCA1 consists of N-terminal RING domain and C-terminal tandem BRCT domains. The RING domain mediates its interaction with BARD1. Through the BRCT domains, it forms several distinct complexes including BRCA1-Abraxas, BRCA1-BACH1 and BRCA1-CtIP that perform key roles during initiation of recombination [48]. In addition, it functions in other DNA repair pathways such as non-homologous end joining (NHEJ) and nucleotide excision repair pathways, and is also part of BASC in genome surveillance [49,50]. Several studies implicate BRCA1 in telomere maintenance [51–53]. BRCA1 deficiency results in telomere dysfunction, as evidenced by elevated chromosome fusions and translocations involving telomeres and telomere shortening [52,54]. $Brca1^{-/-}$ murine T-cells display a high incidence of telomere instability [54], while expression of dominant-negative BRCA1 in human cells results in telomere dysfunction [55]. BRCA1 interacts with the telomere binding proteins TRF1 and TRF2 and is localized to telomeres. Its over-expression inhibits telomerase transcription and promotes shortening of telomeres in telomerase-positive breast and prostate cancer cell lines [56]. Interestingly, BRCA1 knockdown increases telomere length in some telomerase-positive cells [53]. An essential role of BRCA1 in telomere length maintenance is further emphasized by recent reports on telomere length measurements in those with familial breast cancer (those carrying mutations in *BRCA1*) indicating a correlation between telomere shortening in these affecteds and age of breast cancer onset [57].

The biochemical mechanisms by which BRCA1 mediates telomere maintenance are undefined. Although BRCA1 interacts with the recQ-like helicases WRN and BLM to facilitate intra-strand cross-link repair and DSB repair [58], BRCA1 interaction with BLM in the context of telomere metabolism is unclear. This study explores the role of BLM and BRCA1 in telomere metabolism in ALT cells.

Results, Discussion and Conclusions

BLM and BRCA1 co-localize at ALT telomeres

Our recent study demonstrated that telomerase-negative tumor cell lines utilize different ALT mechanisms to maintain telomeres [59]. Some of these mechanisms depend on BRCA1 and depletion of BRCA1 in these cells results in a modest decrease in telomeric sister-chromatid exchange [59]. Depletion of BLM results in a dramatic reductions in APB formation and telomere length in all cell lines utilizing ALT, confirming the role of BLM in telomere maintenance in ALT and/or induction of ALT [59,60]. Both BLM and BRCA1 are essential components of DNA damage-

induced replication/recombination foci and are independently associated with telomere maintenance. To test for a cooperative role of BRCA1 and BLM in telomere maintenance, *in situ* localization studies were performed using telomerase-positive (TA+) cells (HeLa and MG63) and telomerase-negative/ALT cells (Saos-2 and U2OS). Cells were synchronized by double thymidine block and release to assess cell cycle-dependent localization of BRCA1 and a telomeric Cy3-(CCCTAA)$_3$ PNA probe using immunofluorescence and telomere FISH. Asynchronous cells were used as controls. BRCA1 localizes to telomeres primarily in the G2 phase of the cell cycle in ALT cells (Figure 1A, B). Quantitation shows a 2.5-fold increase in telomeric localization of BRCA1 in ALT cells (~5 foci per nucleus) compared to telomerase-positive cells (~2 foci per nucleus) (Figure 2). Knock-down of *BRCA1* by *siRNAs* eliminates co-localization, demonstrating staining specificity (Figure S1). These results are consistent with a role for BRCA1 in telomere metabolism.

BLM is critical for telomere maintenance and its loss results in telomere dysfunction, often yielding increase in telomeric associations [38]. BLM is found with BRCA1 in a variety of protein complexes associated with DNA damage. In order to assess its role in the context of telomeres, cells were synchronized as above and assessed for co-localization of BLM and BRCA1 at telomeres using the telomeric Cy3- (CCCTAA)$_3$ PNA probe (Figure 3, 4A). Our results show that BLM and BRCA1 co-localize at telomeres only in ALT cells and that this interaction increases during G2. Furthermore, almost all BRCA1 foci at ALT telomeres include BLM (Figure 3, 4A). Telomerase-positive cells (HeLa) also contained BLM-BRCA1 co-localized foci (Fig 3, 4A), but none are found at telomeres. Similar results were obtained with another telomerase-positive cell line, MG63 (data not shown). These results demonstrate specific associations of BLM and BRCA1 at telomeres in ALT cells.

Since APB formation is thought to be integral to telomere maintenance in ALT cells, we assessed whether BLM and BRCA1 co-localize with PML at telomeres. While BLM commonly co-localizes with PML at telomeres, BRCA1 does not (Figure S2). As BRCA1 localization is dependent upon initiation of recombination events including DNA strand breaks, the absence of significant co-localization with PML at telomeres may indicate a transient association or exclusion of BRCA1 association from APBs during telomere metabolism. Association of BLM and BRCA1 was confirmed by co-immunoprecipitation of these proteins from total cell extracts made from ALT-positive U2OS cells at different stages of the cell cycle (Figure 4B). Our results show that BRCA1 co-immunoprecipitation with BLM is more pronounced at G2 compared to earlier stages. Extracts prepared from BLM-deficient cells served as a negative control. These data corroborate our immunofluorescence studies.

The MRN (MRE11-RAD50-NBS) complex plays a central role in recruitment of BRCA1 to DNA double strand breaks (DSBs) [42,48,53,61,62], followed by the recruitment of other recombination proteins to initiate end-resection and strand exchange during recombination. MRN also promotes recruitment of BLM to DSBs to participate in early recombination events [63–65]. Our data show that BLM and BRCA1 physically interact and the BLM-BRCA1-telomere co-localized foci are specific to ALT cells (Figures 1-4). In order to discern whether BLM is present during early recombination events in ALT cells, U2OS cell extracts were prepared at different stages of the cell cycle and proteins immunoprecipitated using anti-RAD50. As expected, BRCA1 and RAD50 co-immunoprecipitate from these extracts predominantly in S-phase (Figure 5A). BLM also co-immunoprecipitates with RAD50 with an interaction that is more pronounced in G2-

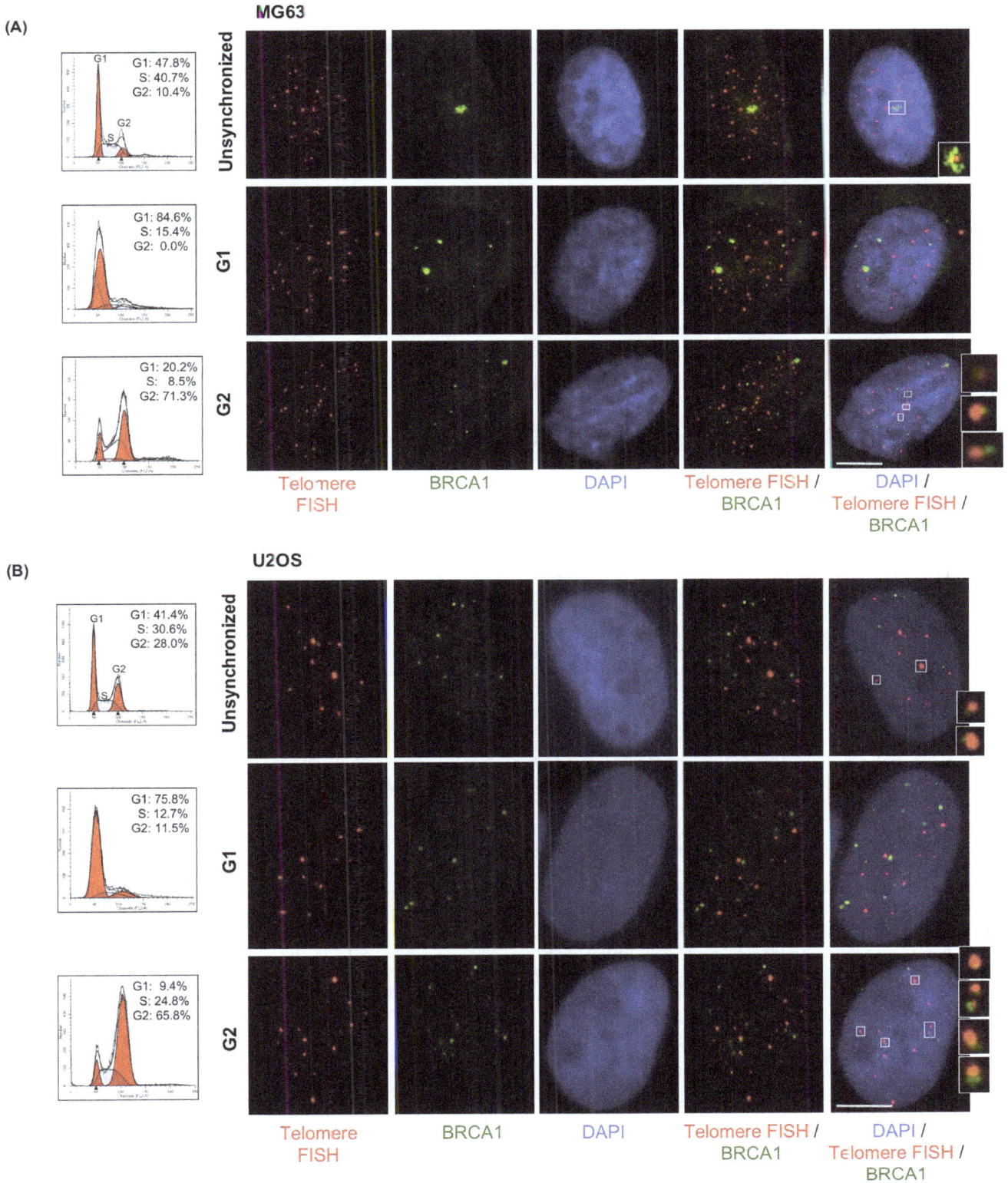

Figure 1. BRCA1 localizes to ALT cell telomeres primarily in G2 of the cell cycle. (A) MG63 and (B) U2OS cells were synchronized by double thymidine block. Asynchronous and synchronized cells were collected and analyzed by flow cytometry to determine cell cycle distribution. Cells were fixed at corresponding phases of cell cycle and stained with antibodies to BRCA1 (green); telomeres were labeled by FISH with a PNA probe (red); nuclei were stained with DAPI (blue). Images shown are a single maximum intensity projection (MIP) image. Enlargements of co-localizations are shown at the right. Scale bar: 10 µm.

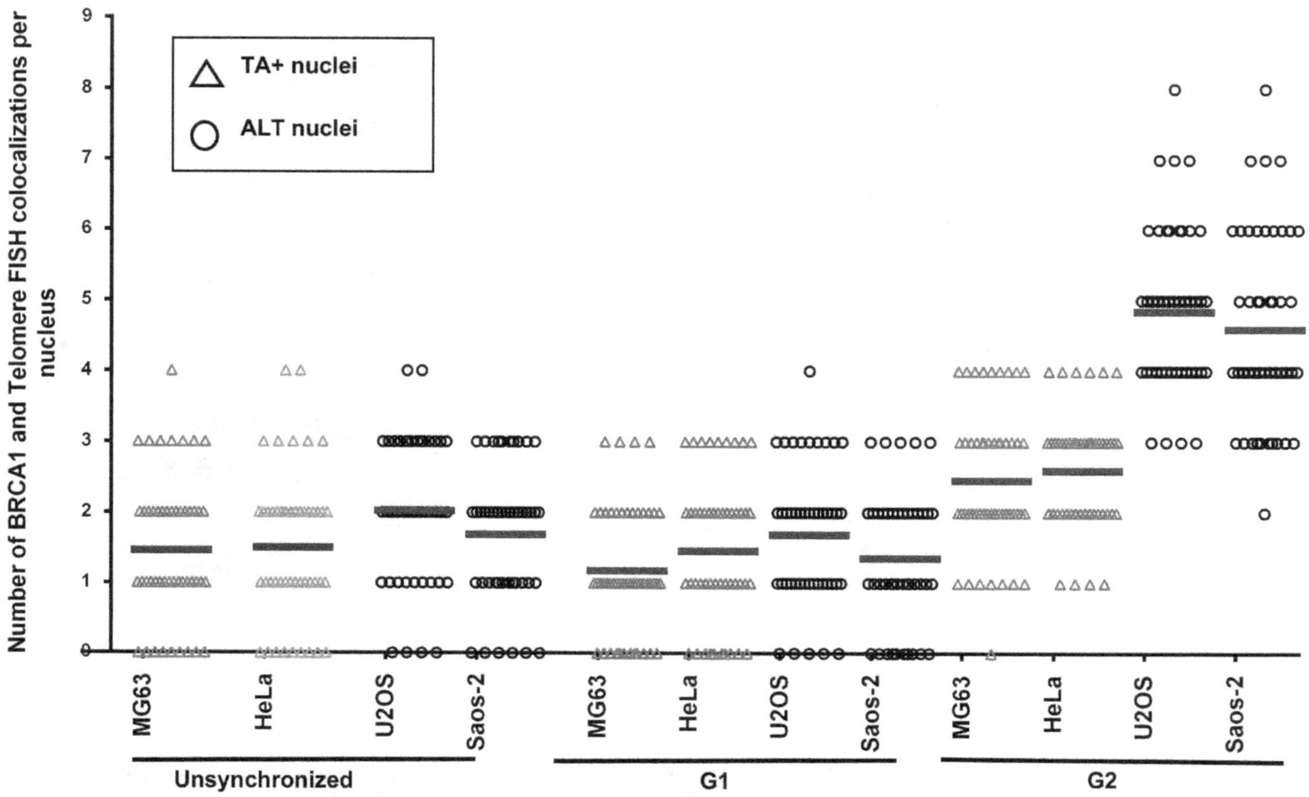

Figure 2. Telomeric localization of BRCA1 is increased in ALT cells. BRCA1 and telomere co-localizations in Figure 1 were quantitated per nucleus in unsynchronized, G1- and G2-synchronized MG63 (telomerase positive, TA+), HeLa (TA+), U2OS (ALT) and Saos-2 (ALT) cells. Each triangle (TA+) or open circle (ALT cells) represents an individual cell. Red bars indicate mean values.

phase (Figure 5B,C). In order to confirm these interactions in the context of telomeres, U2OS cells were synchronized as before and assessed for co-localization of BRCA1 or BLM with RAD50 at telomeres using immunofluorescence and telomere FISH with a telomeric probe (Figures 6–8). Quantitation of co-localized foci confirmed association of BRCA1 with RAD50 at telomeres predominantly at S-phase (Figure 6, Figure 8A) and that of BLM with RAD50 at telomeres predominantly at G2-phase (Figure 7, Figure 8B). These results suggest that BLM and BRCA1 may be part of complexes distinct from those with BRCA1-MRN and may function at different stages of telomeric recombination [62]. In summary, cytological data suggest that BLM and BRCA1 co-localize to telomeres with other recombination proteins in ALT cells and at times during the cell cycle when ALT is thought to occur.

BRCA1 stimulates BLM unwinding activity on a telomeric fork

We asked whether there is any functional significance of BLM-BRCA1 using helicase assays with purified full-length BRCA1 and BLM proteins and telomeric substrates containing one, two or four telomeric repeats (TTAGGG). As unwinding by BLM was most prominent on the telomeric fork substrate (data not shown), it was used for further experiments (Figure 9A). Different concentrations of BLM were tested for unwinding of telomeric fork substrates in 12 minutes (Figure 9B). The fork substrate containing one telomeric repeat was unwound very effectively (>80%) at the

lowest concentration of protein, whereas the fork substrate containing four telomeric repeats was unwound the least (Figure 9B). Subsequently, the fork substrate containing two telomeric repeats was used to measure the effect of BRCA1 on BLM unwinding (Figure 9C). The concentration of BLM was adjusted (1.2 nM) to achieve ≤30% unwinding in 12 minutes. The effect of BRCA1 on BLM helicase activity was then measured by addition of increasing concentrations of purified full-length BRCA1 (0–4 nM). DNA products were resolved by 10% native polyacrylamide gel electrophoresis (PAGE), and the percent of substrate unwound calculated and represented graphically as a function of BRCA1 concentration (Figure 9C). BLM activity is significantly enhanced approximately three-fold by BRCA1 in a protein concentration-dependent manner (Figure 9C). BRCA1 alone did not have a significant unwinding activity even at high concentrations (Figure 9C gel inset). Our data indicate that BRCA1 increases BLM unwinding activity on telomeric fork substrates. The effect of BRCA1 on BLM helicase activity was also tested using a non-telomeric fork. Our data indicate that full-length BRCA1 stimulates BLM on a non-telomeric fork albeit less than that on a telomeric fork (Figure 9D; ~3.6-fold increase for telomeric substrate vs ~1.9-fold increase for non-telomeric substrate). Stimulation of BLM activity by BRCA1 on a non-telomeric fork agrees with previously published work using an internal truncated fragment (amino acids 452–1079) of BRCA1 [58]. These data also suggest that the stimulation of BLM using non-telomeric substrates is independent of the RING and BRCT domains of BRCA1 and by extension, of BARD1 or other protein

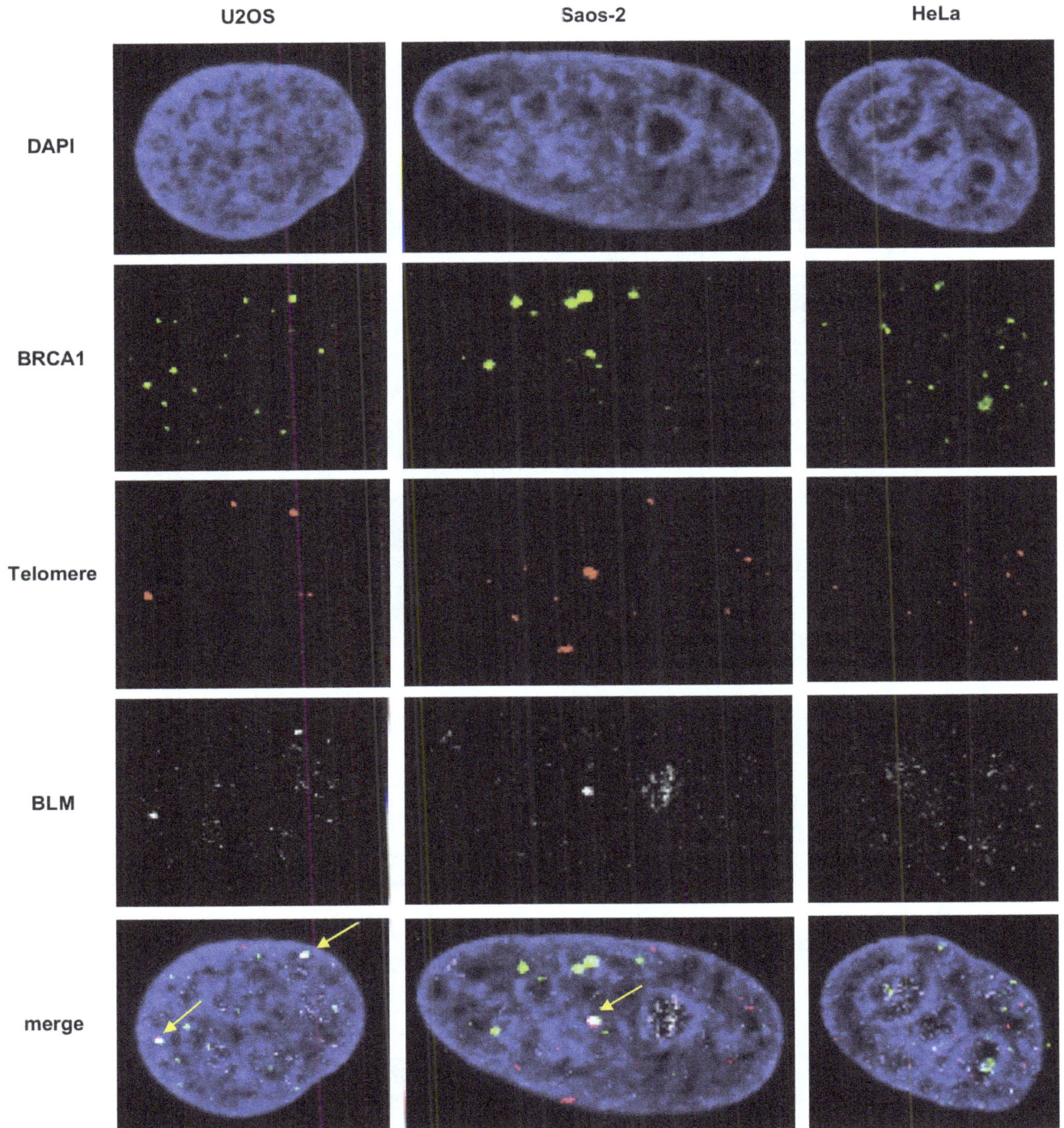

Figure 3. BRCA1 and BLM co-localize at telomeres in ALT cells. (A) Cells were synchronized to G2 (7h post release after double thymidine block) and stained with antibodies to BRCA1 and BLM and telomeres labeled by FISH with a PNA probe (upper panel) as in Figure 1. Yellow arrows indicate foci with BLM-BRCA1-telomere co-localization.

partners that utilize the BRCT domain to interact with BRCA1 [46,58]. These results indicate that full length BRCA1 is sufficient to stimulate BLM unwinding of telomeric forked DNA although it is unknown whether this would be enhanced by BARD1 or other BRCA1 partners.

BRCA1 increases the BLM unwinding rate on a telomeric fork

Finally, to understand the mechanism of action of BRCA1 on BLM, we assessed unwinding kinetics. Reactions were assembled on ice in the presence of BRCA1, started by BLM addition, stopped at regular time intervals and unwinding analyzed by

(A)

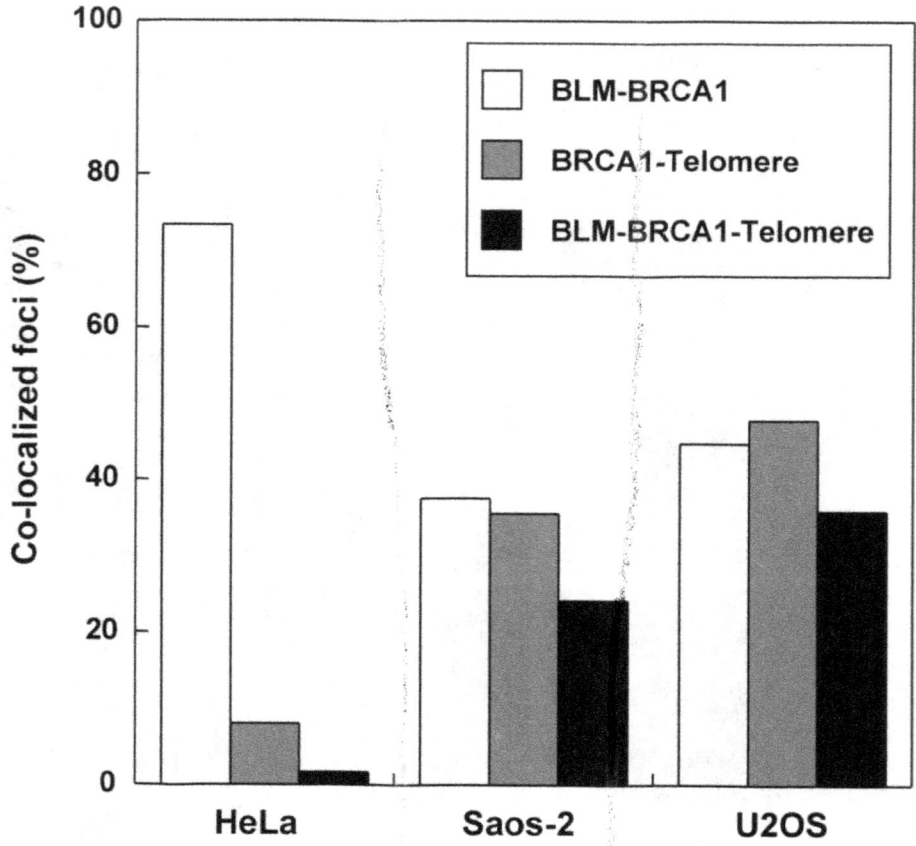

(B)

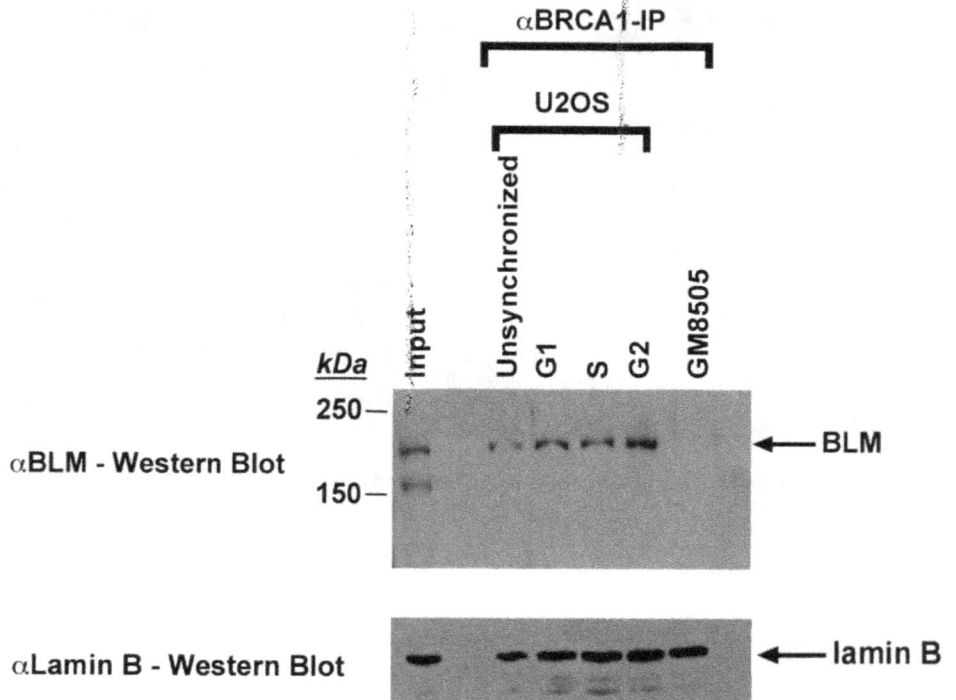

Figure 4. BRCA1 and BLM co-localize at telomeres only in ALT cells and physically interact predominantly during G2. (A) Quantitation of percent of cells with BLM-BRCA1, BRCA1-telomere, and BLM-BRCA1-telomere co-localized foci in Figure 3. **(B)** Upper panel: Co-immunoprecipitation of BLM with BRCA1 from U2OS cells. Cellular extracts (20 μg each) prepared at different stages of cell cycle were immunoprecipitated with an αBRCA1 antibody, separated on an 8% SDS-PAGE and analyzed by western blotting with αBLM antibody. Lower panel: Cellular extracts (20 μg each) used in upper panel corresponding to each stage were separated on an 8% SDS-PAGE and analyzed by western blotting with αLamin B antibody to show equivalent loading. The arrow mark indicates the position of BLM or Lamin B on the blot. Extracts from BLM-deficient cell line GM8505 served as a control.

native PAGE. BRCA1 stimulates BLM in a time-dependent manner (Figure 9E). The respective rates of reaction were calculated by plotting the substrate unwound in the initial stages of reaction against time. The BLM initial unwinding rate was increased by 1.7-fold in the presence of BRCA1.

These biochemical experiments indicate that BRCA1 effectively increases the rate of unwinding by BLM to resolve fork substrates

that contain small stretches of telomeric repeats. The lack of resolution of fork substrates containing four repeats may reflect the lack of processivity of BLM rather than an effect of BRCA1 or a possible requirement of additional factors to overcome the energetic barrier imposed by a stretch of G-rich duplex regions. Our data do not address the temporal requirements of the BLM-BRCA1 interaction. However, their enhanced association at G2

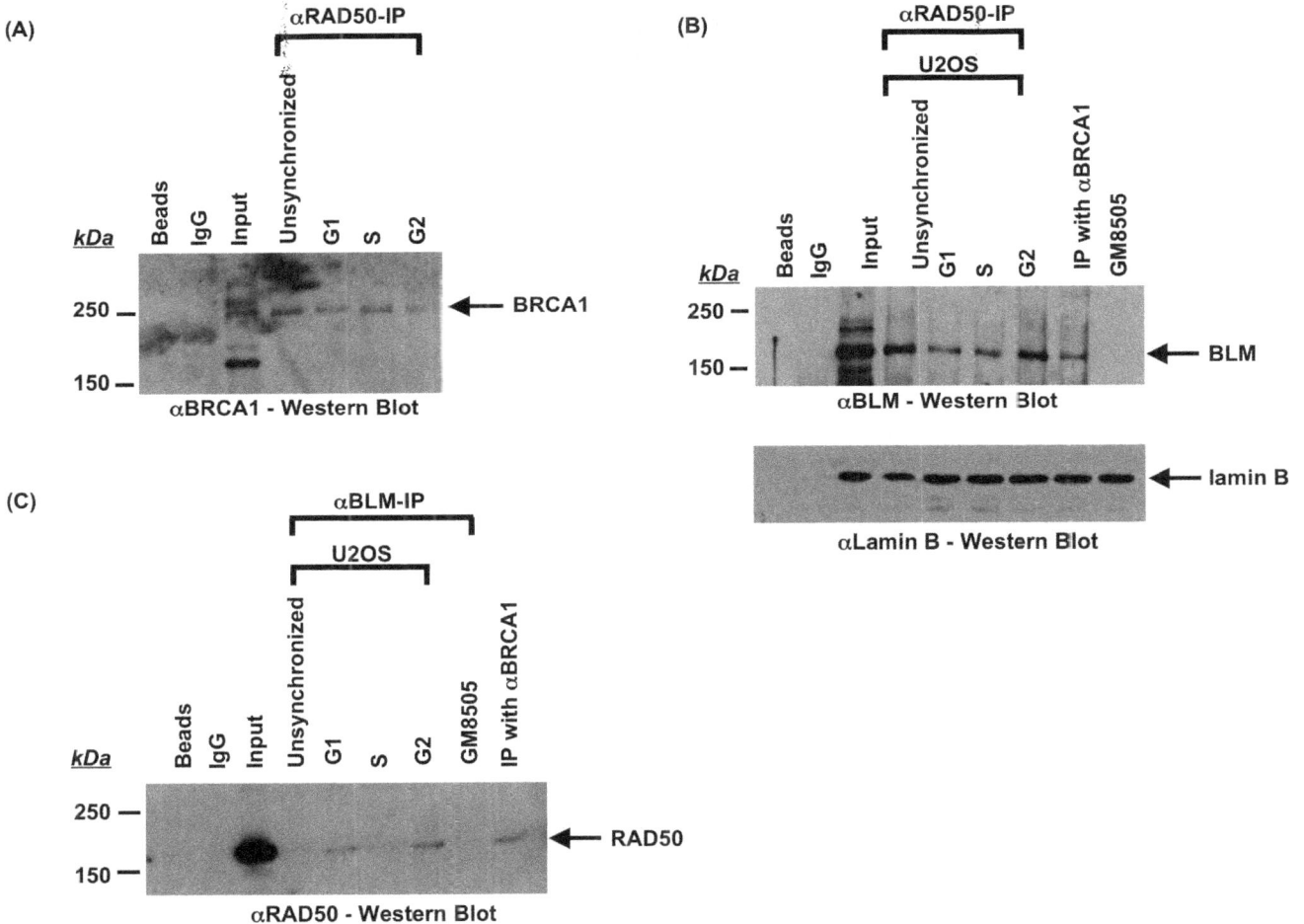

Figure 5. Co-immunoprecipitations of BRCA1, RAD50 and BLM from U2OS cells at different phases of the cell cycle. Cells were synchronized by double-thymidine block and extracts made at different cell cycle phases. Extracts were immunoprecipitated using indicated antibodies, separated by 8% SDS-PAGE and analyzed by western blotting using indicated antibodies. **(A and B) Immunoprecipitation of BRCA1 and BLM by RAD50.** Immunoprecipitation was performed using αRAD50 antibody on extracts representing unsynchronized cells or cells at G1-, S- and G2-phases of cell cycle. Controls included immunoprecipitation in the absence of αRAD50 antibody (Beads) or immunoprecipitation using IgG. Extracts in the absence of immunoprecipitation were included in the gels as input. Western blotting was performed using αBRCA1 (panel A) or αBLM antibody (panel B). Cellular extracts used for immunoprecipitation corresponding to each stage were separated on an 8% SDS-PAGE and analyzed by western blotting with αLamin B antibody to show equivalent loading (panel B lower blot). **(C) Immunoprecipitation of RAD50 by BLM.** Immunoprecipitation was performed using αBLM antibody on extracts representing unsynchronized cells or cells at G1-, S- and G2-phases of cell cycle. Controls included immunoprecipitation in the absence of αRAD50 antibody (Beads), immunoprecipitation using IgG or immunoprecipitation of extracts from a BLM-deficient cell line (GM8505). Extracts in the absence of immunoprecipitation were included in the gel as input. Western Blotting was performed using αRad50 antibody.

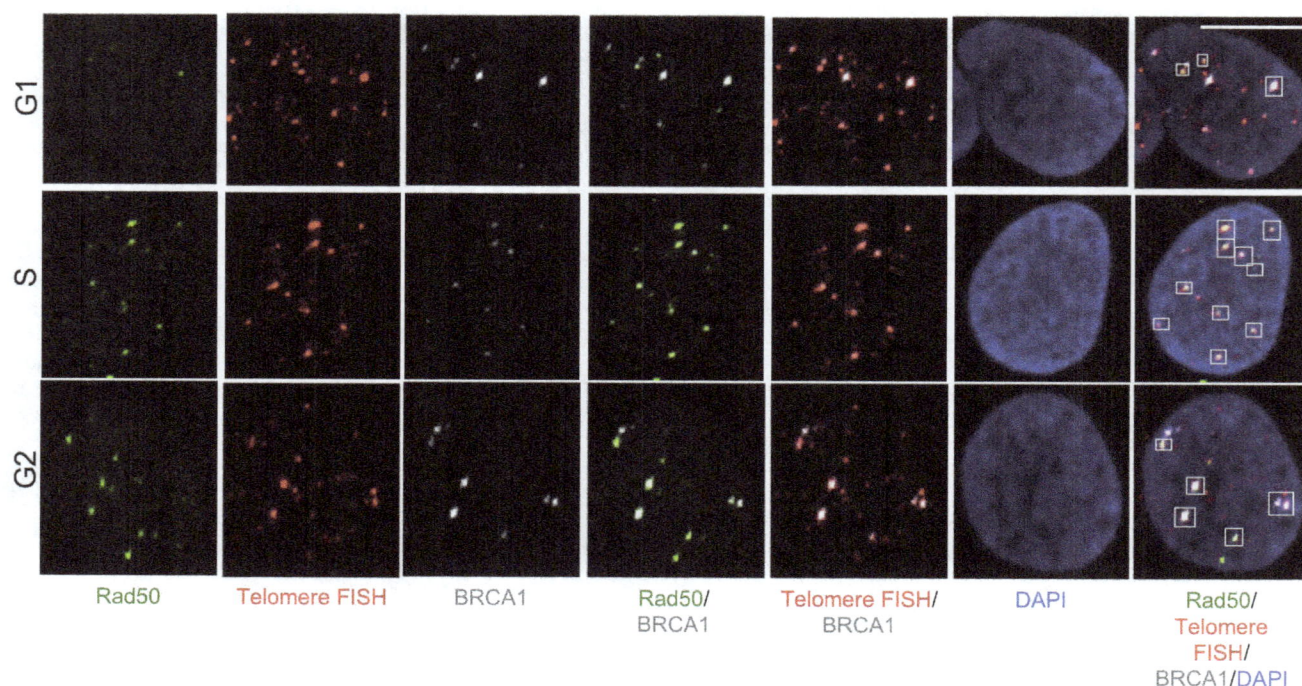

Figure 6. Co-localization of BRCA1 and RAD50 at telomeres at different stages of cell cycle in ALT cells. U2OS cells were synchronized by double thymidine block in G1-, S- and G2-stages of the cell cycle. Cells were fixed and stained with antibodies to BRCA1 (grey), Rad50 (green) and telomeres labeled by FISH with a PNA probe (Red). Nuclei are stained with DAPI. Images are shown as MIP image. White boxes indicate co-localizations of BRCA1, Rad50 and telomere FISH. Scale bar: 10 μm.

suggests a function during late replication or during recombination-associated events at the telomere [38,66]. While BRCA1 is essential for recruitment of recombination proteins to promote strand processing and invasion, and to form recombination intermediates, its recruitment to telomeres requires RAD50 during S-phase [42,53,61]. Our data indicate that BLM is also part of stable complexes with RAD50, albeit predominantly in G2 and suggest that BLM-BRCA1 complexes may be distinct from BRCA1-RAD50 complexes required during recombination initiation (Figures 5–8). It is also unclear whether resolution of the intermediates by BLM requires the recruitment of BRCA1 or the realignment of existing BRCA1-containing complexes. The apparent opposing effects of BRCA1 in promoting recombination to resolve DNA damage through formation of recombination intermediates and preventing recombination by facilitating repair through resolution of recombination intermediates with BLM is intriguing. Given the importance of recombination in ALT, an inhibitory activity of BRCA1 might be essential to limit recombination at telomeric regions resulting from a strand break due to damage or replicative stress. Such a function is consistent with an increase in telomeric chromosomal end-to-end fusions and telomere dysfunction that is seen with deficiency of BRCA1 [25,28,38-40,51,52,54]. Our data implicate both BRCA1 and BLM in alternative telomere length maintenance mechanisms and provide an explanation for how recombination of telomeric repeats could be regulated by BLM and BRCA1 interactions at telomeres.

Materials and Methods

Cell lines

MG63 (osteosarcoma, ATCC), HeLa (cervical adenocarcinoma, ATCC), U2OS (osteosarcoma, ATCC) and Saos-2 (osteosarcoma, ATCC) cells were cultured in Dulbecco's modified Eagle's minimal essential medium (DMEM) (Invitrogen) supplemented with 10% fetal bovine serum (FBS) (Hyclone). All cultures were grown without antibiotics in a humidified incubator at 37°C with 5% CO_2.

Antibodies and *siRNA*

Antibodies for immunofluorescence included: BRCA1 (A301-378A, Bethyl Laboratories; OP92, Calbiochem), and PML (PG-M3, Santa Cruz; ab53773, Abcam). Antibodies for western blot included: BRCA1, RAD50 (Santa Cruz), TRF2 (Imgenex) and lamin B (C-20, Santa Cruz). The BLM antibody was a generous gift from Dr. Albert Davalos. *BRCA1 siRNA* (ON target plus Human *BRCA1* (672) *siRNA* SMARTpool) was purchased from Thermo Scientific.

Cell synchronization

Cells were plated at 30% confluence and treated with 2 mM thymidine (Sigma) for 18 h (first block). After the first thymidine block, cells were washed with PBS and released for 9 h by adding DMEM containing 10% FBS. After release, cells were again treated with 2 mM thymidine for 17 h (second block). After the second block, cells were washed with PBS and released by adding DMEM containing 10% FBS. Cells for G1 analysis were collected at this point; cells for S-phase analysis were typically collected after 3 h post release and G2 analysis were collected after 7 h post release.

Cell cycle analysis

Cells were collected and fixed with ice-cold 80% (v/v) ethanol for 30 min on ice. Cell were washed twice with PBS containing 0.1% EDTA (w/v) and collected by centrifugation. Cells were re-

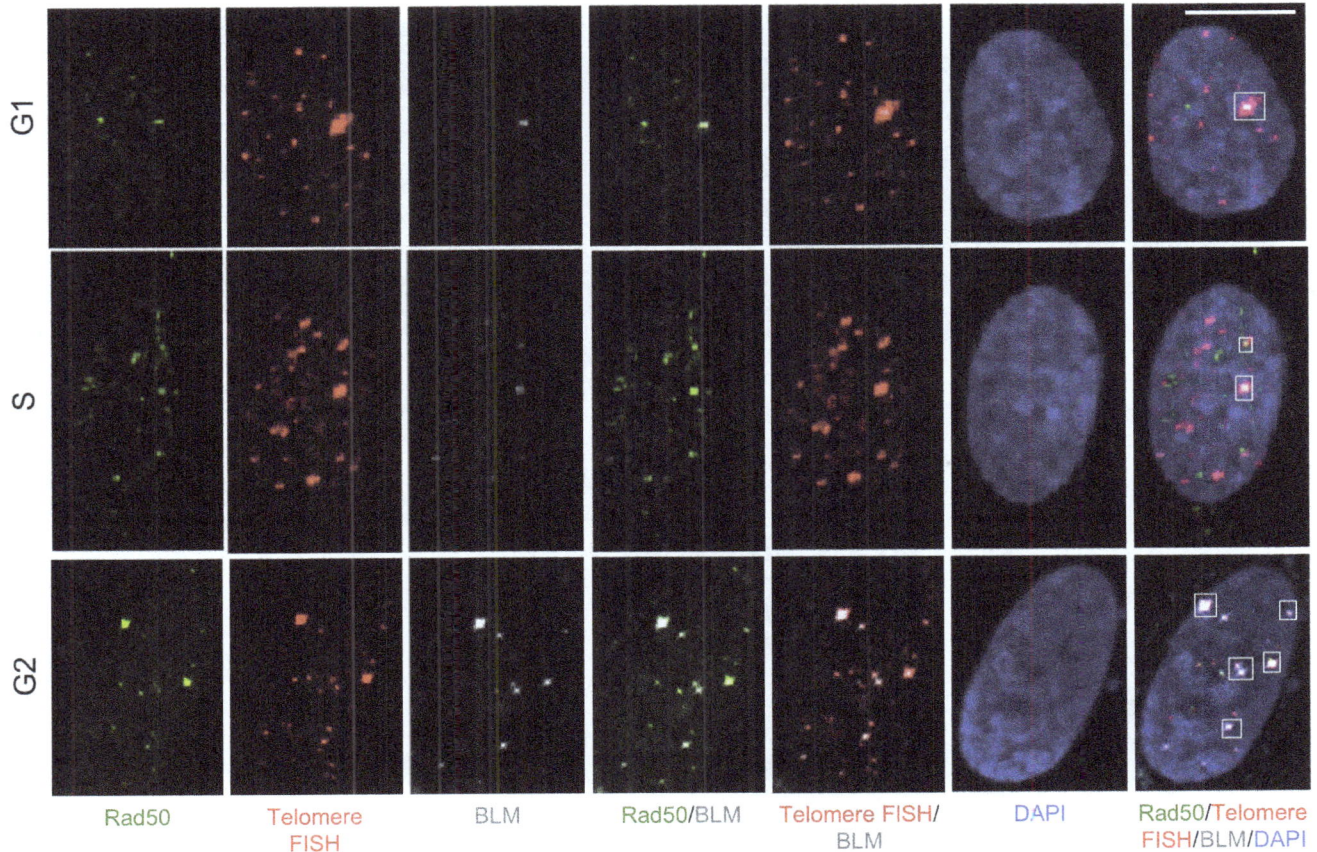

Figure 7. Co-localization of BLM and RAD50 at telomeres at different stages of cell cycle in ALT cells. U2OS cells were synchronized by double thymidine block in G1-, S- and G2-stages of the cell cycle. Cells were fixed and stained with antibodies to BLM (grey), Rad50 (green) and telomeres labeled by FISH with a PNA probe (red). Nuclei are stained with DAPI. Images are shown as MIP image. White boxes indicate co-localizations of BLM, Rad50 and telomere FISH. Scale bar: 10 μm.

suspended in 0.03 mg/ml propidium iodide (Sigma) and 0.3 mg/ml RNAse A (Sigma) and incubated at 4°C for 1 h. DNA content was analyzed using a FACSCalibur flow cytometer (BD Biosciences).

Immunofluorescence and telomere FISH

Unsynchronized, synchronized and *siRNA*-treated cells were grown on coverslips and fixed for 10 min in PBS with 4% (v/v) paraformaldehyde. Cells were dehydrated in a graded ethanol series (70% (v/v) for 3 min, 90% (v/v) for 2 min and 100% for 2 min) and rehydrated for 30 minutes in consecutive washes with PBS and 2X SSC. Cells were overlaid with 0.6 μg/ml Cy3-(CCCTAA)$_3$ PNA probe (Panagene) in *in situ* hybridization solution (Enzo Life Sciences), denatured at 80°C for 3 min and hybridized at 37°C for 3 h. Cells were washed with 2X SSC and PBST. Cells were then permeabilized for 10 min in PBS with 0.5% Triton X-100 (v/v) and blocked for 30 min in 10% goat serum/PBST (0.1% Tween-20 in PBS) (v/v) at room temperature. Cells were incubated with primary antibody diluted in 1% BSA/PBST for 1 h at room temperature or at 4°C overnight, washed with PBST, incubated with secondary antibody diluted in 1% BSA/PBST for 1 h at room temperature and washed with PBST. Finally, cells were rinsed in PBS and mounted onto glass slides in mounting media with DAPI (Vector Laboratories, Inc.). Slides were analyzed with an Olympus FV 1000 spectral confocal system at the Ohio State Campus Microscopy and Imaging Facility or

with a Zeiss Axioskop. Four color imaging was performed using Olympus FV1000 Filter confocal system. Nuclei were captured in 15–20 Z plane increments of 0.44 μm and merged using the extended focus maximum intensity projection (MIP) settings. The 3D co-localization rendering of multiple channels (volume rendering) was created using Metamorph analysis software. At least 50 cells per group were analyzed to generate the percentage of cells with co-localized foci. Similar results were observed in several independent experiments.

Western blot and immunoprecipitation

Western blot analysis was performed using standard methods [67,68]. Immunoprecipitation (IP) was performed at 4°C. For the co-immunoprecipitation assay, protein lysates were prepared from unsynchronized and synchronized U2OS cells in NP40 lysis buffer (50 mM Tris.HCl pH 8.0, 150 mM NaCl, 2 mM EDTA, 1% NP40 + protease inhibitors). Equal amount of protein lysate (20 μg) was pre-cleared using protein-A sepharose beads (GE Healthcare Biosciences) for 30 minutes, then applied to protein-A beads that were incubated with either 10 μl of anti-BRCA1, anti-BLM, anti-Rad50 antibody, rabbit-IgG or mouse-IgG. Protein-A-bound immune complexes were washed three times with IP wash buffer (20 mM Tris.HCl pH 8.0, 2 mM EDTA, 50 mM NaCl); suspended in SDS-sample buffer followed by boiling for 5 minutes. Immunoprecipitates were separated on 6% SDS-PAGE gel and transferred to a PVDF membrane. The membrane was blotted

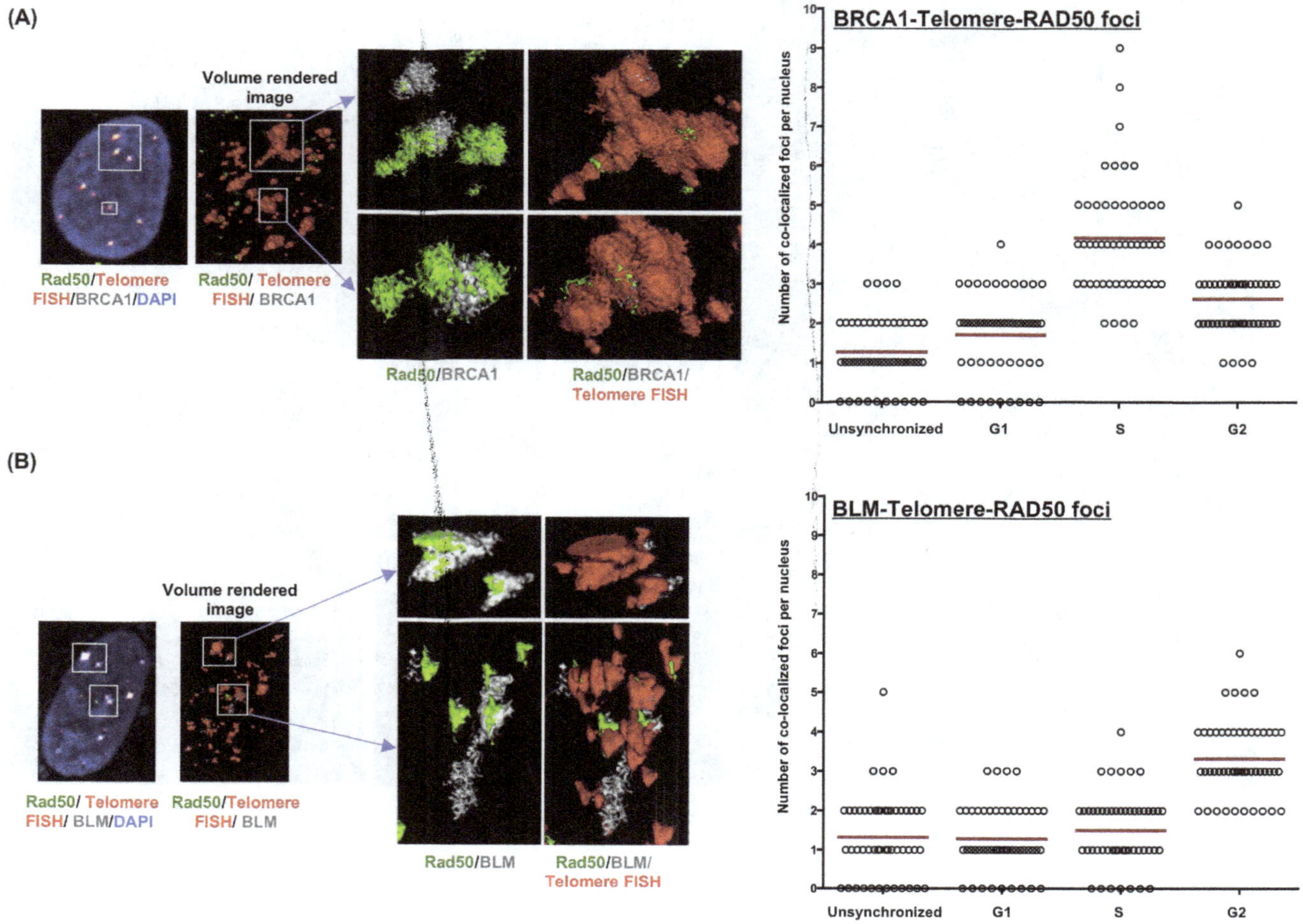

(A)

(B)

Figure 8. BRCA1 and BLM co-localize at telomeres along with RAD50 at different phases of cell cycle in ALT cells. U2OS cells were synchronized and stained with antibodies to BRCA1 or BLM (grey), Rad50 (green) and telomeres were labeled by FISH with a PNA probe (Red); nuclei were stained with DAPI. Representative images are shown as MIP image. White boxes indicate co-localizations of BRCA1 (**panel A**) or BLM (**panel B**) with Rad50 and telomere FISH. Co-localizations were confirmed by 3D rendering of multiple channels (volume rendering) using Metamorph analysis software. Enlargements of rendered co-localizations are shown at the right side and indicated by arrow. Co-localized foci of BRCA1 (or BLM), Rad50 and telomere were quantified per nucleus in unsynchronized, G1, S and G2 synchronized U2OS cells and represented graphically (right side of each panel). Each open circle represents an individual cell. Red bar indicate mean values.

overnight at 4°C with either anti-BRCA1, anti-BLM or anti-Rad50.

Analyses

Dot plots were generated using Graph Pad Prism.

Protein purification

His-tagged human BLM was expressed in yeast and purified as described previously [67,68]. Recombinant full length BRCA1 was purchased from Active Motif.

Oligonucleotides

Oligonucleotides containing different telomeric repeat units and the corresponding complementary strands were designed as described and purchased from Operon [69]. The non-telomeric substrate was made by annealing the following strands: 5′-TTT-TTTTTTTTTTTTT**TTCAGTAGATCA**CATGCACTAC-3′ and 5′-GTAGTGCATG**TGATCTACTGAA**TTTTTTTTTTTTTTT-T-3′.

Helicase assays

The repeat-containing oligonucleotide of each substrate was labeled, annealed with its complementary oligonucleotide and purified on 10% native PAGE. Helicase assays were performed as described [67,68] in the following buffer: 20 mM Tris-HCl pH7.5, 5 mM $MgCl_2$, 1 mM DTT, 2 mM ATP, 100 mM NaCl and 100 µg/ml BSA. Reactions (20 µl) were assembled on ice in the presence (or absence) of BRCA1 and 5fmol of respective labeled substrate. Reactions were started with the addition of BLM and incubated at 37°C for 12 minutes (or as indicated for kinetics). Reactions were stopped by addition of 20 µl of 2X stop buffer containing 1 pmol/ul unlabeled oligonucleotide (corresponding to the labeled oligonucleotide). Reactions were analyzed by a 10% native PAGE in 1X TBE. Gels were dried, exposed on a phosphorimager plate and analyzed by ImageQuant software on a Typhoon phosphorimager. Bands were quantitated, amount of substrate unwound calculated and plotted as a function of protein concentration or time as indicated. Plots were fitted to Michaelis-Menton kinetics as indicated using Kaleidagraph software.

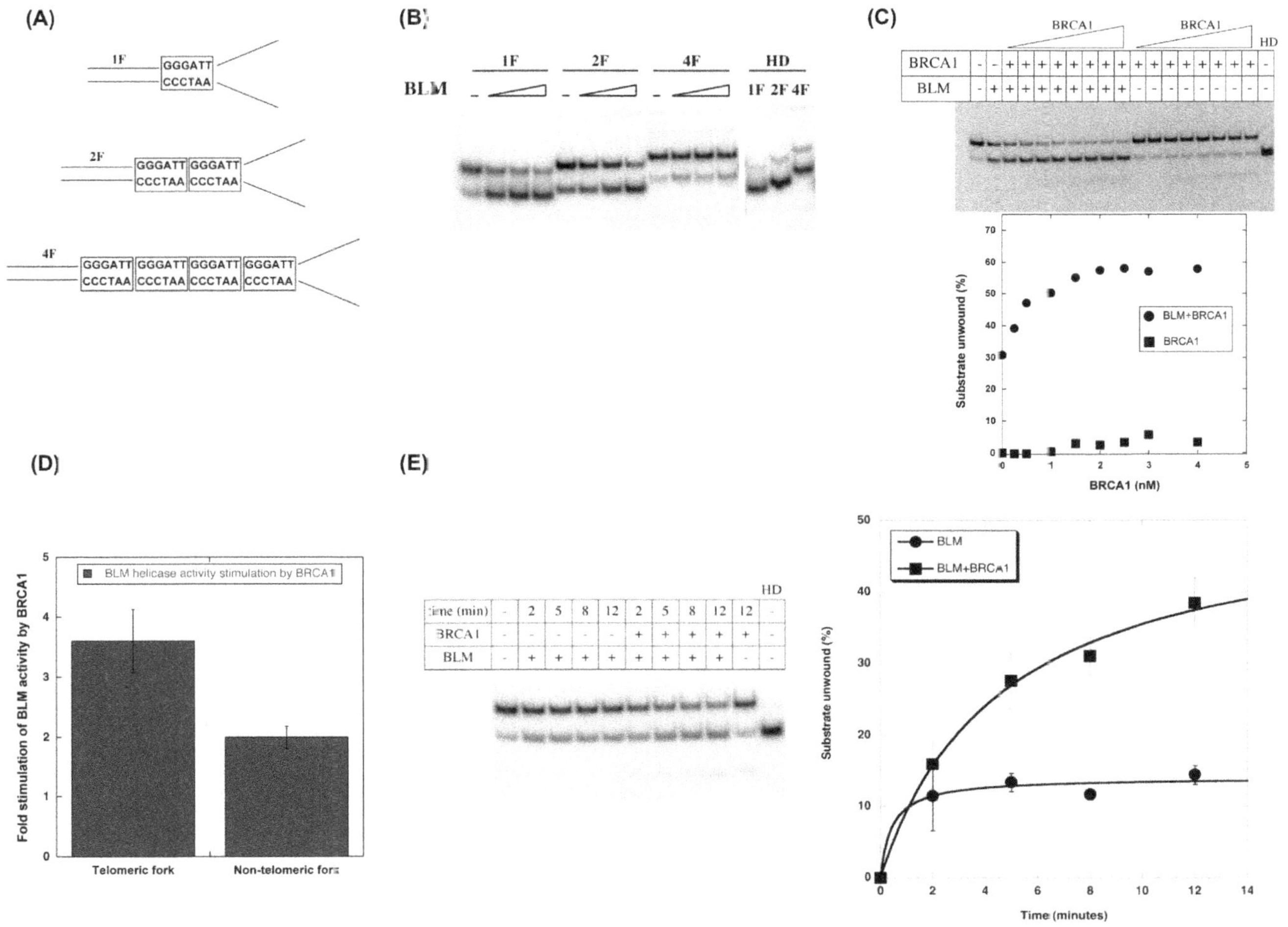

Figure 9. BRCA1 stimulates BLM helicase activity on telomeric repeat forks. (A) Fork substrates (1F, 2F and 4F) used for the study. The number of telomeric repeat units (GGGATT) are boxed in each fork substrate – 1F contains one repeat, 2F contains two repeats and 4F contains four repeats. **(B)** BLM helicase activity on fork substrates. Increasing amounts of BLM (0.6 nM, 1.2 nM and 4.2 nM) were used for each substrate, reactions were terminated after 12 minutes and analyzed by native PAGE. HD refers to heat-denatured substrate. **(C)** Effect of BRCA1 on BLM helicase activity on 2F substrate. Helicase reactions were performed for 12 minutes with 1.2 nM BLM and increasing concentrations of BRCA1 (0–4 nM). Reactions were terminated and analyzed by native PAGE. The amount of substrate unwound (%) was plotted as a function of BRCA1 (nM). A representative gel and corresponding graph are shown. **(D)** Stimulation of BLM activity by BRCA1 on telomeric and non-telomeric substrates. BLM helicase activity was tested in the presence of 3 nM BRCA1 on fork substrates that contained two telomeric repeats (panel A) or a non-telomeric sequence instead of the repeat units. Reactions were analyzed by native PAGE and quantitated on a phosphorimager. The fold stimulation of BLM activity by BRCA1 for each substrate is shown as histogram. **(E)** BRCA1 enhances the rate of unwinding of telomeric fork by BLM. Kinetics of BLM unwinding was analyzed in the presence of 1.2 nM BLM and 3 nM BRCA1. Reactions were analyzed as in C. The amount of substrate unwound (%) was plotted as a function time (minutes) and fitted to Michaelis-Menton kinetics using Kaleidagraph. A representative gel and corresponding graph are shown.

Supporting Information

Figure S1 *BRCA1 siRNA* reduces BRCA1 staining and localization at telomeres. **(A)** Western blot analysis of BRCA1 and lamin B (loading control) in 25 μg of protein extracted from MG63 and U2OS cells treated with mock, scrambled or BRCA1 siRNAs. **(B)** MG63 and U2OS cells were stained with antibodies to BRCA1 (green), telomeres labeled by FISH with a PNA probe (red), nuclei were labeled with DAPI (blue) after 72 hours of *BRCA1 siRNA* knockdown. **(C)** Quantitation of BRCA1 and telomere co-localizations per nucleus in scrambled and BRCA1 siRNA-treated MG63, HeLa, U2OS and Saos-2 cells. Each triangle (TA+ cells) or open circle (ALT cells) represents an individual cell. Red bars indicate mean values.

Figure S2 PML co-localizes with BLM but not BRCA1 at ALT telomeres. Cells were synchronized and stained with antibodies to BRCA1 (green), BLM (white) or PML (top: white; bottom: green), telomeres were labeled by FISH with a PNA probe (red), and nuclei were stained with DAPI (blue). Yellow arrows indicate foci with all three signals.

Acknowledgments

The authors thank Dr. Michael Mcilhatton for critical reading of the manuscript. We thank Dr. Sarah Cole from the Campus Microscopy and Imaging Facility at The Ohio State University for assistance with microscopy. Images presented in this report were generated using the instruments and services at the Campus Microscopy and Imaging Facility at The Ohio State University.

Author Contributions

Conceived and designed the experiments: SA JG. Performed the experiments: SA ZK ASG. Analyzed the data: SA JG JDP. Contributed reagents/materials/analysis tools: SA ZK ASG ARM JH. Contributed to the writing of the manuscript: SA.

References

1. Shampay J, Szostak JW, Blackburn EH (1984) DNA sequences of telomeres maintained in yeast. Nature 310: 154–157.
2. Allshire RC, Dempster M, Hastie ND (1989) Human telomeres contain at least three types of G-rich repeat distributed non-randomly. Nucleic Acids Res 17: 4611–4627.
3. de Lange T, Shiue L, Myers RM, Cox DR, Naylor SL, et al. (1990) Structure and variability of human chromosome ends. Mol Cell Biol 10: 518–527.
4. de Lange T (1992) Human telomeres are attached to the nuclear matrix. EMBO J 11: 717–724.
5. Griffith JD, Comeau L, Rosenfield S, Stansel RM, Bianchi A, et al. (1999) Mammalian telomeres end in a large duplex loop. Cell 97: 503–514.
6. Lundblad V, Blackburn EH (1993) An alternative telomere maintenance rescues est1- senescence. Cell 73: 347–360.
7. Wyllie FS, Jones CJ, Skinner JW, Haughton MF, Wallis C, et al. (2000) Telomerase prevents the accelerated cell ageing of Werner syndrome fibroblasts. Nat Genet 24: 16–17.
8. Bailey SM, Brenneman MA, Goodwin EH (2004) Frequent recombination in telomeric DNA may extend the proliferative life of telomerase-negative cells. Nucleic Acids Res 32: 3743–3751.
9. Laud PR, Multani AS, Bailey SM, Wu L, Ma J, et al. (2005) Elevated telomere-telomere recombination in WRN-deficient, telomere dysfunctional cells promotes escape from senescence and engagement of the ALT pathway. Genes Dev 19: 2560–2570.
10. Bryan TM, Englezou A, Gupta J, Bacchetti S, Reddel RR (1995) Telomere elongation in immortal human cells without detectable telomerase activity. EMBO J 14: 4240–4248.
11. Bryan TM, Englezou A, Dalla-Pozza L, Dunham MA, Reddel RR (1997) Evidence for an alternative mechanism for maintaining telomere length in human tumors and tumor-derived cell lines. Nat Med 3: 1271–1274.
12. Bryan TM, Reddel RR (1997) Telomere dynamics and telomerase activity in in vitro immortalised human cells. Eur J Cancer 33: 767–773.
13. Niida H, Shinkai Y, Hande MP, Matsumoto T, Takehara S, et al. (2000) Telomere maintenance in telomerase-deficient mouse embryonic stem cells: Characterization of an amplified telomeric DNA. Mol Cell Biol 20: 4115–4127.
14. Dunham MA, Neumann AA, Fasching CL, Reddel RR (2000) Telomere maintenance by recombination in human cells. Nat Genet 26: 447–450.
15. Grobelny JV, Godwin AK, Broccoli D (2000) ALT-associated PML bodies are present in viable cells and are enriched in cells in the G(2)/M phase of the cell cycle. J Cell Sci 113: 4577–4585.
16. Montgomery E, Argani P, Hicks JL, DeMarzo AM, Meeker AK (2004) Telomere lengths of translocation-associated and nontranslocation-associated sarcomas differ dramatically. Am J Pathol 164: 1523–1529.
17. Nabetani A, Ishikawa F (2011) Alternative lengthening of telomeres pathway: Recombination-mediated telomere maintenance mechanism in human cells. J Biochem 149: 5–14.
18. Yeager TR, Neumann AA, Englezou A, Huschtscha LI, Noble JR, et al. (1999) Telomerase-negative immortalized human cells contain a novel type of promyelocytic leukemia (PML) body. Cancer Res 59: 4175–4179.
19. Schulz VP, Zakian VA, Ogburn CE, McKay J, Jarzebowicz AA, et al. (1996) Accelerated loss of telomeric repeats may not explain accelerated replicative decline of Werner syndrome cells. Hum Genet 97: 750–754.
20. Hande MP, Samper E, Lansdorp P, Blasco MA (1999) Telomere length dynamics and chromosomal instability in cells derived from telomerase null mice. J Cell Biol 144: 589–601.
21. Reddel RR (2003) Alternative lengthening of telomeres, telomerase, and cancer. Cancer Lett 194: 155–162.
22. Londono-Vallejo JA, Der-Sarkissian H, Cazes L, Bacchetti S, Reddel RR (2004) Alternative lengthening of telomeres is characterized by high rates of telomeric exchange. Cancer Res 64: 2324–2327.
23. Tahara H, Tokutake Y, Maeda S, Kataoka H, Watanabe T, et al. (1997) Abnormal telomere dynamics of B-lymphoblastoid cell strains from Werner's syndrome patients transformed by Epstein-Barr virus. Oncogene 15: 1911–1920.
24. Opresko PL, von Kobbe C, Laine JP, Harrigan J, Hickson ID, et al. (2002) Telomere-binding protein TRF2 binds to and stimulates the Werner and Bloom syndrome helicases. J Biol Chem 277: 41110–41119.
25. Schawalder J, Paric E, Neff NF (2003) Telomere and ribosomal DNA repeats are chromosomal targets of the bloom syndrome DNA helicase. BMC Cell Biol 4: 15.
26. Opresko PL, Otterlei M, Graakjaer J, Bruheim P, Dawut L, et al. (2004) The Werner syndrome helicase and exonuclease cooperate to resolve telomeric D loops in a manner regulated by TRF1 and TRF2. Mol Cell 14: 763–774.
27. Crabbe L, Verdun RE, Haggblom CI, Karlseder J (2004) Defective telomere lagging strand synthesis in cells lacking WRN helicase activity. Science 306: 1951–1953.
28. Lillard-Wetherell K, Machwe A, Langland GT, Combs KA, Behbehani GK, et al (2004) Association and regulation of the BLM helicase by the telomere proteins TRF1 and TRF2. Hum Mol Genet 13: 1919–1932.
29. Opresko PL, Mason PA, Podell ER, Lei M, Hickson ID, et al. (2005) POT1 stimulates RecQ helicases WRN and BLM to unwind telomeric DNA substrates. J Biol Chem 280: 32069–32080.
30. Bhattacharyya S, Keirsey J, Russell B, Kavecansky J, Lillard-Wetherall K, et al. (2009) Telomerase-associated protein 1, HSP90, and topoisomerase IIalpha associate directly with the BLM helicase in immortalized cells using ALT and modulate its helicase activity using telomeric DNA substrates. J Biol Chem 284: 14966–14977.
31. Wang Y, Cortez D, Yazdi P, Neff N, Elledge SJ, et al. (2000) BASC, a super complex of BRCA1-associated proteins involved in the recognition and repair of aberrant DNA structures. Genes Dev 14: 927–939.
32. Wu L, Davies SL, Levitt NC, Hickson ID (2001) Potential role for the BLM helicase in recombinational repair via a conserved interaction with RAD51. J Biol Chem 276: 19375–19381.
33. Chaudhury I, Sareen A, Raghunandan M, Sobeck A (2013) FANCD2 regulates BLM complex functions independently of FANCI to promote replication fork recovery. Nucl Acids Res 41: 6444–6459.
34. Sun H, Karow JK, Hickson ID, Maizels N (1998) The Bloom's syndrome helicase unwinds G4 DNA. J Biol Chem 273: 27587–27592.
35. Stavropoulos DJ, Bradshaw PS, Li X, Pasic I, Truong K, et al. (2002) The Bloom syndrome helicase BLM interacts with TRF2 in ALT cells and promotes telomeric DNA synthesis. Hum Mol Genet 11: 3135–3144.
36. Temime-Smaali N, Guittat L, Wenner T, Bayart E, Douarre C, et al. (2008) Topoisomerase IIIa is required for normal proliferation and telomere stability in alternative lengthening of telomeres. EMBO J 27: 1523–1524.
37. Bhattacharyya S, Sandy A, Groden J (2010) Unwinding protein complexes in ALTernative telomere maintenance. J Cell Biochem 109: 7–15.
38. Barefield C, Karlseder J (2012) The BLM helicase contributes to telomere maintenance through processing of late-replicating intermediates. Nucl Acids Res 40: 7358–7367.
39. Mendez-Bermudez A, Hidalgo-Bravo A, Cotton VE, Gravani A, Jeyapalan JN, et al. (2012) The roles of WRN and BLM RecQ helicases in the alternative lengthening of telomeres. Nucl Acids Res 40: 10809–10820.
40. Hagelstrom RT, Blagoev KB, Niedernhofer LJ, Goodwin EH, Bailey SM (2010) Hyper-telomere recombination accelerates replicative senescence and may promote premature aging. Proc Natl Acad Sci U S A 107: 15768–15773.
41. Moynahan ME, Chiu JW, Koller BH, Jasin M (1999) Brca1 controls homology-directed DNA repair. Mol Cell 4: 511–518.
42. Davalos AR, Campisi J (2003) Bloom syndrome cells undergo p53-dependent apoptosis and delayed assembly of BRCA1 and NBS1 repair complexes at stalled replication forks. J Cell Biol 162: 1197–1209.
43. Cao L, Li W, Kim S, Brodie SD, Deng C-X (2003) Senescence, aging, and malignant transformation mediated by p53 in mice lacking the Brca1 full-length isoform. Genes & Dev 17: 201–213.
44. Wu G, Jiang X, Lee W-H, Chen P-L (2003) Assembly of functional ALT-associated promyelocytic leukemia bodies requires Nijmegen breakage syndrome. Cancer Res 63: 2589–2595.
45. Zhang J, Powell SN (2005) The role of the BRCA1 tumor suppressor in DNA double-strand break repair. Mol Cancer Res 3: 531–539.
46. Simons AM, Horwitz AA, Starita LM, Griffin K, Williams S, et al. (2006) BRCA1 DNA-binding activity is stimulated by BARD1. Cancer Res 66: 2012–2018.
47. Lowndes NF (2010) The interplay between BRCA1 and 53BP1 influences death, aging, senescence and cancer. DNA Repair 9: 1112–1116.
48. Ohta T, Sato K, Wu W (2011) The BRCA1 ubiquitin ligase and homologous recombination repair. FEBS Lett 585: 2836–2844.
49. Zhong Q, Chen CF, Chen PL, Lee WH (2002) BRCA1 facilitates microhomology-mediated end joining of DNA double strand breaks. J Biol Chem 277: 28641–28647.
50. Hartman AR, Ford JM (2002) BRCA1 induces DNA damage recognition factors and enhances nucleotide excision repair. Nat Genet 32: 180–184.
51. McPherson JP, Hande MP, Poonepalli A, Lemmers B, Zablocki E, et al (2006) A role for Brca1 in chromosome end maintenance. Hum Mol Genet 15: 831–838.
52. Cabuy E, Newton C, Slijepcevic P (2008) BRCA1 knock-down causes telomere dysfunction in mammary epithelial cells. Cytogenet Genome Res 122: 336–342.
53. Ballal RD, Saha T, Fan S, Haddad BR, Rosen EM (2009) BRCA1 Localization to the telomere and its loss from the telomere in response to DNA Damage. J Biol Chem 284: 36083–36098.
54. Mak TW, Hakem A, McPherson JP, Shehabeldin A, Zablocki E, et al (2000) Brca1 required for T cell-lineage development but not TCR loci rearrangement. Nat Immunol 1: 77–82.

55. French JD, Dunn J, Smart CE, Manning N, Brown MA (2006) Disruption of BRCA1 function results in telomere lengthening and increased anaphase bridge formation in immortalized cell lines. Genes Chromosomes Cancer 45: 277–289.

56. Xiong J, Fan S, Meng Q, Schramm L, Wang C, et al. (2003) BRCA1 inhibition of telomerase activity in cultured cells. Mol Cell Biol 23: 8668–8690.

57. Martinez-Delgado B, Yanowsky K, Inglada-Perez L, Domingo S, Urioste M, et al. (2011) Genetic anticipation is associated with telomere shortening in hereditary breast cancer. PLoS Genet 7: e1002182.

58. Cheng WH, Kusumoto R, Opresko PL, Sui X, Huang S, et al. (2006) Collaboration of Werner syndrome protein and BRCA1 in cellular responses to DNA interstrand cross-links. Nucl Acids Res 34: 2751–2760.

59. Gocha AR, Acharya S, Groden J (2014) WRN loss induces switching of telomerase-independent mechanisms of telomere elongation. PLoS One 9: e93991.

60. O'Sullivan RJ, Arnoult N, Lackner DH, Oganesian L, Haggblom C, et al. (2014) Rapid induction of alternative lengthening of telomeres by depletion of the histone chaperone ASF1. Nat Struct Mol Biol 21: 167–174.

61. Zhong Q, Chen CF, Li S, Chen Y, Wang CC, et al. (1999) Association of BRCA1 with the hRad50-hMre11-p95 complex and the DNA damage response. Science 285: 747–750.

62. Chiba N, Parvin JD (2001) Redistribution of BRCA1 among four different complexes following replication blockage. J Biol Chem 276: 38549–38554.

63. Gravel S, Chapman JR, Magill C, Jackson SP (2008) DNA helicases Sgs1 and BLM promote DNA double-strand break resection. Genes & Dev 22: 2767–2772.

64. Nimonkar AV, Genschel J, Kinoshita E, Polaczek P, Campbell JL, et al. (2011) BLM-DNA2-RPA-MRN and EXO1-BLM-RPA- MRN constitute two DNA end resection machineries for human DNA break repair. Genes & Dev 25: 350–362.

65. Thompson LH (2012) Recognition, signaling, and repair of DNA double-strand breaks produced by ionizing radiation in mammalian cells: The molecular choreography. Mutat Res 751: 158–246

66. Dutertre S, Ababou M, Onclercq R, Delic J, Chatton B, et al. (2000) Cell cycle regulation of the endogenous wild type Bloom's syndrome DNA helicase. Oncogene 19: 2731–2738.

67. Grierson PM, Acharya S, Groden J (2013) Collaborating functions of BLM and DNA topoisomerase I in regulating human rDNA transcription. Mutat Res 743–744: 89–96.

68. Grierson PM, Lillard K, Behbehani GK, Combs KA, Bhattacharyya S, et al. (2012) BLM helicase facilitates RNA polymerase I-mediated ribosomal RNA transcription. Hum Mol Genet 21: 1172–1183

69. Opresko PL, Laine JP, Brosh RM, Seidman MM, Bohr VA (2001) Coordinate action of the helicase and 3′ to 5′ exonuclease of Werner syndrome protein. J Biol Chem 276: 44677–44687.

6

Expression of XPG Protein in the Development, Progression and Prognosis of Gastric Cancer

Na Deng[1,2], Jing-wei Liu[1], Li-ping Sun[1], Qian Xu[1], Zhi-Peng Duan[1], Nan-Nan Dong[1], Yuan Yuan[1]*

1 Tumor Etiology and Screening Department of Cancer Institute and General Surgery, the First Affiliated Hospital of China Medical University, and Key Laboratory of Cancer Etiology and Prevention (China Medical University), Liaoning Provincial Education Department, Shenyang, China, 2 Department of Oncology, The Fourth Affiliated Hospital of China Medical University, Liaoning, Shenyang, China

Abstract

Background: Xeroderma pigmentosum group G (XPG) plays a critical role in preventing cells from oxidative DNA damage. This study aimed to investigate XPG protein expression in different gastric tissues and in patients with diverse prognoses, thus providing insights into its role in the development, progression and prognosis of gastric cancer (GC).

Methods: A total of 176 GC, 131 adjacent non-tumour tissues, 53 atrophic gastritis (AG) and 49 superficial gastritis (SG) samples were included. Immunohistochemical staining was used to detect XPG protein expression.

Results: XPG expression was significantly higher in GC tissues compared with adjacent non-tumour tissues. In the progressive disease sequence SG→AG→GC, XPG expression was significantly higher in AG and GC compared with SG. Analysis of clinicopathological parameters and survival in GC patients demonstrated a significant association between XPG expression level and depth of tumour invasion, macroscopic type, Lauren's classification, smoking, *Helicobacter pylori* infection and family history. Cox multivariate survival analysis indicated that patients with positive XPG expression had significantly longer overall survival (P = 0.020, HR = 0.394, 95%CI 0.179–0.866), especially in aged younger than 60 years (P = 0.027, HR = 0.361, 95%CI 0.147–0.888) and male patients (P = 0.002, HR = 0.209, 95%CI 0.077–0.571).

Conclusions: This study demonstrated that XPG protein expression was related to the development, progression and prognosis of GC, and might thus serve as a potential biomarker for its diagnosis and prognosis.

Editor: Kapil Mehta, University of Texas MD Anderson Cancer Center, United States of America

Funding: This work is supported by grants from the National Key Basic Research Program of China (973 Program ref no. 2010CB529304), and the Foundation of Science and Technology in Liaoning Province (ref no. 2011225002). The funders had no role in study design, data collection and analysis, decision to publish, or preparation of the manuscript.

Competing Interests: The authors have declared that no competing interests exist.

* Email: yyuan@mail.cmu.edu.cn

Introduction

Gastric cancer (GC) is the world's fourth most common cancer and the second main cause of cancer-related death [1]. Despite recent advances in the diagnosis and therapy of GC, its incidence and associated mortality remain relatively high [2]. The risk factors for GC include genetic predisposition, *Helicobacter pylori* infection, and diet and lifestyle factors, etc, which can effect the development, progression and prognosis of GC.

Cellular DNA is constantly at risk of damage by endogenous and exogenous stimuli, leading to a dynamic balance between damage and repair. An imbalance between DNA damage and repair contributes to the initiation of cancer [3]. Oxidative DNA damage may lead to defects in transcription, and to duplication, mutation and genomic instability, which may in turn lead to cell dysfunction [4]. DNA-repair ability thus plays an essential role in maintaining the physiological functions of normal cells. The DNA-repair system consists of nucleotide excision repair (NER), base excision repair and mistmach repair. NER monitors and repairs a variety of DNA damages, such as ultraviolet-induced cyclobutane pyrimidine dimers, bulky adducts and DNA cross-links [5,6,7]. The process involves various enzymes including excision repair cross-complementing group (ERCC)1, XPD (ERCC2), XPF (ERCC4), XPG (ERCC5), XPC and ERCC6 (Cockayne syndrome B protein) [8]. It has been suggested that genomic instability is involved in tumour initiation, and multistep mutations occur throughout life [9]. NER is a versatile system able to repair multiple DNA damages caused by genetic instability, and thus plays an important role in the early formation of tumours.

Xeroderma pigmentosum group G (XPG) is a structure-specific nuclease belonging to the Fen1 family, which is encoded by *ERCC5* (excision repair cross-complementing group 5) [10,11,12]. XPG is an indispensable member of the NER pathway responsible for the 3′ excision of DNA damage in mammals [13]. Recent investigations have focused on the association between XPG and chemotherapeutic sensitivity. However, few studies have detected the expression of XPG protein in normal tissues and tumours. Although previous studies have been performed in the peripheral blood or metastatic cell lines, without considering expression profiles in paired tissues. In addition, no study to date has investigated the expression of XPG in cancer by immunohistochemical staining, especially in GC, atrophic gastritis (AG) and superficial gastritis (SG), and the association between XPG expression and the biological behaviour and prognosis of GC remains largely unknown.

In the present study, we detected XPG protein expression levels in tissues from patients with different gastric diseases by immunohistochemical staining, and explored its expression profiles in the disease sequence SG→AG→GC. We also investigated the relationships between XPG protein expression and clinicopathological parameters and survival in GC patients to shed light on the potential roles of XPG in the development, progression and prognosis of GC.

Materials and Methods

Patients and tissue specimens

A total of 278 patients were enrolled from the Department of Surgical Oncology of the First Affiliated Hospital of China Medical University and from individuals who participated in a health-check program involving gastroscopy for GC screening in hospitals located in Zhuanghe and Shenyang in Liaoning Province, China, between 2008 and 2011. Tissue samples were obtained from 176 patients with histologically confirmed GC (including coupled adjacent non-tumour tissues from 131 cases), 49 patients with SG, and 53 patients with AG. Patients who (i) had synchronous or metachronous malignant tumours, (ii) XP disease, or (iii) underwent preoperative radiotherapy or chemotherapy were excluded from this study. Follow-up was completed by August 2013. All patients underwent endoscopic gastric mucosal biopsy. Biopsy specimens were paraffin embedded and stained with haematoxylin and eosin for histological diagnosis, which was accomplished by two experienced pathologists. There were no significant differences among the GC, SG, AG and adjacent non-tumour groups in terms of gender or age composition ($P = 0.330$ and $P = 0.431$, respectively) (Table 1). Patients were surgically staged according to the current Borrmann classification system. Histological results was determined on the basis of the World Health Organization criteria, and tumours were staged using the 7th edition of the TNM staging system of the International Union Against Cancer (UICC)/American Joint Committee on Cancer (AJCC) (2010), based on postoperative pathologic examination. A total of 176 patients was histologically confirmed with gastric adenocarcinoma; most cases could be classified according to Lauren classification, but 17 could not. Among the 176 GC cases, 63 were intestinal type, 96 were diffuse type and 17 were mixed type. History of drinking was defined as an average alcohol daily intake ≥50 g and continued ≥1 year. The end of the follow-up time is August 2013. In 176 cases patients, 169 cases completed follow-up information, and follow-up time ranged from 22 month to 38 months. 41 of the 169 patients (24.3%) with gastric cancer had died and the median overall survival time of all patients was 29 months. This study was approved by the Institute Research Medical Ethics Committee of the First Affiliated Hospital of China Medical University. Written informed consents were obtained from participants. Medical histories (including age, sex, smoking, and alcohol consumption) were obtained by questionnaire and the records were computerized.

Immunohistochemistry

Formalin-fixed, paraffin-embedded tissues were cut into 4-μm-thick sections and mounted on poly-L-lysine-coated glass slides.

Briefly, slides were deparaffinized in xylene, rehydrated in a graded alcohol series and washed in tap water. The tissue sections were incubated in boiling sodium citrate buffer (pH 6.0) for 100 s in a steam pressure cooker for antigen retrieval. Endogenous peroxidase was blocked using 3% hydrogen peroxide for 10 min, and the sections were then washed with phosphate-buffered saline (PBS), pH 7.4. Tissue collagen was blocked to avoid nonspecific binding by the addition of 10% normal goat serum at 37°C for 10 min. The polyclonal antibody anti-XPG (ab-99248, 1:300 dilution; Abcam, Cambridge, UK) was used as the primary antibody to detect XPG protein expression, and incubated for 4°C overnight. After rinsing three times with PBS for 5 min each, the sections were incubated with biotinylated secondary antibody (goat anti-rabbit antibody, Maixin Inc., Fujian, China) and streptavidin-biotin peroxidase for 10 min each at 37°C. The slides were then washed in PBS and stained with 3, 3-diaminobenzidine tetrahydrochloride and counterstained with haematoxylin. Finally, the sections were dehydrated and mounted. Primary antibodies were replaced with PBS buffer as a negative control.

Evaluation of immunohistochemistry

The immunohistochemical results were evaluated and scored independently by two investigators who were blinded to the patients' clinicopathological characteristics. Nuclear positivity for XPG protein was evaluated using a semi-quantitative scoring criterion based on the staining intensity (0, no staining; 1, light brown staining; 2, brown staining; and 3, heavy brown staining) and proportion of stained epithelial cells (0, ≤5%; 1, 5–25%; 2, 25–50%; 3, 50–75%; and 4, ≥75%) Staining intensity was measured at the sites of the antrum of the stomach and gastric body gland. The percentage positivity of epithelial cells and staining intensity were then multiplied to generate an immunoreactivity score (IS) for each specimen [14]. The expression was graded as: negative(−), score = 0; weak expression(+), score = 1–4; moderate expression(++), score = 5–8; and strong expression(+++), score = 9–12.

Statistical analysis

Statistical analysis was performed using SPSS (16.0) statistical software (SPSS, Chicago, IL, USA). Non-parametric tests were used to analyse the differences in XPG expression in the SG-AG-GC sequence, and differences between GC and adjacent non-tumour tissues. Correlations between clinicopathological factors and XPG expression were analysed by the χ^2 test or the Fisher's exact probability test. Survival analysis was performed using Kaplan–Meier curves, and differences between the groups were analysed using the log-rank test. Cox regression analysis was conducted for multivariate analysis. Two-tailed P values < 0.05 were considered statistically significant.

Results

Expression of XPG protein in gastric cancer and non-tumour tissues

XPG immunostaining demonstrated a predominantly nuclear localization (Figures 1 and 2). In the progression of gastric diseases, there were significant differences in XPG expression levels between AG and SG ($P1 < 0.001$), and between GC and SG ($P2 = 0.031$). XPG expression was significantly higher in AG and GC than in SG, respectively (Mann–Whitney U-test test, Table 2). In addition, we found the expression levels of XPG in GC were significantly higher than in adjacent non-tumour tissues (P < 0.001). At the same time, we classified adjacent non-tumour tissues

Table 1. Clinicopathological parameters in adjacent, AG, SG, GC and survival in GC.

Variable	Categories	Adjacent (131)	AG (53)	SG (49)	GC (176)	P	Cases of Events	MST	P
Gender						0.330			0.837
	Male	90	31	28	118		31	37	
	Female	41	22	21	58		16	31.308*	
Age						0.431			0.548
	<60	75	29	29	100		28	31.374*	
	≥60	56	24	20	76		19	37	
Smoking						0.720			0.457
	Yes	53	18	18	74		18	33.202*	
	No	78	35	31	102		29	37	
Drinking						0.335			0.297
	Yes	39	12	9	52		17	37	
	No	92	41	40	124		30	32.823*	
HP infection status						**0.001**			0.817
	positive	21	35	13	7		2	37	
	negetive	5	18	36	30		8	33.429*	
Macroscopic Type									**<0.001**
	Early stage				29		1	36.619*	
	Borrmann I–II				23		3	34.25*	
	Borrmann III–IV				115		43	37	
Lauren's classification									0.154
	intestinal-type				63		14	37	
	Diffuse-type				96		31	37	
TNM stage									**<0.001**
	I–II				80		9	35.380*	
	III				87		38	36	
Lymph node metastasis									**<0.001**
	Positive				105		39	37	
	Negative				61		8	35.053*	
T stage									**<0.001**
	T1				27		1	36.579*	
	T2				27		3	34.630*	
	T3				23		5	31.145*	
	T4				90		38	36	

Table 1. Cont.

Variable	Categories	Adjacent (131)			P	Cases of Events	MST	P
		AG (53)	SG (49)	GC (176)				
Growth pattern								0.201
	Expanding			23		3	37	
	Intermediate			78		23	36	
	Infiltrative			66		21	30.216*	
Lymphatic invasion								0.184
	Negative			33		12	36	
	Positive			134		33	32.076*	
family history								0.204
	Positive			32		6	32.924*	
	Negative			135		41	37	

MST median survival time.
*mean survival time.

into 41 cases AG and 88 cases SG. The results suggested that XPG expression was significantly higher in GC than its adjacent SG tissues (P<0.001); no significant association was observed between GC and its adjacent AG tissues (P = 0.244). The relationship of XPG expression in the samples of adjacent tissue and coupled GC were displayed in Table 3.

Associations between XPG staining and clinicopathological characteristics

We analysed the associations between XPG expression and various clinicopathological parameters using Mann-Whitney U-tests (Table 4). XPG expression in intestinal-type GC (98.4%) was significantly higher than in diffuse-type GC. XPG expression levels were also significantly correlated with drinking ($P = 0.031$) (75.0%), depth of tumour invasion (pT stage, $P = 0.012$), macroscopic type ($P = 0.032$) (Table 4), *H. pylori* infection status ($P = 0.039$) and family history of cancer ($P = 0.019$) (Table S1). High XPG expression was observed in patients who drank, T4 cases, intestinal-type GC, *H. pylori* infection-positive, and family history-positive groups. However, there was no significant correlation between XPG expression and Borrmann classification, TNM stage, lymph node metastasis, growth pattern or lymphatic invasion (Table 4).

Relationship between XPG expression and overall survival in patients with GC

We investigated the relationship between XPG expression and survival in patients with GC. According to univariate survival analysis, the expression level of XPG was not an independent prognostic factor ($P = 0.491$), while macroscopic type ($P = 0.002$), TNM stage ($P<0.001$), lymph node metastasis ($P<0.001$) and depth of invasion ($P<0.001$) were all significant prognostic factors (Table 1). Because TNM stage already included information on lymph node metastasis and depth of invasion, we performed multivariate analysis using Cox's proportional hazards model adjusted by sex, age, TNM stage and macroscopic type. Interestingly, the results indicated that XPG expression level was an independent prognostic factor ($P = 0.020$, HR = 0.394, 95%CI 0.179–0.866). Patient with positive expression had a longer survival. We stratified the patients according to age and sex to elucidate more detailed relation between XPG and GC prognosis. Stratification analysis suggested patients aged younger than 60 years, who had positive XPG expression was significantly more favorable in terms of survival than that of patients with negative XPG expression (Figure S1); XPG expression was a protective factor no matter univariate survival analysis or Cox's proportional hazards model ($P = 0.021$, HR = 0.373, 95%CI 0.154–0.901; $P = 0.021$, HR = 0.361, 95%CI 0.147–0.888 respectively), and male patients with XPG positive expression had significantly favorable overall survival ($P = 0.021$ HR = 0.373, 95%CI 0.154–0.901) (Table 5).

Discussion

In the current study, we detected XPG protein expression in tissues from patients with SG, AG and GC, and in adjacent non-tumour tissues, by immunohistochemical staining. Moreover, we investigated the relationships between XPG protein expression and clinicopathological parameters and survival in GC patients, to provide insights into its roles in the development, progression and prognosis of GC. To our best of our knowledge, this is first report of a relationship between XPG protein expression and the development, progression and prognosis of GC.

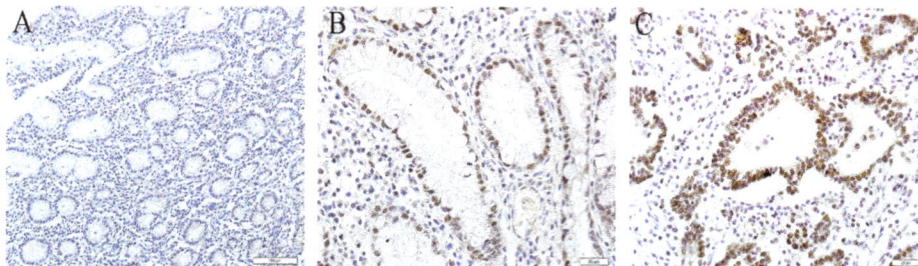

Figure 1. Representative photomicrographs of immunohistochemical staining of XPG in different gastric specimens. Low nuclear expression of XPG was observed in the antrum of the stomach in SG (a). XPG expression levels in AG (b) and GC (c) were higher than in SG. Original magnification, ×400.

A variety of underlying mechanisms might influence the expression of XPG, including *ERCC5* gene mutation, regulation of transcription and translation, protein degradation and promoter methylation [15]. The physiological regulation of XPG expression requires external stimulation of DNA damage. For example, UVC-induced DNA damage may up-regulate XPG expression [16]. In normal individuals DNA damage is rare, and the DNA repair gene *ERCC5* is therefore expressed at low levels. However, various types of environmental carcinogens and endogenous metabolic products may cause DNA damage, thus enhancing the DNA-repair activity of cells and the activities of transcription

and translation [17]. The current study explored the XPG protein expression profile in the SG→AG→GC disease sequence and found XPG expression in SG was relatively lower than GC and AG. The results indicated that XPG protein was induced and activated during the process of carcinogenesis, thereby repairing damaged DNA and maintaining the integrity of the genome. XPG was up-regulated in GC tissues, revealing a potential role for XPG protein as a biomarker to predict the risk of GC and its precancerous lesions. A few studies to date have reported on the relationships between XPG protein expression and other cancers, and the results differed from our findings. For instance, Cheng

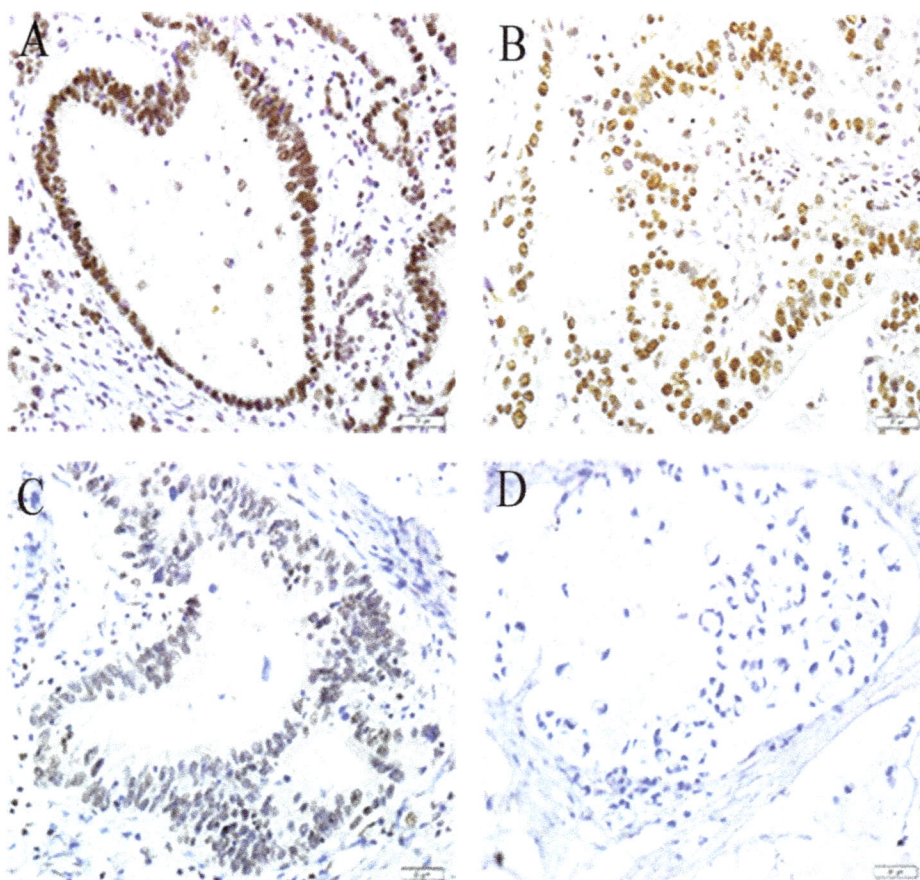

Figure 2. XPG expression in GC tissues. XPG staining in the nucleus was strongly positive (+++) in (a), moderately positive (++) in (b), weakly positive (+) in (c) and negative (−) in (d). Magnification, ×400.

Table 2. XPG expression in SG, AG, GC.

Group	Cases	(-) n (%)	(+) n (%)	(++) n (%)	(+++) n (%)	PR (%)	
SG	49	9(18.4)	27(55.1)	9(18.4)	4(8.2)	81.6	ref.
AG	53	1(1.9)	17(32.1)	15(28.3)	20(37.7)	98.1	**P1<0.001**
GC	176	26(14.8)	69(39.2)	53(30.1)	28(15.9)	85.2	**P2=0.031**

-; +weak; ++moderate; +++strong staining.
PR, Positive rate.
ref., reference.
P1:SG as ref. AG vs. SG.
P2:SG as ref. GC vs. SG.

Table 3. XPG expression in SG, AG of adjacent tissue and GC.

Group	Group1		Group2		Group3		Group4	
	Adjacent	GC	coupled-SG	coupled-GC	Adjacent-SG	AdjacentAG	coupled-AG	coupled-GC
Cases	131	176	88	88	88	41	41	41
(-)	74(56.5)	26(14.8)	69(78.4)	14(15.9)	69(78.4)	3(7.3)	3(7.3)	4(9.8)
(+)	27(20.6)	69(39.2)	15(17.0)	35(39.8)	15(17.0)	12(29.3)	12(29.3)	19(46.3)
(++)	18(13.7)	53(30.1)	2(2.3)	26(29.5)	2(2.3)	16(39.0)	16(39.0)	8(19.5)
(+++)	12(9.2)	28(15.9)	2(2.3)	13(14.8)	2(2.3)	10(24.4)	10(24.4)	10(24.4)
PR (%)	43.5	85.2	21.6	84.1	21.6	92.7	92.7	90.2
P	ref.	<0.001	ref.	<0.001	ref.	<0.001	ref.	0.244

-; +weak; ++moderate; +++strong staining.
PR, Positive rate.
ref. reference.

Table 4. Association between XPG expression and clinicopathological parameters in GC.

Variability	Cases(n)	XPG expression				PR (%)	p
		(−)	(+)	(++)	(+++)		
Macroscopic Type							0.032
Early stage	29	8	12	7	2	72.4	
Borrmann I–IV	138	18	54	43	23	87	
Borrmann classification							0.296
Borrmann I–II	23	4	10	6	3	82.6	
Borrmann III–IV	115	14	44	37	20	87.8	
Lauren's classification							<0.001
intestinal-type	63	1	20	22	20	98.4	
Diffuse-type	96	24	41	25	6	75.0	
TNM stage							0.111
I–II	80	15	32	26	7	81.3	
III	87	11	34	24	18	87.4	
Lymph node metastasis							0.290
Positive	105	13	43	31	18	87.6	
Negative	61	12	23	19	7	80.3	
Depth of invasion							0.012
T1	27	7	12	7	1	74.1	
T2	27	5	10	10	2	81.5	
T3	23	4	13	4	2	82.6	
T4	9	10	31	29	20	88.9	
Growth pattern							0.191
Expanding	23	2	10	7	4	91.3	
Intermediate	78	10	30	23	15	87.2	
Infiltrative	66	14	26	20	6	78.8	
lymphatic invasion							0.480
Positive	33	4	18	6	5	87.9	
Negative	134	22	48	44	20	83.6	
family history							0.019
Positive	32	2	10	13	7	93.8	
Negative	135	24	56	37	18	82.2	

PR, Positive rate.

Table 5. Correlation between XPG expression and survival in GC.

	Cases	Cases of Events	MST	Univariate			Multivariate		
				P	HR	95%CI	P	HR	95%CI
XPG expression									
negative	26	8	29.070*		1(ref)			1(ref)	
positive	143	33	32.784*	0.296	0.666	0.307–1.442	0.020	0.394	0.179–0.866
Stratification									
Age <60									
Negative	16	7	31.000		1(ref)			1(ref)	
Positive	81	17	32.366*	0.021	0.373	0.154 0.901	0.027	0.361	0.147–0.888
Age ≥60									
Negative	10	1	34.714*		1(ref)			1(ref)	
Positive	62	16	32.306*	0.300	2.772	0.368–20.911	0.960	1.060	0.108–10.372
Gender									
Male									
Negative	14	5	27.571*		1(ref)			1(ref)	
Positive	99	21	33.454*	0.135	0.484	0.182–1.285	0.002	0.209	0.077–0.571
Female									
Negative	12	3	30.562*		1(ref)			1(ref)	
Positive	44	12	30.979*	0.859	1.120	0.316–3.970	0.800	0.841	0.219–3.225

MST median survival time.
*mean survival time.
HR: hazard radio, CI: confidence interval.

et al. observed low XPG expression in peripheral blood leukocytes in patients with lung, head and neck, and breast cancers [18,19,20,21,22,23]. XPG was deficient or downregulated in carcinoma of the testis and breast cancer [9,24]. The controversial conclusions from these different studies might result from the diverse biological characteristics of the tumors studied, or from differences in detecting methods and sample sizes. Further large-scale investigations of XPG expression in different cancers are needed to confirm its role.

We further investigated the relationships between XPG expression and clinicopathological parameters including TNM stage, depth of invasion, nodal metastasis, macroscopic type, lymph vessel invasion and growth pattern. The results suggested that XPG protein expression was associated with depth of invasion and macroscopic type; Invasion of cancer cells into the subserous adjacent tissue and more advanced macroscopic type were both key factors with great impacts on disease progression. Previous studies reported that overexpression of DNA repair gene was positively related to deeper invasion and a more developed classification of GC. Ganzinelli M et al. suggested that malignant transformation was associated with the upregulation of genes involved in DNA repair and maintaining genomic stability [25]. It was suggested that long-term hypoxia and inflammation in the tissue microenvironment may be responsible for inducing DNA damage [26]. Furthermore, it has been reported that XPG genes were significantly less expressed in stage III than in stage I ovarian carcinoma [25]. Liu et al. suggested that ERCC1 mRNA expression levels was correlated with age, with high ERCC1 expression being more common in younger patients [27]. The different outcomes of diverse investigations might result from differences in cancer types, ethnicities, sample sizes and environmental factors. Our results indicated that strong expression was frequently detected in T4 and advanced cancer. Considering XPG was less expressed in diffuse-type GC than in intestinal-type GC, poorly differentiated cancer cells may lack the ability to generate XPG which was responsible for tissue repair. Diffuse-type GC might therefore have a poorer prognosis. The above evidence indicates that XPG expression was positively associated with a number of clinicopathological parameters reflecting GC development, and might thus play important roles in the initiation and progression of GC and serve as a biomarker for GC development, predicting biological activities and degree of progression. In addition, XPG overexpression was also associated with family history, *H. pylori* infection and drinking. Alcohol consumption and *H. pylori* infection may induce oxidative damage, thus increasing expression of DNA-repair proteins such as XPG. XPG was more highly expressed in patients with a family history of cancer, suggesting that it might also be a genetic biomarker of cancer.

We further investigated the relationships between XPG expression and overall survival. There was a significant association between XPG protein expression and GC prognosis in multivariate analysis, especially in patients aged younger than 60 years. Positive expression levels of XPG protein could predict longer survival according to the present study. Similarly, high expression of DNA-repair family proteins, such as *ERCC1*, predicted longer overall survival compared with low ERCC1 expression [27]. High XPG expression was associated with longer survival in patients with ovarian cancer [28]. In terms of mRNA levels, high XPG

mRNA levels were an independent prognostic factor predicting longer survival in patients with non-small-cell lung cancer and sarcoma [29,30]. In contrast, XPG has recently been reported to have prognostic value in ovarian cancer; low XPG expression predicted longer survival [31], in accordance with our current findings. Low expression levels of some genes for DNA-repair family proteins, such as *ERCC1*, have been reported to predict longer relapse-free survival and overall survival in GC. High XPF expression was related to early progression; patients with high XPF expression had shorter progression-free survival than patients with low XPF expression [32]. Liu et al. demonstrated that patients with low ERCC1 mRNA expression levels had longer relapse-free and overall survival times than patients with high ERCC1 levels. Different types of cancers have distinct mechanisms of carcinogenesis and their control thus differs between different populations. The prognostic role of XPG is therefore also likely to vary among different types of cancers. In addition, XPG expression might be influenced by various factors, and further large-scale multicentre investigations with a long follow-up are required to clarify the relevance of XPG in cancer prognosis. Nevertheless, XPG expression appears to have potential prognostic value in GC, especially in patients aged younger than 60 years, though further studies are needed to clarify the underlying mechanisms.

In conclusion, we demonstrated for the first time that XPG protein expression was significantly higher in GC than non-tumour tissues, and significantly higher in AG and GC than in SG in the disease sequence SG→AG→GC. The level of XPG expression was also significantly associated with depth of tumour invasion, macroscopic type, Lauren's classification, smoking, *H. pylori* infection and family history of cancer. Multivariate survival analysis indicated that patients with XPG positive expression had significant longer overall survival, especially in patients younger than 60 years. Our results suggest that XPG protein expression is related to the development, progression and prognosis of GC, and may therefore serve as a potential biomarker for the diagnosis and prognosis of this disease.

Supporting Information

Figure S1 A, correlation of XPG expression with survival curves of patients with gastric cancer by univariate survival analysis; B, correlation of XPG expression with survival curves of patients younger than 60 years in gastric cancer by univariate survival analysis; C, correlation of XPG expression with survival curves of patients olderer than 60 years in gastric cancer by univariate survival analysis.

Table S1 **Baseline characteristics of the study population and expression of XPG.**

Author Contributions

Conceived and designed the experiments: YY. Performed the experiments: ND JW-L LP-S. Analyzed the data: ZP-D QX. Contributed to the writing of the manuscript: ND JW-L.

References

1. Brenner H, Rothenbacher D, Arndt V (2009) Epidemiology of stomach cancer. Methods Mol Biol 472: 467–477.

2. Crew KD, Neugut AI (2006) Epidemiology of gastric cancer. World J Gastroenterol 12: 354–362.

3. Iyama T, Wilson DM 3rd (2013) DNA repair mechanisms in dividing and non-dividing cells. DNA Repair (Amst) 12: 620–636.

4. Halliwell B, Gutteridge JM (1990) Role of free radicals and catalytic metal ions in human disease: an overview. Methods Enzymol 186: 1–85.

5. Charames GS, Bapat B (2003) Genomic instability and cancer. Curr Mol Med 3: 589–596.

6. Kim IJ, Ku JL, Kang HC, Park JH, Yoon KA, et al. (2004) Mutational analysis of OGG1, MYH, MTH1 in FAP, HNPCC and sporadic colorectal cancer patients: R154H OGG1 polymorphism is associated with sporadic colorectal cancer patients. Hum Genet 115: 498–503.

7. Kuraoka I, Bender C, Romieu A, Cadet J, Wood RD, et al. (2000) Removal of oxygen free-radical-induced 5′,8-purine cyclodeoxynucleosides from DNA by the nucleotide excision-repair pathway in human cells. Proc Natl Acad Sci U S A 97: 3832–3837.

8. Sancar A, Lindsey-Boltz LA, Unsal-Kacmaz K, Linn S (2004) Molecular mechanisms of mammalian DNA repair and the DNA damage checkpoints. Annu Rev Biochem 73: 39–85.

9. Latimer JJ, Johnson JM, Kelly CM, Miles TD, Beaudry-Rodgers KA, et al. (2010) Nucleotide excision repair deficiency is intrinsic in sporadic stage I breast cancer. Proc Natl Acad Sci U S A 107: 21725–21730.

10. Costa RM, Chigancas V, Galhardo Rda S, Carvalho H, Menck CF (2003) The eukaryotic nucleotide excision repair pathway. Biochimie 85: 1083–1099.

11. Berneburg M, Lehmann AR (2001) Xeroderma pigmentosum and related disorders: defects in DNA repair and transcription. Adv Genet 43: 71–102.

12. Lehmann AR (2003) DNA repair-deficient diseases, xeroderma pigmentosum, Cockayne syndrome and trichothiodystrophy. Biochimie 85: 1101–1111.

13. Sugasawa K (2008) Xeroderma pigmentosum genes: functions inside and outside DNA repair. Carcinogenesis 29: 455–465.

14. Agarwal R, D'Souza T, Morin PJ (2005) Claudin-3 and claudin-4 expression in ovarian epithelial cells enhances invasion and is associated with increased matrix metalloproteinase-2 activity. Cancer Res 65: 7378–7385.

15. Sabatino MA, Marabese M, Ganzinelli M, Cacola E, Geroni C, et al. (2010) Down-regulation of the nucleotide excision repair gene XPG as a new mechanism of drug resistance in human and murine cancer cells. Mol Cancer 9: 259.

16. Tomicic MT, Reischmann P, Rasenberger B, Meise R, Kaina B, et al. (2011) Delayed c-Fos activation in human cells triggers XPF induction and an adaptive response to UVC-induced DNA damage and cytotoxicity. Cell Mol Life Sci 68: 1785–1798.

17. Kamileri I, Karakasilioti I, Garinis GA (2012) Nucleotide excision repair: new tricks with old bricks. Trends Genet 28: 566–573.

18. Cheng L, Spitz MR, Hong WK, Wei Q (2000) Reduced expression levels of nucleotide excision repair genes in lung cancer: a case-control analysis. Carcinogenesis 21: 1527–1530.

19. Cheng L, Sturgis EM, Eicher SA, Spitz MR, Wei Q (2002) Expression of nucleotide excision repair genes and the risk for squamous cell carcinoma of the head and neck. Cancer 94: 393–397.

20. Wei Q, Wang LE, Sturgis EM, Mao L (2005) Expression of nucleotide excision repair proteins in lymphocytes as a marker of susceptibility to squamous cell carcinomas of the head and neck. Cancer Epidemiol Biomarkers Prev 14: 1961–1966.

21. Kovacs E, Stucki D, Weber W, Muller H (1986) Impaired DNA-repair synthesis in lymphocytes of breast cancer patients. Eur J Cancer Clin Oncol 22: 863–869.

22. Kovacs E, Almendral A (1987) Reduced DNA repair synthesis in healthy women having first degree relatives with breast cancer. Eur J Cancer Clin Oncol 23: 1051–1057.

23. Ramos JM, Ruiz A, Colen R, Lopez ID, Grossman L, et al. (2004) DNA repair and breast carcinoma susceptibility in women. Cancer 100: 1352–1357.

24. Skotheim RI, Autio R, Lind GE, Kraggerud SM, Andrews PW, et al. (2006) Novel genomic aberrations in testicular germ cell tumors by array-CGH, and associated gene expression changes. Cell Oncol 28: 315–326.

25. Ganzinelli M, Mariani P, Cattaneo D, Fossati R, Fruscio R, et al. (2010) Expression of DNA repair genes in ovarian cancer samples: biological and clinical considerations. Eur J Cancer 47 1086–1094.

26. Aracil M, Dauffenbach LM, Diez MM, Richeh R, Moneo V, et al. (2013) Expression of XPG protein in human normal and tumor tissues. Int J Clin Exp Pathol 6: 199–211.

27. Liu YP, Ling Y, Qi QF, Zhang YP, Zhang CS, et al. (2013) The effects of ERCC1 expression levels on the chemosensitivity of gastric cancer cells to platinum agents and survival in gastric cancer patients treated with oxaliplatin-based adjuvant chemotherapy. Oncol Lett 5: 935–942.

28. Jian-Wei B, Yi-Min M, Yu-Xia S, Shi-Qing L (2013) Expression levels of ERCC1 and RRM1 mRNA and clinical outcome of advanced non-small cell lung cancer. Pak J Med Sci 29: 1158–1161.

29. Bartolucci R, Wei J, Sanchez JJ, Perez-Roca L, Chaib I, et al. (2009) XPG mRNA expression levels modulate prognosis in resected non-small-cell lung cancer in conjunction with BRCA1 and ERCC1 expression. Clin Lung Cancer 10: 47–52.

30. Schoffski P, Taron M, Jimeno J, Grosso F, Sanfilipio R, et al. (2011) Predictive impact of DNA repair functionality on clinical outcome of advanced sarcoma patients treated with trabectedin: a retrospective multicentric study. Eur J Cancer 47: 1006–1012.

31. Walsh CS, Ogawa S, Karahashi H, Scoles DR, Pavelka JC, et al. (2008) ERCC5 is a novel biomarker of ovarian cancer prognosis. J Clin Oncol 26: 2952–2958.

32. Vaezi A, Wang X, Buch S, Gooding W, Wang L, et al. (2011) XPF expression correlates with clinical outcome in squamous cell carcinoma of the head and neck. Clin Cancer Res 17: 5513–5522.

7

Rad51 Activates Polyomavirus JC Early Transcription

Martyn K. White*, Rafal Kaminski, Kamel Khalili*, Hassen S. Wollebo

Center for Neurovirology, Department of Neuroscience, Temple University School of Medicine, Philadelphia, Pennsylvania, United States of America

Abstract

The human neurotropic polyomavirus JC (JCV) causes the fatal CNS demyelinating disease progressive multifocal leukoencephalopathy (PML). JCV infection is very common and after primary infection, the virus is able to persist in an asymptomatic state. Rarely, and usually only under conditions of immune impairment, JCV re-emerges to actively replicate in the astrocytes and oligodendrocytes of the brain causing PML. The regulatory events involved in the reactivation of active viral replication in PML are not well understood but previous studies have implicated the transcription factor NF-κB acting at a well-characterized site in the JCV noncoding control region (NCCR). NF-κB in turn is regulated in a number of ways including activation by cytokines such as TNF-α, interactions with other transcription factors and epigenetic events involving protein acetylation – all of which can regulate the transcriptional activity of JCV. Active JCV infection is marked by the occurrence of rapid and extensive DNA damage in the host cell and the induction of the expression of cellular proteins involved in DNA repair including Rad51, a major component of the homologous recombination-directed double-strand break DNA repair machinery. Here we show that increased Rad51 expression activates the JCV early promoter. This activation is co-operative with the stimulation caused by NF-κB p65, abrogated by mutation of the NF-κB binding site or siRNA to NFκB p65 and enhanced by the histone deacetylase inhibitor sodium butyrate. These data indicate that the induction of Rad51 resulting from infection with JCV acts through NF-κB via its binding site to stimulate JCV early transcription. We suggest that this provides a novel positive feedback mechanism to enhance viral gene expression during the early stage of JCV infection.

Editor: Michael Nevels, University of Regensburg, Germany

Funding: This study was supported by MW NIH/National Institute of Allergies and Infectious Diseases R01, AI077460, KK NIH/National Institute of Mental Health P30 MH092177, KK NIH/ National Institute of Mental Health R01 MH093271, KK NIH/ National Heart, Lung, and Blood Institute R01 HL123093. The funders had no role in study design, data collection and analysis, decision to publish, or preparation of the manuscript.

Competing Interests: The authors have declared that no competing interests exist.

* Email: martyn.white@temple.edu (MKW); kamel.khalili@temple.edu (KK)

Introduction

The human neurotropic polyomavirus JC (JCV) causes the fatal demyelinating disease of the central nervous system (CNS) known as progressive multifocal leukoencephalopathy (PML) [1]. Primary infection by JCV is very common, usually occurs early in life and appears to be subclinical so that the only evidence for infection is the appearance of serum antibodies to the virus (reviewed in [2]). However, it is clear that the virus persists after infection since it may be shed episodically in the urine and the virus can reappear under conditions of severe immune impairment and productively infect the astrocytes and oligodendrocytes in the CNS giving rise to multiple regions of demyelination and causing PML. PML is almost always associated with some form of impaired immune function including HIV-1/AIDS [3], treatment with Natalizumab [4–7] Rituximab [8], Efalizumab [9] or immunosuppressive drugs administered to prevent transplant rejection [10,11] as well as lymphoproliferative and myeloproliferative disorders [12] and other instances of chronic immunosuppression (reviewed in [13,14]). Our understanding of the pathogenesis of PML and the molecular events of the JCV life cycle remains incomplete. For example, the molecular basis and site(s) within which latent/persistent virus exists and the mechanism whereby the virus reactivates to cause PML remain controversial (reviewed in [2,15]).

JCV is a small DNA tumor virus belonging to the Polyomavirus family that has a circular, closed, supercoiled DNA genome and is small in size (~5.1 Kbp). Both JCV and Polyomavirus BK (BKV), which causes BKV-associated nephropathy, were discovered in 1971 and for many years they were the only known human polyomaviruses, until about 6 years ago when a series of novel polyomaviruses were discovered and now there are at least ten [16]. The genome of JCV is comprised of two coding regions, early and late, which are transcribed in opposite directions [17,18]. The coding regions are separated by the noncoding control region (NCCR), which functions as a bidirectional promoter and contains the binding sites for many transcription factors that regulate JCV gene expression as well as the origin of viral DNA replication. The NCCR co-ordinates the expression of the early proteins (large T-antigen and small t-antigen) and late proteins (VP1, VP2, VP3 and agnoprotein) during the stages of the viral life cycle. The binding of various cellular and viral transcription factors to the NCCR regulates these transcription programs [19].

Our earlier work implicated the NF-κB signaling pathway as a key regulator of the transcriptional status of JCV [20–25]. A unique binding site for NF-κB is located in the early proximal side of the JCV NCCR and is positively regulated by NF-κB p65 binding and negatively regulated by isoforms of the C/EBPβ protein, which bind to an adjacent site [22]. We have also found that TNF-α stimulated JCV transcription through this element [24] and that it is also a target of calcineurin/NFAT4 signaling [25]. The histone deactylation inhibitor trichostatin A (TSA) and expression of the transcriptional coactivators/acetyltransferase p300 were also found to activate transcription via the NF-κB binding site indicating that epigenetic events involving protein acetylation are also important [26]. Our recent data reported here indicate the involvement of Rad51 in this signaling axis.

Rad51 is a highly conserved protein that functions in the homologous recombination-directed DNA double-strand break repair pathway [27]. Infection of astrocyte cultures by JCV results in the induction of DNA and genome damage as evidenced by changes in ploidy, increased micronuclei formation and an induction of the levels of phospho-histone2AX (γH2AX), a marker for double-strand breaks. Concomitantly, JCV infection also causes an induction in the levels of some DNA repair enzymes, notably a large elevation in Rad51 [28]. In other experiments, we have also found that Rad51 is able to bind and activate NF-κB p65 in HIV-1-infected human microglial cells [29] and interplay of Rad51 with the NF-κB signaling pathway stimulates HIV-1 gene expression while inhibition of Rad51 function represses HIV-1 infection [30]. In the light of these findings, we investigated a role for Rad51 on the transcription and replication of JCV. Rad51 was found to act through NF-κB via its binding site in the JCV NCCR to activate JCV early transcription suggesting a positive feedback mechanism to enhance viral gene expression during the early stage of JCV infection. The function of Rad51 in cellular DNA repair and maintenance of cell homeostasis is well established and it is tightly regulated throughout the cell cycle. However in the context of JCV infection, Rad51 may be co-opted by the virus to facilitate the events that ultimately lead to cell lysis.

Materials and Methods

Cell culture and plasmids

The human TC620 oligodendroglioma cell line [24] and SVG-A, a human cell line which was derived from primary human fetal glial cells transformed by origin-defective SV40 and expresses SV40 T-Ag [31], were maintained in Dulbecco's Modified Eagle's Medium (DMEM) supplemented with 10% fetal bovine serum (FBS) line as we have previously described [24]. Reporter plasmids for the wild-type JCV early promoter (JCV$_E$-LUC) and promoter mutants m1 and m2, which contained mutations at two adjacent sites within the KB site, have been described previously [22]. The expression plasmids pCMV-p65, pCMV-LIP [22] and pCMV-Rad51 [29] were described previously. Dominant negative IκBα expression plasmid (DN-IαKB) was from Clontech (pCMV-IκBαM, where IκBαM differs from IκBα by Ser-to-Ala mutations at residues 32 and 36). pJCV has the JCV Mad-1 wild-type whole genome DNA cloned into the BamHI site of pBluescript KS.

Antibodies

Rabbit polyclonal anti-p65 (c-20, sc-372, Santa Cruz Biotechnology Inc., Santa Cruz, CA) and mouse monoclonal anti-C/EBPβ (H7, sc-7962, Santa Cruz) which recognizes all three C/EBPβ isoforms were used for Western blots. Rabbit polyclonal anti-Rad51 antibody (D4B10) was from Cell Signaling Technology, Inc. except for immunocytochemistry where mouse monoclonal anti-Rad51 antibody was used (14B4, GeneTex Inc.) Mouse monoclonal anti-α-tubulin (clone B512) was from Sigma (St. Louis, MO). Rabbit monoclonal antibody (C5811) to acetyl-histone H3 (K9) was from Cell Signaling, Inc., Danvers MA. We have previously described mouse monoclonal antibody against JCV VP1 [32].

Western blots

Western blots were as previously described [33] except antibody was detected with the LI-COR system. Blots were incubated with IRDye 800CW Goat Anti-Rabbit and IRDye 680RD Goat Anti-Mouse Li-COR dyes and visualized with an Odyssey CLx Imaging System (LI-COR, Inc., Lincoln, NE) using LI-COR Odyssey software. Band intensities were quantified using the Quantity One software (Bio-Rad, Hercules CA).

Transient transfection and reporter assays

Experiments involving co-transfection of reporter plasmids and expression plasmids were performed as we have previously described [22,24]. Briefly, TC620 cells were transfected with reporter constructs alone (200 ng) or in combination with expression plasmid(s) at 48 h prior to harvesting. When p65 siRNA was used, 50 pmol of Smartpool p65 siRNA (Dharmacon, Lafayette, CO) was included in the transfection as we have previously described [22]. Treatment with sodium butyrate (SB: 2 mM and 4 mM) was performed for 24 h prior to harvesting. Assay for luciferase was as previously described [24,25].

JCV infection assay

SVG-A is a human fetal glial cell line transformed by an origin-defective SV40 that expresses large T-antigen and supports JCV replication. SVG-A cells were transfected/infected with pJCV linearized by BamHI digestion and harvested after 7 days for Western blot for viral VP1 and agnoprotein. In experiments to investigate the effect of dominant negative IκB, pCMV-IκBαM was included in the transfection with the total amount of DNA kept constant between samples. In experiments to investigate the effect of Rad51 inhibition, 15 μM RI-1 [34] was added following transfection.

Immunocytochemistry (ICC)

TC620 cells were serum-starved overnight with 0.5% BSA and then either untreated or treated with 10 ng/ml TNF-α for 20 min. Cells were fixed in 4% paraformaldehyde in PBS for 10 min, washed, permeabilized for 5 min with 0.1% TritonX-100, blocked for 30 min with 5% normal goat serum and incubated 3 h at 37°C with rabbit anti-NF-κB p65 and mouse anti-Rad51 at a 1:100 dilution in PBS. Cells were then washed, incubated for 2 h with secondary FITC-conjugated goat anti-rabbit and rhodamine-conjugated anti-mouse secondary antibodies at a 1:200 dilution, washed, mounted with DAPI-containing mounting medium (VECTASHIELD, Vector Laboratories Inc. Burlingame, CA) and viewed by fluorescence microscopy.

Cell fractionation

TC620 were transfected with pCMV-p65 and pCMV-Rad51 and the following day serum-starved overnight with 0.5% BSA and then either untreated or treated with 10 ng/ml TNF-α for 20 min. Nuclear and cytoplasmic fractions were prepared using the NE-PER nuclear and cytoplasmic reagents according to the Manufacturers protocol (Pierce Biotechnology, Rockford, IL) as we have previously described [33].

ChIP assay

TC620 cells were transfected with JCV$_E$-LUC, which contains the Mad-1 JCV NCCR in the presence or absence of expression plasmid for DN-IκB. The medium was changed to DMEM with 0.5% BSA and no serum. After overnight serum starvation, cells were stimulated with 10 ng/ml TNF-α for 20 min and ChIP performed at 48 h after transfection as we have previously

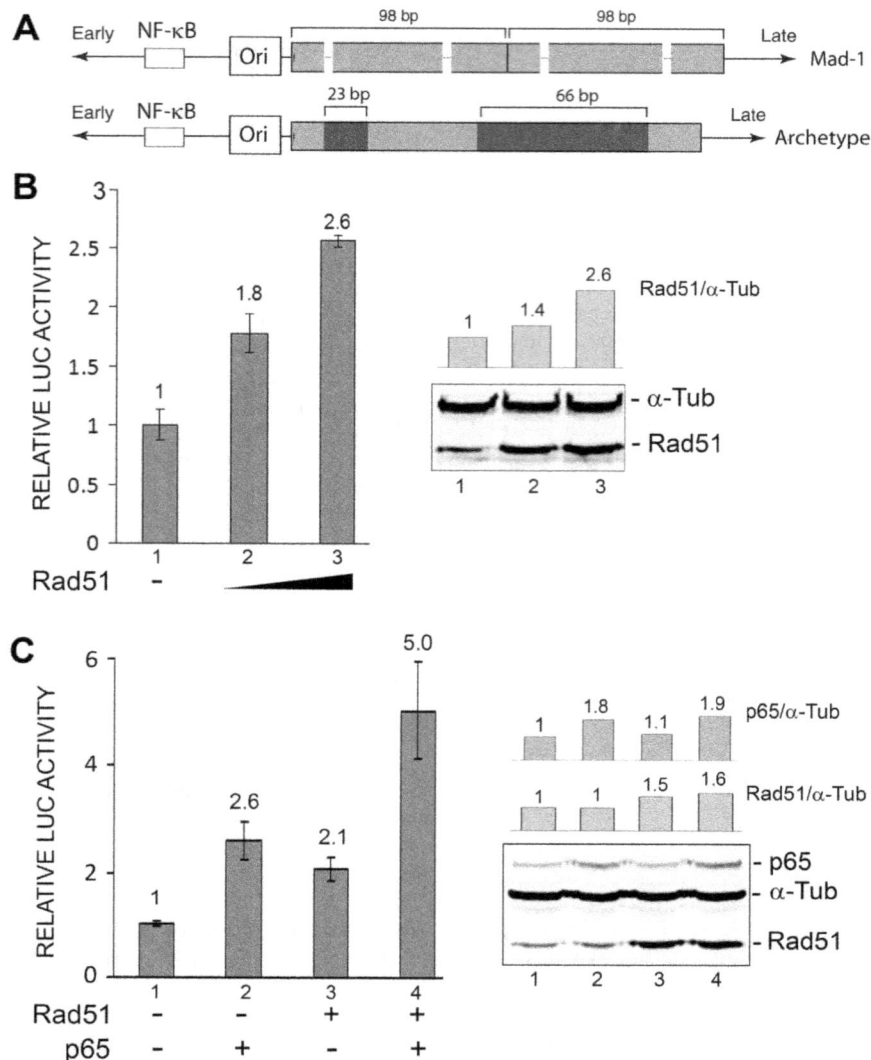

Figure 1. Effect of ectopic expression of Rad51 and NF-κB p65 on JCV early promoter reporter expression. A. Schematic representation (not to scale) of the Mad-1 neurovirulent form of JCV that was isolated from the brain of a PML patient and the archetypal form of JCV, which is found in the environment and may be the transmissible form of the virus. Relative to the archetype, Mad-1 contains 23 bp and 66 bp deletions (black boxes) in the late proximal region followed by a duplication of the remaining 98 bp sequence. Note that the NF-κB site lies in the highly conserved early proximal region of the JCV NCCR that lies between the early coding region (far left) and the viral origin of DNA replication (Ori). This region is highly conserved, not involved in rearrangements and present in all known strains of JCV. **B.** TC620 cells were transfected with luciferase reporter plasmid for the early promoter, JCV$_E$-LUC in the presence or absence of increasing amounts of Rad51 expression plasmid (0, 0.5 and 1 μg). After 48 h, cells were harvested and assayed for luciferase activity. Activities were normalized to the activity for reporter alone (lane 1). The error bars represent one standard deviation. Expression of Rad51 was verified by Western blot as shown on the right-hand side of the panel with α-tubulin (α-Tub) as a loading control. Note the lane numbering in the Western blot corresponds to the numbering in the luciferase assay histogram on the left-hand side of the panel. The intensity of the Rad51 and α-Tub bands were measured for each lane and the ratio shown as a histogram above the Western. **C.** TC620 cells were transfected JCV$_E$-LUC (left) in the presence or absence of Rad1 (0.5 μg) and/or NF-κB p65 (0.5 μg) expression plasmids. Expression of Rad51 and p65 were confirmed by Western blot with α-tubulin as a loading control, and this is shown on the right-hand side of the panel. Again, the lane numbering in the Western blot corresponds to the numbering in the luciferase assay histogram on the left-hand side of the panel. The intensity of the Rad51 and α-Tub bands were measured for each lane and the ratio shown as a histogram above the Western. The intensity of the Rad51, p65 and α-Tub bands were measured for each lane and the ratio of p65/α-Tub and Rad51/α-Tub are shown as histograms above the Western.

described [22] using the ChIP assay kit (Upstate Cell Signaling Solutions). Cross-linking was performed with formaldehyde and the DNA sheared by sonication. The cells were lysed and immunoprecipitation was performed with antibody to Rad51, nonimmune rabbit serum or beads alone as indicated. DNA was extracted and PCR performed using primers spanning the JCV NCCR.

Results

Rad51 and NF-κB p65 cooperate to stimulate JCV early transcription

The JCV noncoding control region (NCCR) contains a binding site for NF-κB that is conserved in all strains of JCV (Fig. 1A) including the archetype and the rearranged neurovirulent strains of JCV that cause PML including the prototypical Mad-1 strain,

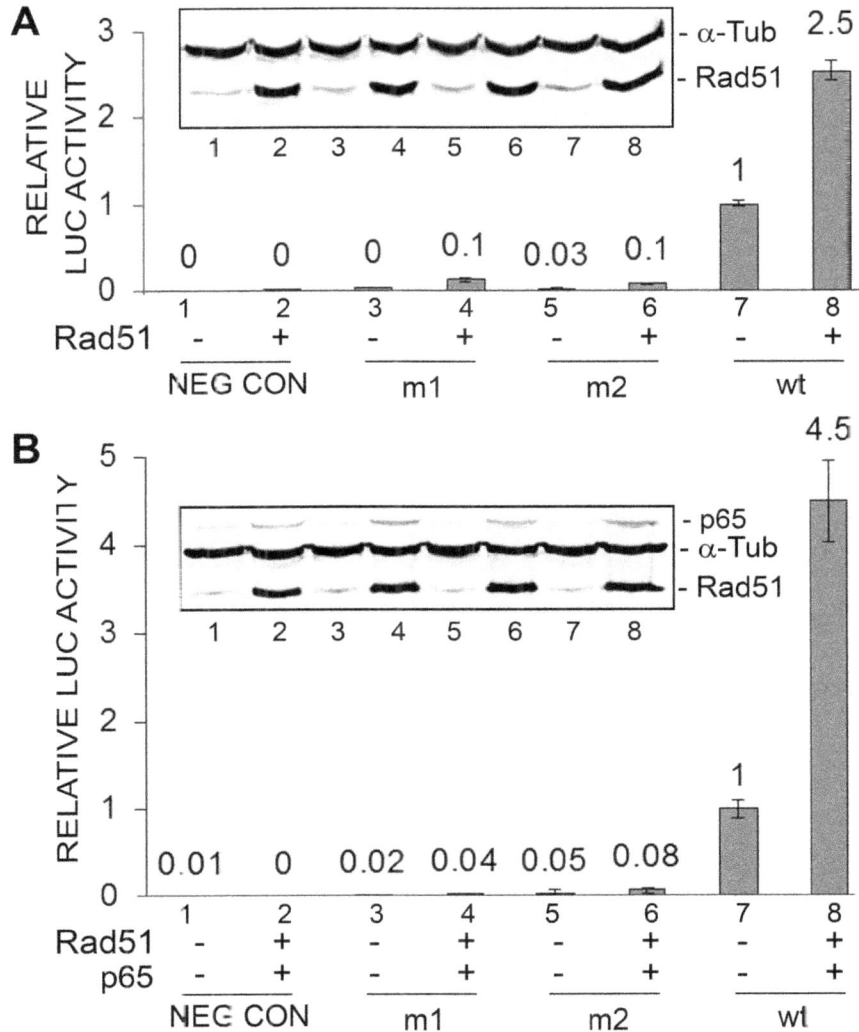

Figure 2. Effect of ectopic expression of Rad51 and p65 on JCV early promoter mutant reporters expression. A. TC620 cells were transfected with JCV_E-LUC reporter plasmid containing either the m1 or m2 NF-κB site mutation or with wild-type (wt) promoter in the presence or absence of Rad51 (1 µg). After 48 h, cells were harvested and assayed for luciferase activity. Activities were normalized to the activity for wild-type alone (lane 7). The error bars represent standard deviation. Western blot is shown as an inset subpanel within the luciferase activity histogram. The lane numbering in the Western blot corresponds to the numbering in the luciferase assay histogram. The intensity of the Rad51 and α-Tub bands were measured for each lane and the ratio shown as a histogram above the Western. **B.** TC620 cells were transfected as in Panel A except that expression plasmids for Rad51 (0.5 µg) and p65 (0.5 µg) were used together.

which was used in this study. This unique NF-κB site mediates the stimulation of transcription caused by NF-κB p65 expression and treatment of cells with PMA or TNF-α [21–24]. This site is also regulated by the calcineurin/NFAT4 signaling pathway [25] and histone acetylation [26]. We now examine a role for the DNA repair protein Rad51 at this site. As shown in Fig. 1B, transient transfection of increasing amounts of Rad51 expression plasmid proportionately stimulated JCV early transcription measured using a luciferase reporter plasmid at 0.5 ($p < 0.05$) and 1 µg ($p < 0.05$). No effect was observed in the case of JCV late transcription (data not shown). An increasing level of Rad51 was verified by Western blot. As we have reported before [22], expression of NF-κB p65 also stimulated JCV early transcription (Fig. 1C, lane 2, $p < 0.05$). When p65 was expressed with Rad51, there was an additive enhancement of JCV early transcription (Fig. 1C, lane 4, $p < 0.05$). Each experiment was performed twice.

Early promoter mutants defective in NF-κB binding fail to respond to Rad51

In earlier studies, we produced two mutant early promoters (m1 and m2) defective at the NF-κB p65-binding site [22]. The two mutants had lower rates of basal transcription and response to Rad51 (Fig. 2A, lanes 3–6) while the wild-type promoter had a higher basal rate of transcription (lane 7) and was robustly inducible by Rad51 (lane 8). The activity of the basal wild-type JCV early LUC reporter promoter was significantly higher (about four-fold) than either m1 or m2 (Fig. 2A, lane 7) as was the activity of wild-type in the presence of Rad51 (Fig. 2A, lane 8). Similarly, the same pattern of response was seen when Rad51 was added together with p65 (Fig. 2B). This experiment was performed twice.

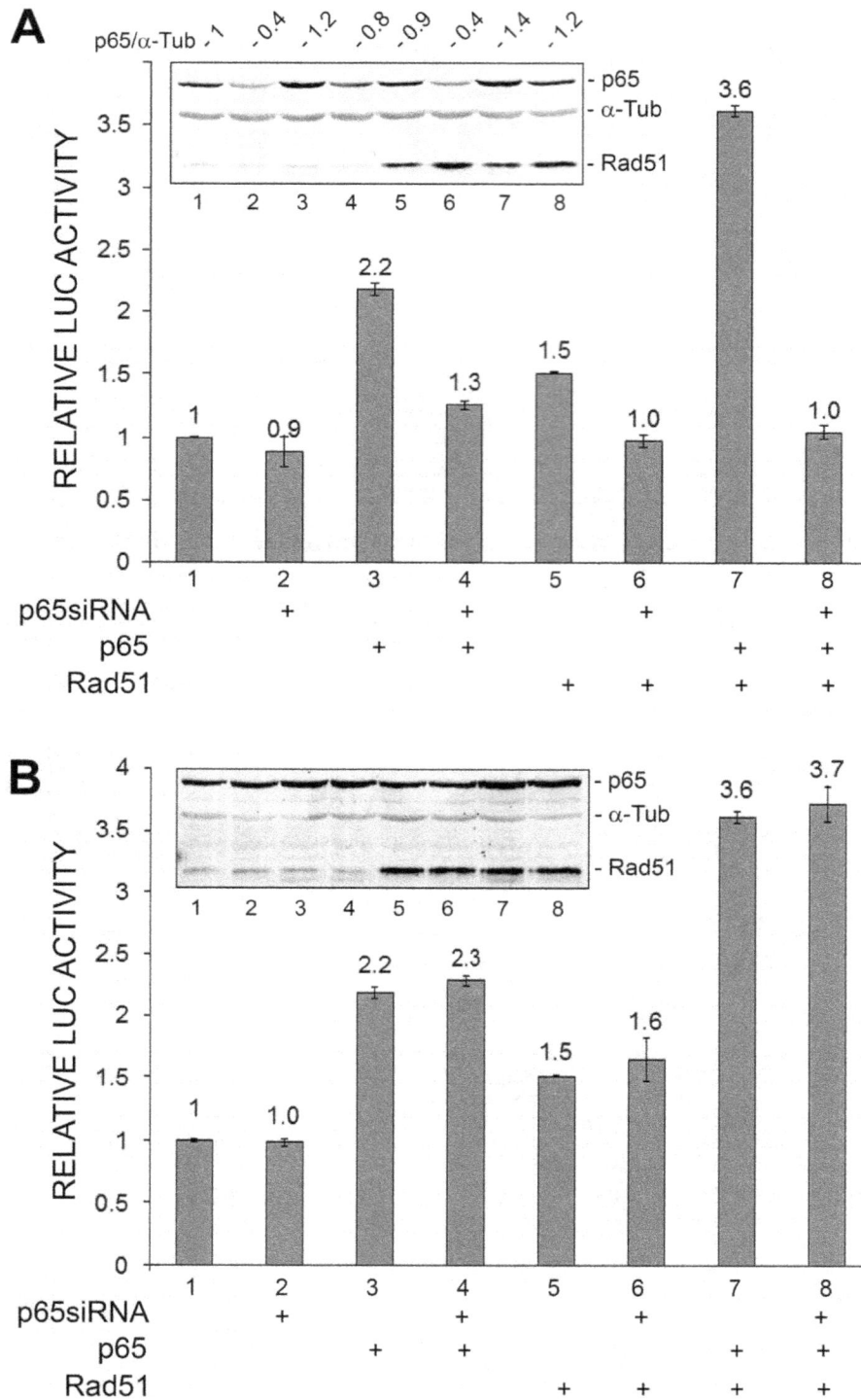

Figure 3. Effect of ectopic expression of Rad51 and siRNAs on JCV early promoter reporter expression. A. TC620 cells were transfected with JCV$_E$-LUC reporter plasmids and expression plasmids for Rad51 (0.5 μg) and p65 (0.5 μg) and/or siRNA for p65 (200 nmol) in various combinations as indicated. After 48 h, cells were harvested and assayed for luciferase activity. Activities were normalized to the activity for reporter alone. The error bars represent standard deviation. Western blot is shown as an inset subpanel within the luciferase activity histogram. The lane numbering in the Western blot corresponds to the numbering in the luciferase assay histogram. The ratio of the quantified relative intensities of the p65 to the α-tubulin bands for each lane are given above the blot to indicate the extent of p65 knockdown. **B.** As for Panel A except that non-targeting (NT) siRNA (200 nmol) replaced p65 siRNA. This was performed in the same experiment as Panel A but is shown separately for clarity of presentation.

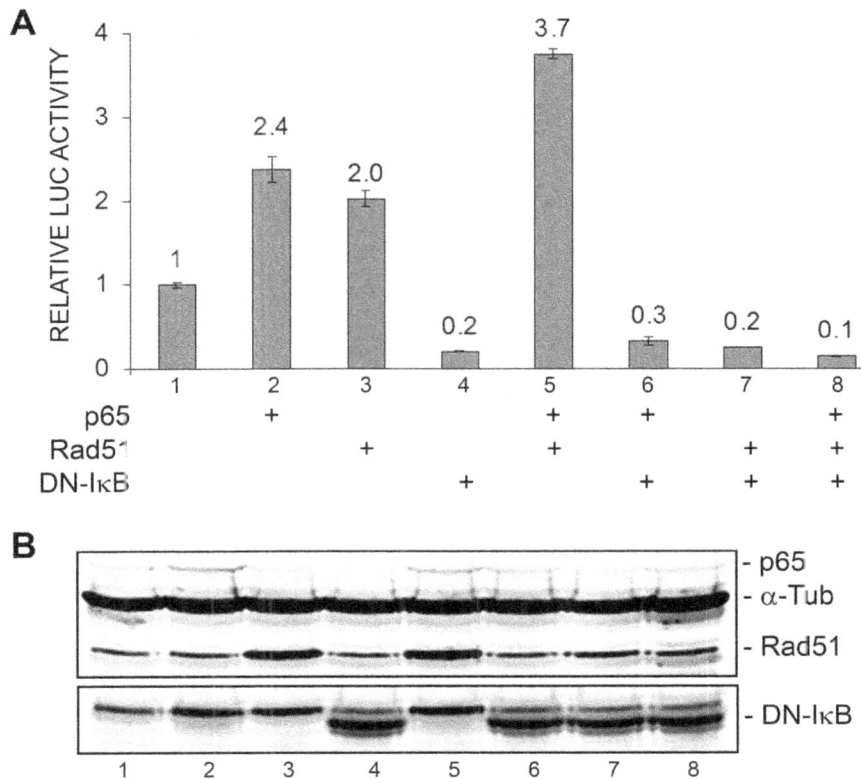

Figure 4. Effect of ectopic expression of dominant negative ΔN-IκB on Rad51 and p65 stimulation of JCV early promoter reporter expression. A. TC620 cells were transfected with JCV$_E$-LUC in the presence or absence of Rad51 (0.5 μg), p65 (0.5 μg) and/or DN-IκB (0.5 μg) expression plasmid in various combinations as indicated. After 48 h, cells were harvested and assayed for luciferase activity. Activities were normalized to the activity for reporter alone. The error bars represent standard deviation. **B.** Expression of Rad51, p65 and ΔN-IκB in this experiment was confirmed by Western blot with α-tubulin as a loading control (lower panel). The lane numbering in the Western blot corresponds to the numbering in the luciferase assay histogram.

Small interfering RNA to NF-κB p65 inhibits Rad51-stimulated and Rad51/NF-κB p65-stimulated transcription of the JCV early promoter

To confirm a role for NF-κB in the stimulation of JCV early transcription, we employed siRNA to p65 (Fig 3). Stimulation of JCV early transcription by p65 or Rad51 or both was inhibited (Fig. 3A) but a non-targeting siRNA used in the same experiment was without effect (Fig. 3B). This experiment was performed twice.

A dominant negative mutant of IκBα inhibits p65 and Rad51 stimulation of JCV$_E$ transcription

IκBα is a cytoplasmic proteins that binds and sequesters inactive NF-κB. Phosphorylation of IκBα by an upstream kinase renders it susceptible to ubiquitination and subsequent degradation by the proteasome, which thus frees active NF-κB to translocate to the nucleus. In the dominant negative IκB mutant, DN-IκB, substitution for alanine of the two serine residues that are phosphorylated by upstream kinase render it resistant to phosphorylation, ubiquitination and degradation by the proteasome thus preventing activation NF-κB [35]. As expected, DN-IκB inhibited p65-stimulated transcription (Fig. 4A, compare lanes 2 and 6). It also inhibited Rad51-stimulated transcription (lanes 3 and 7) and transcription stimulated by both (lanes 5 and 8). Expression of p65, Rad51 and DN-IκB was confirmed by Western blot (Fig. 4B). These data support a role for NF-κB p65 in

mediating the stimulation of JCV early transcription by Rad51. This experiment was performed twice.

C/EBPβ LIP isoform inhibits basal, Rad51-stimulated and Rad51/NF-κB p65-stimulated transcription of the JCV early promoter

In addition to the positive effect of p65 at the NF-κB site, we have reported that the transcription factor C/EBPβ, especially the LIP isoform, binds near to the same site and inhibits JCV transcription [22]. Thus it was of interest to investigate the effects of C/EBPβ LIP and Rad51, each alone and in combination on JCV early transcription. We found that C/EBPβ LIP inhibited both Rad51- and p65-stimulated of JCV early promoter (Fig. 5). This experiment was performed twice.

Rad51 and sodium butyrate cooperate to stimulate JCV early transcription

Since we recently found that the activity of the JCV early promoter is stimulated by histone deacetylase inhibitors such as sodium butyrate (SB) and trichostatin A and this effect is mediated through the NF-κB site [26], it seemed possible that Rad51 and sodium butyrate might act together to enhance JCV early transcription since they act at the same site. We next examined the effect of SB treatment on the Rad51 stimulation of the early promoter. The effect of SB on transcription was markedly more pronounced in the presence of Rad51 (Fig. 6A). We conclude that

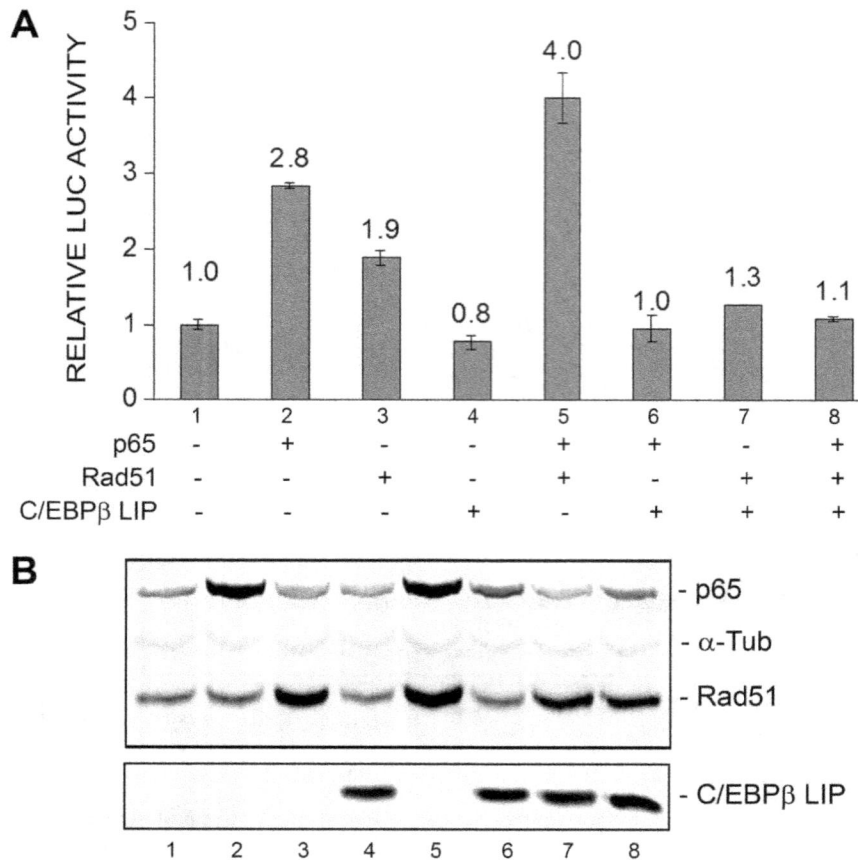

Figure 5. Effect of ectopic expression of Rad51 and C/EBPβ on JCV early promoter reporter expression. A. TC620 cells were transfected with JCV$_E$-LUC in the presence or absence of Rad51 (0.5 μg), p65 (0.5 μg) and/or C/EBPβ LIP (0.5 μg) expression plasmid in various combinations as indicated. After 48 h, cells were harvested and assayed for luciferase activity. Activities were normalized to the activity for reporter alone. The error bars represent standard deviation. **B.** Expression of Rad51, p65 and LIP were confirmed by Western blot with α-tubulin as a loading control (lower panel). The lane numbering in the Western blot corresponds to the numbering in the luciferase assay histogram.

Rad51 and sodium butyrate, which both act at the NF-κB site of the JCV NCCR, cooperate to stimulate JCV early transcription. The level of Rad51 was measured by Western blot and was confirmed to increase upon transfection of expression plasmid (Fig. 6B, lanes 2, 5 and 6). Protein acetylation was assessed by Western blot for acetylated Histone H3 (K9) and was markedly increased upon sodium butyrate treatment (Fig. 6B, lanes 3–6) as expected. This experiment was performed twice.

Inhibition of NF-κB by IκBDN expression or Rad51 by RI-1 treatment inhibits JCV infection

To investigate the role of NF-κB in JCV infection, we performed transfection/infection experiments with SVGA (an SV40 T-Ag-transformed human fetal glial cell line) and wild-type JCV Mad-1 genomic DNA in the presence and absence of expression plasmid for IκBDN (Fig. 7A). After 7 days, expression levels of VP1 and agnoprotein were measured by Western blot. The expression of both proteins was reduced in the presence of IκBDN showing that NF-κB is important in the JCV infection. To investigate the role of Rad51 in JCV infection, we performed transfection/infection experiments with SVGA with JCV and treated cells with and without RI-1. RI-1 covalently and irreversibly binds to Rad51 at Cys319, which is essential for filament formation and recombinase activity [34]. After 7 days, expression levels of VP1 and agnoprotein were measured by

Western blot (Fig. 7B). The expression of both proteins was reduced in the presence of RI-1 showing that Rad51 is important in the JCV infection. Note here that Rad51 plays an essential role in cellular proliferation and Rad51 inhibitors are known to slow down cell growth. In the case of SVG-A cells, 15 μM RI-1 that was used in the experiment has no effect on cell viability but causes up to a 45–50% reduction in the rate of cell proliferation as measured by MTT assay depending on cell density (data not shown). However, we normalized all samples for total cell protein before gel loading to compensate for this. Hence, the level of the cellular structural protein α-tubulin is constant and differences in VP1 and agnoprotein are therefore due to specific effects of RI-1 on viral protein expression levels.

Translocation of Rad51 to the nucleus after cytokine induction

Inactive NF-κB resides in the cytoplasm in association with the inhibitory protein I-κB and is released after cell stimulation by pro-inflammatory cytokines to migrate to the nucleus. Since we have found that Rad51 and NF-κB function together, we next performed immunocytochemistry (ICC) to investigate whether there was any correlation between changes in the localization of these two proteins under different conditions. TC620 cells were serum starved overnight, untreated or treated with 10 ng/ml TNF-α for 20 min and subject to ICC as described in Materials

A

B

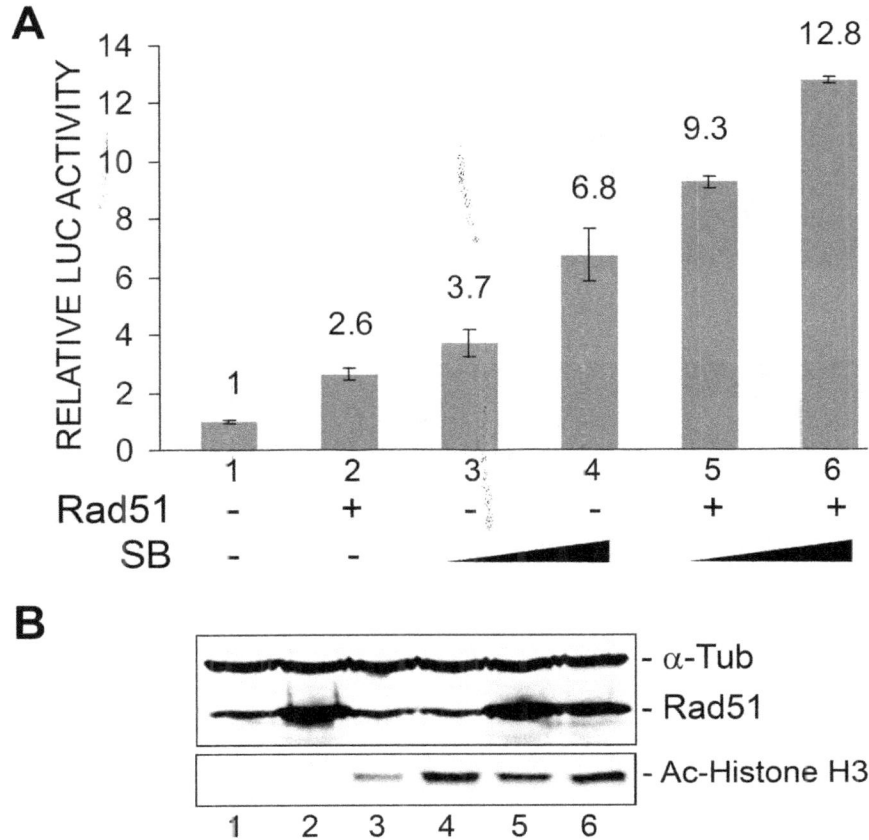

Figure 6. Effect of ectopic expression of Rad51 and sodium butyrate treatment on JCV early promoter reporter expression. TC620 cells were transfected with JCV$_E$-LUC in the presence or absence of Rad51 expression plasmid (1 µg), and/or treated with SB (2 mM and 4 mM) as indicated. **A.** After 48 h, cells were harvested and assayed for luciferase activity. Activities were normalized to the activity for reporter alone. The error bars represent standard deviation. **B.** The Western blots for Rad51, acetyl-histone H3 (K9) and α-tubulin are shown. The lane numbering in the Western blot corresponds to the numbering in the luciferase assay histogram in Panel A.

and Methods (Fig. 8). As expected, treatment with TNF-α resulted in translocation of p65 to the nucleus and this was also found to be the case for Rad51. Thus changes in Rad51 localization correlate with those of NF-κB suggesting the involvement of a common process and this may be important for the costimulation of JCV gene expression by NF-κB and Rad51. Interestingly, the nuclear Rad51 labeling showed a slight degree of speckling reminiscent of Rad51 nuclear foci formation although no DNA damaging agents

were used in this experiment. Similar results were obtained using cell fractionation of TC620 cells that had been transfected with Rad51 and p65 expression plasmids (Fig. 9). Surprisingly, the degree of redistribution of Rad51 to the nucleus in this experiment (compare lanes 2 and 4) was greater than that of NF-κB suggesting other additional mechanisms might exist for Rad51 translocation to the nucleus.

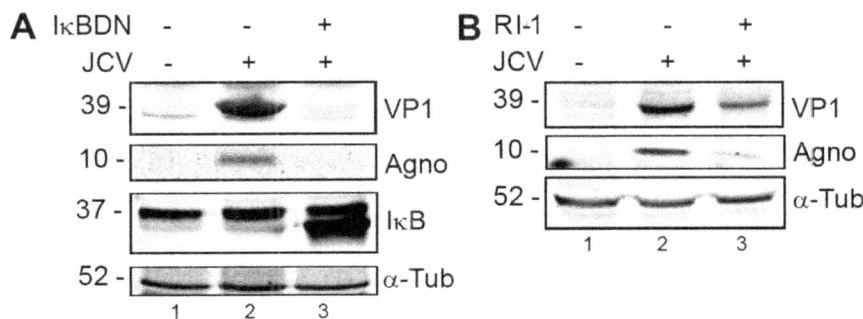

Figure 7. Effect of ectopic expression of IκBDN and RI-1 on JCV infection. **A.** SVGA cells (SV40 T-Ag-transformed human fetal glial cells) were transfected/infected with JCV with and without expression plasmid for IκBDN as indicated and harvested after 7 d for Western blot. **B.** SVGA cells were transfected/infected with JCV with and without 15 µM RI-1 Rad51 inhibitor and harvested after 7d for Western blot.

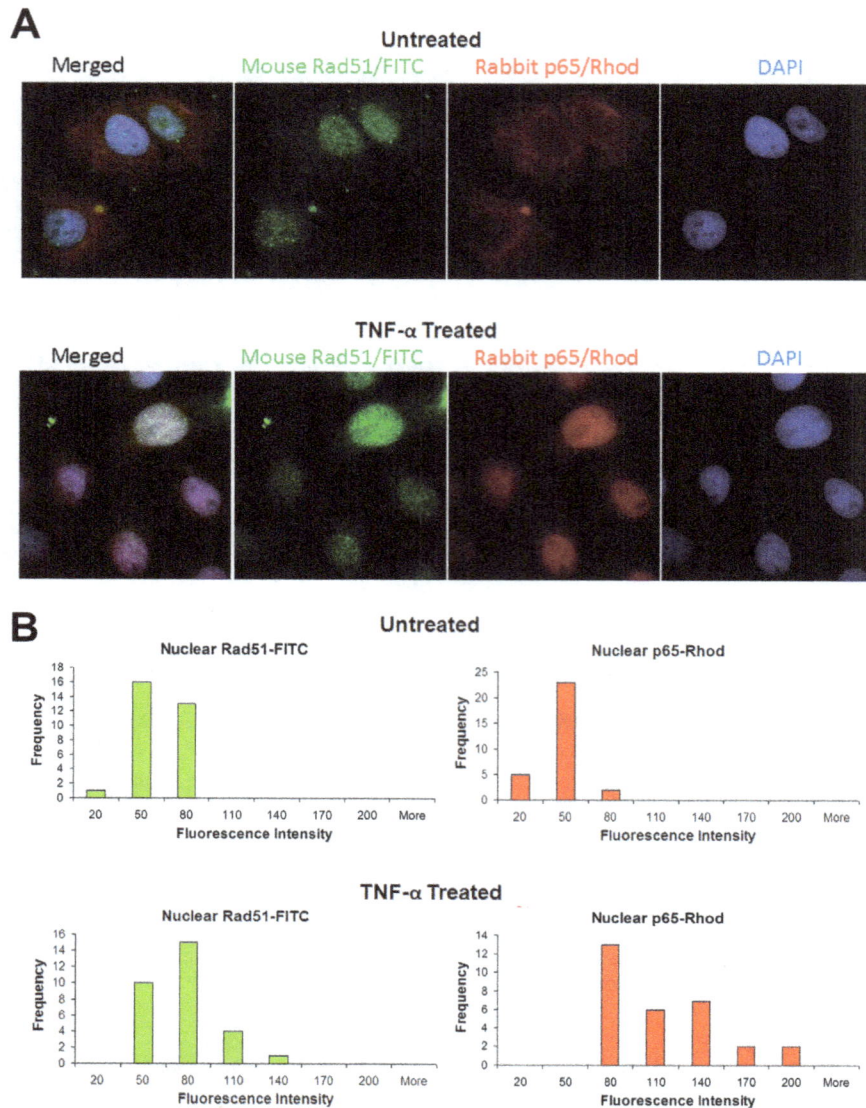

Figure 8. Effect of TNF-α on subcellular localization of NF-κB p65 and Rad51: immunocytochemistry. A. TC620 cells were either untreated or treated with 10 ng/ml TNF-α for 20 min and subject to ICC with antibodies to p65 and Rad51, washed, mounted with DAPI-containing mounting medium and viewed by fluorescence microscopy as described in Materials and Methods. Note, these cells were not transfected so the fluorescence is due to endogenous p65 and Rad51. **B.** Quantification of immunocytochemistry images: Images of labeled cells were analyzed using Adobe Photoshop CS. Nuclear areas of the labeled cells were manually outlined using the lasso selection tool based on DAPI labeling and the average fluorescence intensity levels for the red and green channels were recorded from 30 nuclei for each condition. Next, the fluorescence intensity levels data were converted into histograms using the Analysis Toolpack add-in of Microsoft Excel.

Effect of TNF-α-stimulated binding of Rad51 to the JCV NCCR in vivo by DN-IκB

The translocation of p65 and Rad51 in response to TNF-α suggested that Rad51 might associate with the JCV NCCR after activation of the NF-κB pathway. We stimulated cells with TNF-α in the presence and absence of DN-IκB, which is a dominant negative inhibitor of NF-κB signaling. As shown in Figure 10, Rad51 binds to the JCV NCCR in ChIP assay and this binding is reduced about 2-fold by DN-IκB (compare lane 5 to lane 4). These data indicate that Rad51 that is translocated into the nucleus in response to NF-κB signaling interacts with the JCV NCCR in vivo.

Discussion

Our data indicate that the double-strand DNA break repair protein Rad51 stimulates transcription of the JCV early promoter and evidence is presented for the involvement of the transcription of factor NF-κB in this process. NF-κB is a key regulatory protein in the life cycle of JCV and controls the activation of JCV transcription by cytokines such a TNF-α [24], co-ordinates signaling pathways that converge at the NF-κB-binding site such as calcineurin/NFAT4 [25] and mediates epigenetic control of the virus by protein acetylation/deacetylation [26]. In the present study, the stimulation of JCV early transcription by Rad51 was enhanced when it was co-expressed in the presence of NF-κB p65 and ablated by mutation in the JCV NF-κB binding site. Rad51

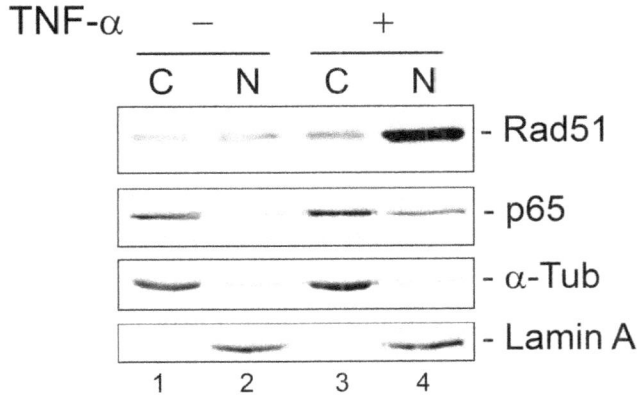

Figure 9. Effect of TNF-α on subcellular localization of NF-κB p65 and Rad51: Cell fractionation. TC520 cells were transfected with expression plasmids for p65 and Rad51, the next day serum-starved overnight and then either untreated or treated with 10 ng/ml TNF-α for 20 min and subject to cell fractionation as described in Materials and Methods.

stimulation of JCV early transcription was also inhibited by transfection of siRNA to p65 or expression of a dominant negative form of IκBα, which sequesters NF-κB in an inactive state in the cytoplasm. Taken together, these data implicate NF-κB as the mediator of the effects of Rad51 on JCV early transcription.

Interestingly, we have also found that Rad51 has a similar role on the HIV-1 virus and acts to stimulate HIV-1 transcription by binding to NF-κB p65 and activating the NF-κB site in the HIV-1 LTR [29,30]. In these studies, we found that there was association of Rad51 with NF-κB as detected by immunoprecipitation/ Western blot with cell extracts expressing endogenous levels of both proteins. Results from GST pull-down protein-binding assays showed that p65/NF-κB interacts with Rad51 protein while analysis of a series of GST-Rad51 deletion mutants demonstrated the importance of the region of Rad51 between amino acids 40–80 in this interaction [29].

What is the importance of this interaction in the regulation of the JCV life cycle? In earlier studies, we found that infection of glial cells by JCV causes extensive DNA damage and elicits the cellular DNA damage response (DDR). JCV-infected cells exhibit increased ploidy in metaphase spreads correlating with duration of infection as well as increased micronuclei formation and the

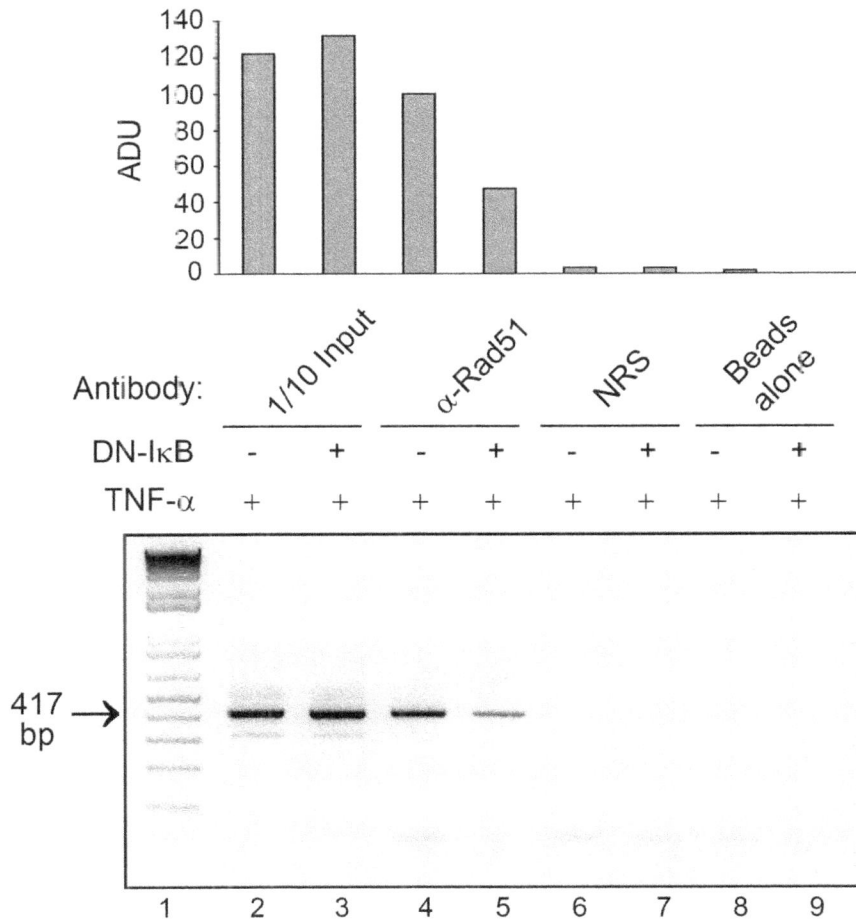

Figure 10. Effect of DN-IκB on TNF-α-stimulated binding of Rad51 to the JCV NCCR in vivo. TC620 cells were transfected with JCV_E-LUC plasmid containing the JCV NCCR in the presence and absence of expression plasmid for DN-IκB, starved of serum and stimulated with TNF-α as described in Materials and Methods. Following cross-linking, ChIP assay was performed using primers flanking the JCV NCCR and antibody to Rad51, normal rabbit serum or no antibody (beads alone). The position of the 417 base pair band corresponding to the amplified NCCR is indicated by an arrow. Lane 1 - molecular weight markers. The top panel shows quantification of the intensity of each band expressed as absorption density units (ADU) after normalizing the density for Rad51 in the absence of DN-IκB (lane 4) to 100%.

presence of γH2AX, which are indicative of DNA damage [28]. Western blot analysis revealed that JCV infection perturbed the expression of some DNA repair proteins including a large elevation in the level of Rad51 [28]. This induction of Rad51 was detected in Western blot of JCV-infected primary glial cell cultures and also in immunohistochemistry of PML clinical samples. Since Rad51 stimulates JCV gene expression, the induction of Rad51 expression by DDR following JCV infection may be a positive feedback mechanism whereby viral activity is boosted after infection.

We have been investigating the role of NF-κB in JCV reactivation and provided evidence to support our hypothesis that extracellular cytokines that initiate signal transduction through pathways that activate NF-κB, which turns on JCV gene expression. Normally, NF-κB is sequestered in an inactive form in the cytoplasm by an inhibitory molecule, IκB, but is released upon cellular stimulation and enters the nucleus [36]. In the case of JCV, active NF-κB strongly stimulates both early and late transcription and serves as a control nexus for other signaling pathways to modulate viral activity in response to cytokine stimulation [24], interaction with other transcription factors including C/EBPβ [22] and NFAT4 [25], and epigenetic modulation through protein acetylation [26]. Interestingly, the DNA damage response (DDR) is known to result in the activation of the NF-κB signaling pathway, a phenomenon known as nucleus to cytoplasm or "inside-out" NF-κB signaling [37,38]. Thus, JCV infection can result in both the induction of Rad51 expression and the activation of the NF-κB pathway. Since Rad51 and activated NF-κB act together to stimulate JCV gene expression, this might provide a powerful positive feedback loop in the reactivation of the virus.

In conclusion, our evidence suggests that NF-κB is a crucial control nexus where different signals can converge and may represent a switch for the initiation of viral reactivation. Recently, experimental and mathematical modeling of the NF-κB signaling module have provided evidence for the existence of a threshold level of input giving a switch-like response [39] and it is possible that such a mechanism triggers the switch between silent JCV and JCV reactivation. This would be an interesting area for future research to advance our understanding of the JCV life cycle, PML pathogenesis and possible novel targets for therapeutic intervention.

Acknowledgments

We thank past and present members of the Center for Neurovirology for their insightful discussion and sharing of ideas and reagents.

Author Contributions

Conceived and designed the experiments: KK HW. Performed the experiments: HW RK. Analyzed the data: KK MW RK HS. Contributed to the writing of the manuscript: MW HW.

References

1. Padgett BL, Walker DL, ZuRhein GM, Eckroade RJ, Dessel BH (1971) Cultivation of papova-like virus from human brain with progressive multifocal leukoencephalopathy. Lancet i: 1257–1260.
2. White MK, Khalili K (2011) Pathogenesis of progressive multifocal leukoencephalopathy – revisited. J Infect Dis 203: 578–586.
3. Berger JR, Concha M (1995) Progressive multifocal leukoencephalopathy: the evolution of a disease once considered rare. J Neurovirol 1: 5–18.
4. Kleinschmidt-DeMasters BK, Tyler KL (2005) Progressive multifocal leukoencephalopathy complicating treatment with natalizumab and interferon beta-1a for multiple sclerosis. N Engl J Med 353: 369–374.
5. Langer-Gould A, Atlas SW, Green AJ, Bollen AW, Pelletier D (2005) Progressive multifocal leukoencephalopathy in a patient treated with natalizumab. N Engl J Med 353: 375–381.
6. Van Assche G, Van Ranst M, Sciot R, Dubois B, Vermeire S, et al. (2005) Progressive multifocal leukoencephalopathy after natalizumab therapy for Crohn's disease. N Engl J Med 353: 362–368.
7. Khalili K, White MK, Lublin F, Ferrante P, Berger JR (2007) Reactivation of JC virus and development of PML in patients with multiple sclerosis. Neurology 68: 985–990.
8. Clifford DB, Ances B, Costello C, Rosen-Schmidt S, Andersson M, et al. (2011) Rituximab-Associated Progressive Multifocal Leukoencephalopathy in Rheumatoid Arthritis. Arch Neurol 68: 1156–1164.
9. Kothary N, Diak IL, Brinker A, Bezabeh S, Avigan M, et al. (2011) Progressive multifocal leukoencephalopathy associated with efalizumab use in psoriasis patients. J Am Acad Dermatol 65: 546–551.
10. Kumar D (2010) Emerging viruses in transplantation. Curr Opin Infect Dis 23: 374–378.
11. Mateen FJ, Muralidharan R, Carone M, van de Beek D, Harrison DM, et al. (2011) Progressive multifocal leukoencephalopathy in transplant recipients. Ann Neurol 70: 305–322.
12. D'Souza A, Wilson J, Mukherjee S, Jaiyesimi I (2010) Progressive multifocal leukoencephalopathy in chronic lymphocytic leukemia: a report of three cases and review of the literature. Clin Lymphoma Myeloma Leuk 10, E1–9.
13. Berger JR (2007) Progressive multifocal leukoencephalopathy. Curr Neurol Neurosci Rep 7: 461–469.
14. Khalili K, Safak M, Del Valle L, White MK (2008) JC virus molecular biology and the human demyelinating disease, progressive multifocal leukoencephalopathy. In Shoshkes Reiss C, editor. Neurotropic virus infections. Cambridge University Press, Cambridge, UK. 190–211.
15. Berger JR (2011) The basis for modeling progressive multifocal leukoencephalopathy pathogenesis. Curr Opin Neurol 24: 262–267.
16. White MK, Gordon J, Khalili K (2013) Human Polyomaviruses: A rapidly expanding family and the challenges in elucidating their roles in human pathology. PLOS Pathogens 9: e1003206.
17. Frisque RJ, Bream GL, Cannella MT (1984) Human polyomavirus JC virus genome. J Virol 51: 458–469.
18. DeCaprio JA, Imperiale MJ, Major EO (2013) Polyomaviruses. In: Knipe DM, Howley PM, editors. Fields Virology, Sixth Edition. Lippincott, Williams & Wilkins, Philadelphia. 6133–1661.
19. White MK, Safak M, Khalili K (2009) Regulation of gene expression in primate polyomaviruses. J Virol 83: 10846–10856.
20. Mayreddy RP, Safak M, Razmara M, Zoltick P, Khalili K (1996) Transcription of the JC virus archetype late genome: importance of the kappa B and the 23-base-pair motifs in late promoter activity in glial cells. J Virol 70: 2387–2393.
21. Ranganathan PN, Khalili K (1993) The transcriptional enhancer element, kappa B, regulates promoter activity of the human neurotropic virus, JCV, in cells derived from the CNS. Nucleic Acids Res 21: 1959–1964.
22. Romagnoli L, Wollebo HS, Deshmane SL, Mukerjee R, Del Valle L, et al. (2009) Modulation of JC virus transcription by C/EBPβ. Virus Res 146: 97–106.
23. Safak M, Gallia GL, Khalili K (1999) A 23-bp sequence element from human neurotrophic JC virus is responsive to NF-kappa B subunits. Virology 262: 178–189.
24. Wollebo HS, Safak M, Del Valle L, Khalili K, White MK (2011) Role for tumor necrosis factor-alpha in JC virus reactivation and progressive multifocal leukoencephalopathy. J Neuroimmunol 233: 46–53.
25. Wollebo HS, Melis S, Khalili K, Safak M, White MK (2012) Cooperative Roles of NF-κB and NFAT4 in polyomavirus JC regulation at the KB control element. Virology 432: 146–154.
26. Wollebo HS, Woldemichaele B, Khalili K, Safak M, White MK (2013) Epigenetic regulation of polyomavirus JC. Virol J. 10, 264.
27. Baumann P, West SC (1998) Role of the human RAD51 protein in homologous recombination and double-stranded-break repair. Trends Biochem Sci 23: 247–51.
28. Darbinyan A, White MK, Akan S, Radhakrishnan S, Del Valle L, et al. (2007) Alterations of DNA damage repair pathways resulting from JCV infection. Virology 364: 73–86.
29. Rom I, Darbinyan A, White MK, Rappaport J, Sawaya BE, et al. (2010). Activation of HIV-1 LTR by Rad51 in microglial cells. Cell Cycle 9: 3715–3722.
30. Kaminski R, Wollebo HS, Datta PK, White MK, Amini S, et al. (2014) Interplay of Rad51 with NF-κB Pathway Stimulates Expression of HIV-1. PLoS One 9: e98304.
31. Major EO, Miller AE, Mourrain P, Traub RG, de Widt E, et al. (1985) Establishment of a line of human fetal glial cells that supports JC virus multiplication. Proc Natl Acad Sci USA 82: 1257–1261.
32. Del Valle L, Gordon J, Enam S, Delbue S, Croul S, et al. (2002) Expression of human neurotropic polyomavirus JCV late gene product Agnoprotein in human medulloblastoma. J Natl Cancer Inst 94; 267–273.
33. White MK, Skowronska A, Gordon J, Del Valle L, Deshmane SL, et al. (2006) Analysis of a mutant p53 protein arising in a medulloblastoma from a mouse transgenic for the JC virus early region. Anticancer Res 26: 4079–4092.

34. Budke B, Logan HL, Kalin JH, Zelivianskaia AS, McGuire CW, et al. (2012) RI-1: a chemical inhibitor of RAD51 that disrupts homologous recombination in human cells. Nucleic Acids Res 40: 7347–7357.

35. Brown K, Gerstberger S, Carlson L, Franzoso G, Siebenlist U (1995) Control of I kappa B-alpha proteolysis by site-specific, signal-induced phosphorylation. Science 267: 1485–1488.

36. Nabel G, Baltimore D (1987) An inducible transcription factor activates expression of human immunodeficiency virus in T cells. Nature 326, 711–713.

37. Habraken Y, Piette J (2006) NF-kappaB activation by double-strand breaks. Biochem Pharmacol 72: 1132–1141.

38. McCool KW, Miyamoto S (2012) DNA damage-dependent NF-κB activation: NEMO turns nuclear signaling inside out. Immunol Rev 246, 311–326.

39. Shinohara H, Behar M, Inoue K, Hiroshima M, Yasuda T, et al. (2014) Positive feedback within a kinase signaling complex functions as a switch mechanism for NF-κB activation. Science 344: 760–764.

8

FOXM1 Modulates Cisplatin Sensitivity by Regulating EXO1 in Ovarian Cancer

Jinhua Zhou[1,2,3,4,5◊], Yunfei Wang[1,2,3,4◊], You Wang[1,2], Xia Yin[1,2], Yifeng He[1,2], Lilan Chen[1,2], Wenwen Wang[1,2], Ting Liu[1,2], Wen Di[1,2,3,4*]

1 Department of Obstetrics and Gynecology, Renji Hospital, School of Medicine, Shanghai Jiao Tong University, Shanghai, China, 2 Shanghai Key Laboratory of Gynecologic Oncology, Shanghai, China, 3 Focus Construction Subject of Shanghai Education Department, Shanghai, China, 4 Shanghai Health Bureau Key Disciplines and Specialties Foundation, Shanghai, China, 5 Department of Obstetrics and Gynecology, The First Affiliated Hospital of Soochow University, Suzhou, Jiangsu, China

Abstract

Cisplatin is commonly used in ovarian cancer chemotherapy, however, chemoresistance to cisplatin remains a great clinical challenge. Oncogenic transcriptional factor FOXM1 has been reported to be overexpressed in ovarian cancer. In this study, we aimed to investigate the potential role of FOXM1 in ovarian cancers with chemoresistance to cisplatin. Our results indicate that FOXM1 is upregulated in chemoresistant ovarian cancer samples, and defends ovarian cancer cells against cytotoxicity of cisplatin. FOXM1 facilitates DNA repair through regulating direct transcriptional target EXO1 to protect ovarian cancer cells from cisplatin-mediated apoptosis. Attenuating FOXM1 and EXO1 expression by small interfering RNA, augments the chemotherapy efficacy against ovarian cancer. Our findings indicate that targeting FOXM1 and its target gene EXO1 could improve cisplatin effect in ovarian cancer, confirming their role in modulating cisplatin sensitivity.

Editor: Alexander James Roy Bishop, University of Texas Health Science Center at San Antonio, United States of America

Funding: In accomplish of this manuscript, the authors have received the support of the National Natural Science Foundation of China (Grant No. 81272882,81302275, 81072137) and Shanghai Committee of Science and Technology (Grant No. 12411950200). The funders had no role in study design, data collection and analysis, decision to publish, or preparation of the manuscript.

Competing Interests: The authors have declared that no competing interests exist.

* E-mail: diwen163@163.com

◊ These authors contributed equally to this work.

Introduction

Ovarian cancer is the most lethal gynecologic malignancy in the world, with 225,500 new cases and 140,200 deaths estimated for 2008[1]. Most women with epithelial ovarian cancer (EOC) present with advanced disease (stage III or IV) at the time of diagnosis. Current standard treatment of ovarian cancer, in both early and advanced stages, consists of complete cytoreductive surgery followed by chemotherapy, usually based on a platinum and taxane doublet [2]. But the development of chemoresistance still presents a major impediment for the successful treatment. Most patients succumb to chemoresistance and relapse, and the overall 5-year survival rate is about 31%[3]. A better understanding of the molecular basis of cisplatin resistance may lead to new antitumor strategies that will sensitize unresponsive ovarian cancers to cisplatin-based chemotherapy.

Mammalian transcription factor Forkhead Box M1 (FOXM1) belongs to a large family of Forkhead transcription factors. Forkhead family members are involved in a wide range of biological processes including embryogenesis, proliferation, differentiation, apoptosis, transformation, tumorigenesis, longevity, and metabolic homeostasis[4]. Unlike the other FOX-transcription factors, FOXM1 is associated with cell proliferation and is overexpressed in cancer. For example, gene expression profiles in carcinomas, including prostate, breast, lung, ovary, colon, pancreas, stomach, bladder, ovarian, liver, and kidney, revealed that FOXM1 is overexpressed in all carcinomas [5–9]. Overexpression of FOXM1 in various tumors indicates a strong dependence of the tumor cells on FOXM1[10]. Moreover, in ovarian cancer, the integrated pathway analysis showed that FOXM1 transcription factor network is significantly altered in 87% of high-grade serous ovarian cancer[11]. FOXM1 promotes cell proliferation, migration and invasion in ovarian cancer[12]. FOXM1 has also been demonstrated to play a crucial role in drug responsiveness and resistance. For instance, it has been shown that deregulated FOXM1 expression can confer resistance to chemotherapeutic drugs, such as cisplatin and epirubicin[13], and protect cancer cells against DNA-damage induced cell death in breast cancer[14]. However, it remains elusive whether the FOXM1 play a similar role responsible for conferring cisplatin resistance in ovarian cancer.

EXO1 is a protein with 5′ to 3′ exonuclease activity as well as an RNase H activity, which interacts with Msh2 and which is involved in mismatch repair and recombination[15,16]. Recent study shows that EXO1 contributes to the induction of DNA damage checkpoints and participates in DNA damage repair [17,18].

In the present study, we provide the evidences that FOXM1 and its direct downstream DNA repair gene EXO1 might play in increasing the survival of ovarian cancer cells after cisplatin treatment, and targeting FOXM1/EXO1 axis can sensitize ovarian cancer cell to cisplatin treatment.

Materials and Methods

Ethics Statement

The protocols for handling paraffin-embedded ovarian cancer specimens and analyzing patient data were approved by the ethical committees of Renji Hospital, Shanghai Jiao Tong University, China. Written informed consents were signed by each enrolled patient if she was still alive or by her first-degree relative if she has died. All tissue samples were registered by a case number in the database with no patient names or personal information indicated.

Immunohistochemistry

The paraffin-embedded tissue samples were collected from 20 women with primary epithelial ovarian cancer, stages II to IV, who had undergone initial surgery at the department of obstetrics and gynecology, Renji Hospital, School of Medicine, Shanghai Jiao Tong University between 2005–2008. The slides were deparaffinized, rehydrated and placed into citric acid buffer (pH 6.0, 0.1 M) for heating for 10 min. The endogenous peroxidase activity was then blocked by incubation with 3% H_2O_2 for 10 min. Afterwards, sections were incubated with blocking buffer (Beyotime, China) for 1 h and then incubated overnight at 4°C with FOXM1 antibody (1:50, Santa Cruz). Following a 10-min incubation of biotinylated second antibody, the slides were again incubated with streptavidin-peroxidase under the same condition. The immunoreaction was then visualized by incubation with diaminobenzidine chromogen (DAB, Maixin-Bio, China) for 5 min. Finally, the slides were counterstained with hematoxylin, dehydrated, cleared and mounted. Negative controls were incubated in blocking buffer alone. These results were only considered if these control samples demonstrated a negative staining.

Cell lines and Culture

The human ovarian cancer cell lines A2780 and SKOV3 were purchased from the Cell Bank of the Chinese Academy of Science (Shanghai, China). Both cell lines were cultured in RPMI 1640 (Hyclone, USA) supplemented with 10% (v/v) fetal bovine serum, 100 units/ml penicillin and 100 g/ml streptomycin and cells were maintained at 37°C in a humidified atmosphere containing 5% CO2/95% air.

siRNA and plasmid transfection and co-transfection

siRNA duplexes were prepared by RiboBio(Guangzhou,China). SiRNA The sequence of siRNAs were as follows: FOXM1 siRNA-1: 5'- GCCAAUCGUUCUCUGACAGAATT-3', siRNA-2: 5'-GGACCACUUUCCCUACUUUUUTT-3'[19]. EXO1 siRNA-1: 5'-CAAGCCUAUUCUCGUAUUUTT-3', siRNA-2: 5'-UA-GUGUUUCAGGAUCAACAUCAUCU-3'[18]. The sequence of negative control (NC) was: 5'-UUCUCCGAACGUGUCAC-GUTT-3'. Transfection or co-transfection of siRNA and plasmid was performed according to the manufacturer's protocol of lipofectamin (Invitrogen).

Real-time PCR

Total RNA was extracted using Trizol (Invitrogen), and cDNA was synthesized using PrimerScript RT reagent Kit (Takara). For real-time quantative PCR, equal amount of cDNA were added to SYBR premix EX Taq II (Takara) and run in Stepone real-time PCR system (Applied Biosystem). The cycling program was 95°C for 5 s and 60°C for 30 s. Each sample was assayed in triplicates, and β-actin was used as an endogenous control. The forward and reverse primers used were as follows: FOXM1: 5'- GGAGCAGC-GACAGGTTAAGG-3' and 5'- GTTCATGGCGAATTGTAT-CATGG-3'. EXO1: 5'- CCTCGTGGCTCCCTATGAAG-3' and 5'- AGGAGATCCGAGTCCTCTGTAA-3'. PLK4: 5'-AAGCTCGACACTTCATGCACC-3' and 5'- GCATTTT-CAGTTGAGTTGCCAG-3'. XRCC1: 5'-CCTTTGGCTTGAGTTTTGTACG-3' and 5'-CCTCCTTCACACGGAACTGG-3'. BRCA2: 5'-TGCCTGAAAACCAGATGACTATC-3' and 5'- AGGCCAG-CAAACTTCCGTTTA-3'. Rad51: 5'- CAACCCATTT-CACGGTTAGAGC-3' and 5'- TTCTTTGGCGCATAGG-CAACA-3'. β-actin: 5'- CATGTACGTTGCTATCCAGGC-3' and 5'- CTCCTTAATGTCACGCACGAT-3'.

Clonogenic assay

After transfection of NC or gene-specific siRNA, cells were subjected to the indicated concentration of cisplatin for 1 h. Then cells were resuspended in fresh complete medium and plated in 6-well cell culture plate at the density of 500 cells/well. Following incubation at 37°C in a humidified atmosphere containing 5% CO2/95% air for 8–10 days, media was changed every 3 days. At the end of culture, cells were stained with 1% methylene blue in 50% methanol for 20 min, washed with water, and colonies (≥50 cells) were counted.

Western blot

Cells were lysed in RIPA buffer with supplement of PMSF protease inhibitor, followed by centrifugation at 14000 g for 10 min. At the end of centrifugation, cell lysates were collected and protein concentration of cell lysates was measured. Equal amount of proteins (10–20 μg) were resolved by SDS-PAGE, and transferred to PVDF membrane (Millipore). The blots were then incubated with primary antibodies in 5% bovine serum albumin/ Tris-buffered saline Tween-20 at 4°C overnight, followed by incubation with secondary antibodies at room temperature for 1 h. The protein signals were detected by Odessey scanner. The antibodies used in this study included: human FOXM1 (1:100, Santa Cruz Biotechnology), phospho-histone H2A.X (γH2AX, 1:1000, Cell Signaling Technology), caspase-3 (1:1000, Cell Signaling Technology), EXO1 (1:100, Thermo Fisher Scienfitic), β-actin (1:2000, Abcam).

Cell viability assay

Cell viability was measured by Cell Counting Kit-8 assay (Dojindo Molecular Technologies). Briefly, cells were plated at a density of 5×10^3 cells/well on 96-well plates and subjected to different treatment. Following 48 h incubation at 37°C in a humidified atmosphere containing 5% CO_2/95% air, the samples were incubated for another 2 h with CCK8 reagent. The absorbance was determined at 450 nm using FLx800 Fluorescence Microplate Reader (Biotek).

γH2AX immunofluorescent staining

A2780 and SKOV3 cells were transfected with NC or gene-specific siRNA. After 48 h, cells were then treated with the indicated concentration of cisplatin for 1 h, and fresh media were changed. 24 hours later, cells were subjected to anti-γH2AX (Ser139) staining. Briefly, cells were fixed with 10% formalin for 15 min, then permeabilized with 0.1% Triton-100 in 10% FCS for 10 min. Samples were blocked with 5% goat serum in 10% FCS for 1 h and then incubated overnight with the primary rabbit anti-γH2AX (Ser139;1:400; Cell Signaling). Following washes with PBS, secondary goat anti-rabbit IgG-TRITC (1:400; Sigma-Aldrich) was added to the samples for 1 h. Cells were counterstained with DAPI before mounting. Images were captured using a Laser Scanning Confocal microscope TCS SP5 (Leica). For foci quantification, cells with greater than 10 foci were counted as positive according to the standard procedure[20]. Experiments were repeated in triplicate.

Flow cytometry

Apoptosis was exmamined by flow cytometric analysis of Annexin V and PI staining (BD) according to the manufacturer's protocol. Briefly, after the indicated treatment, cells were resuspended at a concentration of 1×10^6 cells/ml, then 5 µl of FITC annexin V and 5 µl of PI were added to 1×10^5 cells (100 µl) and the cells were incubated at room temperature for 15 min. After incubation, cells were analyzed by flow cytometer FC500/FC500-MPL (Beckman Coulter). For cell cycle analysis, cells were trypsinized, pelleted, and then resuspended in propidium iodide solution (50 µg/ml propidium iodide, 0.1 mg/ml RNaseA, and 0.05% Triton-X). All reagents were purchased from Sigma. After 40 min of incubation, cells were analyzed by FC500/FC500-MPL.

Chromatin immunoprecipitation assay

Chromatin immunoprecipitation (ChIP) experiments were performed as previously described [21]. 24 hours after cisplatin treatment, cells were fixed in 1% formaldehyde for 10 min to allow crosslinking and then quenched with glycine. Cells were collected and lysed in SDS lysis buffer. Lysate was sonicated, pre-cleared, incubated with antibodies, and collected with Protein-A+ G agarose/Salmon Sperm DNA. DNA-protein cross-links were reversed and chromatin DNA was purified and subjected to PCR analysis. The primers 5'–AAA TCT GGC AAC CCT ACC TCA-3' and 5'-TTA AGT GTG CCT GTC AGT TCC-3' were used to amplify the EXO1 FHRE1-containing region (−1934/−1575), and the primers 5'-CAA TTT CGA TTT GTA GAG GCA AC-3' and 5'-CGG CTT CCA ACT CAT AGG GT-3' were used to amplify the FHRE2-containing region (−459/−74). After amplification, PCR products were resolved on agarose gel visualized by GelRed (Biotium).

Promoter reporters and luciferase assays

The EXO1 promoter region was PCR-amplified from genomic DNA extracted from A2780 cells using forward and reverse primers containing NheI and HindIII restriction sites (5'-CTA GCT AGC AGG ACC AAA GAG CCA TCA CA-3' and 5'-CCC AAG CTT CAC GGG TAA CTT GCC TAC ACA 3'). After restriction digestion, the fragment was cloned in the pGL-3 basic reporter gene vector to generated the EXO1 promoter construct, pGL3-FHER2 promoter construct −490/−148 was cloned by PCR (primers: 5'- CTA GCT AGC AAA GAA CCC AGC GTG AAC TGA-3', 5'- CCC AAG CTT CAC GGG TAA CTT GCC TAC ACA 3'). Putative Forkhead site mutagenesis was performed using a site-directed mutagenesis kit (ExCell Biology). pGL3-Basic, pGL3-EXO1, wild-type pGL3-FHRE2, wild-type pGL3-FHRE2 plus FOXM1 siRNA, and mutant pGL3-FHRE2 were transfected to cells respectively. Transfected cells were treated with cisplatin for 24 h and their luciferase activities were measured by luciferase assay system (Promega).

Statistical analysis

We used SPSS19.0 software to calculate standard deviations and statistically significant differences between samples. The asterisks in each graph indicate statistically significant changes, with P values calculated by the Student t test as follows: *, $P<0.05$; **, $P \leq 0.01$; ***, $P \leq 0.001$. P values of <0.05 were considered statistically significant.

Results

1. FOXM1 expression was up-regulated in cisplatin resistant ovarian cancer tissues and cells

Previously, it has been shown that FOXM1 is overexpressed in ovarian cancer, and that FOXM1 overexpression was significantly correlated with high-grade ovarian cancers, indicating that FOXM1 may play an oncogenic role in ovarian cancer [12]. Thus far, the role of FOXM1 in cisplatin resistance of ovarian cancer has not been elucidated. To investigate the expression of FOXM1 in cisplatin sensitive or resistant ovarian cancer, ovarian cancer tissue samples were obtained from 10 women with recurrent epithelial ovarian cancer in 6 months after standard therapy, and other 10 women who were chemosensitive. All patients received optimal cytoreductive surgery followed by 6 cycles of systemic chemotherapy with the combination of cisplatin and paclitaxel. Among the 10 chemosensitive patients, 7 of them recurred after 12 months and 3 of them did not recur so far. All the slides were from the ovarian cancer tissues resected in the initial operation. The paraffin-embedded slides were immunohis-tochemically stained with FOXM1 antibody and representative stained slides were shown in Fig.1A and Fig.1B. Moderate to high FOXM1 expression were detected in as much as 8 of 10 resistant cases, but only in 4 of 10 sensitive cases (Fig.1C). Next, we compared cisplatin resistance and FOXM1 expression in three cell lines. SKOV3, which showed highest expression of FOXM1, was also the most resistant to cisplatin, while ES2, which was the most sensitive to cisplatin, expressed FOXM1 at the lowest level (Fig.1D). These results indicate that cisplatin resistant ovarian cancer exhibits higher level of FOXM1 expression compared to cisplatin sensitive ovarian cancer.

2. FOXM1 is up-regulated in ovarian cancer cells after cisplatin treatment

To further determine the expression pattern of FOXM1 in ovarian cancer cells, we treated A2780 and SKOV3 with different concentrations of cisplatin, and discovered the mRNA level of FOXM1 increased only slightly after cisplatin treatment (Fig.2A). We found, however, that FOXM1 protein remarkably increased in a concentration and time dependent manner in both cell lines, and corresponded to the level of γH2AX (Fig.2B and Fig.S1), which is the gold standard of DNA damage quantification[22]. We also performed ON/OFF treatment of cisplatin, elevated level of FOXM1 protein was observed in both cell lines at 24 hours post treatment, and the effect sustained till 96 hours (Fig.2C). Since the increased level of FOXM1 protein does not correspond to the increased level of FOXM1 mRNA, it was possible that elevated FOXM1 protein was largely mediated by protein stabilization [23].

3. Targeting FOXM1 increases cisplatin sensitivity in ovarian cancer

Given that FOXM1 was overexpressed in ovarian cancer, and was further up-regulated in response to cisplatin treatment, we hypothesized that targeting FOXM1 could sensitize ovarian cancer cell to cisplatin. We transiently transfected two siRNAs targeting FOXM1 in A2780 and SKOV3, both siRNAs remark-ably reduced FOXM1 expression and siRNA-2 has a greater silencing effect in the two cell lines (Fig.3A and 3B). 48 h after siRNA-2 transfection, cells were treated with the indicated

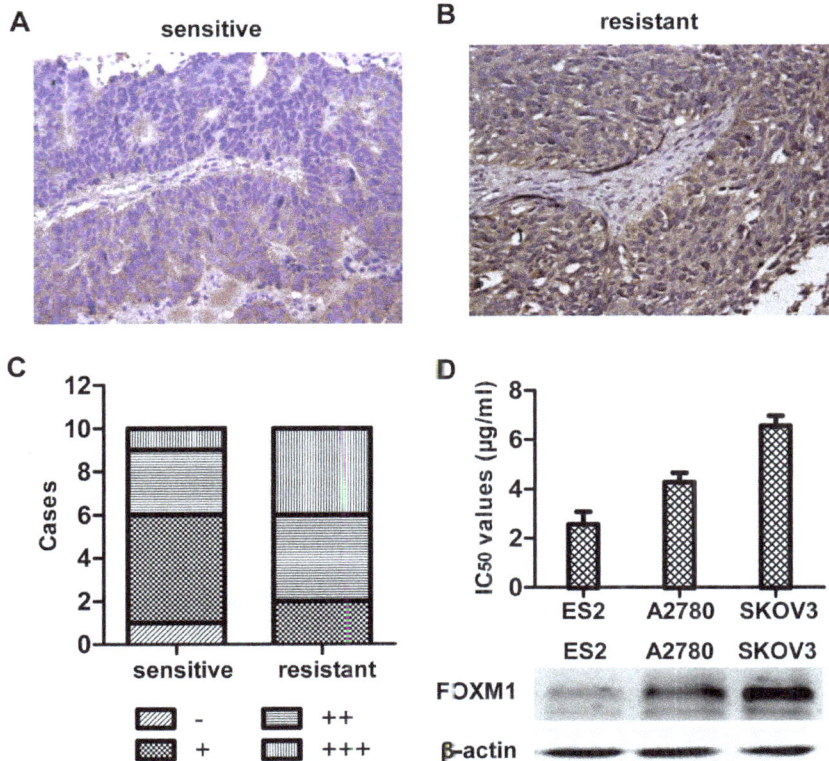

Figure 1. FOXM1 is upregulated in chemoresistant ovarian cancer tissue. (A) Representative FOXM1 immunostained section is shown from the chemosensitive patient group, (B) Representative FOXM1 immunostained section is shown from the chemoresistant patient group. (C) The numbers of cases with the indicated level of FOXM1 expression in chemosensitive and chemoresistant group are shown.(D) The IC_{50} values of different cell lines were shown in the upper panel, and the expression of FOXM1 in cell lines were shown in the lower panel.

concentration of cisplatin. Clonogenic assay was performed at 1 h post-cisplatin treatment, and cellular viability was measured using a CCK8 assay at 48 h post-cisplatin treatment. As expected, FOXM1 siRNA transfection in A2780 and SKOV3 cells rendered both cell lines more sensitive to cisplatin toxicity, as evidenced by a comparison of IC_{50} values between scramble siRNA and FOXM1 siRNA-treated cells ($\sim$1.7 µg/ml vs $\sim$4.1 µg/ml in A2780, $\sim$2.5 µg/ml vs $\sim$6.1 µg/ml in SKOV3) (Fig.3C). Treatment with FOXM1 siRNA and cisplatin also resulted in significant reduction in A2780 and SKOV3 cell numbers as measured by clonogenic assay ($\sim$17% vs $\sim$45% in A2780, $\sim$16% vs $\sim$37% in SKOV3) (Fig.3D). Additionally, we examined whether knockdown of FOXM1 led to increased apoptosis after cisplatin treatment. As shown in Fig.3E, cisplatin combined with FOXM1 siRNA resulted in increased apoptosis rates in both cell lines ($\sim$18% vs $\sim$38% in A2780, $\sim$20% vs $\sim$40% in SKOV3). Corresponding with apoptosis assay, western blot analysis also showed enhanced cleaved caspase-3 after co-treatment with FOXM1 siRNA and cisplatin (Fig.4A). Collectively, these results indicate that targeting FOXM1 provides a strategy for sensitizing ovarian cancer to cisplatin.

4. FOXM1 knocking-down results in DNA repair deficiency

It has been reported that FOXM1 regulated several genes in the DNA repair pathway[14,24], we next examined whether FOXM1 knock-down cells were susceptible to DNA breaks in ovarian cancer. To this end, FOXM1 siRNA-treated cells and scramble-treated cells were treated with cisplatin, and western blotting analysis was performed 24 h post-treatment. Notably increased γH2AX was detected in FOXM1 siRNA-treated cells after same treatment with cisplatin (Fig.4A). Furthermore, we stained for γH2AX 24, 48 and 72 h post cisplatin treatment. γH2AX foci per nucleus was counted in more than 100 cells in each time point. The results were expressed as percent of γH2AX positive cells in each time point. FOXM1 siRNA-treated cells displayed high percentage of unprocessed DNA damages (γH2AX positive cells) at 48 h and 72 h after cisplatin treatment when compared to scramble-treated cells (Fig.4B). Therefore, these data support the conclusion of DNA repair deficiency in the FOXM1 siRNA-treated cells.

5. Screening for FOXM1 target gene involved in cisplatin-induced DSB repair in ovarian cancer

Several target genes of FOXM1, such as *BRCA2*, *XRCC1*, *Rad51*, *EXO1*, *PLK4*, has been reported to be involved in DNA repair after the DNA double strand breaks (DSBs)[14,24]. These results prompted us to determine whether these FOXM1 target genes mediate FOXM1-dependent DNA repair in ovarian cancer. QPCR was employed to determine the expression profile of the above genes after cisplatin treatment. *EXO1* mRNA showed the most robust change and corresponded with the change of FOXM1 protein after cisplatin treatment in A2780 and SKOV3 (Fig.5A). The other genes, however, were slightly or moderately induced after the same treatment (data not shown). Interestingly, we also found that EXO1 protein was not only highly expressed in A2780

A

B

C

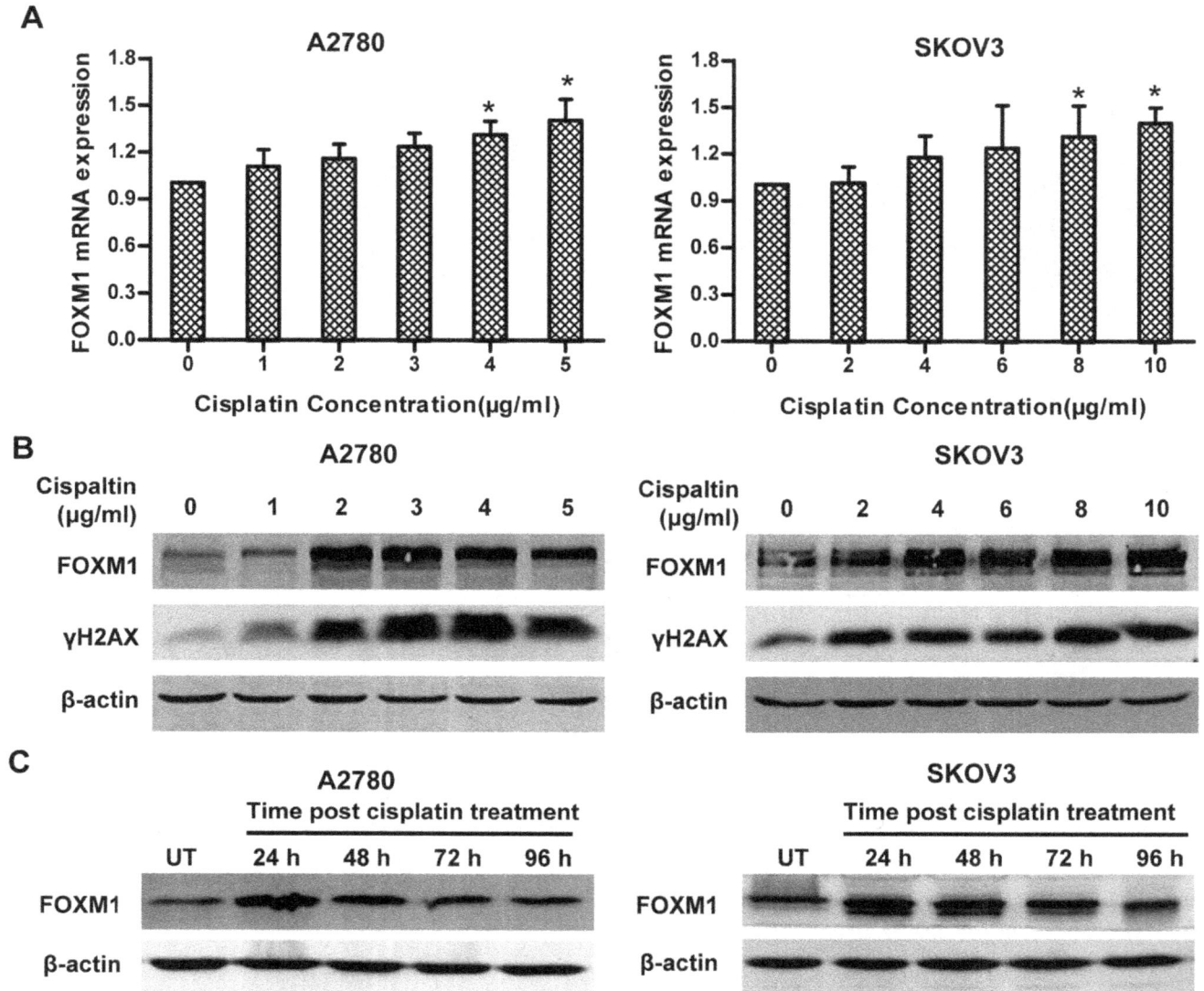

Figure 2. Cisplatin induces FOXM1 expression in ovarian cancer cells. (A) A2780 and SKOV3 cells were treated with the indicated concentration of cisplatin for 24 h. After treatment, FOXM1 mRNA transcription levels were determined by real-time PCR and β-actin was used as an endogenous control. Each column and bar represents mean±s.d. of triplicate determinations. (B) Cell lysates were prepared after the same treatment as in (A), resolved by SDS-PAGE and subjected to immunoblotting analysis using anti-FOXM1, anti-γH2AX, or anti-β-actin, respectively. (C) A2780 and SKOV3 cells were treated with 2 µg/ml and 4 µg/ml cisplatin for 12 h respectively, then were cultured in fresh complete medium for indicated time points (the time when complete medium was added was set as 0 h). Western blot was performed to determine the expression of FOXM1 and β-actin.

and SKOV3 compared to ES2 cell (Fig.S2A), but was up-regulated in a dose and time dependent fashion in A2780 and SKOV3 when treated with cisplatin, just like FOXM1 protein (Fig.5B and Fig.S2B). ON/OFF treatment of cisplatin also resulted in increased expression of EXO1 till 96 h (Fig.5C). It was not surprising that knockdown of FOXM1 was accompanied by 60–70% reduction in EXO1 mRNA expression (Fig.5D). However, FOXM1 knocking-down did not result in profound cell cycle arrest (Fig.S2D), suggesting that reduction of EXO1 was not an indirect effect of cell cycle change. In addition, FOXM1 silencing not only attenuated EXO1 protein expression in response to cisplatin treatment (Fig.S2C), but also after ON/OFF cisplatin treatement (Fig.5E). These results indicate that EXO1 is a candidate target gene of FOXM1 in DNA repair pathway in ovarian cancer.

6. FOXM1 directly binds to the EXO1 promoter and regulates its activity

We postulated that FOXM1 could enhance EXO1 transcription in response to cisplatin treatment. Sequence analysis identified two consensus Forkhead response elements (FHREs) in the promoter region (Fig.6A)[25,26]. To demonstrate that FOXM1 directly binds to endogenous EXO1 promoter sequence after cisplatin treatment, we performed chromotatin immunoprecipitation assays in A2780 and SKOV3 cells. The anti-FOXM1 antibody, but not the control antibody (IgG), precipitated the FHRE2-containing region (−459/−74) (Fig.6B), however, the FHRE1-containing region (−1934/−1575) was not precipitated (data not shown). To assess the functional role of the FHRE2 in EXO1 regulation, we performed site-specific mutagenesis within FHRE2 of EXO1 promoter pGL3-FHRE2 (Fig.6C). As shown in

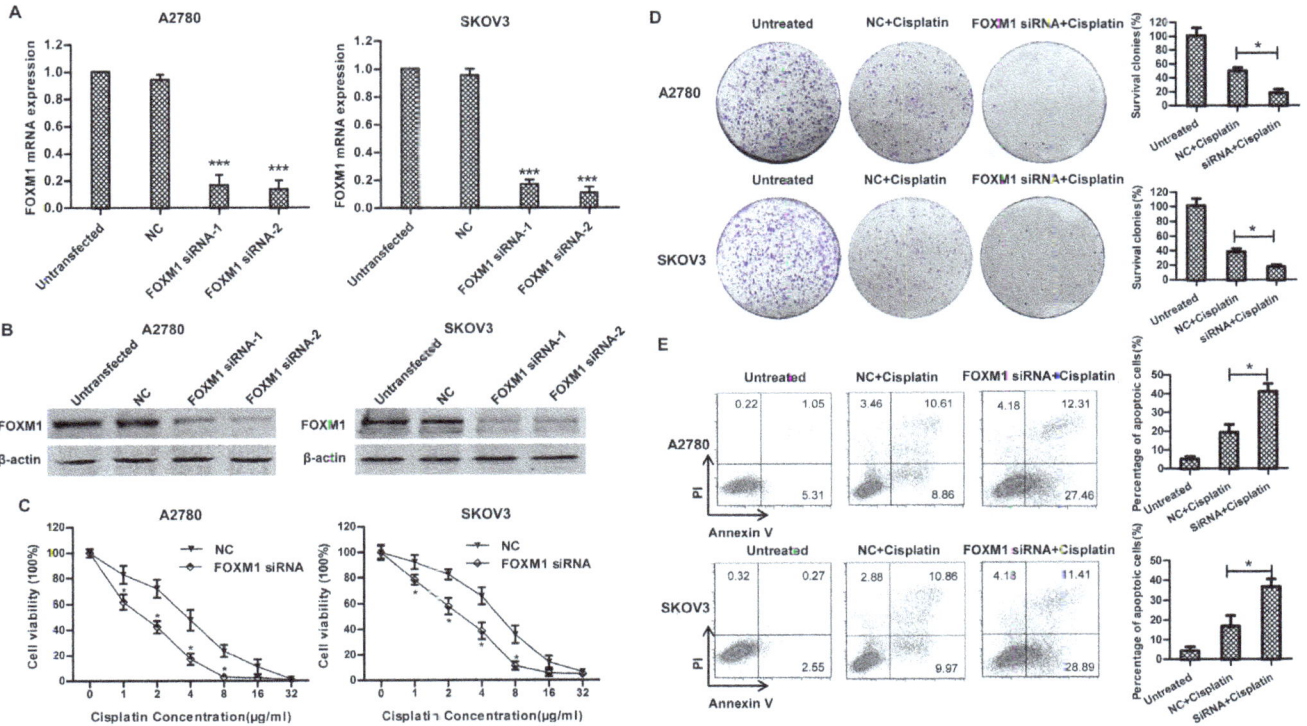

Figure 3. Targeting FOXM1 increases cisplatin sensitivity in ovarian cancer. A2780 and SKOV3 cells were transiently transfected with siRNA (100 nM) directed against FOXM1. Control cells were left untransfected, or negative control siRNA(100 nM)-transfected. 48 h after transfection, FOXM1 mRNA level (A) and protein level (B) was determined by real-time PCR and western blotting, respectively. Each column and bar represents mean±s.d. of triplicate determinations. (C) 48 h after transfection, A2780 and SKOV3 cells were treated with increasing concentrations of cisplatin for another 48 h and their rates of viability were measured by CCK8 and compared to cells without cisplatin treatment. (D) 48 h after siRNA transfection, A2780 and SKVO3 cells were treated for 1 h with 1 µg/ml and 2 µg/ml cisplatin, respectively. Then cells were plated in 6-well plate, colonies were stained and counted after incubation for 8–10 d. Results shown are representative of three independent experiments. The graphs provide quantification as a percentage of the non-treated wells. Each column and bar represents mean±s.d. of triplicate determinations. (E) 48 h after transfection, A2780 and SKOV3 cells were treated for another 48 h with 1 µg/ml and 2 µg/ml cisplatin, respectively. After treatment, apoptosis was determined by flow cytometric analysis of Annexin V and PI staining. The right panel shows means±s.d. of three independent experiments.

Fig.6D, mutation of the FHRE2 abrogated the ability of FOXM1 to activate the reporter construct after cisplatin treatment in A2780 and SKVO3, in addition, co-transfection of FOXM1 siRNA and wild-type pGL3-FHRE2 also resulted in low luciferase activity. Interestingly, pGL3-FHRE2 has stronger transcriptional activity than full promoter sequence. These results suggest that FHRE2 mediates the transcriptional effect of FOXM1 on the EXO1 promoter and that there might be some other sites which can be recognized by transcription inhibiting factors in the upstream region of FHRE2.

7. DNA repair regulation of FOXM1 is partially mediated by EXO1

EXO1 has been proven to be directly involved in DNA repair mechanism[18,27,28]. Thus, we next explored whether EXO1 accounts for FOXM1-mediated cisplatin resistance. We transiently knocked down the expression of EXO1 in A2780 and SKOV3 cells by siRNA transfection. Both siRNAs targeting EXO1 effectively reduced mRNA and protein expression in A2780 and SKOV3 cell lines (Fig.7A and 7B). Knockdown of EXO1 also sensitized cells to cisplatin, as evidenced by a comparison of IC_{50} values (~2.3 µg/ml vs ~4.2 µg/ml in A2780, ~4.1 µg/ml vs ~6.4 µg/ml in SKVO3) and clone numbers (~23% vs ~42% in A2780, ~21% vs ~38% in SKOV3) between scramble siRNA and EXO1 specific siRNA-treated cells (Fig.7C and 7D). In

accordance with the above, the same treatment with cisplatin resulted in more apoptotic cells in EXO1 specific siRNA-transfected cells (~18% vs ~27% in A2780, ~21% vs ~33% in SKVO3) compared to scramble-treated cells (Fig.7E). Although EXO1 knock-down did not affect the expression of FOXM1, it did partly recapitulate the cisplatin sensitization effect of FOXM1 silencing in ovarian cancer cells. EXO1 siRNA-treated cells also showed more DNA damages, enhanced apoptosis signaling pathways and impaired DNA repair efficacy, as detected by immunoblotting for γH2AX and cleaved caspase-3 (Fig.7F), and γH2AX quantification (Fig.7G). These results indicate that DNA repair regulation of FOXM1 is at least partially mediated by EXO1.

Discussion

FOXM1 transcription factor is a regulator of a variety of biological processes including cell cycle progression, apoptosis, angiogenesis, tissue homeostasis and DNA repair[24,29]. Elevated FOXM1 expression has been reported in many tumor types including ovarian cancer[5,11]. These findings suggest that FOXM1 plays a key role in tumorigenesis and is a good therapeutic target for human cancer[30]. We explored whether FOXM1 plays any role in modulating cisplatin sensitivity in ovarian cancer in vitro. We show that FOXM1 is up-regulated in

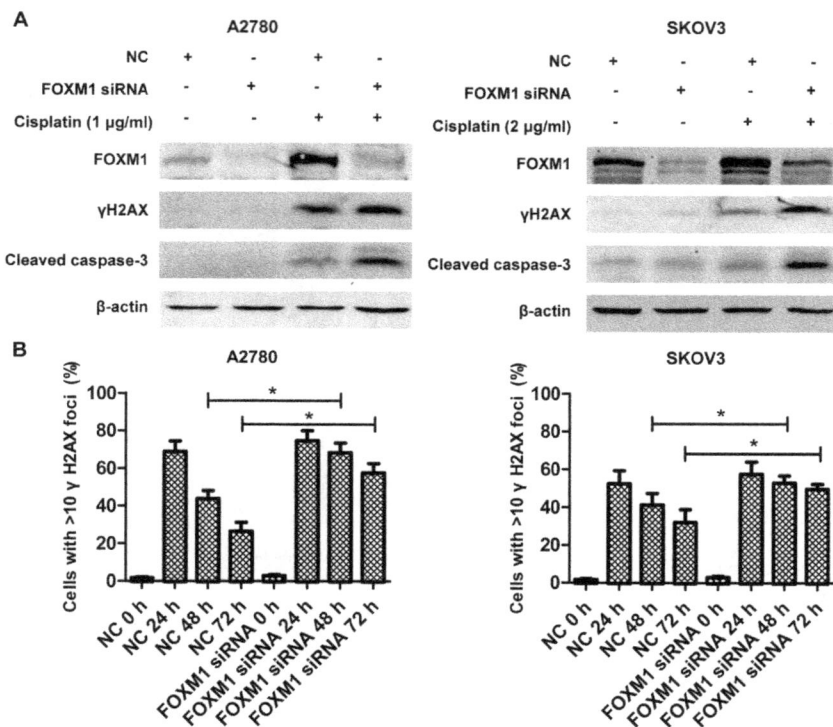

Figure 4. FOXM1 knocking-down leads to DNA repair deficiency. (A) 48 h after transfection, A2780 and SKOV3 cells were treated for 24 h with 2 µg/ml and 4 µg/ml cisplatin, respectively. After treatment, cell lysates were prepared, resolved by SDS-PAGE and subjected to immunoblotting analysis of FOXM1, γH2AX, cleaved caspase-3 and β-actin. (B) A2780 and SKOV3 cells with or without silencing of FOXM1 expression, were treated with 1 µg/ml and 2 µg/ml cisplatin for 1 h, respectively. γH2AX foci of A2780 and SKOV3 cells were quantified at different time point: 24, 48 and 72 h after cisplatin treatment. Percentage of γH2AX positive cells was plotted. Untreated cells were used as control.

chemoresistant ovarian cancer compared to chemosensitive ovarian cancer (Fig.1). Besides, treatment with cisplatin stimulates FOXM1 expression (Fig.2), and gene silencing of FOXM1 sensitizes ovarian cancer cells to cisplatin (Fig.3), through blocking the activation of the DNA repair pathway (Fig.4). We discover that EXO1 is a potential downstream gene of FOXM1 in ovarian cancer (Fig.5), FOXM1 directly binds to EXO1 promoter and enhances EXO1 expression (Fig.6). Finally, we demonstrate that EXO1 plays an important role in the DNA repair pathway activated by FOXM1 in ovarian cancer (Fig.7). Our studies therefore uncover that the FOXM1/EXO1 axis protects ovarian cancer cells after cisplatin treatment by enhancing the DNA damage repair pathway.

In response to DNA damage, the checkpoint network which contains ATM, ATR, chk1 and chk2, is activated and subsequently phosphorylated the downstream proteins, resulting in cell cycle arrest, DNA damage repair, and apoptosis induction[31,32]. In response to DNA damage caused by IR or UV irradiation, FOXM1 can be directly phosphorylated by chk2, and this modification leads to FOXM1 protein stabilization[23]. In this study, we discovered that FOXM1 expression was elevated at both the transcriptional level and the protein level, and that the elevation of FOXM1 protein was more significant than that of FOXM1 mRNA. This result might indicate that phosphorylation and stabilization of FOXM1 by chk2 contributes largely to FOXM1 expression elevation after cisplatin-induced DNA damage.

Cisplatin is a commonly used chemotherapeutic agent against ovarian cancer. Cisplatin treatment caused intrastrand and interstrand DNA crosslinks (ICLs) formation and DSBs[33],

triggering a subset of DNA repair machinery, such as nucleotide excision repair and homologous recombination pathways[34,35]. Recent study also showed that EXO1 is involved in the repair of DSBs [18]. Our data suggests that EXO1 mediate FOXM1-activated DSB repair in ovarian cancer. FOXM1 regulates XRCC1 and BRCA2 in HER positive breast cancer [14], in triple-negative breast cancer, however, FOXM1 transactivates EXO1 and PLK4 in response to doxorubicin[24]. Besides, targeting FOXM1 also sensitized resistant glioblastoma cells to temozolomide by downregulating Rad51[36]. These studies show FOXM1 can regulate multi-steps of the DNA repair pathway in a context dependent manner in different cancer cells.

Intense research conducted during the past years has revealed that multiple mechanisms account for the cisplatin resistant phenotype of tumor cells, including increased efflux of cisplatin, enhanced ability to repair adducts, and evasion of apoptotic pathways in resistant cells [37]. FOXM1 regulates a variety of downstream genes involved in DNA repair and anti-apoptotic pathway[10]; therefore, it would be more effective to target oncogenic transfactor FOXM1 than targeting only the DNA repair pathway. In accordance with this hypothesis, we found that FOXM1 knockdown seems more efficient than EXO1 silencing in sensitizing ovarian cancer cells to cisplatin treatment.

Cisplatin has been proven to have many adverse effects such as nephrotoxicity, neurotoxicity, ototoxicity [38–40]. Novel treatments, such as FOXM1 inhibitor co-treatment with platinum, are potential therapeutic strategies to reduce the necessary dosage of cisplatin and enhance the therapeutic efficacy in treating ovarian cancer. Since FOXM1 is a key regulator of cisplatin response in ovarian cancer, FOXM1 could be a new therapeutic target in

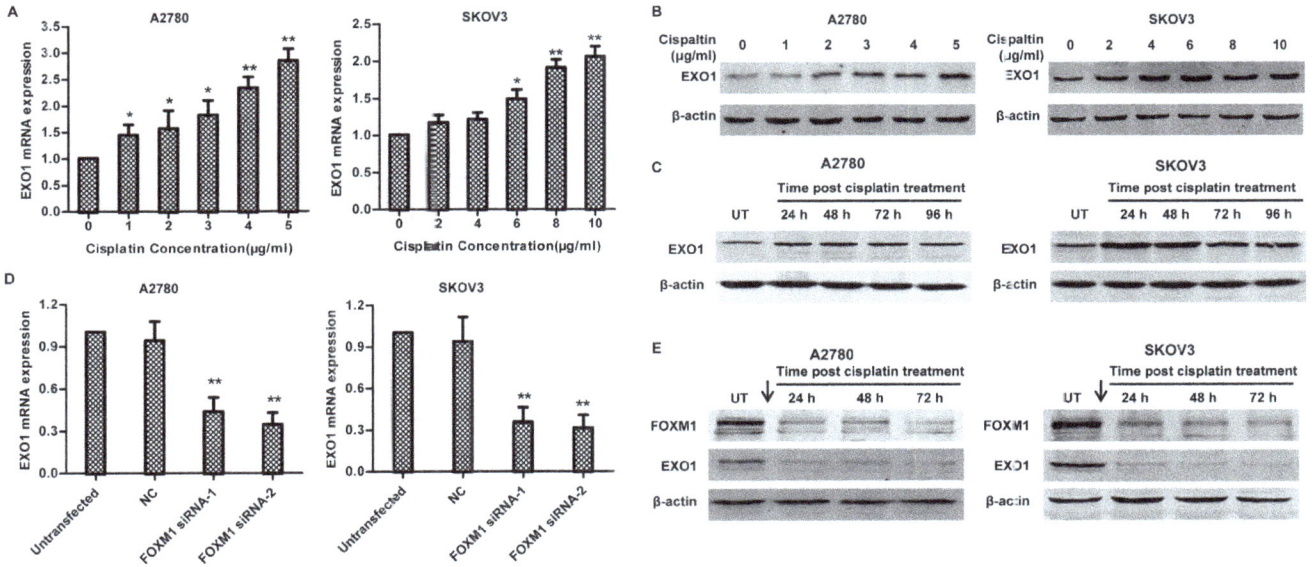

Figure 5. Expression of FOXM1 target genes in response to cisplatin in A2780 and SKVO3 cells. A2780 and SKOV3 cells were treated with the indicated concentration of cisplatin for 24 h, and the expression of EXO1 was determined by real-time PCR analysis (A) and western blotting (B). Results are shown from three independent experiments in triplicates. Columns, mean; bars, SD. (C) A2780 and SKOV3 cells were treated with 2 µg/ml and 4 µg/ml cisplatin for 12 h respectively, then were cultured in fresh complete medium for indicated time points (the time when complete medium was added was set as 0 h). Western blot was performed to determine the expression of EXO1 and β-actin. (D) A2780 and SKO3 cells were transfected with FOXM1 siRNA, 48 h later, EXO1 expression was determined by real-time PCR analysis. Results are shown from three independent experiments in triplicates. Columns, mean; bars, SD. (E) 24 h after FOXM1 siRNA transfection, A2780 and SKOV3 cells were treated with 2 µg/ml and 4 µg/ml cisplatin for 12 h respectively, then were cultured in fresh complete medium for indicated time points (the time when complete medium was added was set as 0 h). The arrow (↓) indicates transfection and subsequent cisplatin treatment. Western blot was performed to determine the expression of FOXM1, EXO1 and β-actin.

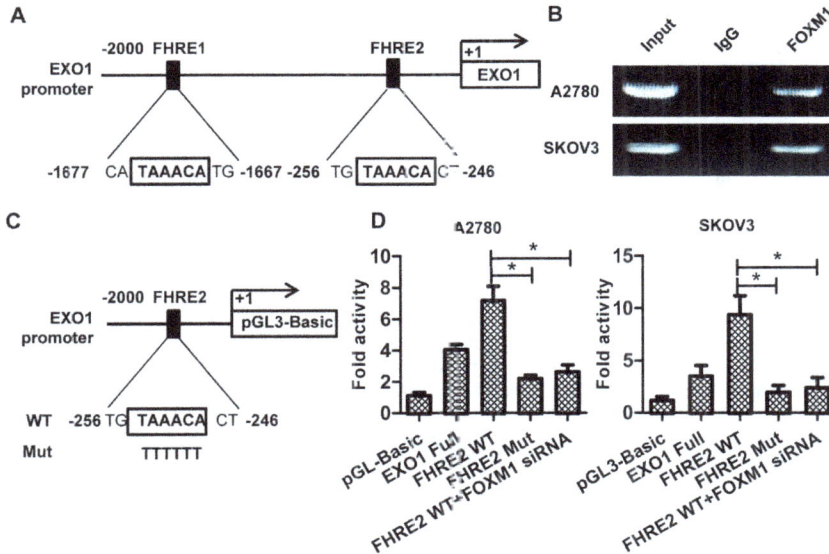

Figure 6. FOXM1 induces the transcriptional activity of the human EXO1 gene through a consensus FHRE site. (A) Sequence and position of the consensus FHRE sequence on the EXO1 promoter. (B) ChIP assays were done in A2780 and SKOV3 cells. Chromatin fragments of the cells were immunoprecipitated with anti-FOXM1 antibody and negative control IgG and subjected to PCR. 1% of the total cell lysates were subjected to PCR before immunoprecipitation as inputs. (C) Schematic structure of wild-type (WT) and mutant (Mut) forms of FHRE2-containing promoter reporters. (D) Luciferase activity with or without mutation in EXO1 promoter. A2780 and SKOV3 cells were transfected with wild-type or mutant FRHE2-containing reporter, or co-transfected with FOXM1 siRNA and wild-type reporter (pGL-3-Basic and pGL3-EXO1 were used as negative and positive control, respectively), then treated with cisplatin for 24 h. Afterwards, luciferase activity in cells were measured. Three independent experiments were conducted.

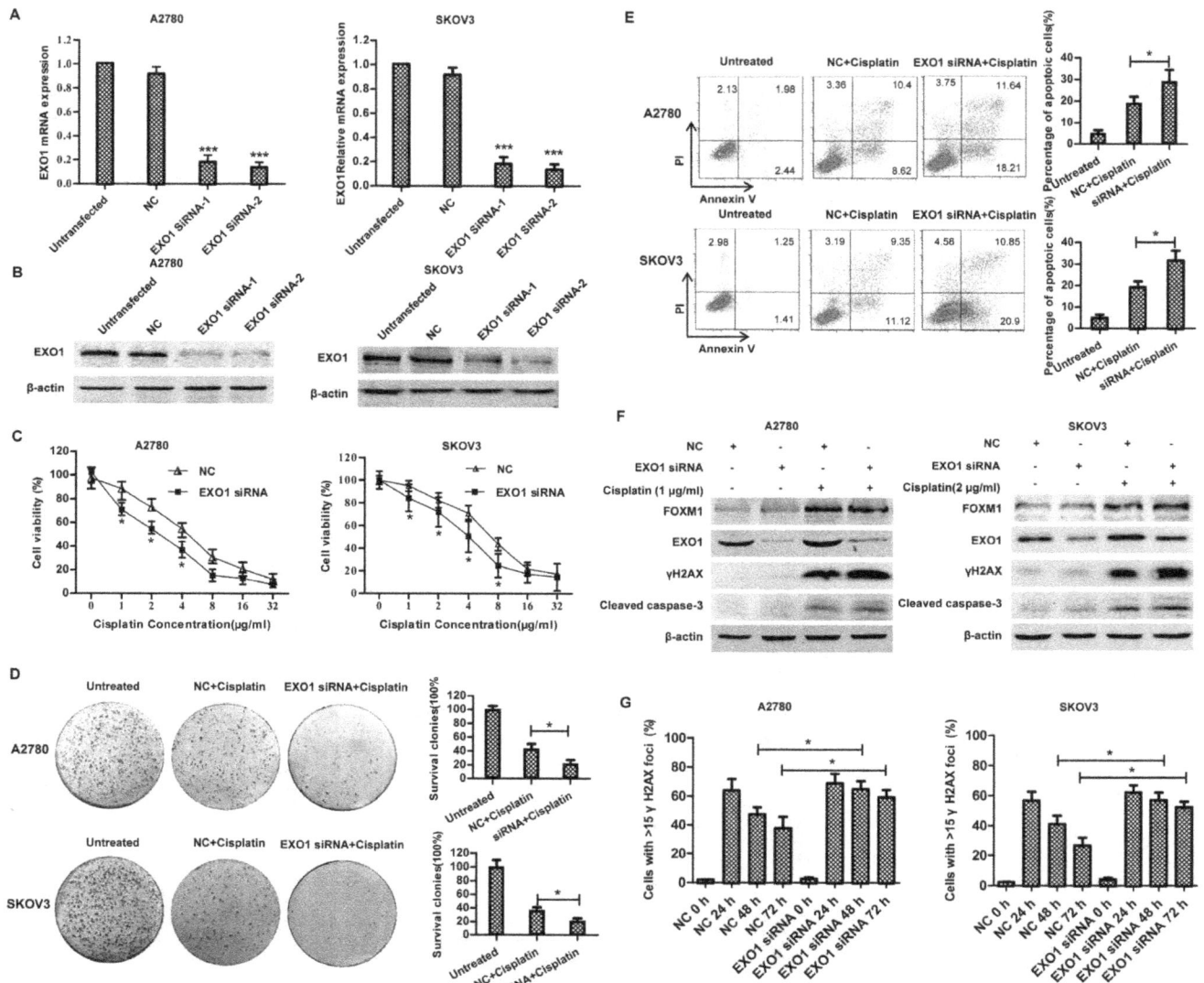

Figure 7. DNA repair regulation of FOXM1 is partially mediated by EXO1. A2780 and SKOV3 cells were transfected with EXO1 specific siRNA or NC siRNA. (A)The expression of EXO1 was determined by real-time PCR analysis 48 h after transfection. (B) Western blotting analysis was done to determine the expression level of EXO1. (C) 48 h after transfection, A2780 and SKOV3 cells were treated with increasing concentrations of cisplatin for another 48 h and their rates of viability were measured by CCK8 and compared to cells without cisplatin treatment. (D) 48 h after siRNA transfection, A2780 and SKVO3 cells were treated for 1 h with 1 μg/ml and 2 μg/ml cisplatin, respectively. Then cells were plated in 6-well plates and incubated for 8–10 d. Then colonies were stained and counted. Results shown are representative of three independent experiments. Graphs provide quantification as a percentage of the nontreated wells. Each column and bar represents mean±s.d. of triplicate determinations. (E) 48 h after transfection, A2780 and SKOV3 cells were treated for 48 h with 1 μg/ml and 2 μg/ml cisplatin, respectively. After treatment, apoptosis was determined by flow cytometric analysis of Annexin V and PI staining. The right panel shows means±s.d. of three independent experiments. (F) 48 h after transfection, A2780 and SKOV3 cells were treated for 24 h with 2 μg/ml and 4 μg/ml cisplatin, respectively. After treatment, cell lysates were prepared, resolved by SDS-PAGE and subjected to immunoblotting analysis of FOXM1, EXO1, γH2AX, cleaved caspase-3 and β-actin. (G) A2780 and SKOV3 cells with or without silencing of EXO1 expression, were treated with 1 μg/ml and 2 μg/ml cisplatin for 1 h, respectively. γH2AX foci of A2780 and SKOV3 cells were quantified at different time point: 24, 48 and 72 h after cisplatin treatment. The percentage of γH2AX positive cells were plotted. Untreated cells were used as control.

ovarian cancer, and inhibition of FOXM1 would overcome cisplatin resistance. In the future, we would like to investigate whether cisplatin combined with FOXM1 inhibitor (thiostrepton or siomycin A) may be good choice to enhance therapeutic response. However, it has been reported that effective inhibition of FOXM1 by thiostrepton requires p53(wild-type or mutated)[12]. These results may indicate that an inhibitor of FOXM1 should be used individually according to p53 status in ovarian cancer.

In conclusion, we found that FOXM1 directly regulated EXO1 expression to promote the DNA repair pathway upon cisplatin treatment, and demonstrated that FOXM1 knockdown can enhance sensitivity of ovarian cancer cells to cisplatin. Thus, FOXM1 might be explored as a candidate of therapeutic target for modulating cisplatin sensitivity in ovarian cancer.

Supporting Information

Figure S1 FOXM1 expression at different time point after cisplatin treatment. A2780 and SKOV3 cells were treated with 1 µg/ml and 2 µg/ml cisplatin respectively, cell lysates were collected at the indicated time point and western blot analysis was performed to determine the protein expression levels of FOXM1, γH2AX and β-actin.

Figure S2 EXO1 expression after cisplatin treatment and FOXM1 knocking-down. (A) EXO1 protein in different cell lines was analyzed by western blotting, β-actin was used us endogenous control. (B) A2780 and SKOV3 were treated for the indicated time with 1 µg/ml and 2 µg/ml cisplatin, respectively. EXO1 were examined by western blot after treatment. (C) A2780

and SKOV3 cells with or without FOXM1 silencing were treated with the indicated concentration of cisplatin for 24 h. After treatment, cell lysates were prepared, resolved by SDS-PAGE and subjected to western blot analysis of EXO1 and β-actin. (D) A2780 and SKO3 cells were transfected with FOXM1 siRNA or negative control siRNA, 48 h later, cell cycle were analyzed by flow cytometry.

Author Contributions

Conceived and designed the experiments: JHZ WD. Performed the experiments: JHZ YFW YW. Analyzec the data: JHZ YFH. Contributed reagents/materials/analysis tools: XY LLC WWW TL. Wrote the paper: JHZ.

References

1. Jemal A, Bray F, Center MM, Ferlay J, Ward E, et al. (2011) Global cancer statistics. CA Cancer J Clin 61: 69–90.
2. Miller DS, Blessing JA, Krasner CN, Mannel RS, Hanjani P, et al. (2009) Phase II evaluation of pemetrexed in the treatment of recurrent or persistent platinum-resistant ovarian or primary peritoneal carcinoma: a study of the Gynecologic Oncology Group. J Clin Oncol 27: 2686–2691.
3. Jemal A, Siegel R, Ward E, Hao Y, Xu J, et al. (2009) Cancer statistics, 2009. CA Cancer J Clin 59: 225–249.
4. Laoukili J, Stahl M, Medema RH (2007) FoxM1: at the crossroads of ageing and cancer. Biochim Biophys Acta 1775: 92–102.
5. Pilarsky C, Wenzig M, Specht T, Saeger HD, Grutzmann R (2004) Identification and validation of commonly overexpressed genes in solid tumors by comparison of microarray data. Neoplasia 6: 744–750.
6. Kalin TV, Wang IC, Ackerson TJ, Major ML, Detrisac CJ, et al. (2006) Increased levels of the FoxM1 transcription factor accelerate development and progression of prostate carcinomas in both TRAMP and LADY transgenic mice. Cancer Res 66: 1712–1720.
7. Kim IM, Ackerson T, Ramakrishna S, Tretiakova M, Wang IC, et al. (2006) The Forkhead Box m1 transcription factor stimulates the proliferation of tumor cells during development of lung cancer. Cancer Res 66: 2153–2161.
8. Yoshida Y, Wang IC, Yoder HM, Davidson NO, Costa RH (2007) The forkhead box M1 transcription factor contributes to the development and growth of mouse colorectal cancer. Gastroenterology 132: 1420–1431.
9. Kalin TV, Ustiyan V, Kalinichenko VV (2011) Multiple faces of FoxM1 transcription factor: lessons from transgenic mouse models. Cell Cycle 10: 396–405.
10. Halasi M, Gartel AL (2013) FOX(M1) news—it is cancer. Mol Cancer Ther 12: 245–254.
11. The Cancer Genome Atlas Research Network (2011) Integrated genomic analyses of ovarian carcinoma. Nature 474: 609–615.
12. Lok GT, Chan DW, Liu VW, Hui WW, Leung TH, et al. (2011) Aberrant activation of ERK/FOXM1 signaling cascade triggers the cell migration/invasion in ovarian cancer cells. PLoS One 6: e23790.
13. Carr JR, Park HJ, Wang Z, Kiefer MM, Raychaudhuri P (2010) FoxM1 mediates resistance to herceptin and paclitaxel. Cancer Res 70: 5054–5063.
14. Kwok JM, Peck B, Monteiro LJ, Schwenen HD, Millour J, et al. (2010) FOXM1 confers acquired cisplatin resistance in breast cancer cells. Mol Cancer Res 8: 24–34.
15. Tran PT, Erdeniz N, Symington LS, Liskay RM (2004) EXO1-A multi-tasking eukaryotic nuclease. DNA Repair (Amst) 3: 1549–1559
16. Eccleston J, Yan C, Yuan K, Alt FW, Selsing E (2011) Mismatch repair proteins MSH2, MLH1, and EXO1 are important for class-switch recombination events occurring in B cells that lack nonhomologous end joining. J Immunol 186: 2336–2343.
17. Sperka T, Wang J, Rudolph KL (2012) DNA damage checkpoints in stem cells, ageing and cancer. Nat Rev Mol Cell Biol 13: 579–590
18. Bolderson E, Tomimatsu N, Richard DJ, Boucher D, Kumar R, et al. (2010) Phosphorylation of Exo1 modulates homologous recombination repair of DNA double-strand breaks. Nucleic Acids Res 38: 1821–1831
19. Halasi M, Gartel AL (2012) Suppression of FOXM1 sensitizes human cancer cells to cell death induced by DNA-damage. PLoS One 7: e31761.
20. Ziebarth AJ, Nowsheen S, Steg AD, Shah MM, Katre AA, et al. (2013) Endoglin (CD105) contributes to platinum resistance and is a target for tumor-specific therapy in epithelial ovarian cancer. Clin Cancer Res 19: 170–182.
21. Zhu H, Xia L, Zhang Y, Wang H, Xu W, et al. (2012) Activating transcription factor 4 confers a multidrug resistance phenotype to gastric cancer cells through transactivation of SIRT1 expression. PLoS One 7: e31431.
22. Olive PL (2011) Retention of gammaH2AX foci as an indication of lethal DNA damage. Radiother Oncol 101: 18–23.
23. Tan Y, Raychaudhuri P, Costa RH (2007) Chk2 mediates stabilization of the FoxM1 transcription factor to stimulate expression of DNA repair genes. Mol Cell Biol 27: 1007–1016.
24. Park YY, Jung SY, Jennings NB, Rodriguez-Aguayo C, Peng G, et al. (2012) FOXM1 mediates Dox resistance in breast cancer by enhancing DNA repair. Carcinogenesis 33: 1843–1853.
25. Korver W, Roose J, Clevers H (1997) The winged-helix transcription factor Trident is expressed in cycling cells. Nucleic Acids Res 25: 1715–1719.
26. Zhao R, Han C, Eisenhauer E, Kroger J, Zhao W, et al. (2014) DNA Damage-Binding Complex Recruits HDAC1 to Repress Bcl-2 Transcription in Human Ovarian Cancer Cells. Mol Cancer Res 12: 370–380.
27. Zhu Z, Chung WH, Shim EY, Lee SE, Ira G (2008) Sgs1 helicase and two nucleases Dna2 and Exo1 resect DNA double-strand break ends. Cell 134: 981–994.
28. Tomimatsu N, Mukherjee B, Deland K, Kurimasa A, Bolderson E, et al. (2012) Exo1 plays a major role in DNA end resection in humans and influences double-strand break repair and damage signaling decisions. DNA Repair (Amst) 11: 441–448.
29. Myatt SS, Lam EW (2008) Targeting FOXM1. Nat Rev Cancer 8: 242.
30. Costa RH (2005) FoxM1 dances with mitosis. Nat Cell Biol 7: 108–110.
31. Abraham RT (2001) Cell cycle checkpoint signaling through the ATM and ATR kinases. Genes Dev 15: 2177–2196.
32. Ciccia A, Elledge SJ (2010) The DNA damage response: making it safe to play with knives. Mol Cell 40: 179–204.
33. Siddik ZH (2003) Cisplatin: mode of cytotoxic action and molecular basis of resistance. Oncogene 22: 7265–7279.
34. Furuta T, Ueda T, Aune G, Sarasin A, Kraemer KH, et al. (2002) Transcription-coupled nucleotide excision repair as a determinant of cisplatin sensitivity of human cells. Cancer Res 62: 4899–4902.
35. Chang IY, Kim MH, Kim HB, Lee DY, Kim SH, et al. (2005) Small interfering RNA-induced suppression of ERCC1 enhances sensitivity of human cancer cells to cisplatin. Biochem Biophys Res Commun 327: 225–233.
36. Zhang N, Wu X, Yang L, Xiao F, Zhang H, et al. (2012) FoxM1 inhibition sensitizes resistant glioblastoma cells to temozolomide by downregulating the expression of DNA-repair gene Rad51. Clin Cancer Res 18: 5961–5971.
37. Galluzzi L, Senovilla L, Vitale I, Michels J, Martins I, et al. (2012) Molecular mechanisms of cisplatin resistance. Oncogene 31: 1869–1883.
38. dos Santos NA, Carvalho Rodrigues MA, Martins NM, dos Santos AC (2012) Cisplatin-induced nephrotoxicity and targets of nephroprotection: an update. Arch Toxicol 86: 1233–1250.
39. Ruggiero A, Trombatore G, Triarico S, Arena R, Ferrara P, et al. (2013) Platinum compounds in children with cancer: toxicity and clinical management. Anticancer Drugs 24: 1007–1019.
40. Carozzi VA, Marmiroli P, Cavaletti G (2010) The role of oxidative stress and anti-oxidant treatment in platinum-induced peripheral neurotoxicity. Curr Cancer Drug Targets 10: 670–682.

9

Precise Gene Modification Mediated by TALEN and Single-Stranded Oligodeoxynucleotides in Human Cells

Xiaoling Wang[1], Yingjia Wang[1,3], He Huang[3], Buyuan Chen[2,4], Xinji Chen[2,4], Jianda Hu[4], Tammy Chang[1], Ren-Jang Lin[2], Jiing-Kuan Yee[1]*

1 Department of Virology, Beckman Research Institute of City of Hope, Duarte, California, United States of America, 2 Department of Molecular and Cellular Biology, Beckman Research Institute of City of Hope, Duarte, California, United States of America, 3 Bone Marrow Transplantation Center, The First Affiliated Hospital, Zhejiang University, Hangzhou, Zhejiang, China, 4 Department of Hematology, Union Hospital of Fujian Medical University, Fuzhou, Fujian, China

Abstract

The development of human embryonic stem cells (ESCs) and induced pluripotent stem cells (iPSCs) facilitates *in vitro* studies of human disease mechanisms, speeds up the process of drug screening, and raises the feasibility of using cell replacement therapy in clinics. However, the study of genotype-phenotype relationships in ESCs or iPSCs is hampered by the low efficiency of site-specific gene editing. Transcription activator-like effector nucleases (TALENs) spurred interest due to the ease of assembly, high efficiency and faithful gene targeting. In this study, we optimized the TALEN design to maximize its genomic cutting efficiency. We showed that using optimized TALENs in conjunction with single-strand oligodeoxynucleotide (ssODN) allowed efficient gene editing in human cells. Gene mutations and gene deletions for up to 7.8 kb can be accomplished at high efficiencies. We established human tumor cell lines and H9 ESC lines with homozygous deletion of the microRNA-21 (miR-21) gene and miR-9-2 gene. These cell lines provide a robust platform to dissect the roles these genes play during cell differentiation and tumorigenesis. We also observed that the endogenous homologous chromosome can serve as a donor template for gene editing. Overall, our studies demonstrate the versatility of using ssODN and TALEN to establish genetically modified cells for research and therapeutic application.

Editor: Linzhao Cheng, Johns Hopkins Univ. School of Medicine, United States of America

Funding: This work is supported by grant RB3-02161 from California Institute of Regenerative Medicine to JKY, grants from Nesvig Foundation and Beckman Research Institute Excellence Award to RJL. YJW was supported by grants from National Natural Science Foundation of China, Zhejiang Provincial Natural Science Foundation of China, Zhejiang Provincial Major Science and Technology Project and China Scholarship Council. BC and XC were supported in part by the P.R.C. National and Fujian Provincial Key Clinical Specialty Discipline Construction Program. The funders had no role in study design, data collection and analysis, decision to publish, or preparation of the manuscript.

Competing Interests: The authors have declared that no competing interests exist.

* E-mail: JYee@coh.org

Introduction

Developments in site-specific gene editing technologies such as zinc finger nucleases (ZFNs), transcription activator-like effector nucleases (TALENs) and clustered regularly interspaced short palindromic repeats (CRISPRs) have greatly facilitated disease modeling in animals and in pluripotent stem cells [1–8]. Among these technologies, CRISPRs have spurred great interest due to the ease of construction. However, recent findings about the off-target effects of CRISPRs confound their wide-spread application [9-11]. In contrast, TALENs exhibit high targeting specificity with little off-target effect except in one study [8,12,13]. Transcription activator-like effectors (TALEs) are important virulence factors first identified in plant pathogenic bacteria *Xanthomonas spp.*[5,14,15]. They directly bind to DNA via a central domain of tandem repeats and function as transcriptional activators [16,17]. Each repeat consists of a 33- to 35- amino acid motif. The amino acid sequences of the repeats are nearly identical except for residues 12 and 13, the so-called repeat variable diresidues (RVD), which determine the DNA targeting specificity with one RVD targeting one nucleotide [18]. This relationship allows the engineering of specific DNA binding domains by assembling repeats with the appropriate RVDs. TALENs are derived from fusing the engineered TALE DNA binding domain to the Fok1 nuclease domain, which generates double-strand DNA breaks (DSBs) when two Fok1 nucleases dimerize [8,19,20].

Site-specific gene editing is based mainly on homology-directed recombination (HDR) between a gene locus and an exogenous DNA fragment. The efficiency of HDR in human cells is strongly stimulated by DSBs in the genome created by site-specific nucleases [21]. Non-homologous end joining (NHEJ) and HDR represent two major pathways for repairing DSB. NHEJ is error prone and can introduce mutations at the site of DSB to affect the expression of a protein coding-gene or microRNA as demonstrated in several model systems, including zebrafish, *Xenopus*, pig, mouse, and rat [4,22–31]. In contrast, HDR is largely error-free and is typically accomplished with a sister chromatid, a homologous chromosome, or an exogenously provided donor template containing homology arms flanking the DSB [32]. However, construction of the donor template, the selection of clones with the desired gene modification, and subsequent removal of the selection marker constitute a lengthy process which unavoidably increases the stress and the risk of generating additional genome instability in human embryonic stem cells (ESCs) or induced pluripotent stem cells (iPSCs). Previous studies have demonstrated that single-strand oligodeoxynucleotide (ssODN) can be used as a template to generate point mutations and short sequence insertions in human cells and animal models [4,22,27]. In this study, we optimized the TALEN design to maximize its genomic cutting efficiency. We showed that using optimized TALENs in conjunction with ssODN as donor templates for HDR could mediate efficient gene editing in human cells. Gene mutations and gene deletions for up to 7.8 kb were accomplished at high efficiencies. Using this approach, we successfully established human tumor cell lines and H9 ESC lines with homozygous deletion of the microRNA-21 (miR-21) gene and miR-9-2 gene. These cell lines provide a robust platform to dissect the roles these genes play during cell differentiation and tumorigenesis. Our study also showed that homologous chromosome could serve as a donor template for gene editing. Taken together, our data demonstrates the versatility of using ssODN and TALEN to establish gene-edited human cell lines for research and therapeutic application.

Materials and Methods

Cell culture

H9 cells were obtained from National Stem Cell Bank (Madison, WI) and cultured on irradiated mouse embryonic fibroblasts (MEF) (GlobalStem, Inc., Rockville, Maryland). H9 cells were grown in ESC medium containing α-MEM/F12 supplemented with 20% knockout serum replacement, 0.1 mM nonessential amino acids, 0.1 mM 2-mercaptoethanol, and 1 mM L-glutamine. Basic fibroblast growth factor (bFGF) was added to a final concentration of 4 ng/ml prior to medium change. The culture medium was changed daily. HEK293T cells (CRL 3216, ATCC, Manassas,VA) were cultured in DMEM medium supplemented with 10% FBS, 2 mM L-glutamine, 100 U/ml penicillin and 100 mg/ml streptomycin. The K562 cell line (CCL 243, ATCC, Manassas,VA) was maintained in RPMI 1640 medium complemented with 10% FBS and 2 mM L-glutamine. The cells were cultured at 37°C in a humidified chamber with 5% CO_2 in air, and passaged 1:10 twice a week.

TALEN design and construction

TAL Effector -Nucleotide Targeter 2.0 (https://tale-nt.cac. cornell.edu/) was used to find TALEN target sites [33]. Golden Gate TALEN and TAL Effector Kit from Addgene were used for TALEN repeats assembly [5].

TALEN cutting efficiency evaluation

HEK293T cells were plated at 40% confluence in 48-well plates and were transfected with 0.2 μg of each TALEN plasmid using Lipofectamine 2000. Forty eight hours after transfection, genomic DNA was extracted with Epicentre QuickExtract solution (Epicentre Biotechnologies, Madison, WI) Approximately 8000 genome equivalents were used as input for PCR. TALEN activity was assayed via Surveyor nuclease following the manufacturer's protocol (Transgenomic, Omaha, NE). Image J was used to quantify the percent gene modification by measuring the intensity of bands separated by agarose gel post digestion. The following formula was used to calculate the percentage of gene modification: % gene modification $= 100 \times [1-(1-\text{fraction cleaved})^{1/2}]$; % cutting efficiency (NHEJ) $= 100 \times$ sum of the cleavage product peak/(cleavage product+ parent peak). Primers used for monitoring gene modification at miR-9, miR-21, TAT intron 3, TAT exon 12 and SF3b1 locus were as follows: M9F2 (5′- tcctggacgaccactcttcggt-3′) and M9R2 (5′- gcagctgcaacaaccctctca-3′) for miR-9, TATF2 (5′-tggggacactactgaggggctg-3′) and TATR2 (5′-tcccgagacccggttcccaa-3′) for TAT intron 3, TATF3(5′-gcatcccagt-

catgggagctgaat-3′) and TATR3 (5′-acctgcctggagagagcgtgt-3′), Surveyor L1 (5′-tggggttcgatcttaacagg-3′)and Surveyor R1 (5′-ctgcattgtgggttttgaaa-3′)for miR-21 and for SF3B1. The amplification was carried out with Hotstar Taq (Qiagen, Valencia, CA), using the following cycling conditions: 95°C for 15 min for initial denaturation; 35 cycles of 94°C for 30 s, 60°C for 30 s and 72°C for 30 s; and a final extension at 72°C for 5 min. Statistical significance was calculated using a paired Student's t test.

ssODN mediated gene editing

The sequence of ssODN used in the TAT point mutation, 7.8 kb deletion, miR-21 and miR-9 gene modification study is as follows: 5′-ataatggctatgccccatccatcggtaagctcctcctgagacccatacctggatcctgccaaatctttagtgctcttataacaggactaaatgtctagc-3′, 5′-ataatggctatgccccat ccatcggtaagctcctcctgagactccatacctggatcctgccaaatctttagtgctcttataacaggactaaatgtctagc-3′, 5′- accatcgtgacatctccatggctgtaccaccttgtcggatcccagcatcattgtttataatcagaaactctggtccttct-3′, and 5′-aaggatcaggacctggagtctggcaagaggaagacagaggatccttcaagatcgccggggagcgtgtga gaatgaaagac-3′. 125 ng of each TALEN plasmid and 2.5 μl 1 μM ssODN were transfected into HEK293T cells using Lipofectamine 2000. Limiting dilution was performed at the following day. Ten days later, genomic DNA was extracted for genotyping using QuickExtract solution. TAT gene mutant clones were first screened with mutation-specific PCR primers: TATR2 & TATBAMF3 (5′-cctgagactccatacctggatc-3′). Genotypes were further confirmed by PCR with primers TATF2 and TATR2 followed by a BamHI digestion. The two expected DNA fragments were 274 bp and 140 bp. TAT, miR-21 and miR-9 deletion mutation clones were screened via deletion PCR assay with primersTATF2 and TATR3, Surveyor L1 and R1, M9F2 and M9R2. The amplification was carried out with JumpStart Taq (Sigma, St. Louis, MO), using the following cycling conditions: 94°C for 1 min for initial denaturation; 35 cycles of 94°C for 30 s, 58°C for 30 s and 72°C for 30 s; and a final extension at 72°C for 5 min. The wild-type band for miR-21 was 430 bp and the targeted deletion resulted in a 310 bp band. A heterozygous clone, #84 was transfected and screened using the methods described above. The homozygous mutation was confirmed by digesting the PCR product with BamHI, which gave rise to 170 and 140 bp fragments.

Electroporation, isolation of targeted clonal cell population and neural differentiation

The K562 cells were suspended in RPMI 1640 without FBS or antibiotics, at a concentration of 10^7 cells per ml. A volume of 0.4 ml was transferred to a sterile electroporation cuvette (Bio-Rad Gene Pulser cuvette, 0.4 cm), and kept at room temperature for 15 min in presence of 16 μg of pPB-e-GFP plasmid to analyze the efficiency of transfection to analyze the efficiency of electroporation, or 20 μg each TALEN pair and 250 nM ssODN. Electroporation was performed with a Bio-Rad Gene Pulser Transfection Apparatus (350 V, 500 μF).

Before electroporation, H9 cells were grown in feeder-free adherent culture in chemically defined mTeSR1 (STEMCELL Technologies, Vancouver, Canada) on plates coated with Matrigel (BD Bioscience) for one generation. The cells were pretreated with 10 μM Rock Inhibitor for 2 hours and dissociated into a single cell suspension with 1 mg/ml Accutase (Invitrogen). Two million cells were mixed with 1 μg of each TALEN plasmid, 1.5 μg GFP plasmid and 2 μg ssODN, and then electroporated with program B-016 using Nucleofector (Lonza AG). Cells were cultured in mTeSR1 supplemented with 10 μM Rock Inhibitor for 48 hours and dissociated by Accutase. GFP-positive cells were collected by FACS (FACS Aria II; BD Biosciences) and replated on irradiated

MEF feeder cells at 1000 cells per well. Ten days after sorting, single colonies were recovered. Half of each colony was manually picked and transferred into QuickExtract DNA extract solution (Epicentre). DNA extractions were done according to manufacturer's protocol. PCR screening was conducted as mentioned above. Neural differentiation was performed following the protocols of Hu et al [34].

Real-time PCR

To test the expression of miR-21 and miR-9, total RNA was isolated using mirVana microRNA extraction kit (Life Technology, Carlsbad, CA). 0.5 μg of total RNA was used for reverse transcription (RT) with the miScript II RT kit (Qiagen, Hercules, CA). miScript primer assay and precursor assay were used for miR-21 and miR-9 quantification. Quantitative PCR was carried out with the miScript SYBR PCR kit (Qiagen, Hercules, CA). Haploid copy number variation in miR-9-2 locus was calculated as previously described [35]. qPCR was conducted in triplicate in a 20 ul reaction using the iQ SYBR Green Supermix and iQ5 multicolor real-time detection system (Biorad, Hercules, CA). Primers used were as follows: M9F5 (5′- ggaatcttaagcgcggcaag -3′) and M9R5 (5′- aacaactcgcttcccacaca-3′), M9F6 (5′-ggggagcgtgt-gagaatgaa-3′) and M9R6 (5′-tttctctcatcccacctttaatca-3′). Wild type H9 cells were used as a calibrator sample and GAPDH was used as a reference gene with primers: GAPDHF1 (5′- gcaaggtcatccct-gagctg -3′) and GAPDHR1(5′- ggcaggttttctagacggc -3′). All reactions were run at 40 cycles using standard condition following manufacturer's protocol. Haploid copy number was calculated based on the observed Ct values: $2^{-\Delta\Delta Ct} = (1+E)^{-\Delta Ctgene} / (1+E)^{-\Delta Ctreferencegene}$. E = efficiency of the PCR reaction (set at default value 0.95), ΔCt_{gene} = difference in the Ct value between test sample and calibrator sample. $\Delta Ct_{referencegene}$ = difference in the Ct value between test sample and the calibrator sample for reference gene.

Immunofluorescence

For immunofluorescence staining, cells were fixed in 4% paraformaldehyde for 10 min at room temperature. After PBS washing, cells were permeabilized with 0.3% Triton X-100 for 45 min at room temperature. After removal of the Triton X-100 solution, cells were washed with PBS and stained at 4°C overnight with primary antibodies at appropriate dilutions. Primary antibodies used include Tra-1-81 (1:200, eBioscience, San Diego, CA), Tra-1-60 (1:100, Stemgent, Cambridge, MA), Oct4 (1:100, Stemgent, Cambridge, MA), Sox2 (1:100, Neuromics, Minneapolis, MN), β III-tubulin (1:2000, Covance, Princeton, NJ), HB9 (1:10, Hybridoma Bank, Iowa City, Iowa). Cells were stained at room temperature with the secondary antibody for 2 hours at 1:800 dilution, including Cy3-conjugated goat anti-rabbit IgG (Chemicon, Temecula, CA) or Cy3-conjugated rabbit anti-mouse IgG antibody (Millipore). Nuclei were stained with DAPI (Life Technology, Carlsbad, CA) at a concentration of 1 μg/ml.

Results

Optimization of TALEN design

We generated multiple TALEN pairs specific for different loci in the human genome (Table 1). Since a defined rule for TALEN design remains unclear, we arbitrarily searched for the TALEN target site preceded by a T, a feature identified within naturally occurring TALE recognition sites [36,37]. We designed our TALENs with their target sites ranging between 15 and 30 bases (Table 1). The spacer between the two TALEN binding sites ranged from 15 to 29 bases. With the 22 TALEN pairs specific for different genes, we found that TALEN pairs with spacers larger than 20 bases generally were less efficient in cutting compared to those with smaller spacers (Table 1 and Figure S1). To exclude the possibility that the difference in cutting efficiency is due to the chromatin position effect, we designed three additional 5′ TALENs and six 3′ TALENs flanking the same cutting site in the miR-9-2 gene (Figure 1A). Cross matching individual TALENs generated 18 additional TALEN pairs with variable spacer lengths. We observed that TALEN pairs with spacer length of 14-20 bases were more effective than others (Figure1B and 1C). Together, data from these 40 TALEN pairs demonstrated that a spacer length of 14-20 bases was optimal for TALEN DNA cutting (Figure 1D). To further improve the TALEN cutting efficiency, we tested the GoldyTALEN scaffold which carried N- and C-terminal truncations of the native TALE protein [23]. Consistent with previous publications [7,8,22,23], the GoldyTALEN scaffold enhanced gene cutting at the TAT and miR-9-2 loci relative to the native TALEN scaffold (Figure 1E). Our subsequent studies were therefore based on the use of the GoldyTALEN scaffold for TALEN construction.

TALEN-mediated gene editing with ssODN in human cell lines

We sought to use ssODN instead of a donor plasmid for gene editing to avoid the lengthy process of drug selection and subsequent removal of the selectable marker. We used a TALEN pair, Tat-7, which cut at intron 3 of the tyrosine aminotransferase (TAT) gene (Table 1 and Figure 2A). We synthesized a 99-base ssODN with a BamHI site flanked by 50- and 46-base homology arms corresponding to the sequences 5′ and 3′ of Tat-7 TALEN cutting site (Figure 2A). K562 cells were electroporated with the Tat-7 expression plasmids and the ssODN. PCR amplification of the TAT locus in individual clones followed by BamHI digestion showed that out of 150 randomly picked clones, 4 (2.7%) carried ssODN mediated HDR, which were further confirmed by sequencing (Figure 2B, 2C). This represents an underestimation of the homologous recombination efficiency since the transfection efficiency in K562 cells in around 50%. Our results suggest that ssODN is well-suited for generating point mutations at the DSB created by TALEN.

Generating deletion is of great interest for loss-of-function studies. To determine whether ssODN can mediate small gene deletions, a BamHI-containing ssODN sharing 38- and 40-base sequence homology flanking the stem-loop structure of the miR-21 gene was synthesized (Figure 3A). Successful gene editing with the ssODN is expected to create a 120-bp deletion that removes the entire stem-loop structure of the miR-21gene and silences its expression. The M21-3 TALEN expression plasmids and the ssODN were co-transfected into HEK293T cells and PCR analysis of individual clones showed that 13 out of 110 clones (11.8%) exhibited a PCR product with reduced fragment size (Figure 3B). Sequence analysis confirmed the expected deletion in these clones with clone 103 containing a triallelic knockout of the miR-21 gene (Table 2).

To obtain more homozygous miR-21 knockout clones, we chose clone 84 to carry out a second round of gene knockout. This clone had one allele derived from ssODN-mediated HDR and the other derived from a NHEJ-mediated 18-bp deletion (Table 2). Since the 18-bp deletion abolished the binding of the original TALEN pair M21-3, we adopted a different TALEN pair, M21-1, for knocking out the remaining allele (Figure 3A). We identified 6 homozygous knockout clones out of 60 clones screened (10%) (Table 2 and Figure 3C). The level of miR-21 in these clones was determined by RT-PCR and the result showed that miR-21

A

```
CTTCATAAAGCTAGAT (M9-5-1)
   CATAAAGCTAGATAAC  (M9-5-2)
      AAAGCTAGATAACCGA (M9-5-3)
CTTCATAAAGCTAGATAACCGAAAGTAAAAACTCCTTCAAGATCGCCGGGGAGCGTGTGAGAATG
                              CTCCTTCAAGATCGCCGGGG (M9-3-1)
                                CCTTCAAGATCGCCGGGG (M9-3-2)
                                  TTCAAGATCGCCGGGG (M9-3-3)
                                    CAAGATCGCCGGGG (M9-3-4)
                                        CGCCGGGGAGCGTGTG (M9-3-5)
                                          CGGGGAGCGTGTGAGA (M9-3-6)
```

B

TALEN spacer length (bp)

	M9-5-1	M9-5-2	M9-5-3
M9-3-1	15	12	9
M9-3-2	17	14	11
M9-3-3	19	16	13
M9-3-4	21	18	15
M9-3-5	27	24	21
M9-3-6	30	27	24

C

Percent NHEJ (%)

	M9-5-1	M9-5-2	M9-5-3
M9-3-1	5.34	0.00	0.00
M9-3-2	7.91	7.35	0.00
M9-3-3	5.52	11.26	1.16
M9-3-4	0.93	5.56	3.94
M9-3-5	0.00	0.00	0.00
M9-3-6	0.00	0.00	0.00

D

E

% NHEJ   14.6 7.7   7.8 5   16.4 13.8

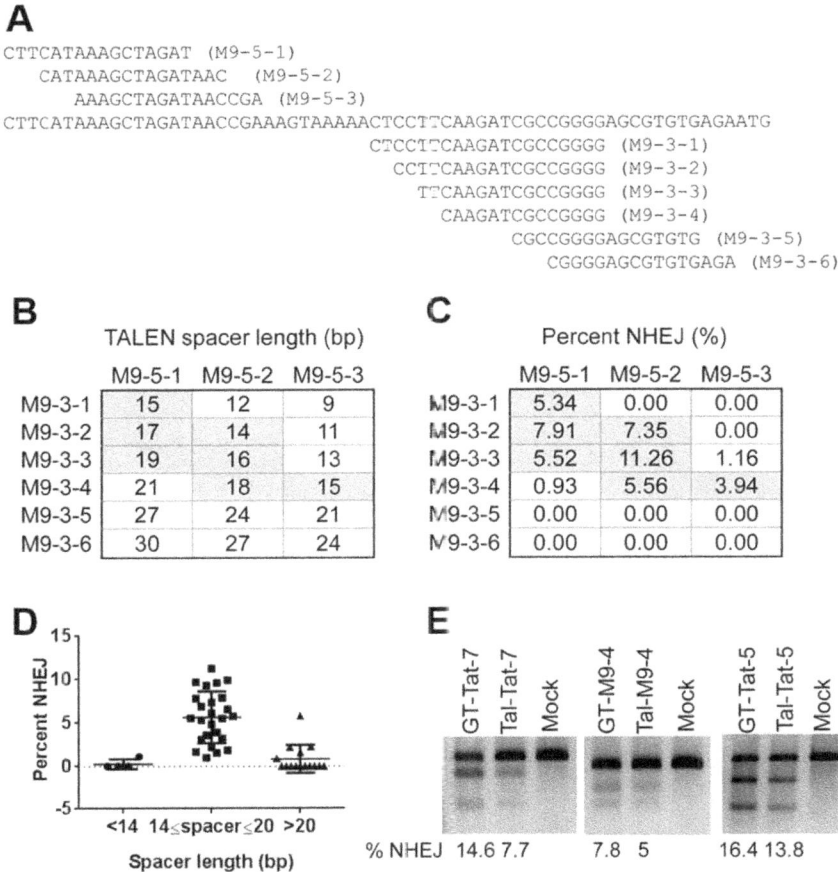

Figure 1. Optimization of TALEN design. (A) Target sequences of TALENs in the miR-9-2 locus. Target sequences for the three 5' TALENs and six 3' TALENs were shown. (B) Spacer lengths of the 18 TALEN pair combinations. (C) Percentage of NHEJ induced by the 18 TALEN pair combinations. Each TALEN pair shown in (B) was transfected into HEK293T cells and the Surveyor assay was carried out 72 h later. (D) Target cutting efficiencies of 40 TALEN pairs with various spacer lengths. Bar: average ± standard deviation, $p<0.05$, two tailed p value, student's T test. (E) Increased cutting efficiencies with the GoldyTALEN scaffold. Indicated TALEN pairs were transfected into HEK293T cells and NHEJ was measured by the Surveyor assay 72 hours later. GT: Goldy TALEN. Tal: wild-type TALEN.

expression was reduced in the heterozygous clones and completely silent in the homozygous knockout clones (Figure 3D), confirming the complete knockout of all three miR-21 alleles from HEK293T cells.

A TALEN-mediated large genomic deletion in the TAT locus

Introduction of a small deletion or frame-shift mutation may not be sufficient to completely inactivate the gene function since RNA splicing or alternate transcription start sites can skip the deletion or mutation and produce a protein with partial function. Deletion of more than two critical exons or even the entire gene may be required to completely abolish the gene function. To evaluate whether ssODN could induce large genomic deletions, we synthesized a BamHI-containing ssODN that shared sequence homology with intron 3 and exon 12 of the TAT gene (Figure 4A). HDR mediated by this ssODN was expected to remove a 7.8-kb genomic fragment spanning the majority of the TAT gene. Initially, we screened individual HEK293T clones transfected by the TALEN pair Tat-7 and the ssODN with primer pair L1/R2 located outside of the deleted region (Figure 4A) We found that none of the 96 clones screened showed the expected deletion (data not shown). We then sought to test whether applying two TALEN

pairs, Tat-5 and Tat-7 (Figure 4A), could cooperatively induce the deletion. HEK293T cells were transiently transfected with the TALEN pairs and the ssODN. PCR was used to semi-quantify the overall deletion events in pooled cells. We observed that deletions induced by a single TALEN pair and the ssODN were detectable but the signal was weak (Figure 4B). Cells treated with the two TALEN pairs exhibited a much stronger PCR band both with and without the ssODN (Figure 4B). Screening individual clones showed that 24 out of 59 clones (40.7%) transfected by the two TALEN pairs and the ssODN exhibited a 729-bp PCR fragment expected from the deletion of the 7.8-kb genomic fragment (Figure 4C, upper panel). Out of these 24 positive clones, the PCR product from 12 clones (20.4%) was cut by BamHI into the expected 447- and 282-bp fragments (Figure 4D), indicating the presence of at least one HDR-derived allele in these clones. The other 12 clones that could not be cut by BamHI were most likely derived from NHEJ (Figure 4C and D). These observations were further confirmed by cloning and sequencing the PCR products (data not shown). We then used L1 and R1, a primer positioned within the deleted region, to screen for the presence of the wild-type allele among these clones. Out of the 12 clones with HDR-mediated deletion, 3 clones (5.1%) failed to show the expected 414 bp wild-type band (Figure 4C, lower panel), suggesting

Table 1. Summary of the design and cutting efficiency of TALEN pairs.

Gene	Name	Spacer (nt)	%NHEJ	TALEN-A sequence	TALEN-B sequence	
miR-9-2	M9-1	15	1	CCTGGACGACCACTCT	GCCAGACTCCAGGTCCTGATCCT	
	M9-2	29	2.29	ATCTAGCTGTATGAGT	CCCCGGCGATCTTGAAGGAGTTTTTACTTT	
	M9-3	22	5.82	CTTCATAAAGCTAGAT	CTCACACGCTCCCCGGCGATCTT	
	M9-4	19	9.6	CTTCATAAAGCTAGAT	CCCCGGCGATCTTGAA	X
	M9-5	16	3.24	GGCAAGAGGAAGACAG	AGATAACCAAAGATAA	
TAT	Tat-1	19	6.13	GTGAGCAGCACTACCAT	AGGAGTGTGATAAAT	
	Tat-2	16	5.78	CTGTGAGCAGCACTACCAT	AGGAGGAGTGTGATAAAT	
	Tat-3	22	0	GTGAGCAGCACTACCAT	AGTGTGATAAATAGGCCTGC	
	Tat-4	19	6.91	CTGTGAGCAGCACTACCAT	AGGAGTGTGATAAAT	
	Tat-5	16	9.95	GTGAGCAGCACTACCAT	AGGAGGAGTGTGATAAAT	X
	Tat-6	22	0	CTGTGAGCAGCACTACCAT	AGTGTGATAAATAGGCCTGC	
	Tat-7	18	4.85	CCTGAGACTCCATACCT	AGTGCTCTTATAACAGG	X
	Tat-8	29	0	GGCTATGCCCCATCCATCGGT	ACTGCCAAATCTTTAGTGCTCTTAT	
	Tat-9	21	0	CCATCGGTAAGCTCCT	ACTGCCAAATCTTTAGTGCTCTTAT	
miR-21	M21-1	16	3.57	CATGGCTGTACCACCT	AGACTGATGTTGACTG	
	M21-3	16	7.83	CCATATCCAATGTTCT	AGCATCATTGTTTAT	X
Sf3b1	Sf-1	19	2.24	AGTTAAAACCTGTGTTT	ATGAGCAGCAGAAAGTTCGG	
	Sf-2	23	1.64	ATTATCTGCTGACAGGCTAT	ATTTTGTTTAATGTGAACAT	
	Sf-3	23	0	AGGACAGCTGTCCTAAAAT	AAATGGAAAGGCATAGCTCT	
	Sf-4	15	1.87	ATGGTATCGAATCTT	AGCCTTTATGGAAGGGT	
	Sf-5	16	6.57	GTTTGGTTTTGTAGGT	AGAAAGTTCGGACC	
	Sf-6	16	9.67	AGTTAAAACCTGTGTT	GTGGATGAGCAGCAG	

TALENs were assembled according to the protocol described by Cermak *et al* [1]. The target sequences of each TALEN pairs (TALEN-A and -B) are listed. Cutting efficiency for each TALEN pair was measured using the Surveyor endonuclease. Percentage NHEJ is indicated. The pairs used for gene editing in this study are indicated with an "X" in the last column. TAT: tyrosine aminotransferase; Sf3b1: Splicing factor 3B subunit 1

homozygous deletion of the TAT gene in these clones. Thus, simultaneous administration of two TALEN pairs can efficiently remove a large genomic sequence between the two TALEN target sites and rejoin the genomic ends together. Although generating two distant cleavages in cis without the ssODN seems sufficient to create a relatively large deletion in the genome (Figure 4B), the presence of the ssODN can mediate the deletion precisely at the single nucleotide level.

TALEN-mediated deletion of the miR-9-2 gene in the human H9 ESC line

We next tested TALEN and ssODN mediated gene deletion in human ESC line. MiR-9 regulates neurogenesis through its action on the proliferation, migration and differentiation of neural progenitor cells [38-43]. Three genes, miR-9-1, miR-9-2 and miR-9-3 located on chromosome 1, 5, 15, respectively, encode miR-9 [44]. Although mature miR-9 from the three genes is identical in sequence, the precursor RNA sequences are different. It was reported that the mature miR-9 in human ESC-derived neuroprogenitors was mostly expressed from the miR-9-2 gene [40]. To determine the role miR-9-2 plays in ESC neuronal differentiation, we designed an ssODN that shared 40 bp and 39 bp sequence homology flanking the stem-loop structure of miR-9-2 gene (Figure 5A). HDR mediated by this ssODN was expected to delete the entire stem-loop structure of the miR-9-2 gene and silence its expression. We first tested this ssODN by co-transfecting HEK293T cells with a TALEN pair, M9-3

(Figure 5A), and the ssODN followed by random clone isolation. Out of 96 clones screened, 5 clones (5.2%) carried the expected 89-bp deletion mediated by HDR (data not shown). We then repeated the same procedure in H9 cells with a GFP expression plasmid included in the nucleofection mix to enrich for the transfected cells via cell sorting. To estimate the overall gene modification rate, we sequenced the miR-9-2 locus in 90 randomly picked H9 clones (clone 2101-2190). We found that 15 clones (16.7%) contained NHEJ-mediated mutations in at least one miR-9-2 allele and 5 of them contained mutations in both alleles (Table S1), suggesting efficient cutting by M9-3 in H9 cells. Based on genomic PCR screening, we identified two clones (clones 2079 and 2247) out of 300 clones (0.67%) carrying HDR-mediated deletion, which was further confirmed by *BamH*I digestion of the PCR product and sequencing (Figure 5B and Table S2). These clones not only retained their self-renewal capacity, but also maintained the ability to differentiate into neurons (Figure 5C, D). In addition to the expected ssODN-mediated deletion, clone 2247 had a NHEJ-mediated 13-bp deletion in one allele (Table S2). This deletion removed the complementary strand of the entire miR-9 seed sequence and presumably would disrupt proper miR-9-2 processing and impair its expression. We measured the expression of mature miR-9 in H9 and clone 2247 before and after neuronal differentiation. As expected, the level of mature miR-9 remained extremely low both in undifferentiated H9 cells and clone 2247 (Figure 5E, Day 0) [40]. Upon differentiation, the level of mature miR-9 was elevated to more than 1000 fold in H9 cells and

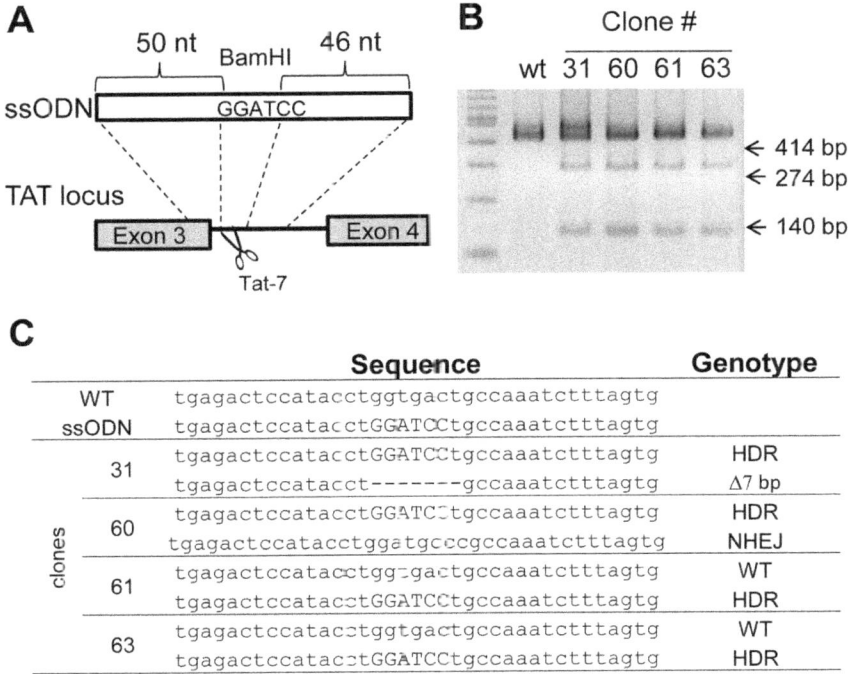

Figure 2. Induction of point mutations in the tyrosine aminotransferase (TAT) gene with ssODN and TALEN. (A) Schematic representation of the TALEN target region in the TAT gene and the ssODN used for HDR. (B) Analysis of randomly picked K562 clones transfected with the TALEN pair and ssODN. Individual clones were isolated by limiting dilution and subjected to genomic PCR using a primer pair flanking the TALEN cutting site. Gene edited clones were identified by BamH1 digestion that generated 274 and 140 bp fragments. (C) Sequence analysis of the TAT locus in the gene-edited clones. The PCR product from individual clones was TA cloned and subjected to sequencing analysis. HDR denotes ssODN-mediated homologous recombination. "Δ" denotes deletion. The deletion of the 7 bp in one of the TAT alleles in clone 31 is also shown.

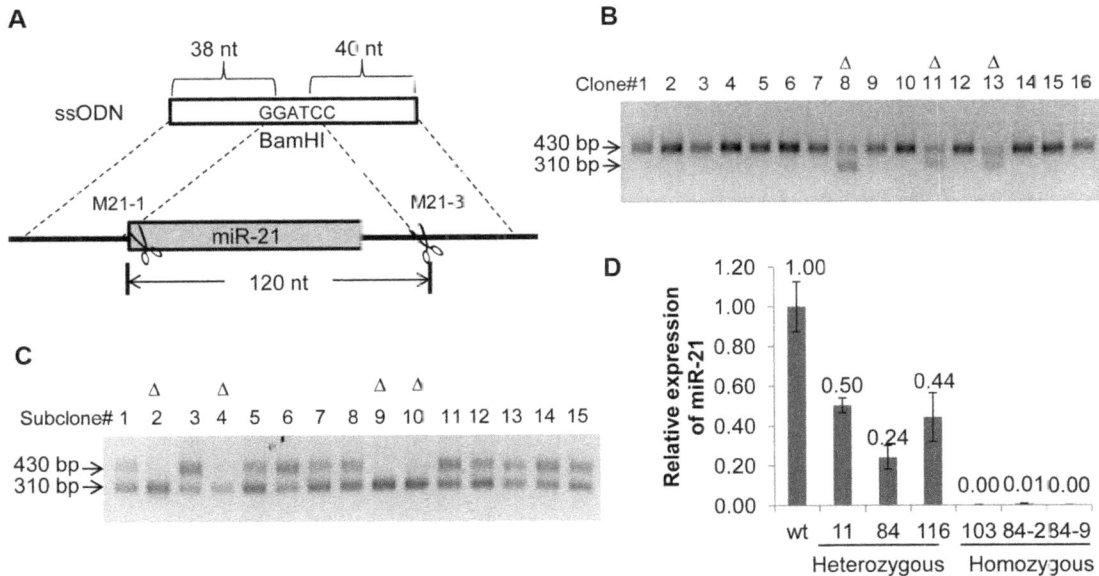

Figure 3. TALEN and ssODN-mediated deletion of the stem-loop structure in the miR-21 locus. (A) Schematic representation of the ssODN and its target in the miR-21 locus. The shaded box denotes the stem-loop structure of the miR-21 gene. The TALEN cutting site and the size of the ssODN-mediated deletion are indicated. (B) Representative picture of PCR screening of individual clones with gene editing in the miR-21 locus. HEK293T cells were transfected by the ssODN and M21-3. Gene edited clones were screened with a pair of PCR primer flanking the TALEN cutting site in the miR-21 gene. Positive clones exhibiting a 120-bp shorter PCR fragment are indicated by "Δ". (C) Representative picture of PCR screening of complete miR-21 knockout clones. Clone 84 was transfected by the ssODN and M21-1, and individual clones were screened as described in b. Clones with homozygous deletion exhibit only a single PCR fragment which is 120-bp shorter than the wild-type fragment. Potential miR-21 homozygous knockouts are indicated by "Δ". (D) Analysis of miR-21 expression in gene edited HEK293T clones. Total RNA from the clones indicated was isolated and subjected to qRT-PCR to assess the level of the mature miR-21 relative to that from parental HEK293T cells (wt). $p < 0.05$.

Table 2. Sequence analysis of selected miR-21 clones used for quantitative RT-PCR (qRT-PCR) studies.

Clone No.	Sequence	Genotype
	ACATCTCCATGGCTGTACCACCTTGTCGG. 106 nt.CATTTAAACATTACCCAGCATCA	wild type
	ACATCTCCATGGCTGTACCACCTTGTCGGATCCCAGCATCA	ssODN
	Selected heterozygous clones	
11	ACATCTCCATGGCTGTACCACCTTGTCGGATCCCAGCATCATTGT	HDR
	ACATCTCCATGGCTGTACCACCTTGTCGG. 94 nt. CATTTAAACATTACCCAGCATCA	Δ 12 bp
	ACATCTCCATGGCTGTACCACCTTGTCGG. 106 nt.CATTTAAACATTACCCAGCATCA	WT
84	ACATCTCCATGGCTGTACCACCTTGTCGGATCCCAGCATCATTGT	HDR
	ACATCTCCATGGCTGTACCACCTTGTCGG. 106 nt. CAT-----------------CA	Δ 18 bp
116	ACATCTCCATGGCTGTACCACCTTGTCGGATCCCAGCATCATTGT	HDR
	ACATCTCCATGGCTGTACCACCTTGTCGG. 106 nt.CATTTAA---TTACCCAGCATCA	Δ 3 bp
	Knockout clones	
103	ACATCTCCATGGCTGTACCACCTTGTCGGATCCCAGCATCATTGT	HDR
	ACA------------------------//---------------CAGCATCA	Δ 150 bp
84-2	ACATCTCCATGGCTGTACCACCTTGTCGGATCCCAGCATCATTGT	HDR
84-4	ACATCTCCATGGCTGTACCACCTTGTCGGATCCCAGCATCATTGT	HDR
84-9	ACATCTCCATGGCTGTACCACCTTGTCGGATCCCAGCATCATTGT	HDR
84-10	ACATCTCCATGGCTGTACCACCTTGTCGGATCCCAGCATCATTGT	HDR
84-27	ACATCTCCATGGCTGTACCACCTTGTCGGATCCCAGCATCATTGT	HDR
84-48	ACATCTCCATGGCTGTACCACCTTGTCGGATCCCAGCATCATTGT	HDR

Genomic PCR of individual miR-21 clones was carried out and the PCR products were TA cloned and sequenced. The sequence of the ssODN and wild-type cells is shown on top of the table. HDR denotes homology directed recombination. "Δ" denotes deletion which is indicated by a dished line.

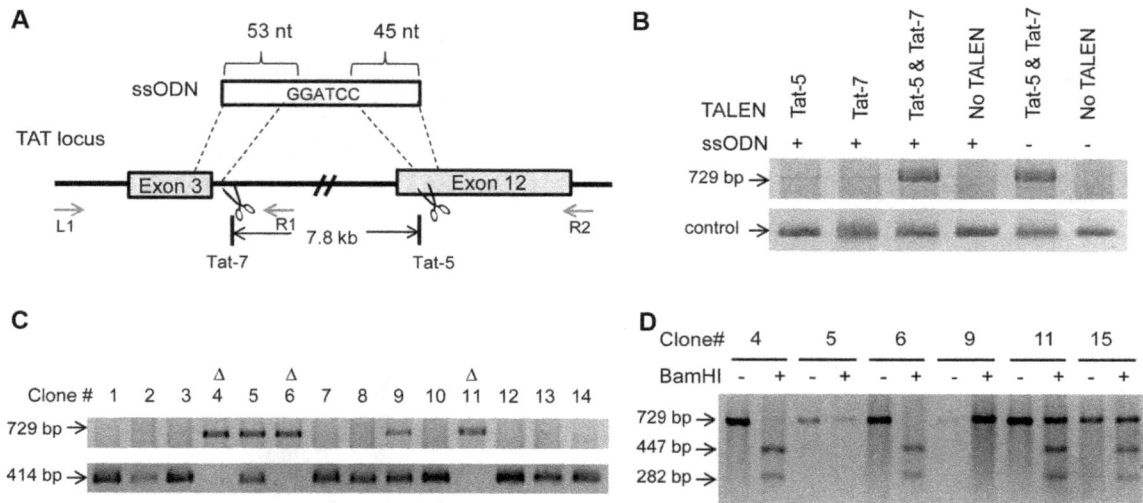

Figure 4. Deletion of a large genomic fragment with two TALEN pairs and an ssODN. (A) Schematic representation of the TALEN target regions in the TAT gene. Tat-7 and Tat-5 cut in intron 3 and exon 12, respectively, resulting in the deletion of a 7.8 kb genomic fragment. A100-mer ssODN used for HDR and the homology regions between the ssODN and the TAT gene are shown. The primers used for PCR screening of isolated clones, L1, R1 and R2, and their positions in the TAT gene are indicated. **(B)** TALEN and ssODN mediated a large genomic deletion in the TAT gene. HEK293T cells were transiently transfected with the TALEN and the ssODN as indicated, and the total genomic DNA harvested was subjected to PCR analysis using primer L1 and R2. A primer pair specific for the miR-9-2 gene was used for PCR as the loading control. **(C)** Representative picture of PCR analysis of individual HEK293T clones transfected with the two TALEN pairs and the ssODN. Top panel: targeted deletion in the TAT gene was amplified with L1 and R2, resulting in a 729 bp PCR fragment. Bottom panel: wild-type TAT locus was amplified with L1 and R1, resulting in a 414 bp PCR fragment. Homozygous knockout clones were indicated by "Δ". **(D)** Validation of HEK293T clones containing HDR-mediated deletion. The PCR product from HDR-mediated deletion was digested by BamHI into two fragments with sizes of 447 bp and 282 bp.

approximately 500 fold in clone 2247 (Figure 5E, Day 45). We also measured the expression of the three miR-9 precursors in H9 and clone 2247 using quantitative RT-PCR. As reported previously [44,45], our data showed that pre-miR-9-1 and pre-miR-9-2 were more abundant, whereas pre-miR-9-3 was barely detectable (data not shown). In clone 2247, pre-miR-9-2 expression was undetectable regardless of the differentiation status consistent with the complete knockout of the miR-9-2 gene (Figure 5F). Based on these results, we concluded that the 13-bp deletion in miR-9-2 had a negative impact on its processing which contributed to the complete absence of miR-9-2 expression in this clone.

Since a homologous chromosome can act as the repair template in a substantial proportion of DSB repair events [46,47], it was of interest to determine whether it could also facilitate the generation of homozygous gene knockout in ESCs. Clone 2287 represents an ideal candidate to test homologous chromosome-mediated HDR as this clone has one wild-type miR-9-2 allele and a 35-bp deletion in the other allele which was generated by NHEJ (Table S2). The 35-bp deletion eliminates the TALEN binding sites and renders the wild-type allele the only target for TALEN cutting. If homologous chromosome-mediated HDR occurred, we would expect to isolate homozygous knockout clones with the 35-bp deletion in both of the miR-9-2 alleles. To test this hypothesis, we co-transfected M9-3 and the ssODN into clone 2287. Out of 196 clones screened, 8 clones (4.1%) no longer exhibited a wild-type PCR band (Figure S2B). Among them 3 clones (1.5%) had the expected ssODN-mediated 89-bp deletion of the wild-type allele, and one clones (0.5%), clone 2287-19, had a 35-bp deletion in the remaining wild-type allele (Figure S2B). This was verified by using PCR to measure the genomic copy near the region of the TALEN cutting site and direct DNA sequencing of the PCR product (Table 3 and Figure S2C). This result therefore suggested that the DSB generated by TALEN in the remaining wild-type miR-9-2 allele was repaired using the homologous chromosome with the 35-bp deletion as a template. The wild-type alleles in the remaining 4 clones were repaired by NHEJ as they showed deletions with variable sizes (Table 3 and Figure S2A). Based on this result, we were able to assess the total HDR efficiency at around 2% (4/196 clones) in H9 cells. We also measured the levels of miR-9 and pre-miR-9-2 in clone 2287-derived homozygous

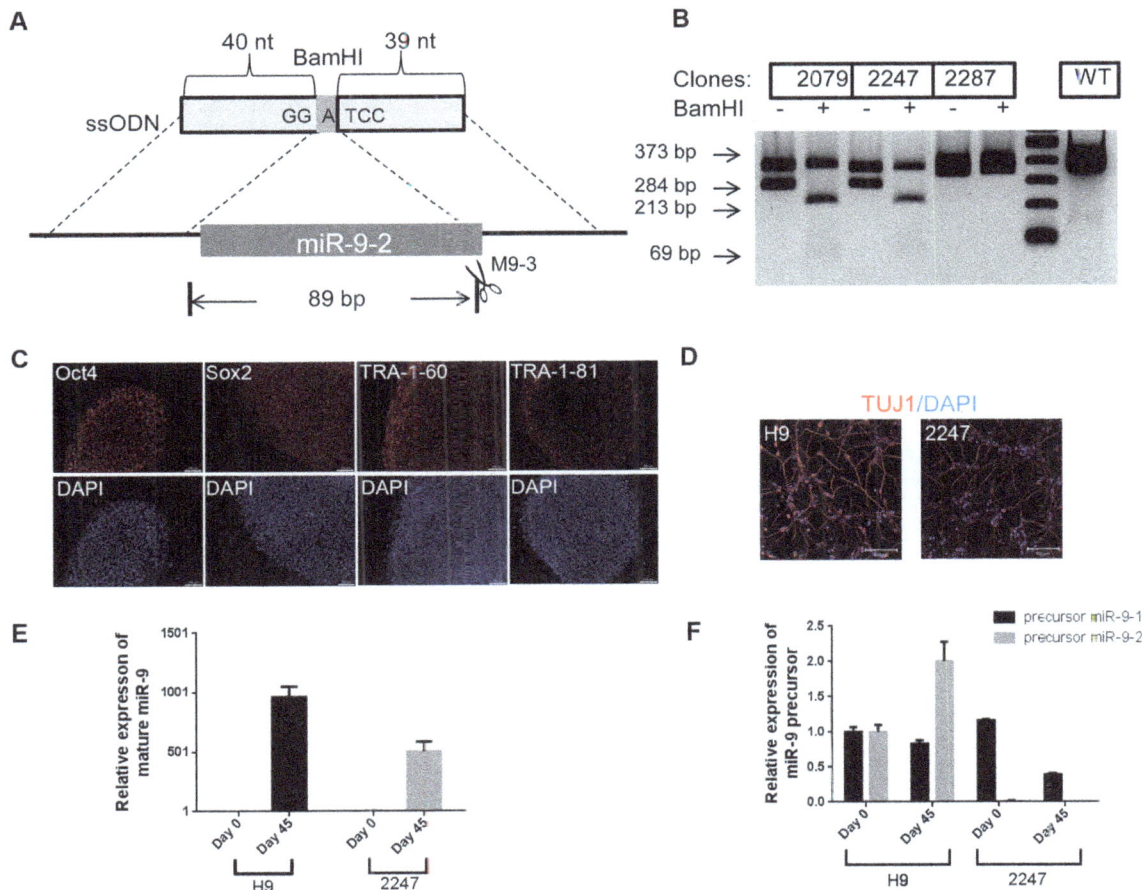

Figure 5. Knockout of the miR-9-2 gene in H9 cells. (**A**) Schematic representation of the miR-9-2 gene and a 100-mer ssODN used for miR-9-2 deletion. The box in the miR-9-2 locus indicates the stem-loop structure of the gene. Homology regions between the ssODN and the miR-9-2 gene are indicated. (**B**) Genomic PCR screening of the miR-9-2 gene deletion. H9 clones transfected with the TALEN and ssODN were isolated. Genomic PCR to amplify the region surrounding the TALEN cutting site followed by BamH1 digestion was carried out. The expected fragment sizes for wild-type and ssODN-mediated HDR are 373 bp and 284 bp, respectively. BamHI cuts the 284 bp fragment into 213 bp and 69 bp fragments. (**C**) Immunofluorescence staining of stem cell markers in undifferentiated clone 2247 cells. Nuclei were counterstained by DAPI. Scale bar = 100 μm. (**D**) Immunofluorescence staining of TUJ1 in neuronal cells derived from differentiated H9 and clone 2247 cells. Scale bar = 100 μm. (**E**) Level of mature miR-9 in H9 and clone 2247. Quantitative RT-PCR was used to measure the level of mature miR-9. Day 0 denotes the undifferentiated cells whereas day 45 denotes neuronal cells. $p < 0.05$. (**F**) Level of precursor miR-9-1 and miR-9-2 in H9 and clone 2247. Pre-miR-9-2 was undetectable in clone 2247.

Table 3. Sequence analysis of miR-9-2 locus in subclones derived from clone 2287.

Clone No.	Sequence	Genotype
	ACAGAGGATCCTTCAAGATCGCCGG	ssODN
Parental clone 2287	ACAGAGG.65 bp. GCTAGATAACCGAAAGTAAAAACTCCTTCAAGATCGCCGG	WT
	ACAGAGG.55 bp. -------------------------CTTCAAGATCGCCGG	Δ 35 bp
2287–114	ACAGAGGaTCCTTCAAGATCGCCGG	HDR
	ACAGAGG.55 bp. -------------------------CTTCAAGATCGCCGG	Δ 35 bp
2287–182	ACAGAGGaTCCTTCAAGATCGCCGG	HDR
	ACAGAGG.55 bp. -------------------------CTTCAAGATCGCCGG	Δ 35 bp
2287–191	ACAGAGGaTCCTTCAAGATCGCCGG	HDR
	ACAGAGG.55 bp. -------------------------CTTCAAGATCGCCGG	Δ 35 bp
2287–19	ACAGAGG.55 bp. -------------------------CTTCAAGATCGCCGG	Δ 35 bp
2287–151	ACAGAGG.55 bp. -------------------------CTTCAAGATCGCCGG	Δ 35 bp
	-----------------------------AAAAACTCCTTCAAGATCGCCGG	Δ 235 bp
2287–50	ACAGAGG.55 bp. -------------------------CTTCAAGATCGCCGG	Δ 35 bp
	ACAGAGG.65 bp. GCTAGA-------------------TTCAAGATCGCCGG	Δ 20 bp
2287–68	ACAGAGG.55 bp. -------------------------CTTCAAGATCGCCGG	Δ 35 bp
	ACAGAGG.62 bp. -------------------AAACTCCTTCAAGATCGCCGG	Δ 22 bp
2287–72	ACAGAGG.55 bp. -------------------------CTTCAAGATCGCCGG	Δ 35 bp
	ACAGAGG.65 bp. GCTAGAT----------AAAACTCCTTCAAGATCGCCGG	Δ 11 bp

Clone 2287 was transfected with the TALEN and ssODN followed by clone isolation as described for Figure 4. Genomic PCR of individual clones was carried out and the PCR products were TA cloned and sequenced. Part of the ssODN sequence is shown on top of the table and the homology regions between the ssODN and the wild-type allele are underlined. HDR denotes homology directed recombination. "Δ" denotes deletion which is indicated by a dished line.

knockout clones and confirmed the complete absence of miR-9-2 expression in those clones (data not shown).

Discussion

In this study, we demonstrated the application of combining ssODN and TALEN to inactivate both of the miR-9-2 alleles in H9 cells. However, the efficiency of precise gene editing remains low (2 out of 300 H9 clones screened). In ESCs, the gene editing efficiency could be modulated by the TALEN cutting efficiency, the intracellular ssODN concentration and the accessibility of the genomic target. Using the GoldyTALEN scaffold, we showed enhanced target cutting which may be due to the additional truncations between the TALE repeats and the FokI nuclease domain in GoldyTALEN that increase the nuclease activity. We observed highly efficient NHEJ events at the miR-9-2 locus in the transfected H9 cells. Up to 17% of the transfected clones had NHEJ in the miR-9-2 locus, suggesting that the TALEN-mediated genomic cutting was not likely to be the rate-limiting step in gene editing. HDR-mediated gene editing also relies on donor template availability. We employed unmodified ssODN as the donor template. Single-stranded ODNs with phosphorothioate (PTO) modification were used to increase the stability of ssODNs [48–50]. However, PTO-protected ssODNs also increased the frequency of cell cycle arrest [51]. Incorporation of other types of nuclease-resistant residues such as 2′-O-methyl-ribonucleoside and locked nucleic acids in ssODN may avoid the adverse effects of PTO and increase the stability of ssODN [52–54].

Currently little information is available regarding TALEN target site accessibility. Bultmann et al. showed that 5-methylated cytosine in the genomic DNA had negative impact on TALE-mediated gene activation [55]. Chen et al. also observed a

significant negative correlation between TALEN-mediated gene editing and the number of CpG repeats in TALEN target sites in zebrafish [56]. However, they found no such correlation in human cells. Our data does not support such a correlation either as some of our most efficient TALEN pairs have multiple CpG in their targets. Our results also showed that TALEN could cleave its genomic target irrespective of the gene activation status as TAT [57] and miR-9-2 genes (unpublished data) were silent in HEK293T cells, and their cutting efficiencies were comparable to actively expressed genes such as miR-21. Thus, target site accessibility could not account for the low gene editing efficiency in H9 cells. Homologous chromosome can also serve as template for DSB repair. Indeed, using clone 2287 containing heterozygous miR-9-2 alleles, we showed homologous chromosome-mediated HDR existed and the frequency was comparable to that of ssODN-mediated HDR. The involvement of homologous chromosome as a repair template for DSB may also explain the low efficiency of gaining the desired miR-9-2 deletion mutant as the wild-type allele in the homologous chromosome may compete against the transfected ssODN as a template to repair the DSB in the other allele.

Several groups have reported the highly efficient generation of germ-line transmittable gene knockouts in multiple species based on TALEN-mediated NHEJ events [22–28,58]. However, small insertion or deletion generated by NHEJ in a gene may not be sufficient to completely abolish the encoded protein function. Precise deletion of multiple exons or even the entire gene may be preferable to ensure complete inactivation of the gene. Using two TALEN pairs in conjunction with an ssODN, we were able to generate the expected 7.8-kb deletion in all three TAT alleles in HEK293T cells at a frequency of 5.1%. This frequency was higher than the 0.3–1% reported previously by Lee et al. using two ZFN pairs without ssODN, and the 0.6% reported by Chen et al. using ssODN and one pair of ZFN [21,59]. Our study therefore demonstrated the capacity of using TALEN and ssODN to create large genomic deletions efficiently. Such a strategy should also be applicable to other gene editing systems, such as CRISPR/Cas9.

The technologies for gene editing are fast evolving. In the recent two years, TALEN and CRISPR/Cas9 is well adopted due to the ease of nuclease assembly and high efficiency in gene editing. While CRISPR design is constrained by the requirement of the protospacer-adjacent motif (PAM) sequence (NGG) following the 20 bp CRISPR RNA target, no such restriction is known for TALENs. These two strategies are therefore complementary to each other for editing most of the genomic sequence. Currently one major concern of using these gene editing systems is the off-target effect on unintended genomic sequences. Off-target mutations can cause genome instability, DNA rearrangement and disruption of normal gene functions. The specificity of CRISPR relies on the 20 base guide sequence, whereas a TALEN pair targets approximately 30–40 bp genomic sequence. Recent studies showed that CRISPR/Cas9 could tolerate up to five mismatches between the guide RNA and its target to varying degree which confounded its application in research and therapeutics[10,60,61]. Although not immune to this problem, TALEN was reported to generate fewer off-target effects in general [13,62]. However, to vigorously address this issue, an unbiased assay such as the use of integration defective lentiviral vectors to tag DSBs generated by TALEN will need to be employed [63].

In summary, our study shows that ssODN can serve as a feasible donor template for HDR in human cell lines including ESCs. Using ssODN in gene editing studies avoids the time-consuming step of constructing the template plasmid. It also avoids prolonged selection and removal of the introduced selectable marker from established ESC or iPSC clones. This novel gene editing technology should create a robust platform for dissecting genotype-phenotype relationships *in vitro*.

Supporting Information

Figure S1 Validation of TALEN cutting in HEK293T cells. Each TALEN pair was transfected into HEK293T cells, and NHEJ was evaluated 48 h later with the Surveyor assay.

Figure S2 Genotyping the miR-9-2 locus in the subclones derived from clone 2287. Clone 2287 was treated with an additional round of gene knockout as described in Figure 4, and the genomic DNA from several subclones was isolated for PCR analysis. (A) Schematic drawing of the miR-9-2 locus and TALEN cutting site. The PCR primer pairs used for genotyping are shown. The two miR-9-2 alleles in clone 2287-19 and clone 2287-151 are also indicated. (B) PCR analysis of the genomic DNA isolated from 2287 subclones to detect miR-9-2 deletions. The primers used for

this analysis are M9F2 and M9R2. The parental clone (clone 2287) is heterozygous for miR-9-2 with one wild-type allele and one deleted allele mediated by NHEJ. PCR amplification of the wild-type allele generates a 373 bp fragment and amplification of the deleted allele generates a 338 bp fragment. Knocking out the wild-type allele with ssODN generates a 284 bp fragment whereas knocking out the wild-type allele with the homologous chromosome generates two fragments with an identical size of 338 bp. Clones with ssODN-mediated HDR in the wild-type allele are indicated by "Δ". The clone with homologous chromosome-mediated HDR is indicated by "*". Both clone 2287-19 and clone 2287-151 exhibit only a single 338 bp PCR fragment. Additional PCR using M9F4 and M9R2 as primers showed that clone 2287-151 had an extended 235-bp deletion in the remaining wild-type allele (Table 3). This deletion, most likely generated by NHEJ, prevents the binding of M9F2 for PCR. (C) Verification of homozygous deletion in the miR-9-2 loci in clone 2287-19. M9F5 & R5, M9F6 & R6 were used in qPCR to measure the haploid copy number in regions flanking the TALEN cutting site in the miR-9-2 gene. The H9 genomic DNA was used as a calibrator. The GAPDH gene on chromosome 2 was used as a reference gene for gene copy normalization. PCR by both primer pairs shows that clone 2287-19 has an equivalent copy number as H9 in this genomic region. Due to NHEJ-induced 235 bp deletion, clone 2287-151 has only half of the copy as clone 2287-19 and H9 when M9F5 & R5 were used.

Table S1 Sequence analysis of H9 clones with NHEJ. Genomic PCR products from randomly isolated H9 clones transfected with the TALEN and ssODN were directly sequenced. The sequence was aligned with the sequence of ssODN and the wild-type miR-9-2 gene shown on top of the table. "Δ" denotes deletion and "I" denotes insertion. Inserted sequences are underlined and deletions are indicated by dashed lines.

Table S2 Sequence analysis of H9 clones with large deletion in the miR-9-2 locus. Genomic PCR products from the H9 clones with deletion in the miR-9-2 locus were TA cloned and sequenced. The sequence was aligned with the sequence of ssODN and the wild-type (WT) miR-9-2 gene shown on top of the table. "Δ" denotes deletion and "I" denotes insertion. The inserted sequence is underlined and deletions are indicated by dashed lines.

Author Contributions

Conceived and designed the experiments: XW JY. Performed the experiments: XW YW TC. Analyzed the data: XW RL JY. Contributed reagents/materials/analysis tools: HH BC XC JH. Wrote the paper: XW JY.

References

1. Urnov FD, Miller JC, Lee YL, Beausejour CM, Rock JM, et al. (2005) Highly efficient endogenous human gene correction using designed zinc-finger nucleases. Nature 435: 646–651.
2. Cong L, Ran FA, Cox D, Lin S, Barretto R, et al. (2013) Multiplex genome engineering using CRISPR/Cas systems. Science 339: 819–823.
3. Wang H, Yang H, Shivalila CS, Dawlaty MM, Cheng AW, et al. (2013) One-step generation of mice carrying mutations in multiple genes by CRISPR/Cas-mediated genome engineering. Cell 153: 910–918.
4. Ding Q, Lee YK, Schaefer EA, Peters DT, Veres A, et al. (2013) A TALEN genome-editing system for generating human stem cell-based disease models. Cell Stem Cell 12: 238–251.

5. Cermak T, Doyle EL, Christian M, Wang L, Zhang Y, et al. (2011) Efficient design and assembly of custom TALEN and other TAL effector-based constructs for DNA targeting. Nucleic Acids Res 39: e82.
6. Reyon D, Tsai SQ, Khayter C, Foden JA, Sander JD, et al. (2012) FLASH assembly of TALENs for high-throughput genome editing. Nat Biotechnol 30: 460–465.
7. Mussolino C, Morbitzer R, Lutge F, Dannemann N, Lahaye T, et al. (2011) A novel TALE nuclease scaffold enables high genome editing activity in combination with low toxicity. Nucleic Acids Res 39: 9283–9293.
8. Hockemeyer D, Wang H, Kiani S, Lai CS, Gao Q, et al. (2011) Genetic engineering of human pluripotent cells using TALE nucleases. Nat Biotechnol 29: 731–734.

9. Hsu PD, Scott DA, Weinstein JA, Ran FA, Konermann S, et al. (2013) DNA targeting specificity of RNA-guided Cas9 nucleases. Nat Biotechnol 31: 827–832.

10. Fu Y, Foden JA, Khayter C, Maeder ML, Reyon D, et al. (2013) High-frequency off-target mutagenesis induced by CRISPR-Cas nucleases in human cells. Nat Biotechnol 31: 822–826.

11. Cho SW, Kim S, Kim Y, Kweon J, Kim HS, et al. (2013) Analysis of off-target effects of CRISPR/Cas-derived RNA-guided endonucleases and nickases. Genome Res.

12. Sanjana NE, Cong L, Zhou Y, Cunniff MM, Feng G, et al. (2012) A transcription activator-like effector toolbox for genome engineering. Nat Protoc 7: 171–192.

13. Osborn MJ, Starker CG, McElroy AN, Webber BR, Riddle MJ, et al. (2013) TALEN-based gene correction for epidermolysis bullosa. Mol Ther 21: 1151–1159.

14. Li T, Huang S, Zhao X, Wright DA, Carpenter S, et al. (2011) Modularly assembled designer TAL effector nucleases for targeted gene knockout and gene replacement in eukaryotes. Nucleic Acids Res 39: 6315–6325.

15. Christian M, Cermak T, Doyle EL, Schmidt C, Zhang F, et al. (2010) Targeting DNA double-strand breaks with TAL effector nucleases. Genetics 186: 757–761.

16. Mak AN, Bradley P, Cernadas RA, Bogdanove AJ, Stoddard BL (2012) The crystal structure of TAL effector PthXo1 bound to its DNA target. Science 335: 716–719.

17. Deng D, Yan C, Pan X, Mahfouz M, Wang J, et al. (2012) Structural basis for sequence-specific recognition of DNA by TAL effectors. Science 335: 720–723.

18. Streubel J, Blucher C, Landgraf A, Boch J (2012) TAL effector RVD specificities and efficiencies. Nat Biotechnol 30: 593–595.

19. Li T, Huang S, Jiang WZ, Wright D, Spalding MH, et al. (2010) TAL nucleases (TALNs): hybrid proteins composed of TAL effectors and FokI DNA-cleavage domain. Nucleic Acids Res 39: 359–372.

20. Mahfouz MM, Li L, Shamimuzzaman M, Wibowo A, Fang X, et al. (2011) De novo-engineered transcription activator-like effector (TALE) hybrid nuclease with novel DNA binding specificity creates double-strand breaks. Proc Natl Acad Sci U S A 108: 2623–2628.

21. Chen F, Pruett-Miller SM, Huang Y, Gjoka M, Duda K, et al. (2011) High-frequency genome editing using ssDNA oligonucleotides with zinc-finger nucleases. Nat Methods 8: 753–755.

22. Bedell VM, Wang Y, Campbell JM, Poshusta TL, Starker CG, et al. (2012) In vivo genome editing using a high-efficiency TALEN system. Nature 491: 114–118.

23. Carlson DF, Tan W, Lillico SG, Stverakova D, Proudfoot C, et al. (2012) Efficient TALEN-mediated gene knockout in livestock. Proc Natl Acad Sci U S A 109: 17382–17387.

24. Huang P, Xiao A, Zhou M, Zhu Z, Lin S, et al. (2011) Heritable gene targeting in zebrafish using customized TALENs. Nat Biotechnol 29: 699–700.

25. Sander JD, Cade L, Khayter C, Reyon D, Peterson RT, et al. (2011) Targeted gene disruption in somatic zebrafish cells using engineered TALENs. Nat Biotechnol 29: 697–698.

26. Tong C, Huang G, Ashton C, Wu H, Yan H, et al. (2012) Rapid and cost-effective gene targeting in rat embryonic stem cells by TALENs. J Genet Genomics 39: 275–280.

27. Wefers B, Meyer M, Ortiz O, Hrabe de Angelis M, Hansen J, et al. (2013) Direct production of mouse disease models by embryo microinjection of TALENs and oligodeoxynucleotides. Proc Natl Acad Sci U S A 110: 3782–3787.

28. Lei Y, Guo X, Liu Y, Cao Y, Deng Y, et al. (2012) Efficient targeted gene disruption in Xenopus embryos using engineered transcription activator-like effector nucleases (TALENs). Proc Natl Acad Sci U S A 109: 17484–17489.

29. Hu R, Wallace J, Dahlem TJ, Grunwald DJ, O'Connell RM (2013) Targeting human microRNA genes using engineered Tal-effector nucleases (TALENs). PLoS One 8: e63074.

30. Takada S, Sato T, Ito Y, Yamashita S, Kato T, et al. (2013) Targeted Gene Deletion of miRNAs in Mice by TALEN System. PLoS One 8: e76004.

31. Kim YK, Wee G, Park J, Kim J, Baek D, et al. (2013) TALEN-based knockout library for human microRNAs. Nat Struct Mol Biol.

32. Moynahan ME, Jasin M (2010) Mitotic homologous recombination maintains genomic stability and suppresses tumorigenesis. Nat Rev Mol Cell Biol 11: 196–207.

33. Doyle EL, Booher NJ, Standage DS, Voytas DF, Brendel VP, et al. (2012) TAL Effector-Nucleotide Targeter (TALE-NT) 2.0: tools for TAL effector design and target prediction. Nucleic Acids Res 40: W117–122.

34. Hu BY, Weick JP, Yu J, Ma LX, Zhang XQ, et al. (2010) Neural differentiation of human induced pluripotent stem cells follows developmental principles but with variable potency. Proc Natl Acad Sci U S A 107: 4335–4340.

35. De Preter K, Speleman F, Combaret V, Lunec J, Laureys G, et al. (2002) Quantification of MYCN, DDX1, and NAG gene copy number in neuroblastoma using a real-time quantitative PCR assay. Mod Pathol 15: 159–166.

36. Boch J, Scholze H, Schornack S, Landgraf A, Hahn S, et al. (2009) Breaking the code of DNA binding specificity of TAL-type III effectors. Science 326: 1509–1512.

37. Moscou MJ, Bogdanove AJ (2009) A simple cipher governs DNA recognition by TAL effectors. Science 326: 1501.

38. Shibata M, Kurokawa D, Nakao H, Ohmura T, Aizawa S (2008) MicroRNA-9 modulates Cajal-Retzius cell differentiation by suppressing Foxg1 expression in mouse medial pallium. J Neurosci 28: 10415–10421.

39. Leucht C, Stigloher C, Wizenmann A, Klafke R, Folchert A, et al. (2008) MicroRNA-9 directs late organizer activity of the midbrain-hindbrain boundary. Nat Neurosci 11: 641–648.

40. Uchida N (2010) MicroRNA-9 controls a migratory mechanism in human neural progenitor cells. Cell Stem Cell 6: 294–296.

41. Dajas-Bailador F, Bonev B, Garcez P, Stanley P, Guillemot F, et al. (2012) microRNA-9 regulates axon extension and branching by targeting Map1b in mouse cortical neurons. Nat Neurosci 15: 697–699.

42. Delaloy C, Liu L, Lee JA, Su H, Shen F, et al. (2010) MicroRNA-9 coordinates proliferation and migration of human embryonic stem cell-derived neural progenitors. Cell Stem Cell 6: 323–335.

43. Yuva-Aydemir Y, Simkin A, Gascon E, Gao FB (2011) MicroRNA-9: functional evolution of a conserved small regulatory RNA. RNA Biol 8: 557–564.

44. Shibata M, Nakao H, Kiyonari H, Abe T, Aizawa S (2011) MicroRNA-9 regulates neurogenesis in mouse telencephalon by targeting multiple transcription factors. J Neurosci 31: 3407–3422.

45. Laneve P, Gioia U, Andriotto A, Moretti F, Bozzoni I, et al. (2010) A minicircuitry involving REST and CREB controls miR-9-2 expression during human neuronal differentiation. Nucleic Acids Res 38: 6895–6905.

46. Gandhi M, Evdokimova VN, K TC, Nikiforova MN, Kelly LM, et al. (2012) Homologous chromosomes make contact at the sites of double-strand breaks in genes in somatic G0/G1-phase human cells. Proc Natl Acad Sci U S A 109: 9454–9459.

47. Richardson C, Moynahan ME, Jasin M (1998) Double-strand break repair by interchromosomal recombination: suppression of chromosomal translocations. Genes Dev 12: 3831–3842.

48. Campbell CR, Keown W, Lowe L, Kirschling D, Kucherlapati R (1989) Homologous recombination involving small single-stranded oligonucleotides in human cells. New Biol 1: 223–227.

49. Radecke S, Radecke F, Peter I, Schwarz K (2006) Physical incorporation of a single-stranded oligodeoxynucleotide during targeted repair of a human chromosomal locus. J Gene Med 8: 217–228.

50. Papaioannou I, Disterer P, Owen JS (2009) Use of internally nuclease-protected single-strand DNA oligonucleotides and silencing of the mismatch repair protein, MSH2, enhances the replication of corrected cells following gene editing. J Gene Med 11: 267–274.

51. Aarts M, te Riele H (2010) Subtle gene modification in mouse ES cells: evidence for incorporation of unmodified oligonucleotides without induction of DNA damage. Nucleic Acids Res 38: 6956–6967.

52. Igoucheva O, Alexeev V, Anni H, Rubin E (2008) Oligonucleotide-mediated gene targeting in human hepatocytes: implications of mismatch repair. Oligonucleotides 18: 111–122.

53. Igoucheva O, Alexeev V, Scharer O, Yoon K (2006) Involvement of ERCC1/XPF and XPG in oligodeoxynucleotide-directed gene modification. Oligonucleotides 16: 94–104.

54. Andrieu-Soler C, Casas M, Faussat AM, Gandolphe C, Doat M, et al. (2005) Stable transmission of targeted gene modification using single-stranded oligonucleotides with flanking LNAs. Nucleic Acids Res 33: 3733–3742.

55. Bultmann S, Morbitzer R, Schmidt CS, Thanisch K, Spada F, et al. (2012) Targeted transcriptional activation of silent oct4 pluripotency gene by combining designer TALEs and inhibition of epigenetic modifiers. Nucleic Acids Res 40: 5368–5377.

56. Chen S, Oikonomou G, Chiu CN, Niles BJ, Liu J, et al. (2013) A large-scale in vivo analysis reveals that TALENs are significantly more mutagenic than ZFNs generated using content-dependent assembly. Nucleic Acids Res 41: 2769–2778.

57. Dvorak Z, Modriansky M, Pichard-Garcia L, Balaguer P, Vilarem MJ, et al. (2003) Colchicine down-regulates cytochrome P450 2B6, 2C8, 2C9, and 3A4 in human hepatocytes by affecting their glucocorticoid receptor-mediated regulation. Mol Pharmacol 64: 160–169.

58. Ding Q, Lee YK, Schaefer EA, Peters DT, Veres A, et al. (2013) A TALEN genome-editing system for generating human stem cell-based disease models. Cell Stem Cell 12: 238–251.

59. Lee HJ, Kim E, Kim JS (2010) Targeted chromosomal deletions in human cells using zinc finger nucleases. Genome Res 20: 81–89.

60. Cradick TJ, Fine EJ, Antico CJ, Bao G (2013) CRISPR/Cas9 systems targeting beta-globin and CCR5 genes have substantial off-target activity. Nucleic Acids Res 41: 9584–9592.

61. Cho SW, Kim S, Kim Y, Kweon J, Kim HS, et al. (2014) Analysis of off-target effects of CRISPR/Cas-derived RNA-guided endonucleases and nickases. Genome Res 24: 132–141.

62. Fine EJ, Cradick TJ, Zhao CL, Lin Y, Bao G (2013) An online bioinformatics tool predicts zinc finger and TALE nuclease off-target cleavage. Nucleic Acids Res.

63. Gabriel R, Lombardo A, Arens A, Miller JC, Genovese P, et al. (2011) An unbiased genome-wide analysis of zinc-finger nuclease specificity. Nat Biotechnol 29: 816–823.

10

A Meta-Analysis Approach for Characterizing Pan-Cancer Mechanisms of Drug Sensitivity in Cell Lines

Kendric Wang[1], Raunak Shrestha[1,2], Alexander W. Wyatt[1], Anupama Reddy[4], Joseph Lehár[4], Yuzhou Wang[1,3], Anna Lapuk[1,9], Colin C. Collins[1,3*,9]

1 Vancouver Prostate Centre, Vancouver General Hospital, Vancouver, Canada, 2 CIHR/MSHFR Bioinformatics Training Program, University of British Columbia, Vancouver, Canada, 3 Department of Urologic Sciences, the University of British Columbia, Vancouver, Canada, 4 Novartis Pharmaceuticals, Oncology Division, Basal, Switzerland

Abstract

Understanding the heterogeneous drug response of cancer patients is essential to precision oncology. Pioneering genomic analyses of individual cancer subtypes have begun to identify key determinants of resistance, including up-regulation of multi-drug resistance (MDR) genes and mutational alterations of drug targets. However, these alterations are sufficient to explain only a minority of the population, and additional mechanisms of drug resistance or sensitivity are required to explain the remaining spectrum of patient responses to ultimately achieve the goal of precision oncology. We hypothesized that a pan-cancer analysis of *in vitro* drug sensitivities across numerous cancer lineages will improve the detection of statistical associations and yield more robust and, importantly, recurrent determinants of response. In this study, we developed a statistical framework based on the meta-analysis of expression profiles to identify pan-cancer markers and mechanisms of drug response. Using the Cancer Cell Line Encyclopaedia (CCLE), a large panel of several hundred cancer cell lines from numerous distinct lineages, we characterized both known and novel mechanisms of response to cytotoxic drugs including inhibitors of Topoisomerase 1 (TOP1; Topotecan, Irinotecan) and targeted therapies including inhibitors of histone deacetylases (HDAC; Panobinostat) and MAP/ERK kinases (MEK; PD-0325901, AZD6244). Notably, our analysis implicated reduced replication and transcriptional rates, as well as deficiency in DNA damage repair genes in resistance to TOP1 inhibitors. The constitutive activation of several signaling pathways including the interferon/STAT-1 pathway was implicated in resistance to the pan-HDAC inhibitor. Finally, a number of dysregulations upstream of MEK were identified as compensatory mechanisms of resistance to the MEK inhibitors. In comparison to alternative pan-cancer analysis strategies, our approach can better elucidate relevant drug response mechanisms. Moreover, the compendium of putative markers and mechanisms identified through our analysis can serve as a foundation for future studies into these drugs.

Editor: Caterina Cinti, Institute of Clinical Physiology, c/o Toscana Life Sciences Foundation, Italy

Funding: The authors have no funding or support to report.
Competing Interests: The co-authors AR and JL are employees of Novartis Pharmaceuticals.

* Email: ccollins@prostatecentre.com

9 These authors contributed equally to this work.

Introduction

Over the past decade, cancer treatment has seen a gradual shift towards 'precision medicine' and making rational therapeutic decisions for a patient's cancer based on their distinct molecular profile. However, broad adoption of this strategy has been hindered by an incomplete understanding for the determinants that drive tumour response to different cancer drugs. Intrinsic differences in drug sensitivity or resistance have been previously attributed to a number of molecular aberrations. For instance, the constitutive expression of almost four hundred multi-drug resistance (MDR) genes, such as ATP-binding cassette transporters, can confer universal drug resistance in cancer [1]. Similarly, mutations in cancer genes (such as EGFR) that are selectively targeted by small-molecule inhibitors can either enhance or disrupt drug binding and thereby modulate cancer drug response [2]. In spite of these findings, the clinical translation of MDR inhibitors have been complicated by adverse pharmacokinetic

interactions [3]. Likewise, the presence of mutations in targeted genes can only explain the response observed in a fraction of the population, which also restricts their clinical utility. As an example of the latter, lung cancers initially sensitive to EGFR inhibition acquire resistance which can be explained by EGFR mutations in only half of the cases. Other molecular events, such as MET proto-oncogene amplifications, have been associated with resistance to EGFR inhibitors in 20% of lung cancers independently of EGFR mutations [4]. Therefore, there is still a need to uncover additional mechanisms that can influence response to cancer treatments.

Historically, gene expression profiling of *in vitro* models have played an essential role in investigating determinants underlying drug response [5–8]. Specifically, cell line panels compiled for individual cancer types have helped identify markers predictive of lineage-specific drug responses, such as associating P27(KIP1) with Trastuzumab resistance in breast cancers and linking epithelial-mesenchymal transition genes to resistance to EGFR inhibitors in lung cancers [9–11]. However, application of this strategy has been limited to a handful of cancer types (e.g. breast, lung) with sufficient numbers of established cell line models to achieve the statistical power needed for new discoveries.

Recent studies addressed the problem of limited sample sizes by investigating *in vitro* drug sensitivity in a pan-cancer manner, across large cell line panels that combine multiple cancer types screened for the same drugs [7,8,12,13]. In this way, pan-cancer analysis can improve the testing for statistical associations and help identify dysregulated genes or oncogenic pathways that recurrently promote growth and survival of tumours of diverse origins [14,15]. The common approach used for pan-cancer analysis directly pools samples from diverse cancer types; however, this has two major disadvantages. First, when samples are considered collectively, significant gene expression-drug response associations present in smaller sized cancer lineages can be obscured by the lack of associations present in larger sized lineages. Second, the range of gene expressions and drug pharmacodynamics values are often lineage-specific and incomparable between different cancer lineages (**Figure 1A**). Collectively, these issues reduce the potential to detect meaningful associations common across multiple cancer lineages.

To tackle the problems introduced through the direct pooling of data, we developed a statistical framework based on meta-analysis called 'PC-Meta'. PC-Meta identifies pan-cancer markers and mechanisms of drug response by testing for gene expression-drug response associations in each cancer lineage individually and combining the results from each lineage. Prior studies have successfully applied meta-analyses to combine incompatible genomic datasets for a single cancer type, and to combine datasets from different cancers to identify common mechanisms of cancer initiation and progression [16–18]. To our knowledge, this is the first study to leverage meta-analysis in the identification of intrinsic pan-cancer determinants of response to cancer therapy.

Materials and Methods

Cancer Cell Line Encyclopaedia (CCLE) Dataset

The CCLE pan-cancer dataset used in this study encompasses 1046 cancer cell lines derived from 24 cancer types and screened for pharmacological sensitivity to 24 anti-cancer compounds [8]. The pre-processed gene expression and drug sensitivity data were directly obtained from the CCLE project (http://www. broadinstitute.org/ccle/home; GSE36139). Cell lines were profiled prior to treatment for gene expression using the Affymetrix U133plus2.0 array, and for mutations in 33 known cancer genes by mass spectrometric genotyping (OncoMap). Inhibitory concentration 50 (IC50) values extrapolated in the original study from dose response data were used as the measure of drug effectiveness.

Meta-analysis Approach to Pan-Cancer Analysis

Our PC-Meta approach for the identification of pan-cancer markers and mechanisms of drug response is illustrated in **Figure 1B**. Initially, each cancer lineage in the pan-cancer dataset was treated as a distinct dataset and independently assessed for associations between baseline gene expression levels and drug response values. These lineage-specific expression-response correlations were calculated using the Spearman's rank correlation test. Lineages that exhibited minimal differential drug sensitivity value (having fewer than three samples or an $\log_{10}(IC50)$ range of less than 0.5) were excluded from analysis.

Then, results from the individual lineage-specific correlation analyses were combined using meta-analysis to determine pan-cancer expression-response associations. We used Pearson's method [19], a one-tailed Fisher's method for meta-analysis.

Fisher's method is a standard technique that aggregates multiple p-values into a single meta P-value where a small meta P-value indicates significant expression-response correlation in one or more cancer lineages. Pearson's method can reduce false associations resulting from conflicting directions of correlation in different lineages. It combines individual lineage p-values for positive and negative correlations separately and returns the more significant of the two combined values (meta P^+ and meta P^-) as the final meta P-value (meta P^*). From this, a multiple-test corrected meta P-value (meta-FDR) was calculated using the Benjamini-Hochberg (BH) method. For each drug, genes with meta-FDR < 0.01 were considered pan-cancer markers of response.

Next, pan-cancer mechanisms of response were revealed by performing pathway enrichment analysis on the discovered pan-cancer markers using the Ingenuity Pathway Analysis software (IPA; Ingenuity Systems, Inc., Redwood City, CA). The statistical over-representation of canonical IPA pathways was calculated using Fischer's exact test and BH multiple-test correction method. A 'pathway involvement (PI) score' was calculated for each pathway as the $-\log_{10}$(BH-corrected pathway enrichment p-value). Pathways with PI score >1.0 were considered significantly associated with drug response.

Finally, since pan-cancer markers may be relevant in only a subset of cancer lineages, we defined sets of genes associated with response in each lineage as lineage-specific markers. Lineage-specific markers were derived as the subset of pan-cancer markers that significantly correlated with response in a given lineage (Spearman's rank correlation test p-value <0.05 and |Spearman's correlation coefficient| >0.3). Since pan-cancer mechanisms may similarly be involved in only a subset of cancer lineages, their involvement in each lineage was delineated through the pathway enrichment analysis of lineage-specific gene markers as described above.

Alternative Approaches to Pan-Cancer Analysis

We evaluated PC-Meta against two alternative approaches commonly used in prior studies for identifying pan-cancer markers and mechanisms. One of them, which we termed 'PC-Pool', identifies pan-cancer markers as genes that correlate with drug response in a pooled dataset of multiple cancer lineages [8,12]. Statistical significance was determined based on the same statistical test of Spearman's rank correlation with BH multiple test correction (BH-corrected p-values <0.01 and |Spearman's rho, r_s| >0.3). Pan-cancer mechanisms were revealed by performing pathway enrichment analysis on these pan-cancer markers.

A second alternative approach, which we termed 'PC-Union', naively identifies pan-cancer markers as the union of response-associated genes detected in each cancer lineage [20]. Response-associated markers in each lineage were also identified using the Spearman's rank correlation test with BH multiple test correction (BH-corrected p-values <0.01 and |r_s| >0.3). Pan-cancer mechanisms were revealed by performing pathway enrichment analysis on the collective set of response-associated markers identified in all lineages.

Results and Discussion

Strategy for Pan-Cancer Analysis

We developed PC-Meta, a two stage pan-cancer analysis strategy, to investigate the molecular determinants of drug response (**Figure 1B**). Briefly, in the first stage, PC-Meta assesses correlations between gene expression levels with drug response values in all cancer lineages independently and combines the results in a statistical manner. A meta-FDR value calculated for

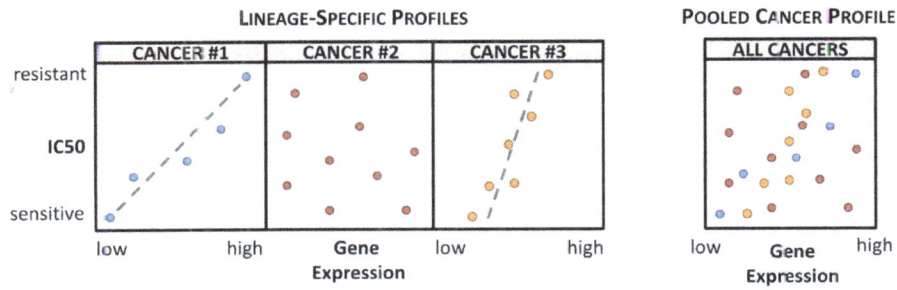

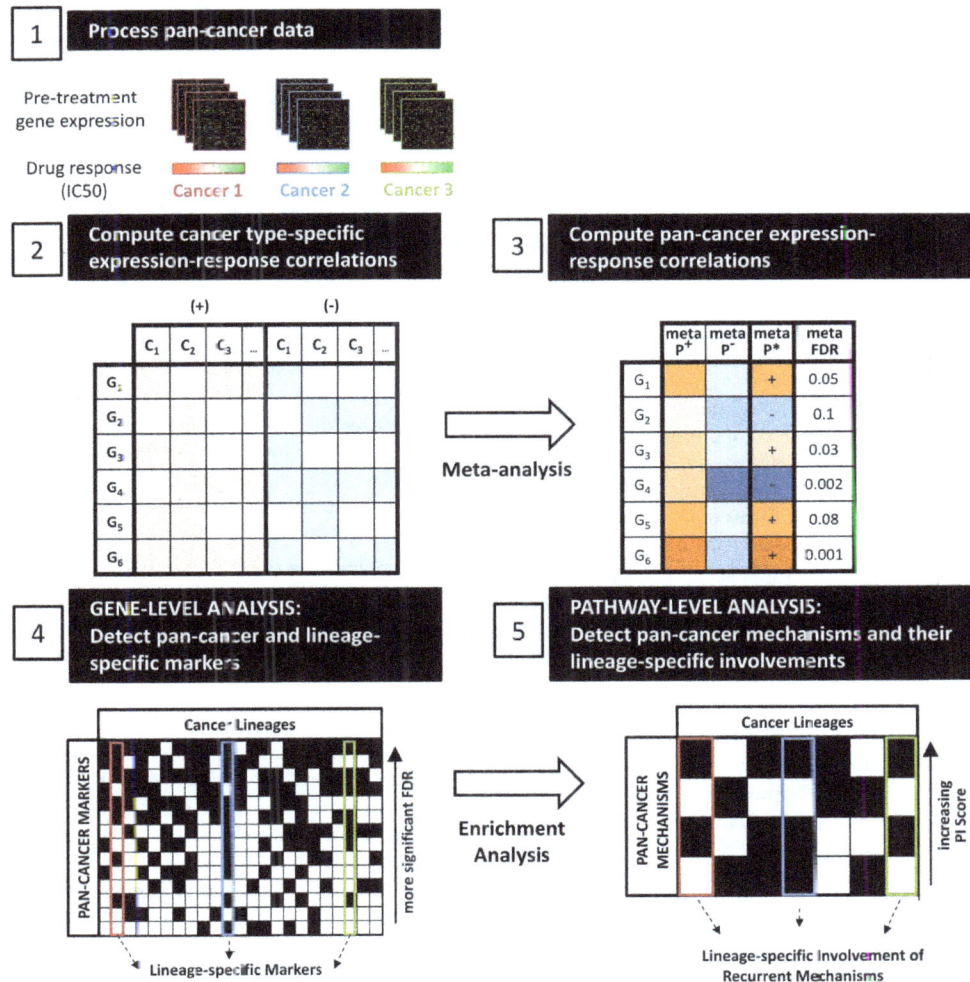

Figure 1. Pan-cancer analysis strategy. (A) Schematic demonstrating a major drawback of the commonly-used pooled cancer approach (PC-Pool), namely that the gene expression and pharmacological profiles of samples from different cancer lineages are often incomparable and therefore inadequate for pooling together into a single analysis. (B) Workflow depicting our PC-Meta approach. First, each cancer lineage in the pan-cancer dataset is independently assessed for gene expression-drug response correlations in both positive and negative directions (Step 2). Then, a meta-analysis method is used to aggregate lineage-specific correlation results and to determine pan-cancer expression-response correlations. The significance of these correlations is indicated by multiple-test corrected p-values (meta-FDR; Step 3). Next, genes that significantly correlate with drug response across multiple cancer lineages are identified as pan-cancer gene markers (meta-FDR <0.01; Step 4). Finally, biological pathways significantly enriched in the discovered set of pan-cancer gene markers are identified as pan-cancer mechanisms of response (PI Score >1.0; Step 5). A subset of the pan-cancer markers correlated with drug response in individual cancer lineages are selected as lineage-specific markers. The involvement levels of pan-cancer mechanisms in individual cancer lineages are calculated from the pathway enrichment analysis of these lineage-specific markers.

each gene is used to pinpoint genes that are recurrently associated with response in multiple cancer types and therefore are potential pan-cancer markers. In the second stage, the pan-cancer gene markers are mapped to cell signaling pathways to elucidate pan-cancer mechanisms involved in drug response. To test our approach, we applied PC-Meta to the CCLE dataset, a large pan-cancer cell line panel that has been extensively screened for pharmacological sensitivity to numerous cancer drugs. PC-Meta was evaluated against two commonly used pan-cancer analysis strategies, which we termed 'PC-Pool' and 'PC-Union'. PC-Pool identifies pan-cancer markers as genes that are associated with drug response in a pooled dataset of cancer lineages. PC-Union, a simplistic approach to meta-analysis (not based on statistical measures), identifies pan-cancer markers as the union of response-correlated genes detected in each cancer lineage. Additional details of PC-Meta, PC-Pool, and PC-Union are provided in the Methods section.

Selecting CCLE Compounds Suitable for Pan-Cancer Analysis

24 compounds available from the CCLE resource were evaluated to determine their suitability for pan-cancer analysis. For eight compounds, none of the pan-cancer analysis methods returned sufficient markers (more than 10 genes) for follow-up and were therefore excluded from subsequent analysis (**Table S1**). Failure to identify markers for these drugs can be attributed to either an incomplete compound screening (i.e. performed on a small number of cancer lineages) such as with Nutlin-3, or the cancer type specificity of compounds such as with Erlotinib, which is most effective in EGFR-addicted non-small cell lung cancers (**Figure S1**). Seven additional compounds, including L-685458 and Sorafenib, exhibited dynamic response phenotypes in only one or two lineages and were also considered inappropriate for pan-cancer analysis (**Figure 2; Figure S1**). Even though the PC-Pool strategy identified numerous gene markers associated with response to these seven compounds, close inspection of these markers indicated that many of them actually corresponded to molecular differences between lineages rather than relevant determinants of drug response. For instance, L-685458, an inhibitor of AβPP γ-secretase activity, displayed variable sensitivity in hematopoietic cancer cell lines and primarily resistance in all other cancer lineages. As a result, the identified 815 gene markers were predominantly enriched for biological functions related to Hematopoetic System Development and Immune Response (**Table S2**). This highlights the limitations of directly pooling data from distinct cancer lineages. Out of the remaining nine compounds, we focused on five drugs that belonged to distinct classes of inhibitors (targeting TOP1, HDAC, and MEK) and exhibited a broad range of responses in multiple cancer lineages (**Figure 2, Table 1**).

Intrinsic Determinants of Response to TOP1 Inhibitors (Topotecan and Irinotecan)

Topotecan and Irinotecan are cytotoxic chemotherapies that inhibit the TOP1 enzyme. They disrupt normal replication and transcription processes to induce DNA damage and apoptosis in rapidly dividing cells. Resistance to TOP1 inhibition can occur as a result of mutations in TOP1 or in cells not undergoing DNA replication; whereas, hypersensitivity can arise due to deficiencies in checkpoint and DNA-repair pathways [21].

In the CCLE panel, these two TOP1 inhibitors showed largely similar pharmacological effects based on IC50 values (**Figure 2**). We applied PC-Meta to each drug dataset and identified 757 and

211 pan-cancer gene markers associated with response to Topotecan and Irinotecan respectively (**Table 1; Table S5**). The discordant number of markers identified for these two drugs may have resulted from differences in drug actions or the different number of cell lines screened for each drug – 480 for Topotecan and 303 for Irinotecan. Nonetheless, 134 out of the 211 (63.5%) gene markers identified for Irinotecan still overlapped with those identified for Topotecan and are likely associated with general mechanisms of TOP1 inhibition (**Table 1**).

Out of the 134 common genes identified for the two drugs by PC-Meta (**Table S3**), many are highly correlated with response (based on meta-FDR values) and have known functions that can affect the cytotoxicity of TOP1 inhibitors. For example, the top gene marker Schlafen family member 11 (SLFN11) showed increased expression in cell lines sensitive to both Topotecan and Irinotecan across ten individual cancer lineages (**Figure 3A**). This significant trend (meta-FDR $= 6.4 \times 10^{-18}$ for Topotecan and 1.9×10^{-10} for Irinotecan; see Methods) agrees with recent studies delineating SLFN11's role in sensitizing cancer cells to DNA-damaging agents by enforcing cell cycle arrest and induction of apoptosis [8,22]. Another top marker, high-mobility group box 2 (HMGB2), is a mediator of genotoxic stress response and showed reduced expression in cell lines resistant to TOP1 inhibitors in multiple lineages (**Figure 3B**; meta-FDR $= 1.7 \times 10^{-07}$ for Topotecan and 3.7×10^{-03} for Irinotecan). This coincides with previous findings showing that abrogated HMGB2 expression results in resistance to chemotherapy-induced DNA damage [23]. Similarly, BCL2-Associated Transcription Factor 1 (BCLAF1), a regulator of apoptosis and double-stranded DNA repair, was also down-regulated in drug-resistant cell lines (meta-FDR $= 4.8 \times 10^{-04}$ for Topotecan and 1.9×10^{-03} for Irinotecan), which is concordant with its previously observed suppression in intrinsically radioresistant cell lines [24].

To investigate pan-cancer mechanisms underlying variations in Topotecan response, we mapped the entire set of pan-cancer gene markers identified by PC-Meta onto corresponding cell signaling pathways (using IPA pathway enrichment analysis). Each pathway was assigned a 'pathway involvement (PI) score' defined as $-\log_{10}$ of the pathway enrichment p-value, and pathways with PI scores $>= 1$ were considered to have significant influence on response. On the Topotecan dataset, PC-Meta detected 15 pan-cancer pathways relevant to drug response (PI scores $= 1.3$–6.6), with the most significant pathways related to cell cycle regulation and DNA damage repair (**Figure 4A; Table 2**). In contrast, the same enrichment analysis yielded only 3 significantly enriched pathways for PC-Pool markers and no significant pathways for PC-Union markers. Clearly, the identification of more significant pathways by PC-Meta can be attributed to the increased power of our approach to pinpoint additional potentially relevant gene markers compared to PC-Pool and PC-Union (757 vs. 474 and 61 respectively; **Table 1**).

The pathways detected by PC-Meta converged onto two major mechanisms that could influence chemotherapy response: cellular growth rate and chromosomal instability (**Figure 4A–B**). All genes involved in cell cycle control, DNA transcription, RNA translation, and nucleotide synthesis processes were down-regulated in chemotherapy-resistant cell lines, which suggested slower growth kinetics as a mechanism of resistance. Most genes involved in DNA damage repair and cell cycle checkpoint regulation were also down-regulated in resistant cell lines. This may appear counter-intuitive because repair pathways typically mitigate DNA damage-induced cell death (as caused by TOP1 inhibitors). However, some of their component genes (such as RAD51, BRCA2, and FANC-family genes) are also key regulators of genomic stability and their

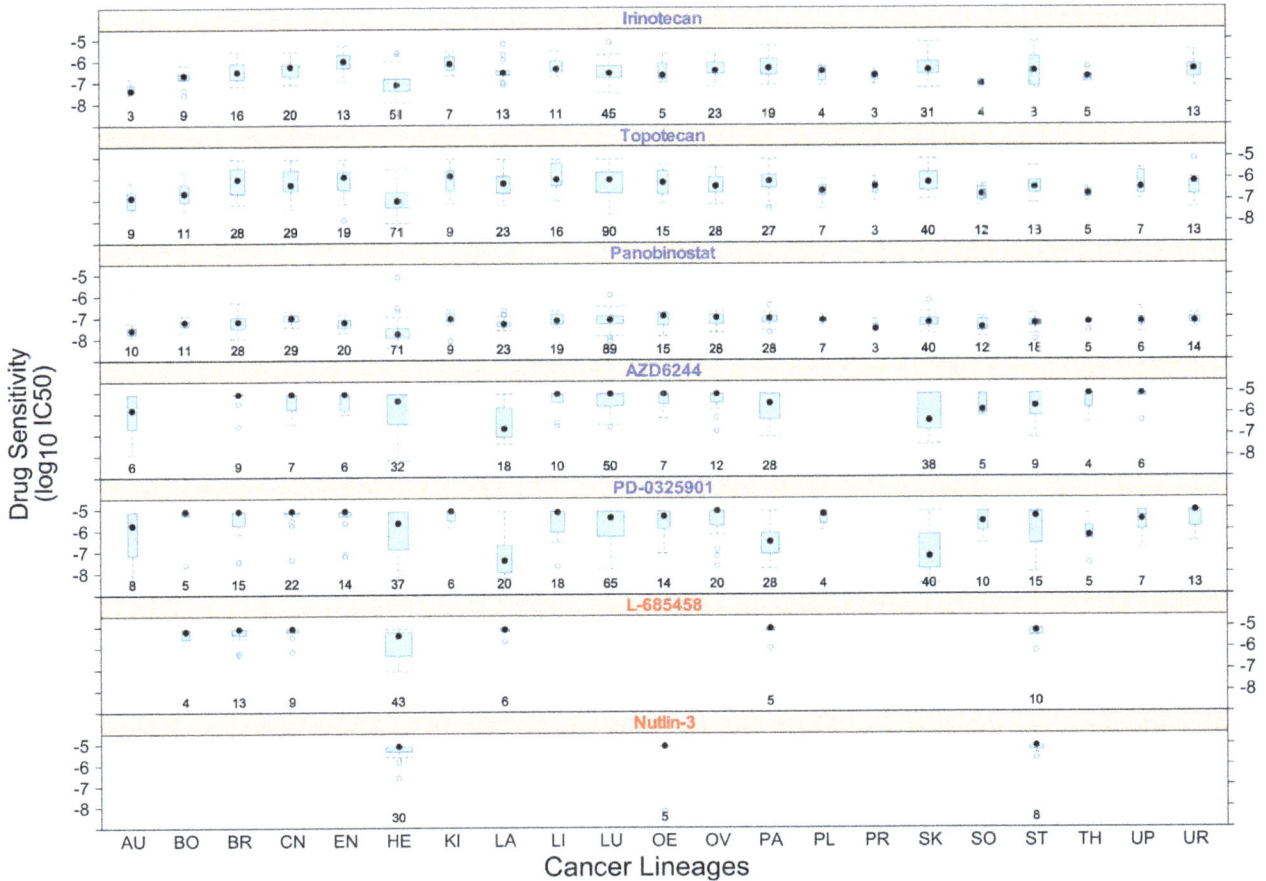

Figure 2. Drug response across different cancer lineages for a subset of CCLE compounds. Boxplots indicate the distribution of drug sensitivity values (based on IC50) in each cancer lineage to each cancer drug. For example, most cancer lineages are resistant to L-685458 (with IC50 around 10^{-5} M) except for haematopoietic cancers (IC50 from 10^{-5} to 10^{-8} M). The number of samples in a cancer lineage screened for drug response is shown under the corresponding boxplot. Compounds denoted in blue text exhibited a broad range of responses in multiple cancer lineages and were selected for analysis in this study, whereas compounds denoted in red text are examples of compounds excluded from analysis. Cancer lineage abbreviations – **AU**: autonomic; **BO**: bone; **BR**: breast; **CN**: central nervous system; **EN**: endometrial; **HE**: haematopoietic/lymphoid; **KI**: kidney; **LA**: large intestine; **LI**: liver; **LU**: lung; **OE**: oesophagus; **OV**: ovary; **PA**: pancreas; **PL**: pleura; **PR**: ?; **SK**: skin; **SO**: soft tissue; **ST**: stomach; **TH**: thyroid; **UP**: upper digestive; **UR**: urinary

disruption can reflect a genome instability phenotype that is inherently resistant to genotoxic stress from chemotherapy [25,26]. In fact, our finding agrees with a recently reported DNA repair gene signature that was predictive of both homologous repair suppression contributing to genome instability as well as sensitivity to chemotherapy in patient studies [27]. Enrichment

analysis performed on the Irinotecan marker set revealed similar dysregulated pathways related to cell cycle control and DNA damage repair (**Table S6**). This suggests these two mechanisms are generally important for managing TOP1 inhibition.

Since recurrent drug response pathways may be involved in only a subset of cancer types, we aimed to delineate the extent of

Table 1. Number of gene markers significantly correlated with response to different drugs identified by PC-Meta, PC-Pool, and PC-Union approaches.

Compound	Target(s)	No. of PC-Meta Markers	No. of PC-Pool Markers (Overlap with PC-Meta)	No. of PC-Union Markers (Overlap with PC-Meta)
Irinotecan	TOP1	211	832 (105; 13%)	30 (19; 63%)
Topotecan	TOP1	757	474 (256; 54%)	61 (57; 93%)
Panobinostat	HDAC	542	723 (200; 28%)	58 (46; 79%)
AZD6244	MEK	10	51 (6; 12%)	7 (1; 14%)
PD-0325901	MEK	171	46 (23; 50%)	156 (29; 19%)

A. SLFN11

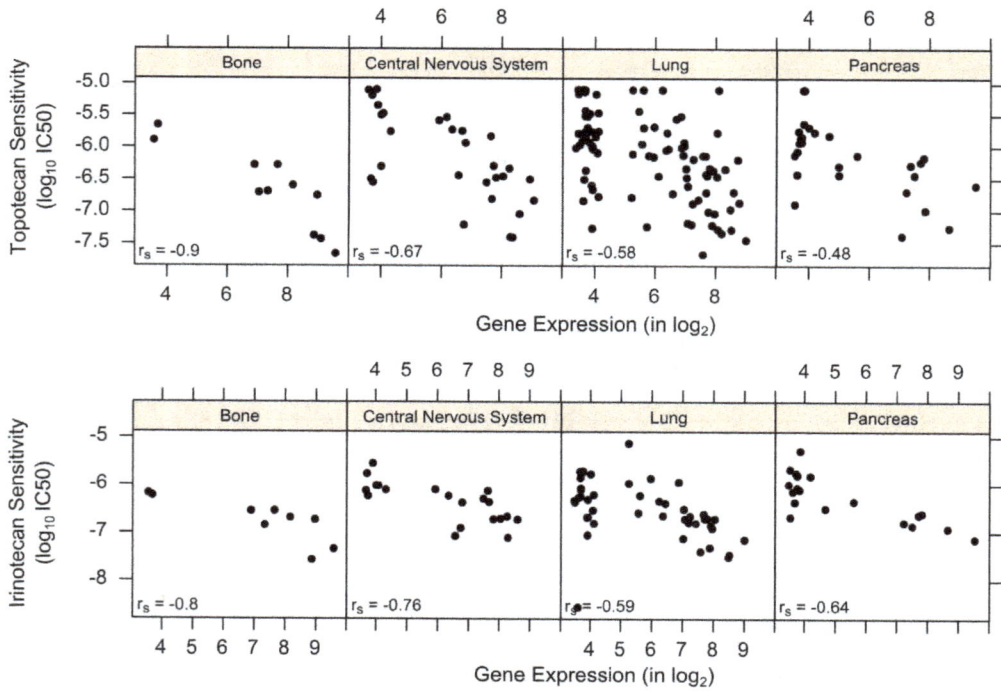

B. HMGB2

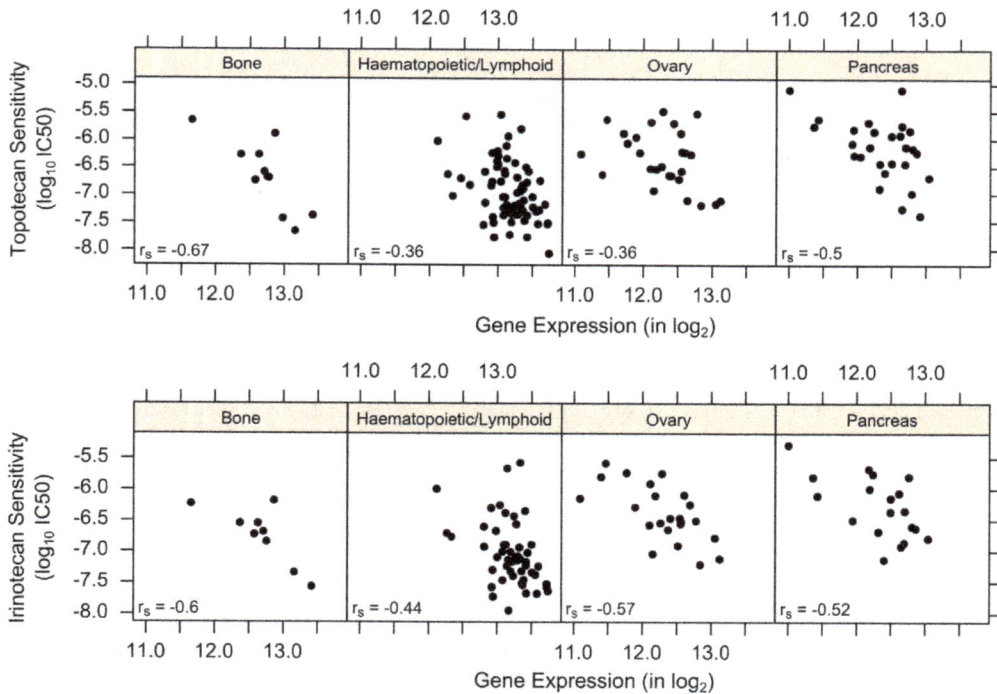

Figure 3. Top markers of response to TOP1 inhibitors: (A) SLFN11 and (B) HMGB2. Scatter plots show correlation between gene expression and pharmacological response values across several cancer lineages, where up-regulation of SLFN11 and HMGB2 correlate with drug sensitivity (indicated by smaller IC50 values).

A

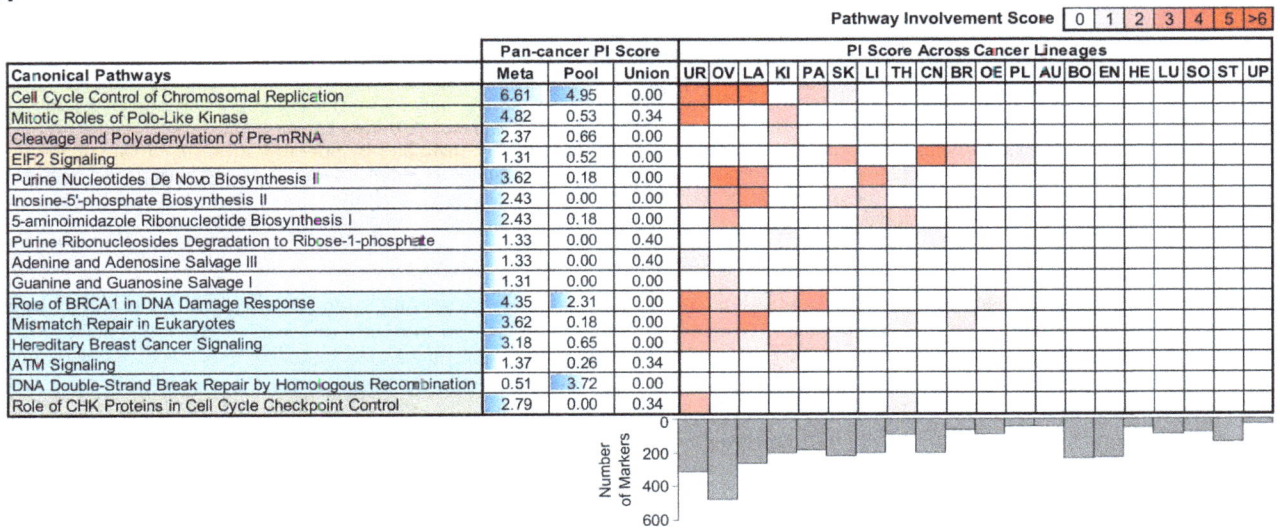

B

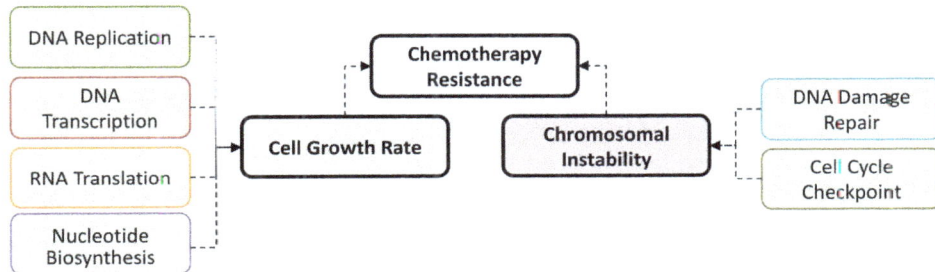

C

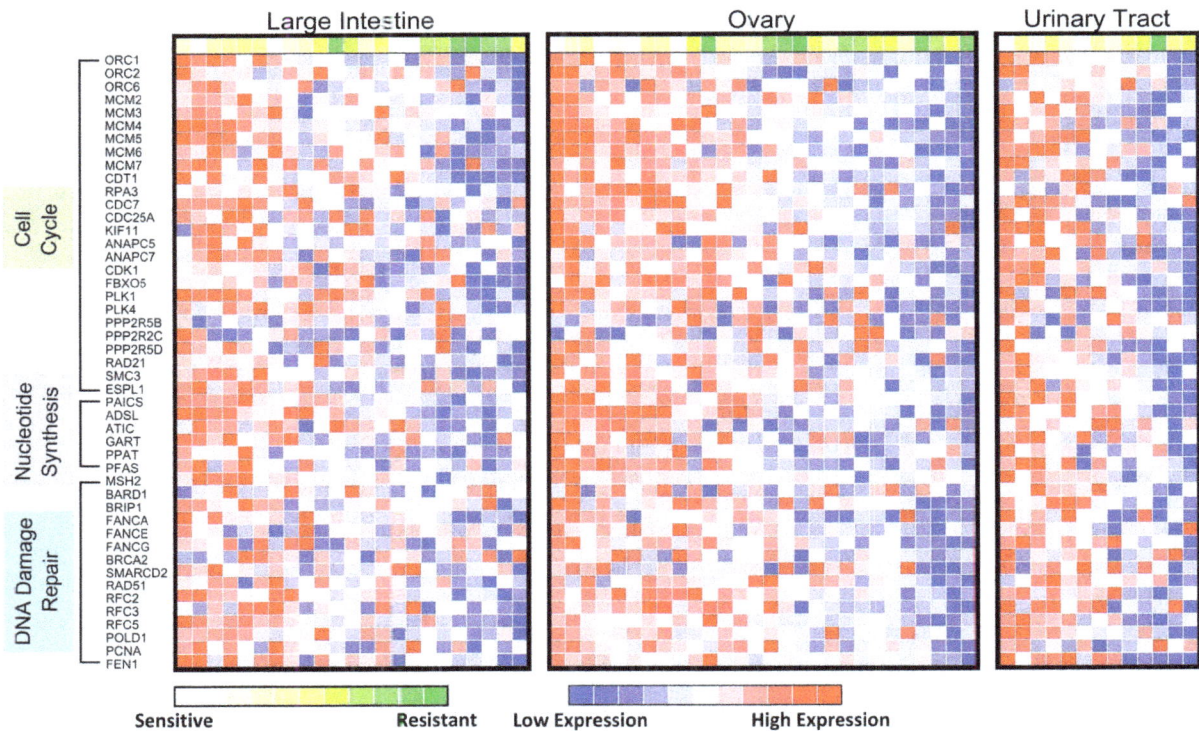

Large Intestine   Ovary   Urinary Tract

Sensitive   Resistant   Low Expression   High Expression

Figure 4. Pan-cancer analysis of TOP1 inhibitor Topotecan. (A) Pan-cancer pathways with significant involvement in drug response detected by PC-Meta, PC-Pool, PC-Union approaches (on the left). These pathways can be grouped into six biological processes (distinguished by background color), which converge on two distinct mechanisms. The involvement level of these pan-cancer pathways predicted by different approaches is illustrated with blue horizontal bars. Pathway involvement in each cancer lineage predicted by PC-Meta is indicated by the intensity of red fills in corresponding table (on the right). Pan-cancer and lineage-specific pathway involvement (PI) scores are derived from pathway enrichment analysis and calculated as -$\log_{10}$(BH-adjusted p-values). Only the top pathways with PI scores >1.3 are shown. Cancer lineage abbreviations – AU: autonomic; BO: bone; BR: breast; CN: central nervous system; EN: endometrial; HE: haematopoetic/lymphoid; KI: kidney; LA: large intestine; LI: liver; LU: lung; OE: oesophagus; OV: ovary; PA: pancreas; PL: pleura; SK: skin; SO: soft tissue; ST: stomach; TH: thyroid; UP: upper digestive; UR: urinary (B) Predicted known and novel mechanisms of intrinsic response to TOP1 inhibition. Red- and green-fill indicate increased and decreased activity in drug-resistant cell-lines respectively. (C) Heatmap showing the expression of genes in the cell cycle, nucleotide synthesis, and DNA damage repair pathways correlated with Topotecan response in multiple cancer lineages.

their roles in each cancer lineage. A subset of pan-cancer markers significantly correlated with response in each cancer type were selected as 'lineage-specific markers'. Then, each set of lineage-specific markers was assessed for enrichment to calculate a PI score for each pan-cancer pathway in each lineage. Interestingly, the pan-cancer pathways relevant to Topotecan response exhibited obvious lineage-specific differences (**Figure 4A**). Intrinsic response

in urinary, ovarian and large intestine cancers appeared prominently influenced through multiple mechanisms including cell cycle regulation, nucleotide synthesis, and DNA repair pathways (**Figure 4C**), whereas response in central nervous system cancers primarily involved EIF2 signaling. One-third of the cancer lineages were not characterized by any pan-cancer response mechanisms. Lineages without significant PI scores generally had

Table 2. Component genes of top pan-cancer pathways associated with drug response.

Topotecan	
Cell Cycle Control of Chromosomal Replication	ORC1(9), MCM6(6), ORC2(6), CDT1(4), MCM2(4), MCM4(4), RPA3(4), MCM5(3), MCM7(3), ORC6(3), CDC7(2), MCM3(2)
Mitotic Roles of Polo-Like Kinase	KIF11(6), ANAPC5(5), ANAPC7(5), CDK1(5), FBXO5(4), CDC25A(3), PLK4(3), PPP2R5D(3), RAD21(3), SMC3(3), CDC7(2), PLK1(2), PPP2R5B(2), ESPL1(1), PPP2R2C(1)
Cleavage and Polyadenylation of Pre-mRNA	CPSF2(5), NUDT21(5), PAPOLA(5), CPSF6(3), CSTF3(3)
EIF2 Signaling	RPL4(7), EIF3H(6), RPL36(6), **EIF2AK3**(5), EIF3A(5), EIF3D(5), EIF3E(5), PPP1CC(5), RPL11(5), **AGO2**(4), EIF2S1(4), EIF3L(4), RPL5(4), RPL8(4), RPLP2(4), RPS6(4)
Purine Nucleotides De Novo Biosynthesis II	PAICS(6), ADSL(5), ATIC(5), GART(5), PPAT(5), PFAS(3)
Adenine and Adenosine Salvage III	HPRT1(4), PNP(4), ADAT3(3)
Role of BRCA1 in DNA Damage Response	MSH2(7), FANCA(6), RFC5(6), BARD1(5), BRIP1(5), FANCG(5), BRCA2(4), SMARCD2(4), FANCE(3), RAD51(3), RFC2(3), RFC3(3), PLK1(2)
Mismatch Repair in Eukaryotes	MSH2(7), RFC5(6), POLD1(5), PCNA(4), FEN1(3), RFC2(3), RFC3(3)
ATM Signaling	CDK1(5), TDP1(5), MAPK8(4), SMC2(4), CDC25A(3), CREB1(3), RAD51(3), SMC3(2)
DNA Double-Strand Break Repair by Homologous Recombination	BRCA2(4), LIG1(4), RAD51(3)
Hereditary Breast Cancer Signaling	MSH2(7), FANCA(6), POLR2D(6), POLR2F(6), RFC5(6), BARD1(5), CDK1(5), FANCG(5), **HDAC11**(5), SMARCD2(5), BRCA2(4), FANCE(3), POLR2I(3), RAD51(3), RFC2(3), RFC3(3)
Role of CHK Proteins in Cell Cycle Checkpoint Control	RFC5(6), CDK1(5), CLSPN(4), PCNA(4), CDC25A(3), PPP2R5D(3), RFC2(3), RFC3(3), PLK1(2), **PPP2R5B**(1)
Panobinostat	
Interferon Signaling	IFIT3(8), IRF1(6), IFIT1(5), IFITM1(5), IRF9(4), PSMB8(4), RELA(4), STAT2(4), TAP1(3)
Hepatic Fibrosis/Hepatic Stellate Cell Activation	FGF2(7), TGFBR2(7), EGFR(6), IL6(6), TIMP1(6), CCL2(5), CCL5(5), IGFBP3(5), MYH9(5), SMAD3(5), VEGFA(5), IL1B(4), RELA(4), TIMP2(4), FGF1(3), IL8(3), MMP1(3), TGFB2(3)
Glucocorticoid Receptor Signaling	SMARCD2(7), TGFBR2(7), IL6(6), NR3C1(6), POU2F1(6), ADRB2(5), CCL2(5), CCL5(5), EP300(5), RRAS2(5), SMAD3(5), HMGB1(4), IL1B(4), MAP3K14(4), PIK3C2B(4), POLR2F(4), RELA(4), TAF3(4), IL8(3), MMP1(3), SERPINE1(3), SLPI(3), TGFB2(3), HLTF(2)
Antigen Presentation Pathway	HLA-C(5), TAP2(5), PSMB8(4), PSMB9(4), TAP1(3)
NF-κB Signaling	TGFBR2(7), EGFR(6), UBE2N(6), EP300(5), FGFR4(5), RRAS2(5), IL1B(4), MAP3K14(4), PIK3C2B(4), RELA(4), TNIP1(4), EIF2AK2(3), NGF(3)
Granzyme A Signaling	ANP32A(6), EP300(5), HIST1H1E(5), NME1(5)
Caveolar-mediated Endocytosis Signaling	EGFR(6), FLNA(6), CAV1(5), HLA-C(5), ITGA5(5), PTRF(4)
PD-0325901	
Human Embryonic Stem Cell Pluripotency	BDNF(8), NGF(6), FZD2(5), MRAS(5), S1PR1(5), TGFB2(5), FGF2(3)
Neurotrophin/TRK Signaling	BDNF(8), SPRY2(7), NGF(6), MRAS(5)

Note: Number in parentheses indicates the number of cancer lineages that each gene was predicted to be involved in. Genes in regular and bolded font are down- and up-regulated in resistant cell lines respectively. For pathways with many overlapping component genes, the best representative pathway is listed. Full list of pathways is available in **Table S6**.

fewer detected lineage-specific markers (**Figure 4A**), but not in all cases – bone and endometrial cancers had a similar number of markers to urinary and large intestine cancers, two lineages with the most significant PI scores.

Intrinsic Determinants of Response to HDAC Inhibitor (Panobinostat)

Panobinostat (LBH-589) is a pan-histone deacetylase (HDAC) inhibitor, which causes the hyperacetylation of histone and non-histone proteins. This triggers a plurality of anti-cancer mechanisms through both transcriptional and post-translational processes, including the activation of apoptotic pathways and the degradation of oncogenic HSP90 client proteins [28]. Resistance to HDAC inhibition has been associated with numerous mechanisms including enforced expression of anti-apoptotic proteins, activation of MAPK/PI3K/STAT3 signaling pathways, and the activation of NFkB pathway [28].

Application of the PC-Meta analysis identified 542 pan-cancer gene markers associated with intrinsic response to Panobinostat (**Table 1; Table S5**). One of the top markers identified by PC-Meta was the histone acetyltransferase (HAT) enzyme EP300, which antagonizes HDACs. It had reduced expression in drug-resistant cell lines across five cancer lineages (Figure 5A; meta-FDR = 8.9×10-3). In previous studies, lower EP300 expression has been shown to boost HDAC influence and attenuate the effects of HDAC inhibition [28]. Another interesting top pan-cancer gene marker, PEA-15, has anti-apoptotic function and was up-regulated

in the resistant cell lines of seven cancer lineages (Figure 5B; meta-FDR = 2.7×10-5). Since PEA-15 overexpression can suppress FAS/TNFα-mediated cell death, it may counteract the effects of HDAC inhibitors on the extrinsic apoptotic pathway [28,29].

To investigate pan-cancer mechanisms of response to Panobinostat, we applied pathway enrichment analysis to the set of PC-Meta pan-cancer gene markers. This revealed 20 pathways significantly associated with response with PI scores ranging from 1.0 to 4.0 (**Figure 6A; Table 2**). In contrast, enrichment analysis based on gene markers derived from PC-Pool and PC-Union identified only 6 and 8 pathways respectively, even though the PC-Pool approach provided greater number of gene markers than PC-Meta (723 vs 542). The PI scores for commonly detected pathways (e.g. Hepatic Stellate Cell Activation) were significantly higher for gene markers derived by PC-Meta compared to the two alternative pan-cancer analysis methods. Similar to our conclusions for the TOP1 inhibitors, PC-Meta performed better than alternative approaches in identifying pathways potentially involved in response to Panobinostat.

The pan-cancer pathways predicted by PC-Meta to be most associated with response were Interferon Signaling, Glucocorticoid Receptor (GR) Signaling, and Hepatic Stellate Cell (HSC) Activation (**Figure 6A**). Transient overexpression of the Interferon signalling pathway has been shown to trigger anti-viral/anti-pathogen immune responses as well as inhibit cell proliferation and induce apoptosis. However, recent studies showed that the constitutive overexpression of Interferon signaling confers resistance to genotoxic stress/damage possibly due to inability of a cell

A. EP300

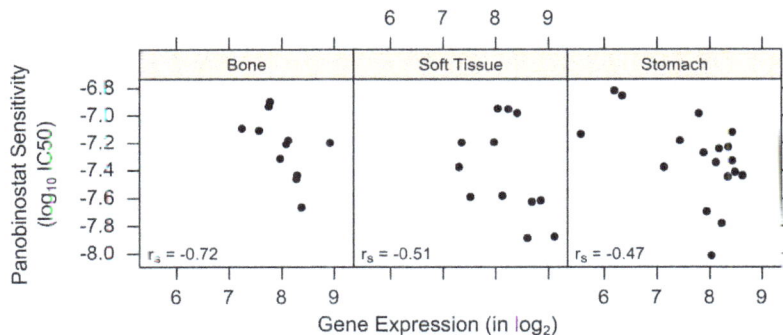

B. PEA15

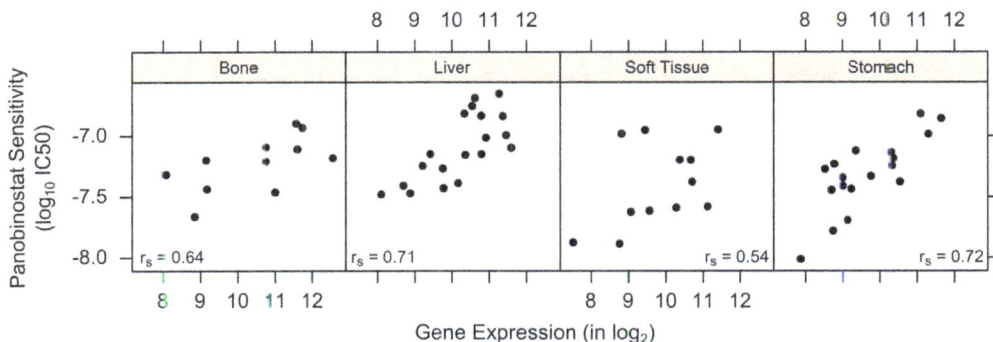

Figure 5. Top gene markers of response to HDAC inhibitor Panobinostat: (A) EP300 and (B) PEA15. Scatter plots show correlation between gene expression and pharmacological response values across several cancer lineages, where down-regulation of EP300 and up-regulation of PEA15 correlate with drug resistance (indicated by greater IC50 values).

A

B

C

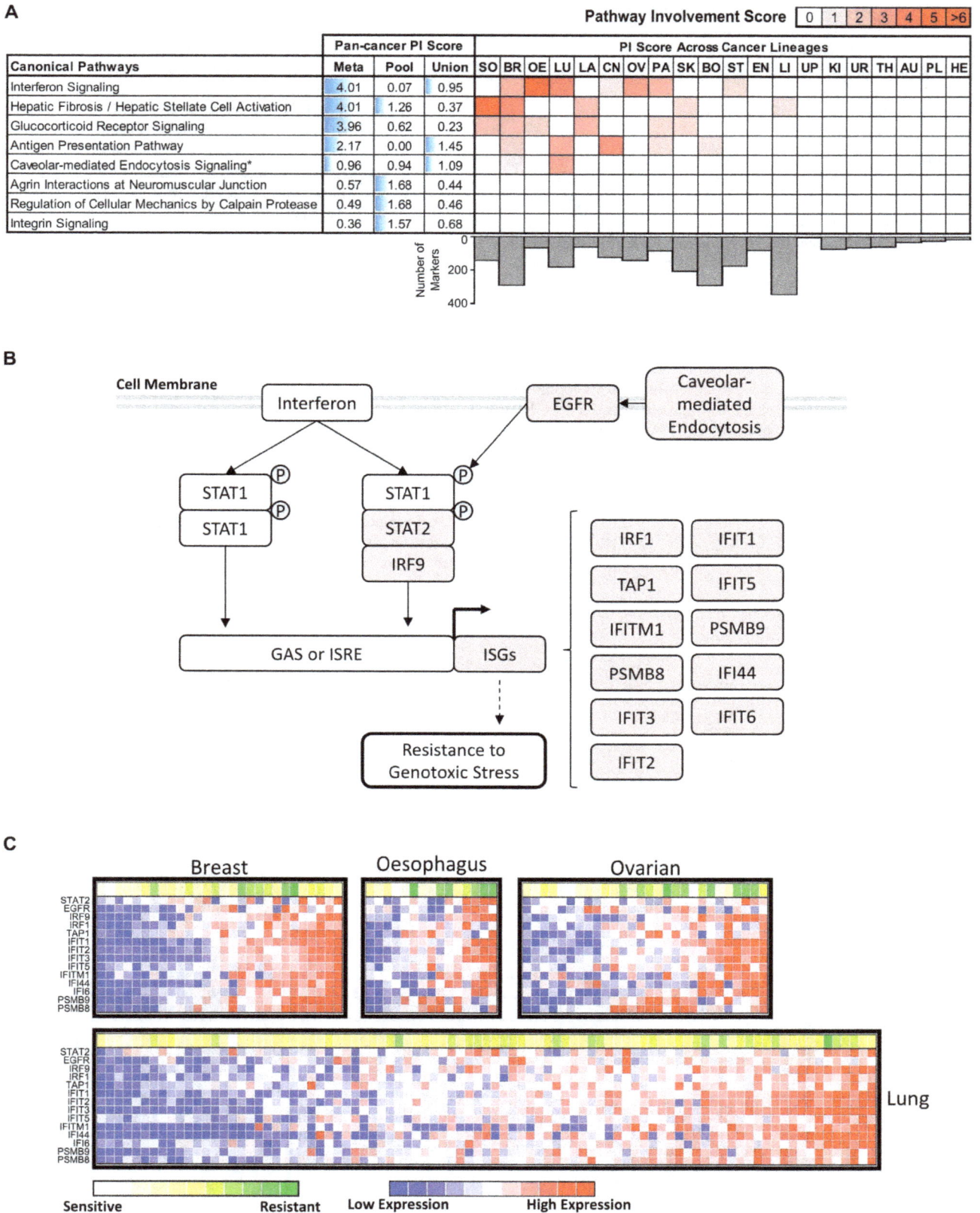

Figure 6. Pan-cancer analysis of HDAC inhibitor Panobinostat. (A) Pan-cancer pathways with significant involvement in drug response detected by PC-Meta, PC-Pool, PC-Union approaches (on the left). The predicted involvement level of these pan-cancer pathways by different approaches is illustrated with blue horizontal bars (in the middle). The involvement of these pan-cancer pathways in each cancer lineage predicted by PC-Meta is indicated by the intensity of red fills in corresponding table (on the right). Pan-cancer and lineage-specific pathway involvement (PI) scores

are derived from pathway enrichment analysis and calculated as -log$_{10}$(BH-adjusted p-values). Only the top pathways with PI scores >1.3 are shown. Cancer lineage abbreviations – AU: autonomic; BO: bone; BR: breast; CN: central nervous system; EN: endometrial; HE: haematopoetic/lymphoid; KI: kidney; LA: large intestine; LI: liver; LU: lung; OE: oesophagus; OV: ovary; PA: pancreas; PL: pleura; SK: skin; SO: soft tissue; ST: stomach; TH: thyroid; UP: upper digestive; UR: urinary (B) The predicted role of STAT/Interferon signaling pathway in Panobinostat inhibition. Red- and green-fills indicates increased and decreased gene expression in drug-resistant cell-lines respectively. (C) Heatmap showing the expression of genes in the STAT/Interferon pathway correlated with Panobinostat response in multiple cancer lineages.

to transmit cytotoxic response signals [30,31]. The latter was in line with our observations that genes in this pathway, such as interferon-stimulated genes (ISG), were overexpressed in drug-resistant cell lines across seven cancer lineages (**Figure 6B–C**). Interestingly, we also observed that the caveolar-mediated endocytosis signaling pathway had significant involvement in response specifically in lung cancers. Caveolar trafficking pathways can internalize various membrane receptors such as EGFR, and thereby strengthen EGFR signaling [32] and downstream activation of Interferon/STAT-1 signaling. Therefore, we speculate that the collective overexpression of caveolar-mediated endocytosis, EGFR, and Interferon/STAT-1 signaling pathway genes can coordinate stronger inherent resistance to Panobinostat in a subset of lung cancers.

GR signaling pathway, the second most enriched pathway in our analysis, is a regulator of immune responses as well as cellular apoptosis and proliferation. It comprises a number of genes that were overexpressed in the drug-resistant cell lines across several cancer lineages (**Table 2**), such as the nuclear hormone receptor GR/NR3C1 and RELA component of NF-kB complex. The expression of nuclear hormone receptor GR/NR3C1 normally drives the induction of anti-apoptotic proteins through the downstream activation of NF-kB signaling; however, this function can be compromised in absence of HDAC6 [33]. Therefore, we speculate that the observed up-regulations of GR/NR3C1 and NF-kB can oppose loss GR function resulting from HDAC inhibition [34]. Several genes with anti-apoptotic functions comprising the HSC Activation pathway, the third most enriched pathway, also had up-regulated expression in drug-resistant cell lines. These included members of the tissue inhibitor of metalloproteinase family (TIMP1 and TIMP2) that mediate cell survival [35], members of the fibroblast growth factor family (FGF1, FGF2) that up-regulate anti-apoptosis proteins and have broad cytoprotective effects across cancer types, and member of the vascular endothelial growth factor (VEGF1) that has also demonstrated pro-survival effects [36]. Collectively, these findings suggest that the up-regulation of cell survival through a complex diversity of molecular regulators is likely to be a primary modulator of response to Panobinostat across diverse cancer lineages.

Intrinsic Determinants of Response to MEK Inhibitors (PD-0325901 and AZD6244/Selumetinib)

MEK inhibitors have shown promise in treating cancers addicted to oncogenic mutations that dysregulate the RAF/MEK/ERK signaling pathway. For example, activating BRAF mutations occur in roughly 7% of all cancers, including up to 70% of melanomas, 22% of colorectal cancers, and 30% of serous ovarian cancers, and can confer sensitivity to MEK inhibition [37]. Resistance to MEK inhibition can occur as a result of molecular alterations upstream in the RAF/MEK/ERK pathway (e.g. KRAS amplifications or EGFR mutations) as well as activating mutations in the PI3K/AKT/MTOR pathway, which regulates similar mechanisms in apoptosis and cell growth [38].

We investigated two experimental MEK inhibitors currently undergoing clinical trials: PD-0325901 and AZD6244 (Selumeti-

nib). Both drugs showed similar patterns of pharmacological sensitivity across the panel of cancer lineages (**Figure 2**). However, these drugs and their response data are characterized by important differences: PD-0325901 is 10-times more potent than AZD6244 as a MEK inhibitor [39] and these drugs were screened on different numbers of cell lines (PD-0325901 on 366 and AZD6244 on 247). Our PC-Meta analysis yielded 171 response markers for the more potent PD-0325901 and only 10 response markers for AZD6244 (**Table S5**). Although this high discrepancy was unexpected, we believe it can be partly attributed to the aforementioned differences. Nevertheless, 8/10 (80%) of the AZD6244 gene markers were shared with PD-0325901 and may represent promising markers of resistance to the family of MEK inhibitors (**Table S4**). In particular, three of the identified genes were previously published as a part of the MEK-response gene signature [12]. These included SPRY2 that was down-regulated in resistant cell lines (meta-FDR $= 1.4 \times 10^{-3}$ for PD-0325901 and 4.0×10^{-3} for AZD6244), FZD2 that was up-regulated (**Figure 7A**; meta-FDR $= 1.5 \times 10^{-4}$ for PD-0325901 and 6.0×10^{-3} for AZD6244) and CRIM1 (meta-FDR $= 1.6 \times 10^{-5}$ for PD-0325901 and 5.0×10^{-3} for AZD6244) that was also up-regulated in resistant cells, consistent with previous findings (**Figure 8**). The observed decrease in expression of other common genes such as SPATA13 (**Figure 7B**), LYZ, and MGST2, to our knowledge, have not yet been implicated in resistance to MEK inhibitors and thus invites further investigation.

We selected the more potent and broadly screened PD-0325901 to further characterize mechanisms of intrinsic response to MEK inhibition. Pathway enrichment analysis of the PC-Meta pan-cancer gene markers resulted in only two significant pathways (**Figure 8A; Table 2**). Strikingly, no significant pathways were detected from PC-Pool or PC-Union gene markers. This result may be partially attributed to the limited number of markers for PC-Pool (46), but not for PC-Union (156), which detected a comparable number of genes as PC-Meta (**Table 1**).

The two pathways discovered by PC-Meta, Neutrophin/TRK signaling and Human Embryonic Stem Cell Pluripotency comprise numerous genes located upstream of the MEK target whose dysregulations can activate the PI3K signaling pathway and drive resistance to MEK inhibition. (**Figure 8B**). The neutrophin growth factors NGF and BDNF and the fibroblast growth factor FGF2 can trigger PI3K signaling through RAS and adaptor protein GRB2 [40]. These growth factors were overexpressed in PD-0325901-resistant cell lines. Additionally, the relevance of FGF2 regulated signaling appears to be reinforced through the suppressed expression of FGF antagonists SPRY1/2 in drug-resistant cell lines [36]. Interestingly, M-RAS, a close relative of classical RAS proteins (e.g. K-RAS, N-RAS), can also activate downstream PI3K/AKT effectors [41], and had elevated expression in resistant cell lines. Finally, in resistant cell lines, we observed up-regulation of gamma-protein coupled receptor S1PR, which can also stimulate the PI3K/AKT pathways [42] as well as the up-regulation of transforming growth factor beta TGFBII, which has been recently implicated in resistance to MEK-inhibitor AZD6244 [43]. Altogether, our findings support existing knowledge of PI3K pathway involvement as a principal mechanism of

A. FZD2

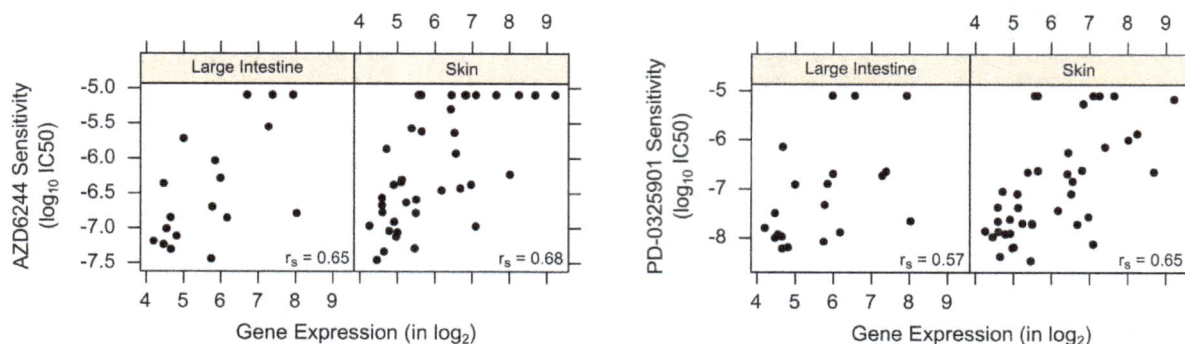

B. SPATA13

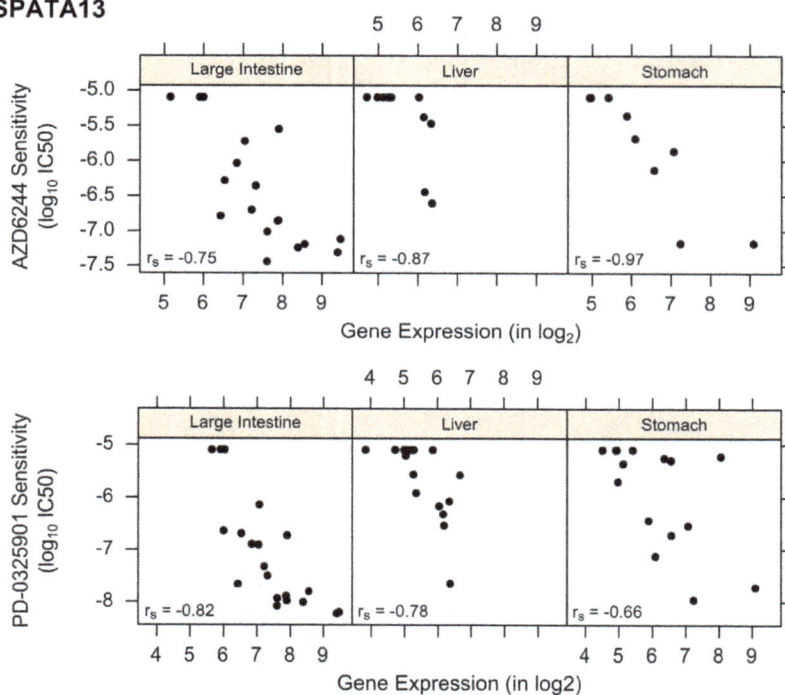

Figure 7. Top gene markers of response to MEK inhibitors PD-0325901 and AZD6244: (A) FZD2 and (B) SPATA13. Scatter plots show correlation between gene expression and pharmacological response values across several cancer lineages, where up-regulation of FZD2 and down-regulation of SPATA13 correlate with drug resistance (indicated by greater IC50 values).

resistance to MEK inhibitors. Additionally, the seven genes identified through our analysis may serve as a useful gene signature of such resistance.

Since mutations in the RAS/MEK/ERK or PI3K/AKT/MTOR pathways have been linked to the response to MEK inhibitors, we evaluated these mutations against our seven-gene signature in predicting drug response (**Figure 8C**). The mean expression of the seven-gene resistance signature was significantly correlated with response values in three cancer lineages: kidney cancers (Spearman's rho = 0.85, p-value = 0.017), large intestine/colorectal cancers (Spearman's rho = 0.61, p-value = 0.002), and soft tissue cancers (Spearman's rho = 0.61, p-value = 0.031). In contrast, individual mutation events were significantly associated with response in fewer cancer lineages. For instance, BRAF

mutations were associated with drug response values in only large intestinal/colorectal cancers (Student's t-test, p-value = 0.024). Of the multiple RAS proteins (KRAS, NRAS, HRAS) whose mutation are known to drive oncogenic MEK pathway activation [44,45], only NRAS mutations were associated with drug response values in soft tissue cancers (Student's t-test, p-value = 0.003). Finally, PIK3CA mutations, which can confer inappropriate activation of the PI3K signaling pathway, were weakly associated with drug-resistance in cancers of the large intestine and upper aerodigestive tract (Student's t-test, p-value = 0.003 in both). Altogether, these findings underscore the fact that known mutations cannot fully explain the response in entire cancer population. Importantly, it illustrates the advantages of our PC-

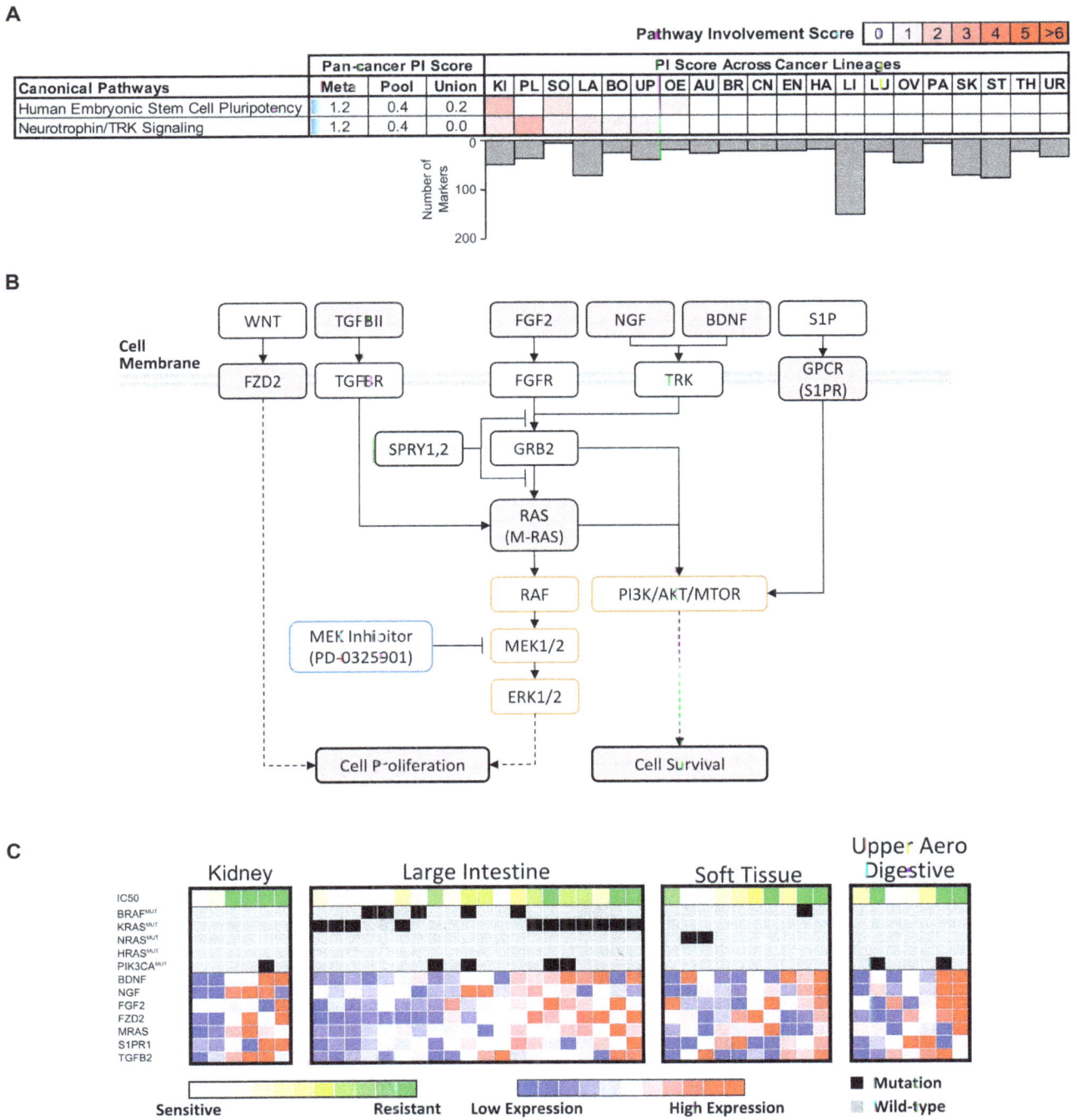

Figure 8. Pan-cancer analysis of MEK Inhibitor PD-0325901. (A) Pan-cancer pathways with significant involvement in drug response detected by PC-Meta, PC-Pool, PC-Union approaches (on the left). The predicted involvement level of these pan-cancer pathways by different approaches is illustrated with blue horizontal bars (in the middle). The involvement of these pan-cancer pathways in each cancer lineage predicted by PC-Meta is indicated by the intensity of red fills in corresponding table (on the right). Pan-cancer and lineage-specific pathway involvement (PI) scores are derived from pathway enrichment analysis and calculated as -log10(BH-adjusted p-values). Cancer lineage abbreviations – AU: autonomic; BO: bone; BR: breast; CN: central nervous system; EN: endometrial; HE: haematopoetic/lymphoid; KI: kidney; LA: large intestine; LI: liver; LU: lung; OE: oesophagus; OV: ovary; PA: pancreas; PL: pleura; SK: skin; SO: soft tissue; ST: stomach; TH: thyroid; UP: upper digestive; UR: urinary (B) The predicted role of PC-Meta identified compensatory mechanisms in MEK inhibition. Red- and green-fills indicates increased and decreased gene expression or activity in drug-resistant cell-lines respectively. Downstream RAF/MEK/ERK and PI3K/AKT/MTOR pathways are indicated in orange boxes and inhibitor is indicated in blue box. (C) Heatmap showing the expression of genes in the PC-Meta detected compensatory pathways correlated with PD-0325901 resistance in multiple cancer lineages.

Meta approach to identify potentially important compensatory mechanisms by which cancers resist targeted therapies.

Conclusions

In this study, we investigated the inherent determinants of cancer drug response across multiple cancer lineages. For this purpose, we developed a pan-cancer analysis strategy based on meta-analysis, PC-Meta, and comprehensively characterized known and novel mechanisms of response to both cytotoxic chemotherapies and targeted therapies in the publically available CCLE resource. Since many CCLE compounds were not amenable to comprehensive analysis due to highly biased pharmacological profiles or lack of reasonable sample sizes, we focused on a subset of five drugs that exhibited a broad range of *in vitro* sensitivity values across numerous cancer lineages. Importantly, compared to alternative approaches, our PC-Meta approach consistently demonstrated higher power in identifying potentially relevant markers and ability to infer the mechanisms of response.

For TOP1 inhibitors that are dependent on DNA replication and transcription rates, our analysis predicted cell lines with slower growth kinetics as inherently more drug-resistant irrespective of cancer lineage. Although this was not unexpected, our predictions suggested that the cellular growth rates in different cancer types can be suppressed through down-regulation of several processes including cell cycle control, nucleotide synthesis, and RNA translation. The degree of involvement of specific pathways in each cancer lineage can guide selection of proper combination therapy to circumvent resistance. We further observed that the overexpression of DNA repair genes may be indicative of a genome instability phenotype that may confer intrinsic resistance to TOP1 inhibition.

For Panobinostat, a pan-HDAC inhibitor that has been hypothesized to act on cancer cells through a number of diverse mechanisms, we identified the up-regulation of STAT-1/interferon signaling as a principal factor of inherent resistance across multiple cancer lineages. The basal overexpression of this pathway has been previously implicated in resistance to both radiotherapy and chemotherapy in lung and breast cancers, where it was suggested to confer resistance to genotoxic stress and damage as a result of failing to transmit cytotoxic signals. Our results expand its importance for additional cancer types such as those arising from ovarian and oesophageal tissue. Interestingly, our approach also identified a set of lung-specific markers involved in the caveolar-mediated endocytosis signaling, suggesting an important role of this pathway in the resistance of lung cancers to Panobinostat.

For MEK inhibitors, our PC-Meta analysis identified multiple determinants of inherent resistance that are upstream of the targeted MEK. These determinants include up-regulation of alternative oncogenic growth factor signaling pathways (e.g. FGF, NGF/BDNF, TGF) in resistant cell lines. In particular, we speculate that the up-regulation of the neutrophin-TRK signaling pathway can induce resistance to MEK-inhibition through the compensatory PI3K/AKT pathway and may serve as a promising new marker. We also identified the overexpression of MRAS, a less studied member of the RAS family, as a new indicator of drug-resistance. Importantly, our analysis demonstrated that gene expression markers identified by PC-Meta provides greater power in predicting *in vitro* pharmacological sensitivity than known mutations (such as in BRAF and RAS-family proteins) that are known to influence response. This emphasizes the importance of continuing efforts to develop gene expression based markers and

warrants their further evaluation on multiple independent datasets.

In conclusion, we have developed a meta-analysis approach for identifying inherent determinants of response to chemotherapy. Our approach avoids the significant loss of signal that can potentially result from using the standard pan-cancer analysis approach of directly pooling incomparable pharmacological and molecular profiling data from different cancer types. Application of this approach to three distinct classes of inhibitors (TOP1, HDAC, and MEK inhibitors) available from the public CCLE resource revealed recurrent markers and mechanisms of response, which were supported by findings in the literature. This study provides compelling leads that may serve as a useful foundation for future studies into resistance to commonly-used and novel cancer drugs and the development of strategies to overcome it. We make the compendium of markers identified in this study available to the research community.

Supporting Information

Figure S1 Drug response across different lineages for 24 CCLE compounds. Boxplots indicate the distribution of drug sensitivity values (based on IC50) in each cancer lineage for each cancer drug. For example, most cancer lineages are resistant to L-685458 (IC50 around 10^{-5} M) except for haematopoietic cancers (IC50 from 10^{-5} to 10^{-8} M). The number of samples in a cancer lineage screened for drug response is indicated under its boxplot. Cancer lineage abbreviations – **AU**: autonomic; **BO**: bone; **BR**: breast; **CN**: central nervous system; **EN**: endometrial; **HE**: haematopoetic/lymphoid; **KI**: kidney; **LA**: large intestine; **LI**: liver; **LU**: lung; **OE**: oesophagus; **OV**: ovary; **PA**: pancreas; **PL**: pleura; **SK**: skin; **SO**: soft tissue; **ST**: stomach; **TH**: thyroid; **UP**: upper digestive; **UR**: urinary.

Table S1 Summary of PC-Meta, PC-Pool, and PC-Union markers identified for all CCLE drugs (meta-FDR <0.01).

Table S2 Functions significantly enriched in the PC-Pool gene markers associated with sensitivity to L-685458.

Table S3 Overlap of PC-Meta markers between TOP1 inhibitors, Topotecan and Irinotecan.

Table S4 Overlap of PC-Meta markers between MEK inhibitors, PD-0325901 and AZD6244, and reported signature in [12].

Table S5 List of significant PC-Meta pan-cancer markers identified for each of 20 drugs.

Table S6 Pan-cancer pathways with predicted involvement in response to TOP1, HDAC, and MEK inhibitors.

Acknowledgments

Phuong Dao, Robert Bell, Fan Mo provided valuable discussions regarding the methodology.

Author Contributions

Conceived and designed the experiments: KW AL. Performed the experiments: KW RS. Analyzed the data: KW AWW AL. Contributed reagents/materials/analysis tools: KW AR JL. Contributed to the writing of the manuscript: KW AL AWW CCC. Algorithm development: KW AR JL. Critical review of manuscript: AWW YW.

References

1. Gillet J, Gottesman MM (2010) Multi-Drug Resistance in Cancer. 596. Available: http://www.springerlink.com/index/10.1007/978-1-60761-416-6. Accessed 25 May 2013.
2. Bianco R, Troiani T, Tortora G, Ciardiello F (2005) Intrinsic and acquired resistance to EGFR inhibitors in human cancer therapy. Endocr Relat Cancer 12 Suppl 1: S159–71. Available: http://www.ncbi.nlm.nih.gov/pubmed/16113092. Accessed 13 June 2013.
3. Szakács G, Paterson JK, Ludwig J a, Booth-Genthe C Gottesman MM (2006) Targeting multidrug resistance in cancer. Nat Rev Drug Discov 5: 219–234. Available: http://www.ncbi.nlm.nih.gov/pubmed/16518375. Accessed 8 November 2013.
4. Bean J, Brennan C, Shih J-Y, Riely G, Viale A, et al. (2007) MET amplification occurs with or without T790M mutations in EGFR mutant lung tumors with acquired resistance to gefitinib or erlotinib. Proc Natl Acad Sci U S A 104: 20932–20937. Available: http://www.pubmedcentral.nih.gov/articlerender.fcgi?artid=2409244&tool=pmcentrez&rendertype=abstract.
5. Shoemaker RH (2006) The NCI60 human tumour cell line anticancer drug screen. Nat Rev Cancer 6: 813–823. Available: http://www.ncbi.nlm.nih.gov/pubmed/16990858.
6. Györffy B, Surowiak P, Kiesslich O, Denkert C, Schäfer R, et al. (2006) Gene expression profiling of 30 cancer cell lines predicts resistance towards 11 anticancer drugs at clinically achieved concentrations. Int J Cancer 118: 1699–1712. Available: http://www.ncbi.nlm.nih.gov/pubmed/16217747. Accessed 2 March 2013.
7. Garnett MJ, Edelman EJ, Heidorn SJ, Greenman CD, Dastur A, et al. (2012) Systematic identification of genomic markers of drug sensitivity in cancer cells. Nature 483: 570–575. Available: http://www.nature.com/nature/journal/v483/n7391/full/nature11005.html#/acknowledgments. Accessed 1 April 2012.
8. Barretina J, Caponigro G, Stransky N, Venkatesan K, Margolin AA, et al. (2012) The Cancer Cell Line Encyclopedia enables predictive modelling of anticancer drug sensitivity. Nature 483: 603–607. Available: http://www.ncbi.nlm.nih.gov/pubmed/22460905. Accessed 1 April 2012.
9. Yauch RL, Januario T, Eberhard D a, Cavet G, Zhu W, et al. (2005) Epithelial versus mesenchymal phenotype determines in vitro sensitivity and predicts clinical activity of erlotinib in lung cancer patients. Clin Cancer Res 11: 8686–8698. Available: http://www.ncbi.nlm.nih.gov/pubmed/16361555. Accessed 13 December 2013.
10. Neve RM, Chin K, Fridlyand J, Yeh J, Baehner FL, et al. (2006) A collection of breast cancer cell lines for the study of functionally distinct cancer subtypes. Cancer Cell 10: 515–527. Available: http://www.pubmedcentral.nih.gov/articlerender.fcgi?artid=2730521&tool=pmcentrez&rendertype=abstract. Accessed 6 July 2011.
11. Minna JD, Girard L, Xie Y (2007) Tumor mRNA expression profiles predict responses to chemotherapy. J Clin Oncol 25: 4329–4336. Available: http://www.ncbi.nlm.nih.gov/pubmed/17906194. Accessed 2 February 2012.
12. Dry JR, Pavey S, Pratilas C a, Harbron C, Runswick S, et al. (2010) Transcriptional pathway signatures predict MEK addiction and response to selumetinib (AZD6244). Cancer Res 70: 2264–2273. Available: http://www.pubmedcentral.nih.gov/articlerender.fcgi?artid=3166660&tool=pmcentrez&rendertype=abstract. Accessed 26 November 2012.
13. Mo Q, Wang S, Seshan VE, Olshen AB, Schultz N, et al. (2013) Pattern discovery and cancer gene identification in integrated cancer genomic data. Proc Natl Acad Sci U S A 110: 4245–4250. Available: http://www.pubmedcentral.nih.gov/articlerender.fcgi?artid=3600490&tool=pmcentrez&rendertype=abstract. Accessed 22 May 2013.
14. Hanahan D, Weinberg R a (2011) Hallmarks of cancer: the next generation. Cell 144: 646–674. Available: http://www.ncbi.nlm.nih.gov/pubmed/21376230. Accessed 21 May 2013.
15. Tamborero D, Gonzalez-Perez A, Perez-Llamas C, Deu-Pons J, Kandoth C, et al. (2013) Comprehensive identification of mutational cancer driver genes across 12 tumor types. Sci Rep 3: 2650. Available: http://www.pubmedcentral.nih.gov/articlerender.fcgi?artid=3788361&tool=pmcentrez&rendertype=abstract. Accessed 31 October 2013.
16. Rhodes DR, Yu J, Shanker K, Deshpande N, Varambally R, et al. (2004) Large-scale meta-analysis of cancer microarray data identifies common transcriptional profiles of neoplastic transformation and progression. Proc Natl Acad Sci U S A 101: 9309–9314. Available: http://www.pubmedcentral.nih.gov/articlerender.fcgi?artid=438973&tool=pmcentrez&rendertype=abstract. Accessed 5 June 2012.
17. Rhodes DR, Kalyana-Sundaram S, Mahavisno V, Varambally R, Yu J, et al. (2007) Oncomine 3.0: Genes, Pathways, and Networks in a Collection of 18,000 Cancer Gene Expression Profiles. Neoplasia 9: 166–180. Available: http://openurl.ingenta.com/content/xref?genre=article&issn=1522-8002&volume=9&issue=2&spage=166. Accessed 21 May 2013.
18. Glinsky G V, Berezovska O, Glinskii AB (2005) Microarray analysis identifies a death-from-cancer signature predicting therapy failure in patients with multiple types of cancer. 115: 1503–1521. doi:10.1172/JCI23412.The.
19. Owen AB (2009) Karl Pearson's meta-analysis revisited. Ann Stat 37: 3867–3892. Available: http://projecteuclid.org/euclid.aos/1256303530. Accessed 2013 March 3.
20. Tseng GC, Ghosh D, Feingold E (2012) Comprehensive literature review and statistical considerations for microarray meta-analysis. Nucleic Acids Res 40: 3785–3799. Available: http://www.pubmedcentral.nih.gov/articlerender.fcgi?artid=3351145&tool=pmcentrez&rendertype=abstract. Accessed 27 February 2013.
21. Pommier Y (2006) Topoisomerase I inhibitors: camptothecins and beyond. Nat Rev Cancer 6: 789–802. Available: http://www.ncbi.nlm.nih.gov/pubmed/16990856. Accessed 3 March 2013.
22. Zoppoli G, Regairaz M (2012) Putative DNA/RNA helicase Schlafen-11 (SLFN11) sensitizes cancer cells to DNA-damaging agents. Proc 11: 2–7. Available: http://www.pnas.org/content/109/37/15030.short. Accessed 2012 November 22.
23. Krynetskaia NF, Phadke MS, Jadhav SE, Krynetskiy EY (2009) Chromatin-associated proteins HMGB1/2 and PDIA3 trigger cellular response to chemotherapy-induced DNA damage. Mol Cancer Ther 8: 864–872. Available: http://www.pubmedcentral.nih.gov/articlerender.fcgi?artid=2684979&tool=pmcentrez&rendertype=abstract. Accessed 2013 December 16.
24. Lee YY, Yu YB, Gunawardena HP, Xie L, Chen X (2012) BCLAF1 is a radiation-induced H2AX-interacting partner involved in γH2AX-mediated regulation of apoptosis and DNA repair. Cell Death Dis 3: e359. Available: http://www.pubmedcentral.nih.gov/articlerender.fcgi?artid=3406578&tool=pmcentrez&rendertype=abstract. Accessed 2013 December 16.
25. McClelland SE, Burrell R a, Swanton C (2009) Chromosomal instability: a composite phenotype that influences sensitivity to chemotherapy. Cell Cycle 8: 3262–3266. Available: http://www.ncbi.nlm.nih.gov/pubmed/19806022.
26. Schlacher K, Wu H, Jasin M (2012) A distinct replication fork protection pathway connects Fanconi anemia tumor suppressors to RAD51-BRCA1/2. Cancer Cell 22: 106–116. Available: http://www.ncbi.nlm.nih.gov/pubmed/22789542. Accessed 2013 July 30.
27. Pitroda SP, Pashtan IM, Logan HL, Budke B, Darga TE, et al. (2014) DNA Repair Pathway Gene Expression Score Correlates with Repair Proficiency and Tumor Sensitivity to Chemotherapy. Sci Transl Med 6: 229ra42–229ra42. Available: http://stm.sciencemag.org/cgi/doi/10.1126/scitranslmed.3008291. Accessed 2014 March 29.
28. Robey RW, Chakraborty AR, Basseville A, Luchenko V, Bahr J, et al. (2011) Histone deacetylase inhibitors: emerging mechanisms of resistance. Mol Pharm 8: 2021–2031. Available: http://www.pubmedcentral.nih.gov/articlerender.fcgi?artid=3230675&tool=pmcentrez&rendertype=abstract.
29. Fiory F, Formisano P, Perruolo G, Beguinot F (2009) Frontiers: PED/PEA-15, a multifunctional protein controlling cell survival and glucose metabolism. Am J Physiol Endocrinol Metab 297: E592–601. Available: http://www.ncbi.nlm.nih.gov/pubmed/19531639. Accessed 2013 July 22.
30. Khodarev NN, Roizman B, Weichselbaum RR (2012) Molecular pathways: interferon/stat1 pathway: role in the tumor resistance to genotoxic stress and aggressive growth. Clin Cancer Res 18: 3015–3021. Available: http://www.ncbi.nlm.nih.gov/pubmed/22615451. Accessed 2013 July 30.
31. Weichselbaum RR, Ishwaran H, Yoon T, Nuyten DS a, Baker SW, et al. (2008) An interferon-related gene signature for DNA damage resistance is a predictive marker for chemotherapy and radiation for breast cancer. Proc Natl Acad Sci U S A 105: 18490–18495. Available: http://www.pubmedcentral.nih.gov/articlerender.fcgi?artid=2587578&tool=pmcentrez&rendertype=abstract.
32. Mosesson Y, Mills GB, Yarden Y (2008) Derailed endocytosis: an emerging feature of cancer. Nat Rev Cancer 8: 835–850. Available: http://www.ncbi.nlm.nih.gov/pubmed/18948996. Accessed 2013 May 21.
33. Vilasco M, Communal L, Mourra N, Couttin A Forgez P, et al. (2011) Glucocorticoid receptor and breast cancer. Breast Cancer Res Treat 130: 1–10. Available: http://www.ncbi.nlm.nih.gov/pubmed/21818591. Accessed 2014 January 30.
34. Kovacs JJ, Murphy PJM, Gaillard S, Zhao X, Wu J-T, et al. (2005) HDAC6 regulates Hsp90 acetylation and chaperone-dependent activation of glucocorticoid receptor. Mol Cell 18: 601–607. Available: http://www.ncbi.nlm.nih.gov/pubmed/15916966. Accessed 2014 January 24.
35. Liu X-W, Bernardo MM, Fridman R, Kim H-RC (2003) Tissue inhibitor of metalloproteinase-1 protects human breast epithelial cells against intrinsic apoptotic cell death via the focal adhesion kinase/phosphatidylinositol 3-kinase and MAPK signaling pathway. J Biol Chem 278: 40364–40372. Available: http://www.ncbi.nlm.nih.gov/pubmed/12904305. Accessed 2013 August 20.
36. Turner N, Grose R (2010) Fibroblast growth factor signalling: from development to cancer. Nat Rev Cancer 10: 116–129. Available: http://www.ncbi.nlm.nih.gov/pubmed/20094046. Accessed 2013 May 22.

37. McCubrey J a, Steelman LS, Abrams SL, Chappell WH, Russo S, et al. (2010) Emerging MEK inhibitors. Expert Opin Emerg Drugs 15: 203–223. Available: http://www.ncbi.nlm.nih.gov/pubmed/20151845.

38. Mccubrey JA, Steelman LS, Chappell WH, Stephen L, Franklin RA, et al. (2012) Ras/Raf/MEK/ERK PI3K/PTEN/Akt/mTOR Cascade Inhibitors: How Mutations Can Result in Therapy Resistance and How to Overcome Resistance Abstract: 3: 1068–1111.

39. Sebolt-Leopold JS (2008) Advances in the development of cancer therapeutics directed against the RAS-mitogen-activated protein kinase pathway. Clin Cancer Res 14: 3651–3656. Available: http://www.ncbi.nlm.nih.gov/pubmed/18559577. Accessed 2013 November 16.

40. Thiele CJ, Li Z, McKee AE (2009) On Trk—the TrkB signal transduction pathway is an increasingly important target in cancer biology. Clin Cancer Res 15: 5962–5967. Available: http://www.pubmedcentral.nih.gov/articlerender.fcgi?artid = 2756331&tool = pmcentrez&rendertype = abstract. Accessed 2013 May 30.

41. Watanabe-Takano H, Takano K, Keduka E, Endo T (2010) M-Ras is activated by bone morphogenetic protein-2 and participates in osteoblastic determination, differentiation, and transdifferentiation. Exp Cell Res 316: 477–490. Available: http://www.ncbi.nlm.nih.gov/pubmed/19800879. Accessed 2013 July 29.

42. O'Sullivan C, Dev KK (2013) The structure and function of the S1P1 receptor. Trends Pharmacol Sci 34: 401–412. Available: http://www.ncbi.nlm.nih.gov/pubmed/23763867. Accessed 2013 July 30.

43. Huang S, Hölzel M, Knijnenburg T, Schlicker A, Roepman P, et al. (2012) MED12 controls the response to multiple cancer drugs through regulation of TGF-β receptor signaling. Cell 151: 937–950. Available: http://www.ncbi.nlm.nih.gov/pubmed/23178117. Accessed 2013 May 23.

44. Wee S, Jagani Z, Xiang KX, Loo A, Dorsch M, et al. (2009) PI3K pathway activation mediates resistance to MEK inhibitors in KRAS mutant cancers. Cancer Res 69: 4286–4293. Available: http://www.ncbi.nlm.nih.gov/pubmed/19401449. Accessed 2013 December 10.

45. Solit DB, Garraway L a, Pratilas C a, Sawai A, Getz G, et al. (2006) BRAF mutation predicts sensitivity to MEK inhibition. Nature 439: 358–362. Available: http://www.pubmedcentral.nih.gov/articlerender.fcgi?artid = 3306236&tool = pmcentrez&rendertype = abstract. Accessed 2013 December 5.

11

ALDH1A1 Maintains Ovarian Cancer Stem Cell-Like Properties by Altered Regulation of Cell Cycle Checkpoint and DNA Repair Network Signaling

Erhong Meng[1], Aparna Mitra[1], Kaushlendra Tripathi[1], Michael A. Finan[1], Jennifer Scalici[1], Steve McClellan[1], Luciana Madeira da Silva[1], Eddie Reed[2], Lalita A. Shevde[3], Komaraiah Palle[1]*, Rodney P. Rocconi[1]*

1 University of South Alabama Mitchell Cancer Institute, Mobile, Alabama, United States of America, **2** National Institutes of Health, National Institute on Minority Health and Health Disparities, Bethesda, Maryland, United States of America, **3** University of Alabama at Birmingham, Birmingham, Alabama, United States of America

Abstract

Objective: Aldehyde dehydrogenase (ALDH) expressing cells have been characterized as possessing stem cell-like properties. We evaluated ALDH+ ovarian cancer stem cell-like properties and their role in platinum resistance.

Methods: Isogenic ovarian cancer cell lines for platinum sensitivity (A2780) and platinum resistant (A2780/CP70) as well as ascites from ovarian cancer patients were analyzed for ALDH+ by flow cytometry to determine its association to platinum resistance, recurrence and survival. A stable shRNA knockdown model for ALDH1A1 was utilized to determine its effect on cancer stem cell-like properties, cell cycle checkpoints, and DNA repair mediators.

Results: ALDH status directly correlated to platinum resistance in primary ovarian cancer samples obtained from ascites. Patients with ALDH^{HIGH} displayed significantly lower progression free survival than the patients with ALDH^{LOW} cells (9 vs. 3 months, respectively $p<0.01$). ALDH1A1-knockdown significantly attenuated clonogenic potential, PARP-1 protein levels, and reversed inherent platinum resistance. ALDH1A1-knockdown resulted in dramatic decrease of KLF4 and p21 protein levels thereby leading to S and G2 phase accumulation of cells. Increases in S and G2 cells demonstrated increased expression of replication stress associated Fanconi Anemia DNA repair proteins (FANCD2, FANCJ) and replication checkpoint (pS317 Chk1) were affected. ALDH1A1-knockdown induced DNA damage, evidenced by robust induction of γ-H2AX and BAX mediated apoptosis, with significant increases in BRCA1 expression, suggesting ALDH1A1-dependent regulation of cell cycle checkpoints and DNA repair networks in ovarian cancer stem-like cells.

Conclusion: This data suggests that ovarian cancer cells expressing ALDH1A1 may maintain platinum resistance by altered regulation of cell cycle checkpoint and DNA repair network signaling.

Editor: Robertus A.M. de Bruin, University College London, United Kingdom

Funding: This work was supported by the Gynecologic Cancer Foundation Sherri's From a Whisper to a Roar, Women's Motorcycle Foundation Ovarian Cancer Research Award and The Eleanor Ruth Frenkel Fund for Ovarian Cancer Research (R.P.R); NIH grant R01GM098956, and Abraham Mitchell Endowment grant (K.P.). The funders had no role in study design, data collection and analysis, decision to publish, or preparation of the manuscript.

Competing Interests: The authors have declared that no competing interests exist.

* Email: kpalle@health.southalabama.edu (KP); rocccni@health.southalabama.edu (RPR)

Introduction

Ovarian cancer is the most lethal of all gynecologic malignancies, affecting over 22,000 lives of women annually in the United States alone. Although the majority of ovarian cancer patients achieve a complete initial clinical response to cytoreductive surgery followed by combination chemotherapy, most will experience a recurrence and unfortunately succumb to progressive disease [1]. Vital to the prognosis of ovarian cancer patients is the disease's varying sensitivity to platinum agents. Although a continuum, patients are stratified by their disease's original response to platinum chemotherapy as either "platinum-sensitive"

or "platinum-resistant" defined by the length of the relapse-free interval. This spectrum is highly predictive of clinical endpoints of when a cancer recurs, the success of surgery and/or chemotherapy at recurrence, and a patient's overall survival.

Considering the heterogeneity of cancer, not all cells within a malignancy would be expected to be resistant to chemotherapy. The cancer stem cells (CSCs) theory proposes that these resistant cells encompass only a minority of cells within a cancer, yet are solely responsible for long-term recurrence [2]. Thereby, irrespective of the initial response rates, if chemotherapy fails to eradicate these resistant CSCs, then cancer will regenerate and a recurrence or progression of disease will occur. The identification of these resistant cells and determining their innate molecular pathways are paramount in finding more effective targeted therapies [3]. Therefore, one strategy to improve the success of ovarian cancer therapy is to enhance CSCs sensitivity to platinum agents. Overcoming platinum resistance would be vital in the treatment of ovarian cancer with the potential benefits of enhanced response rates, longer survival, and more cures.

Recently, aldehyde dehydrogenase (ALDH) activity has been shown to be a very attractive CSCs marker in many cancers such as lung [4], breast [5], prostate [6], thyroid [7], head and neck cancer [8], and ovarian cancer [9–12]. ALDH family comprises cytosolic isoenzymes responsible for oxidizing intracellular alde-hydes, thus contributing to the oxidation of retinol to retinoic acid in early stem cell differentiation [4]. The human ALDH superfamily currently consists of 19 known putatively functional genes in 11 families and 4 subfamilies with distinct chromosomal locations. Of the vast ALDH families and subfamilies, ALDH1A1 has been a valid marker among several malignant tissues. It holds the attractive distinction of not only being a potential marker of stemness but potentially playing a role in the biology of tumor-initiating cells as well [13]. Additionally, the ALDH1A1 subpop-ulation had demonstrated to be associated with chemoresistance in ovarian cancer patients [9,14].

Recent studies in breast cancer models demonstrated an interesting relationship between BRCA1 and stem cell differenti-ation [15,16]. BRCA1 also has been shown to play an important role in breast tissue differentiation by regulating Notch signaling and tumor response to anti-endocrine therapy[14]. Particularly, an inverse relationship between ALDH1A1 expression and BRCA1 is noteworthy in the context of studying cancer stem-like cells and chemoresistance. BRCA1 plays important roles in protecting genome from aberrant DNA lesions, and mutations or deletion in this gene lead to genome instability and increased incidence of breast, ovarian and other cancers [17]. In response to DNA damage it rapidly localizes to the sites of double strand breaks (DSB) and mediates several signaling responses including cell cycle checkpoints and choice of the DNA repair pathway to fix these lesions [17–19]. However, BRCA1 status and ALDH+ ovarian cancer stem-like cells maintenance and their resistance to chemotherapy has not been studied.

We demonstrate that ALDH+ phenotype possesses CSC characteristics of enhanced invasion, colony formation, and stem cell markers. The specific ALDH1A1 isotype appears to be responsible for ALDH-mediated platinum resistance both clini-cally as well as in in-vitro models. Our data supports an ALDH1A1-mediated platinum resistance mechanism in ovarian cancer via an altered regulation of cell cycle checkpoint and DNA repair network signaling.

Materials and Methods

Cell Lines and Cultures

A2780 and an isogenic cisplatin resistant A2780/CP70 cell line was generated as described earlier [20].

ALDEFLUOR Assay and Fluorescence-activated Cell Sorting

To isolate the cell population with a high ALDH enzymatic activity, ALDEFLUOR assay kit (STEMCELL Technologies Inc.) was used according to the manufacturer's instructions. After trypsinization, cells were suspended in ALDEFLUOR assay buffer containing ALDH enzyme substrate BODIPY-aminoacetaldehyde (BAAA), and incubated at 37°C for about 40 minutes. Cells were stained using the identical conditions with the specific ALDH

inhibitor, diethylaminobenzaldehyde (DEAB), to serve as a negative control. Flow cytometry sorting was conducted using a BD Bioscience Aria II SORP cell sorter.

Carcinogenic Properties

After sorting for ALDH phenotypes (ALDH+ vs. ALDH−), Matrigel invasion and soft agar colony formation assays were performed as previously described [21]. To evaluate the effect of chemotherapy on colony formation, cells were treated with fresh media with 20 μM carboplatin added every 3–4 days. Visible colonies (>50 cells) were counted on five randomly selected 40X microscopic fields in each well.

CellTiter-Glo Luminescent Cell Viability Assay

Sorted A2780/CP70 cells were plated at density of 4000 cells per well in 96-well black plate with clear bottom (Corning, NY, USA). The following day, the cells were treated with various concentrations of carboplatin up to 72 hours. After 24, 48 and 72 hours, 100 μl of CellTiter-Glo reagent (Promega) per well were added, incubated for 10 minutes at room temperature and luminescence was recorded on a Synergy H4 Hybrid Reader (BioTek).

Real-time Quantitative RT-PCR

Real-time Quantitative RT-PCR was performed as described previously [21]. Primers and probes for the TaqMan system were selected from the Applied Biosystems website [BMI1 assay ID: Hs00180411_m1, c-myc assay ID: Hs00905030_m1, Kruppel-like factor 4 (KLF4) assay ID: Hs00358836_m1, oct3/4 assay ID: Hs01009568_m1, S100 calcium binding protein A1 (S100A1) assay ID: Hs00984741_m1, ALDH1A1 assay ID: Hs00946916_m1, CDKN1A (p21) assay ID: Hs00355782_m1, internal control glyceraldehyde-3-phosphate dehydrogenase assay ID: Hs99999905_m1]. The relative expression mRNA levels of BMI1, c-myc, Oct3/4, KLF4, S100A1, ALDH1A1, p21, were calculated using the $\Delta\Delta$Ct method and normalization to GAPDH.

Lentiviral shRNA Vector Transfection

Six different pGIPZ Lentiviral shRNA glycerol stocks against ALDH1A1 and one negative control shRNA (Thermo Scientific) were transfected according to the manufacturer's instructions. A2780/CP70 cells were plated at a density of 2×10^5 cells per well of a 6-well plate for 18–24 hours. For each well, 2 μg shRNA plasmid DNA (pGIPZ) were transfected into A2780/CP70 using Arrest-In reagent (Thermo Scientific, USA). Puromycin (0.8 μg/ml) was used to select the transfected cells. After optimization, ALDH1A1-knockdown efficiencies of individual shRNAs were evaluated using real-time quantitative PCR and Western Blot. Vector 398453 demonstrated the most efficient transfection with over 95% knockdown efficacy of ALDH1A1 and was used for all shRNA knockdown experiments.

Western Blot Analysis

Cultured cells were collected in NP-40 lysis buffer with 10 μl/ml protease inhibitor cocktail (Sigma) and subjected to immuno-blotting analysis by standard techniques using antibodies against ALDH1A1, FANCJ, KLF4 (Sigma-Aldrich), FANCD2, PARP-1, XRCC1, β-actin, GAPDH (Santa Cruz Biotechnology, Inc.), and p21, phospho–Chk1 (Ser317), BRCA1 antibodies (Cell Signaling Technology).

RT^2 Profiler PCR Array

The human Cancer Drug Resistance & Cell Cycle RT^2 Profiler PCR Array (Qiagen, USA) was used to profile the expression of 84 genes involved in cancer drug resistance and cell cycle with five housekeeping genes per manufacturer's instructions. Controls for genomic DNA contamination and for the efficiency of the RT-PCR and PCR reactions were also assayed. The PCR arrays were run using a Bio-Rad iQ5 real-time detection system (Bio-Rad).

Cell Cycle Analysis by Flow Cytometry

A2780/CP70 cells were transfected with control or shRNAs targeting to ALDH1A1 using Lipofectamine 2000 (Life Technologies) and cells were collected and stained for cell cycle analysis according to the manufacturer's instructions (BD Biosciences). Cells at 10^6 were re-suspended with 300 µl PBS, and 700 µl ice cold methanol to fix the cells for overnight at −20°C. Cells were washed twice with PBS, and then stained with 500 µl propidium iodide (BD Bioscience) at room temperature for 30 minutes in the dark. Cell cycle profiles were analyzed by flow cytometry.

Apoptosis Assay

A2780/CP70 cells transfected with negative control or shRNA-ALDH1A1 were induced for apoptosis by treating with 1.0 µM staurosporine for 6 hours [22,23]. APC-Annexin V and 7-AAD staining was performed according to the manufacturer's instructions. Each group contains three isotype controls: unstained cells; cells stained with APC Annexin V alone; cells stained with 7-AAD alone. Samples were analyzed by flow cytometry.

PARP Activity Assay

PARP activity was measured using HT PARP in vivo Pharmacodynamic Assay II kit (Trevigen). After treatment with 100 µM carboplatin for 45 minutes, A2780/CP70 cells transfected with negative control or shRNA-ALDH1A1 were washed twice with 5 ml of warm (37°C) PBS. Cells were scraped into 300 µl of cold cell lysis buffer and incubated on ice for 15 minutes. SDS was added to samples to a final SDS concentration of 1% and incubated at 100°C for 5 minutes. When samples cooled to room temperature, 0.01 volume of 100X Magnesium cation and 2 µl of DNase I (2 Units/µl) were added to the samples and incubated for additional 90 minutes at 37°C. After a brief centrifugation, supernatants were collected and polyADP-ribose (PAR) levels in the cell extracts were quantified using ELISA method.

Clinical Correlation

All the participants provided their written informed consent to participate in this study and the institutional review board at the University of South Alabama Health System approved this study, as well as the consent procedure. Ascites from 15 consecutive patients undergoing surgery for advanced stage IIIC/IV papillary serous ovarian cancer as well as 2 patients with benign ascites were collected and was immediately processed to perform ALDE-FLUOR assay after washing them with PBS and removing the erythrocytes using ACK lysing buffer (Lonza, Walkersville, MD, USA). Clinicopathologic data was collected for the respective patients and correlated to percentage of cells exhibited ALDH+ phenotype in their ascites.

Statistical Analysis

Comparisons between two groups were carried out using Student's t-test and ANOVA where appropriate. Statistical significance was determined at $p<0.05$. Kaplan-Meier curve was performed for survival with log-rank for statistical comparison.

Results

ALDH status correlates with ovarian cancer resistance to platinum agents

Isogenic cell lines of platinum sensitive (A2780) and resistant (A2780/CP70) ovarian cancer cells were evaluated for their survival rates in the presence and absence of different doses of carboplatin. Consistent with the previously reported results [24,25], A2780/CP70 cells required up to a 10-fold higher dose of carboplatin to achieve the IC$_{50}$ concentration compared to its platinum sensitive counterpart, A2780 (Figure 1A). Recently, in several cancer models, ALDH status has been implicated in tumor resistance to chemotherapy by maintaining cancer stem-like cells' characteristics such as aggressive growth, increased survival and re-differentiation potential [9]. In order to test the correlation between ALDH status and platinum resistance in ovarian cancer cells, ALDEFLOUR assays were performed on these isogenic cells. Interestingly platinum resistant ovarian cancer cell line A2780/CP70 exhibited at least 110-fold higher percentage of ALDH+ cells (with a range of 22–40%) compared to the platinum sensitive A2780 cells, which had only 0.2% ALDH+ cells (Figure 1B). Likewise, western blot analysis of ALDH1A1 protein levels in these cells revealed similar results, suggesting association of ALDH status with platinum resistance (Figure 1C).

To assess whether ALDH+ cancer stem-like cells are also present in primary tumors and its association with progression free survival of the patients, we have collected ascites from 15 ovarian cancer patients with advanced disease and 2 benign ascites from Meigs syndrome patients and analyzed for the percent of cells with ALDH expression using ALDEFLOUR assay. In agreement with cancer stem-cell hypothesis, ALDH+ cells were present in much greater percentage in malignant ascites compared to their benign counterparts. The percentage of ALDH+ cells in malignant ascites ranged from 1.3 to 25.4% (patients 3–17 compared to 2 benign ascites (patients 1 & 2) (Figure 2A). Most importantly, the percent of ALDH+ cells in patient ascites inversely correlated to progression free survival. Patients that exhibited ALDH^{HIGH} (> 15% ALDH) in their ascites demonstrated significantly lower progression free survival compared to patients with ALDH^{LOW} (< 15% ALDH) (3 vs. 9 months, respectively $p = 0.003$) (Figure 2B). Though it is difficult to draw a meaningful conclusion due to the limited number of ascites used in this study, these data indicates a direct clinical correlation between ALDH status with tumor response to platinum agents and progression free survival of the ovarian cancer patients.

ALDH+ ovarian cancer cells exhibits stem cell-like properties

These results led us to further characterize ALDH as a potential stem-cell marker in ovarian cancer. Tumor progression can be associated with the presence of a subset of cells that express stem cell markers and exhibit aggressive behavioral properties including invasive and increased colony formation potential. To investigate their invasive properties, sorted cells (ALDH+ vs. ALDH−) were assessed using Matrigel invasion assay. As shown in the figures 3A & 3B, ALDH+ cells demonstrated over 1.7 fold increase ($p<0.01$) in invasion through Matrigel compared to ALDH− cells.

Another surrogate measure to characterize cancer stem-like cells is the ability to form colonies, especially in the presence of chemotherapeutics [26]. Consistent with their invasive potential, ALDH+ cells demonstrated enhanced colony formation ability compared with ALDH− phenotypes (2-fold increase, $p<0.01$). Importantly, ALDH+ phenotypes displayed enhanced colony formation ability in the presence of carboplatin (5.4-fold increase,

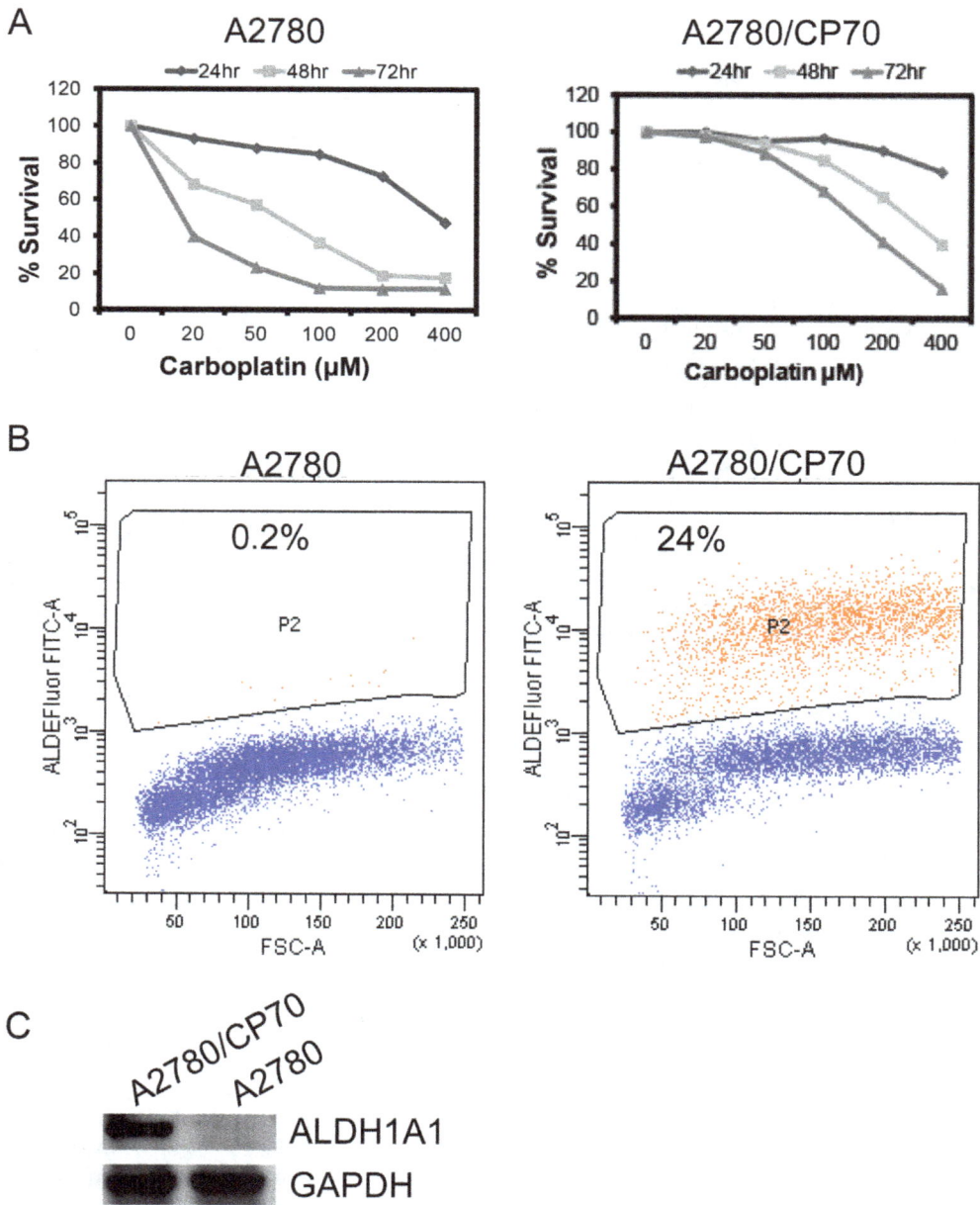

Figure 1. ALDH1A1 status correlates with platinum resistance in ovarian cancer cells. Isogenic cell lines (A2780- platinum sensitive & A2780/CP70- platinum resistant) were evaluated for platinum response using drug sensitivity assay as described in M&M section (A). To assess the percent of ALDH+ cells, in A2780 and A2780/CP70 cells ALDEFLUOR assay was performed by using BODIPY-aminoacetaldehyde (BAAA) as substrate for ALDH enzyme, after 40 minutes incubation at 37°C flow cytometry analysis was performed (B) and western blot data shows representing levels of ALDH1A1 isozyme in these cells (C).

$p<0.01$) (Figure 3C). In order to gain insight into the potential stem-like mechanisms of these cells, we evaluated potential stem cell pathways of interest in these cells. The RT-PCR data showed nearly 3-fold higher level expression of Krüppel-Like Factor 4 (KLF4) in ALDH+ cells compared to their ALDH− counterparts. KLF4 belongs to zinc finger family of transcription factors, which has been reported to be critical for the maintenance of breast cancer stem cells and their aggressive behavior such as migration and invasion ad resistance to cisplatin [27] [28]. However, other stem cell mediators like BMI1, c-myc, Oct3/4 and S100A1 did not show any noticeable changes in their expression compared with ALDH− phenotypes ($p<0.01$) (Figure 3D).

ALDH1A1 isotype promotes ovarian cancer stem-like cells' properties

Consistent with the CSC literature, our data revealed elevated expression of ALDH1A1 isozyme in the platinum resistant A2780/CP70 cells. To further evaluate the role of ALDH1A1 in maintenance of cancer stem-like cells properties of platinum resistant ovarian cancer cells, we have downregulated ALDH1A1 specific isozyme using shRNAs (Figure S1). Contrary to its high expression, downregulation of ALDH1A1 has not shown any considerable differences in invasive properties of these cells (Figure 4A & 4B). However, ALDH1A1 knockdown affected their

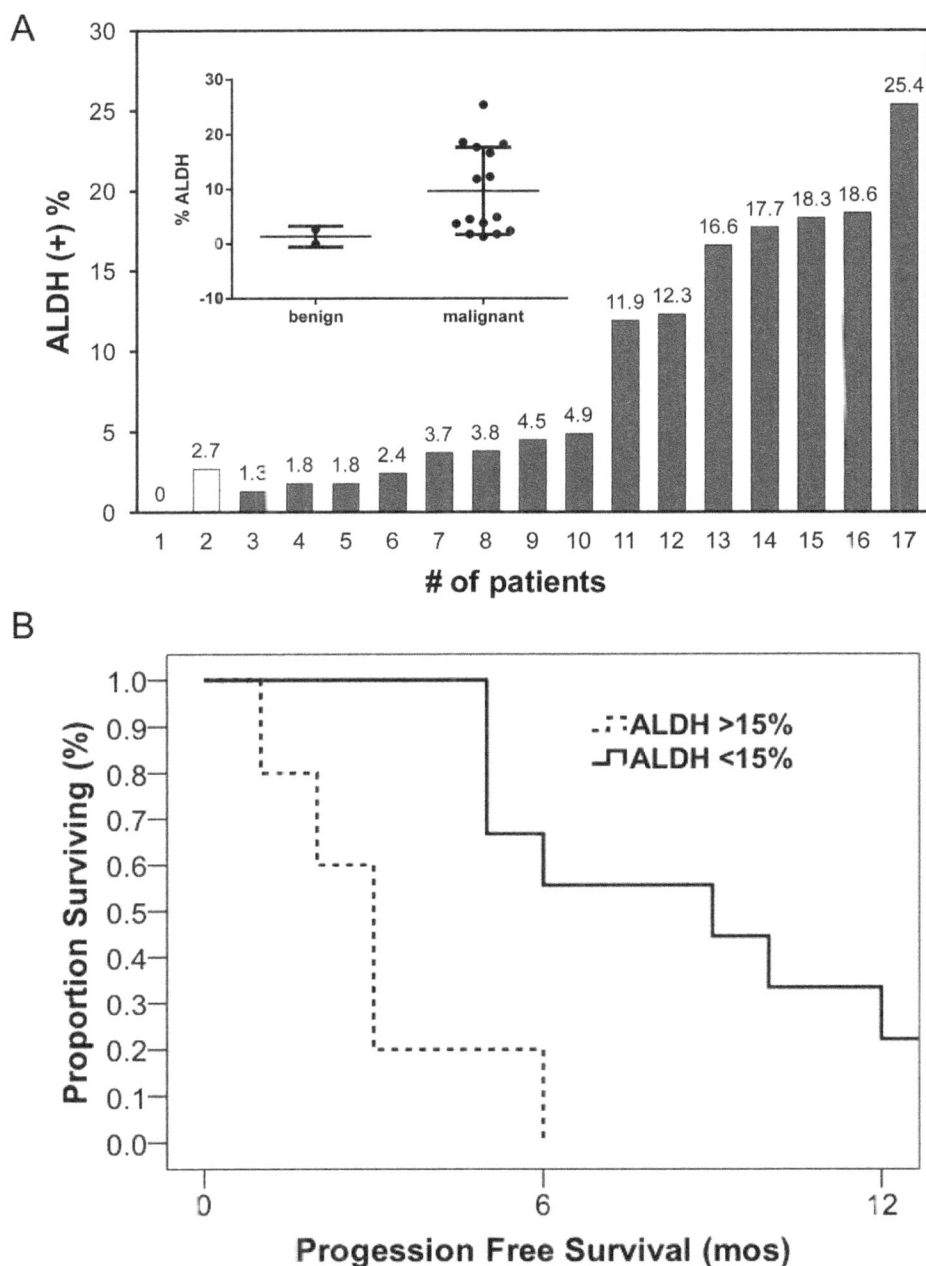

Figure 2. ALDH1A1 status correlates with progression free survival in ovarian cancer patients. Ascites from 15 consecutive patients with primary advanced stage III/IV ovarian cancer and 2 from benign (Miegs syndrome) was obtained and analyzed for percentage of ALDH+ cells through ALDEFLUOR assay. The histogram in inset shows the percent of ALDH+ cells in benign and malignant ascites (A). The clinicopathologic information from the ovarian cancer patients were correlated with the percent of ALDH+ cells in their ascites and evaluated progression free survival with ALDH[HIGH] (>15% ALDH) to ALDH[LOW] (<15% ALDH) patients (3 vs. 9 months, respectively; $p<0.01$) (B).

ability to form colonies in soft agar, demonstrating a 2.5-fold decrease in the colonies ($p<0.01$) (Figure 4C). Similarly, down-regulation of ALDH1A1 alone significantly sensitized inherently platinum resistant A2780/CP70 cells to carboplatin. Considering IC_{50} doses required (82.9 μM and 43.8 μM for negative control and shALDH1A1 cells respectively) for these cells, about 50% reduction in carboplatin dose is evident for ALDH1A1 knockdown cells ($p<0.001$) (Figure 4D). Together, these data suggests that ALDH1A1 status is one of the critical factors in maintaining stem-like cell properties and platinum resistance in ovarian cancer.

ALDH1A1 controls cell cycle checkpoints by regulation of KLF4 and p21 proteins

Increased expression of KLF4 in ALDH+ cells (Figure 3D) led us to evaluate any functional relationship between ALDH1A1 and KLF4. Although ALDH1A1 knockdown did not affect the level of KLF4 mRNA, a significant decrease in KLF4 protein levels was evidenced in these cells (Figure 5A). Considering that the functional status of the cell cycle regulator p21 is intimately related to KLF4's function, the mRNA and protein levels of p21 were also assessed. As expected, both ALDH1A1 transcript and

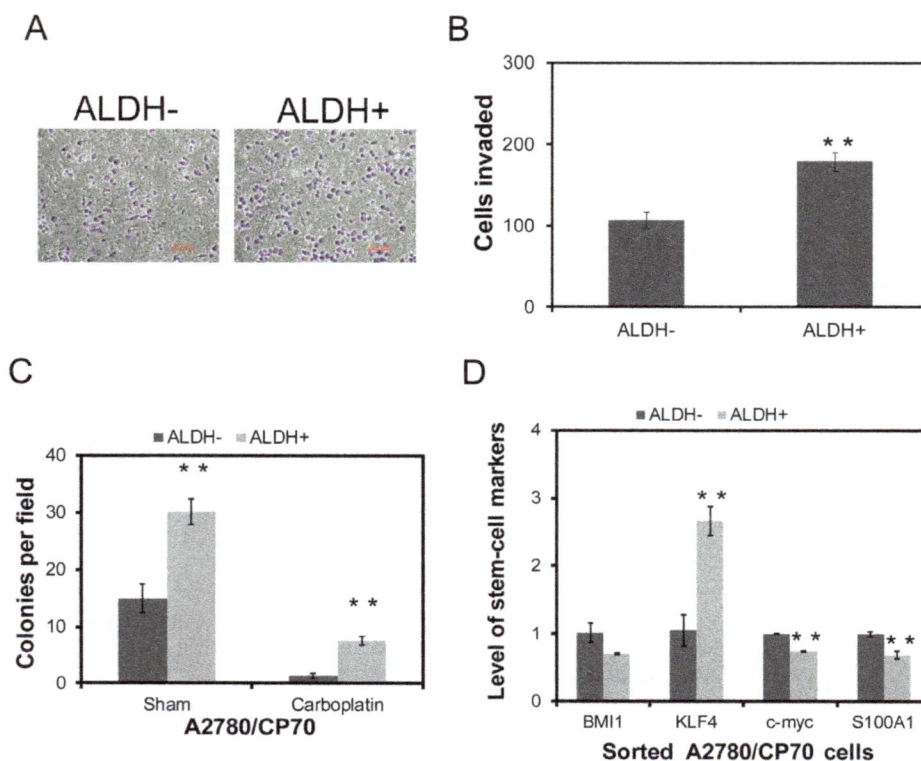

Figure 3. ALDH+ phenotypes demonstrate cancer stem cell properties. A2780/CP70 cells were sorted into ALDH− and ALDH+ phenotypes and evaluated for their abilities for invasion using Matrigel invasion chambers (A), quantitative data as represented (B) and colony formation potential in the presence and absence of carboplatin (20 μM) were assessed using soft agar colony formation assays (C). In order to determine possible mechanism for cancer stem cell characteristics in ALDH+ cells, we evaluated multiple markers of "stemness". A2780/CP70 cells were sorted into ALDH− and ALDH+ phenotypes, total RNA was isolated, cDNA was prepared and real-time quantitative RT-PCR was performed (D). **indicates statistical significance ($p<0.01$).

protein levels of p21 were dramatically decreased in ALDH1A1 deficient A2780/CP70 cells (Figure 5A). Since ALDH1A1 status influenced expression of cell cycle checkpoint proteins p21/CDK4, we further analyzed the cell cycle profiles of these cells. The flow cytometric data clearly indicate decreased G1 cell population (50.25% to 42.10%) and a compensatory increase in accumulation of cells in S and G2 phases (Figure 5B). Due to the fact that cells in active replication (S and G2 phases) are more vulnerable to genotoxic stress compared to their non-dividing or other restive phases (G0 and G1), the re-sensitization of ALDH1A1 deficient cells may be in part attributable to the changes in cell cycle distribution. Furthermore, we have also confirmed that KLF4 status affects p21 expression levels in A2780/CP70 cells (Figure S2A & S2B). However, evaluation of ALDH activity and ALDH1A1 expression in cells did not exhibit any noticeable changes, suggesting KLF4 likely serves downstream to ALDH1A1 (Figure S2C).

To further evaluate the genes responsible for chemoresistance and cell cycle regulation based on the status of ALDH1A1, we have used RT² Profiler PCR Array for the human Cancer Drug Resistance & Cell Cycle (Ambion). The comparative expression profiles of genes in ALDH1A1 knockdown vs. control cells revealed a significant decrease in expression of the cell cycle regulators CDKN1A (p21) (0.27-fold) and CDK4 (0.26-fold), which confirms its role in conjunction with KLF4 (Table 1).

Of note, with restored platinum sensitivity from ALDH1A1 knockdown, expression of the pro-apoptotic factor BAX was up-regulated nearly 3.95-fold. ALDH1A1 knockdown demonstrated

increased number of cells in early apoptotic phase compared to the control. After exposure of cells to 1.0 μM staurosporine for 6 hours, a dramatic increase in early apoptotic cells was observed in ALDH1A1 deficient cells compared to their ALDH1A1 proficient counter parts (35.3% vs. 20.3%) (Figure 5C). These data suggests that ALDH1A1 knockdown cells are more susceptible to BAX-induced apoptosis, which has been well described in the inhibition of p21 cell cycle checkpoint [29].

ALDH1A1-mediated platinum resistance correlates to altered DNA repair networks

Intact cell cycle checkpoints and DNA damage response (DDR) signaling mechanisms are important for the cell's ability to counter with different kinds of genomic insults and orderly progression of cell cycle. However, a common feature of cancer cells is altered regulation of these signaling cascades to acquire additional genetic changes required for re-differentiation and survival thereby display therapeutic resistance. Likewise, ALDH1A1 cells displayed altered regulation of KFL4/p21 mediated cell cycle checkpoint mechanism, which primarily directs the inhibition of G1 to S and G2 to M progression in response to DNA damage to allow more time for the cell to repair. Considering the association of PARP-1 in repair of carboplatin induced DNA damage, we evaluated its involvement in ALDH1A1 cells. PARP-1 levels progressively increased up to 45 minutes following carboplatin treatment (Figure 6A and 6B). However, downregulation of ALDH1A1 resulted in significant decrease (1.8 fold) in total PAR levels (PARP activity) (Figure 6C) compared to ALDH1A1 proficient cells ($p = 0.012$).

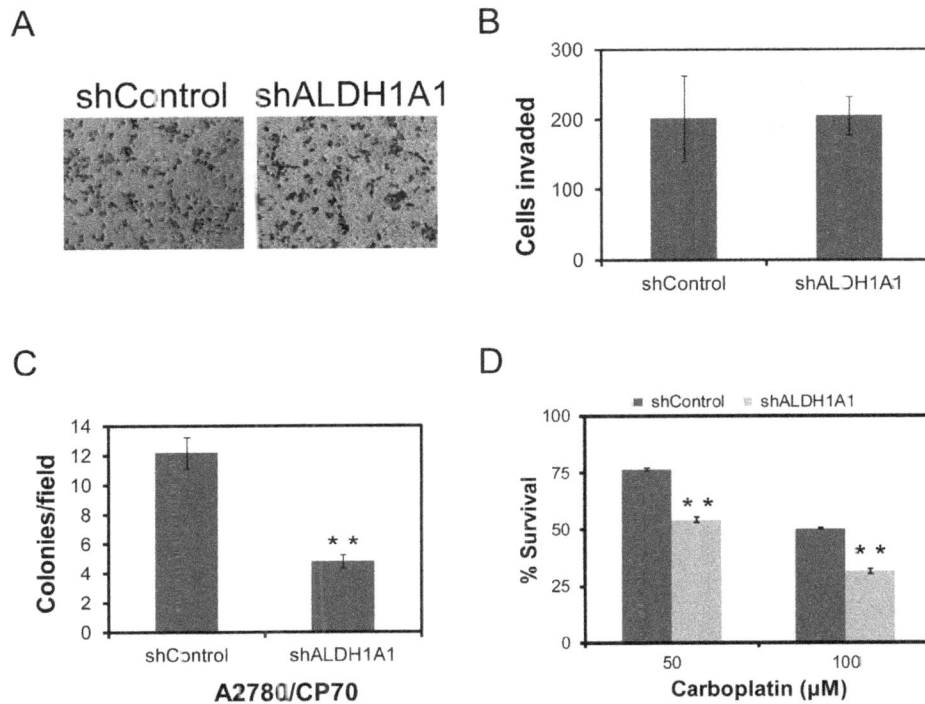

Figure 4. ALDH1A1 down regulation differentially affects on cancer stem cell properties. Lentiviral vectors expressing ALDH1A1 specific shRNAs or nontargeting shRNAs were transfected into A2780/CP70 cells and its effect on stem-like cell properties were evaluated for invasive potential using Matrigel invasion chambers (A), quantitative data as represented (B), clonogenic potential using soft agar colony formation (C, and carboplatin dependent growth inhibition by CellTiter-Glo Luminescent Cell Viability Assay (D). Statistical significance was evaluated using student's *t*-test.

Several recent studies on breast cancer stem-cells indicate altered regulation of DNA repair networks, particularly an inverse relationship between ALDH1A1 status and BRCA1 gene expression [15,16]. Moreover, in response to DNA damage, BRCA1 is known to govern cell cycle checkpoints and choice of the DNA repair pathways to timely repair of these DNA lesions [16]. Consistent with breast cancer stem-cell data, Western blot analysis revealed an inverse relationship between ALDH1A1 and BRCA1 expression in A2780/CP70 cells, suggesting ALDH1A1 expressing ovarian cancer stem-like cells more likely to lose or express low levels of BRCA1. Further analysis revealed down regulation of ALDH1A1 induced spontaneous DNA damage response by expressing γ-H2AX protein (a marker of double strand breaks). This is also coincided with the diminished levels of excision repair protein (XRCC1), replication checkpoint kinase protein 1 (Chk1) and other replication stress associated Fanconi anemia (FA)-BRCA

gene products FANCD2 and FANCJ [30–32]. Together these data suggest that ovarian cancer stem-like cells may maintain therapeutic resistance by expressing ALDH1A1 and depletion of which, abrogates G1 and S-phase checkpoints (Figures 5A and 6C) leading to replication stress (Figure 5B). Though ALDH1A1 depleted cells accumulated in S and G2 phases, the phosphorylation status of replication checkpoint protein Chk1 (Ser317) and expression of replication fork associated FA pathway proteins FANCD2 and FANCJ were affected. This is also conferred by induction of γ-H2AX, a marker for DSB and reduced cell survival. Since Chk1 and FA proteins are important for the replication checkpoint and the stability of stalled replication forks, the spontaneous DNA damage response in these cells can be attributed to defect in these proteins (Figure 6D). To identify the molecular network signals that are differentially expressed in ALDH1A1 expressing cells, we initially assessed the expression of

Table 1. The human Cancer Drug Resistance & Cell Cycle RT^2 Profiler PCR Array results were compared between ALDH1A1 knockdown and controls.

Gene	Function	Fold difference (shRNA/control)
CDKN1A (p21)	A potent cyclin-dependent kinase inhibitor (CKI); A regulator of cell cycle progression at G1.	0.27
CDK4	A part of the cyclin-dependent kinase family; Important for cell cycle G1 phase progression.	0.26
BAX	Accelerating apoptosis.	3.95

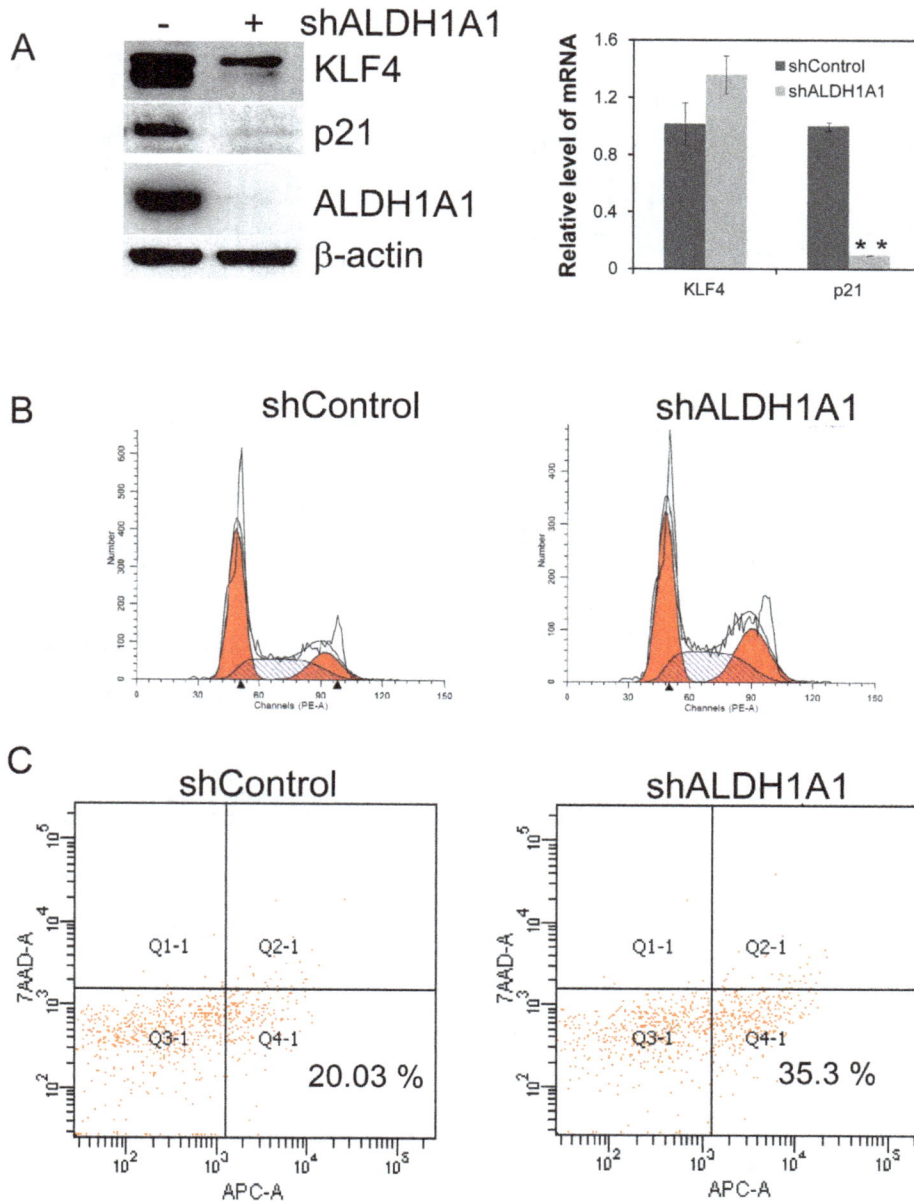

Figure 5. ALDH1A1 downregulation leads to lower KLF4 & p21 expression with altered cell-cycle profile. ALDH1A1 proficient and deficient A2780/CP70 cells were evaluated for expression of stem-like cell marker KLF4 and cell cycle checkpoint protein p21 by RT-PCR and Western blot analysis (A). Cell cycle distributions of cells were analyzed after fixing the cells in 70% methanol and propidium iodide staining followed by flow cytometry (B). Apoptotic cells were detected after staining the cells with APC-Annexin V and 7-AAD according to the manufacturer's instructions and analyzed by flow cytometry (C).

Fanconi anemia pathway and tumor resistance to chemotherapeutic agents. Consistently, our results demonstrated a direct correlation between ALDH1A1 status and FANCD2 expression. Together our data indicates a connection between ALDH1A1 status to stemness and platinum resistance of ovarian cancer cells by altered regulation of DNA repair works.

Discussion

Several potential ovarian CSCs specific surface markers have been described such as CD44+/CD117+ [33], CD44+/MyD88+ [34], CD133+ [35], CD44+/CD24− [21,36] and ALDH/CD133+ [37]. Detecting ALDH1A1 via the ALDEFLUOR assay is a simple and effective approach for identifying and isolating ovarian CSCs from cell lines and primary tissues. Importantly, its detection via a functional assay of stem-cells is advantageous opposed to surface markers that might or might not be actively contributing to stem cell features. Considering the assay of ALDH+ cells are based on their fluorescence, they remain viable and amenable to further in vitro and in vivo research as well as clinical applications.

We demonstrated that ALDH+ phenotypes exhibit cancer stem-like properties of enhanced invasion, colony formation ability, as well as increased expression of stem cell mediator KLF4. Additionally, our data confirmed that platinum resistant cell line

A

Carboplatin

0   15   30   45   60   90   :Time (min)

PARP1

β-actin

C

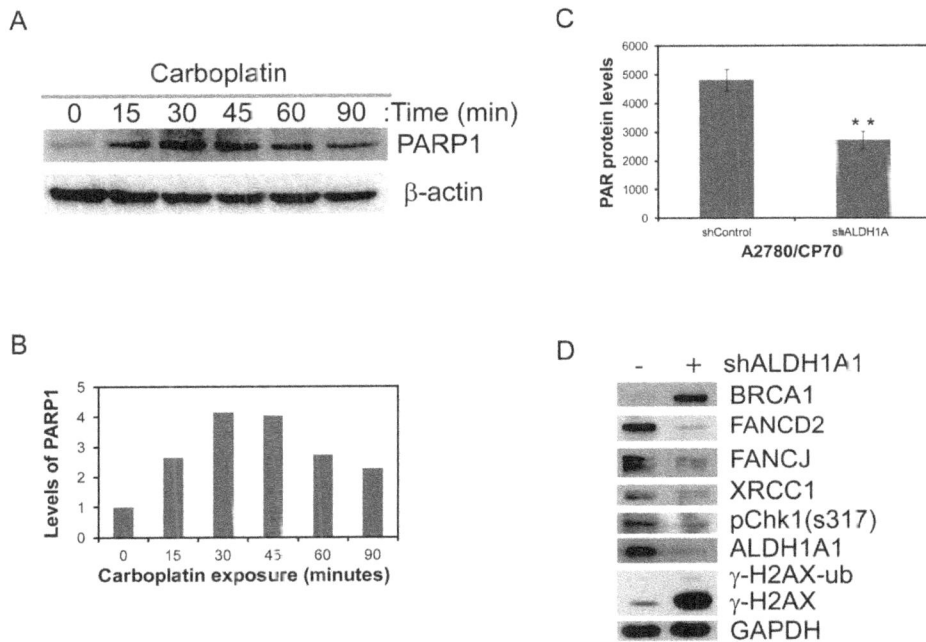

Figure 6. ALDH1A1 status alters cell cycle checkpoints and DNA repair networks. ALDH1A1 proficient (control) and deficient (shALDH1A1) A2780/CP70 cells were assessed for their abilities to repair carboplatin induced single strand breaks by looking at time dependent induction of PARP-1 protein levels by western blots (A), densitometry of blots by Image J (B) and total PARP activity was assayed by measuring PAR levels (C). To assess the ALDH1A1 dependent expression DDR and repair proteins, whole cell lysates were normalized for total proteins and western blot analysis were performed using antibodies as represented (D).

A2780/CP70 exhibits much higher ALDH activity than its isogenic parental platinum sensitive cell line A2780. Importantly, presence of ALDH+ cells also associates with clinical and pathological relevance of tumor ascites, with a direct correlation to worse progression free survival.

ALDH and its expression have been linked to poor prognosis in several cancer models [4]. Particularly, ALDH1A1 isozyme has been shown to play an important functional role in maintaining cancer stem cells. In this study, we further investigated the potential role of ALDH1A1 isozyme in maintenance of ovarian cancer stem-like cells' properties. The stable downregulation of ALDH1A1 isozyme alone dramatically decreased their ability to form colonies. Although ALDH+ cells demonstrated increased invasive properties compared to ALDH− cells, a difference in invasive potential of a single isozyme ALDH1A1 was not seen. This may be attributed to invasive roles for other isoforms of ALDH and other cancer stem cell markers in maintaining certain properties of stem-like cells [38–41].

In regards to platinum-resistance, ALDH1A1 silencing alone sensitized the inherently platinum resistant A2780/CP70 cells to carboplatin. Further exploration of possible chemoresistance pathways in ALDH1A1 positive cells revealed a vital role for KLF4/p21 interaction. KLF are transcriptional regulators that influence several cellular functions, ranging from differentiation to proliferation and apoptosis. Being a potent inhibitor of cell cycle progression, p21 seems to be intimately related to KLF4's function; KLF4 and p21 are context-dependent opposing force in cancer [42]. We found that ALDH1A1 silencing leads to diminished levels of both KLF4 and p21. Yu et al [27] reported knockdown of KLF4 in breast cancer cells decreased the proportion of stem/progenitor cells as demonstrated by expression of stem cell surface markers ALDH. In this study, KLF4 knockdown in A2780/CP70 cells could lead to decreased

expression of p21, but did not affect ALDH activity or ALDH1A1 expression, suggesting differential regulation of stem-cell pathways.

This KLF4/p21 mediation has been well described in the literature with numerous publications demonstrating its ability to control chemoresistance [43,44]. ALDH1A1 knockdown cells show reduced expression of p21 and cyclin-dependent kinase 4 (CDK4). CDK4 is one of the members of cyclin-dependent kinase family while p21 is a potent CDK inhibitor. Both p21 and CDK4 regulate cell cycle progression at G1 phase progression [45] and ALDH1A1 silencing induces A2780/CP70' cell-cycle arrest (S and G2 arrest) which is a more favorable phase for genotoxins induced cell death. Importantly, p21 and CDK4 levels were decreased with knockdown of ALDH1A1, and this was also associated with BAX-mediated apoptosis, where a 4-fold increase in BAX levels was observed (Table 1).

Cancer stem cells may maintain their stem-ness by altered expression of cell cycle checkpoints such that they can become resistant to therapies due to their accumulation at particular cell cycle phase. In response to DNA damage, altered cell cycle and checkpoint signals also differentially regulate DNA repair networks. In our study, consistent with G1-phase accumulation, ALDH1A1 proficient cells exhibited increased expression of G1 checkpoint proteins KLF4/p21 and CDK4. Concomitant down-regulation of ALDH1A1 exhibited increased accumulation of cells in S-phase but decreased S-phase checkpoint leading to DDR as evidenced by γ-H2AX. Likewise, when KLF4 was transiently downregulated in these cells, decreased levels of p21 and CDK4 was observed (Figure S2B). Further systematic evaluation of ALDH1A1/cell cycle axis is needed to confirm the platinum resistance and poor prognosis of ALDH1A1 positive ovarian cancers. Consistent with the altered cell cycle profiles and checkpoint proteins in ALDH1A1 cells, our studies also demonstrated differential expression of DNA repair network proteins.

Although depletion of ALDH1A1 led to G1 checkpoint abrogation and increased S-phase accumulation of the cells, the replication checkpoint (pChk1) and replication stress associated DDR proteins FANCD2 and FANCJ were drastically diminished. Conversely, ALDH1A1 depletion in A2780/CP70 cells resulted in robust increase of BRACA1 protein in association with γ-H2AX induction, demonstrating altered regulation of DNA damage response and repair networks in cancer stem-like cells.

Collectively, these results indicate ALDH over-expression is associated with many properties of ovarian cancer stem-like cells such as enhanced invasion, colony formation, and chemoresistance. Our studies also demonstrated that ALDH1A1 plays a key role in maintenance of ovarian cancer stem-like cells' properties and might mediate carboplatin resistance through altered regulation of cell cycle and DNA repair networks. These new findings offer an important tool for the study of ovarian CSCs and provide a potential prognostic factor and therapeutic target for treatment of patients with ovarian cancer. Despite the fact these results do not explain the mechanistic basis for these altered cell cycle and DNA repair networks, this pilot study reveal an important features of chemoresistance mechanisms adopted by ovarian cancer stem-like cells. Importantly, our data also implicates a novel connection between ALDH1A1 status and altered regulation of cell cycle and DNA repair networks that influences on ovarian cancer stem-like cell properties and platinum resistance. However, molecular basis by which ALDH1A1 regulates cell cycle checkpoint signaling and DNA repair networks needs to be evaluated. Due to their therapeutic importance, further evaluation of molecular networks that govern these DNA repair networks based on ALDH1A1 status is urgently needed.

References

1. Eisenhauer EA, Vermorken JB, van Glabbeke M (1997) Predictors of response to subsequent chemotherapy in platinum pretreated ovarian cancer: a multivariate analysis of 704 patients [seecomments]. Ann Oncol Off J Eur Soc Med Oncol ESMO 8: 963–968.
2. Soltanian S, Matin MM (2011) Cancer stem cells and cancer therapy. Tumour Biol J Int Soc Oncodevelopmental Biol Med 32: 425–440.
3. Bapat SA (2010) Human ovarian cancer stem cells. Reprod Camb Engl 140: 33–41.
4. Jiang F, Qiu Q, Khanna A, Todd NW, Deepak J, et al. (2009) Aldehyde dehydrogenase 1 is a tumor stem cell-associated marker in lung cancer. Mol Cancer Res MCR 7: 330–338.
5. Charafe-Jauffret E, Ginestier C, Iovino F, Tarpin C, Diebel M, et al. (2010) Aldehyde dehydrogenase 1-positive cancer stem cells mediate metastasis and poor clinical outcome in inflammatory breast cancer. Clin Cancer Res Off J Am Assoc Cancer Res 16: 45–55.
6. Li T, Su Y, Mei Y, Leng Q, Leng B, et al. (2010) ALDH1A1 is a marker for malignant prostate stem cells and predictor of prostate cancer patients' outcome. Lab Investig J Tech Methods Pathol 90: 234–244.
7. Todaro M, Iovino F, Eterno V, Cammareri P, Gambara G, et al. (2010) Tumorigenic and metastatic activity of human thyroid cancer stem cells. Cancer Res 70: 8874–8885.
8. Clay MR, Tabor M, Owen JH, Carey TE, Bradford CR, et al. (2010) Single-marker identification of head and neck squamous cell carcinoma cancer stem cells with aldehyde dehydrogenase. Head Neck 32: 1195–1201.
9. Ma I, Allan AL (2011) The role of human aldehyde dehydrogenase in normal and cancer stem cells. Stem Cell Rev 7: 292–306.
10. Landen CN Jr, Goodman B, Katre AA, Steg AD, Nick AM, et al. (2010) Targeting aldehyde dehydrogenase cancer stem cells in ovarian cancer. Mol Cancer Ther 9: 3186–199.
11. He Q-Z, Luo X-Z, Wang K, Zhou Q, Ao H, et al. (2014) Isolation and characterization of cancer stem cells from high-grade serous ovarian carcinomas. Cell Physiol Biochem Int J Exp Cell Physiol Biochem Pharmacol 33: 173–1784.
12. Xiang T, Long H, He L, Han X, Lin K, et al. (2013) Interleukin-17 produced by tumor microenvironment promotes self-renewal of CD133(+) cancer stem-like cells in ovarian cancer. Oncogene.
13. Yokota A, Takeuchi H, Maeda N, Ohoka Y, Kato C, et al. (2009) GM-CSF and IL-4 synergistically trigger dendritic cells to acquire retinoic acid-producing capacity. Int Immunol 21: 361–377.
14. Wang Y-C, Yo Y-T, Lee H-Y, Liao Y-P, Chao T-K, et al. (2012) ALDH1-bright epithelial ovarian cancer cells are associated with CD44 expression, drug resistance, and poor clinical outcome. Am J Pathol 180: 1159–1169.
15. Liu S, Ginestier C, Charafe-Jauffret E, Foco H, Kleer CG, et al. (2008) BRCA1 regulates human mammary stem/progenitor cell fate. Proc Natl Acad Sci U S A 105: 1680–1685.
16. Madjd Z, Gheytanchi E, Erfani E, Asadi-Lari M (2013) Application of stem cells in targeted therapy of breast cancer: a systematic review. Asian Pac J Cancer Prev APJCP 14: 2789–2800.
17. Venkitaraman AR (2002) Cancer susceptibility and the functions of BRCA1 and BRCA2. Cell 108: 171–182.
18. Bunting SF, Callén E, Wong N, Chen H-T, Polato F, et al. (2010) 53BP1 inhibits homologous recombination in Brca1-deficient cells by blocking resection of DNA breaks. Cell 141: 243–254.
19. Kakarougkas A, Jeggo P (2014) DNA DSB repair pathway choice: an orchestrated handover mechanism. Br J Radiol 87(1035): 20130685.
20. Li QQ, Lee RX, Liang H, Wang G, Li JM, et al. (2013) β-Elemene enhances susceptibility to cisplatin in resistant ovarian carcinoma cells via downregulation of ERCC-1 and XIAP and inactivation of JNK. Int J Oncol 43: 721–728.
21. Meng E, Long B, Sullivan P, McClellan S, Finan MA, et al. (2012) CD44+/CD24− ovarian cancer cells demonstrate cancer stem cell properties and correlate to survival. Clin Exp Metastasis 29: 939–9348.
22. Mabuchi S, Hisamatsu T, Kawase C, Hayashi M, Sawada K, et al. (2011) The activity of trabectedin as a single agent or in combination with everolimus for clear cell carcinoma of the ovary. Clin Cancer Res Off J Am Assoc Cancer Res 17: 4462–4473.
23. Cartee L, Kucera GL, Willingham MC (1998) Induction of apoptosis by gemcitabine in BG-1 human ovarian cancer cells compared with induction by staurosporine, paclitaxel and cisplatin. Apoptosis Int J Program Cell Death 3: 439–449.
24. Zhen W, Link CJ Jr, O'Connor PM, Reed E, Parker R, et al. (1992) Increased gene-specific repair of cisplatin interstrand cross-links in cisplatin-resistant human ovarian cancer cell lines. Mol Cell Biol 12: 3689–3698.
25. Parker RJ, Eastman A, Bostick-Bruton F, Reed E (1991) Acquired cisplatin resistance in human ovarian cancer cells is associated with enhanced repair of cisplatin-DNA lesions and reduced drug accumulation. J Clin Invest 87: 772–777.
26. Steg AD, Bevis KS, Katre AA, Ziebarth A, Dobbin ZC, et al. (2012) Stem cell pathways contribute to clinical chemoresistance in ovarian cancer. Clin Cancer Res Off J Am Assoc Cancer Res 18: 869–881.

Supporting Information

Figure S1 Optimization of shRNA against ALDH1A1 in A2780/CP70 cells. Six different pGIPZ Lentiviral shRNA vectors against ALDH1A1 as well as negative control shRNA were transfected into A2780/CP70 cells, respectively. 0.8 μg/ml puromycin was used to select the transfected cells to decrease the background (A). After optimization through real-time quantitative RT-PCR and Western Blot, the ALDH1A1 vector 398453 demonstrated efficient transfection as well as superior knockdown efficacy (B and C).

Figure S2 KLF4 silencing led to significantly decreased p21, without affecting ALDH. A2780/CP70 cells were plated in 6-well plates for 18–24 hours before transfection. 60 pmols of siRNA against KLF4 as well as scramble siRNA was transfected into A2780/CP70 cells through Lipofectamine 2000 reagent (Invitrogen). 36 hours later, cells were harvested to detect KLF4, p21, ALDH1A1 expression through Western Blot and ALDH activity using ALDEFLUOR assay. KLF4 knockdown through siRNA led to significantly lower level of p21 (A and B), but didn't affect ALDH activity or ALDH1A1 expression in A2780/CP70 cells (B and C).

Author Contributions

Conceived and designed the experiments: EM AM KP RPR. Performed the experiments: EM AM KT SM. Analyzed the data: EM AM KT MAF JS SM LM ER LAS KP RPR. Contributed reagents/materials/analysis tools: MAF JS SM LM ER LAS KP RPR. Contributed to the writing of the manuscript: EM LM KP RPR.

27. Yu F, Li J, Chen H, Fu J, Ray S, et al. (2011) Kruppel-like factor 4 (KLF4) is required for maintenance of breast cancer stem cells and for cell migration and invasion. Oncogene 30: 2161–2172.

28. Jia Y, Zhang W, Liu H, Peng L, Yang Z, et al. (2012) Inhibition of glutathione synthesis reverses Krüppel-like factor 4-mediated cisplatin resistance. Cancer Chemother Pharmacol 69: 377–385.

29. Er E, Oliver L, Cartron P-F, Juin P, Manon S, et al. (2006) Mitochondria as the target of the pro-apoptotic protein Bax. Biochim Biophys Acta 1757: 1301–11.

30. Palle K, Vaziri C (2011) Rad18 E3 ubiquitin ligase activity mediates Fanconi anemia pathway activation and cell survival following DNA Topoisomerase 1 inhibition. Cell Cycle Georget Tex 10: 1625–1638.

31. D'Andrea AD (2003) The Fanconi Anemia/BRCA signaling pathway: disruption in cisplatin-sensitive ovarian cancers. Cell Cycle Georget Tex 2: 290–292.

32. Wu Y, Brosh RM Jr (2009) FANCJ helicase operates in the Fanconi Anemia DNA repair pathway and the response to replicational stress. Curr Mol Med 9: 470–4782.

33. Zhang S, Balch C, Chan MW, Lai H-C, Matei D, et al. (2008) Identification and characterization of ovarian cancer-initiating cells from primary human tumors. Cancer Res 68: 4311–4320.

34. Alvero AB, Chen R, Fu H-H, Montagna M, Schwartz PE, et al. (2009) Molecular phenotyping of human ovarian cancer stem cells unravels the mechanisms for repair and chemoresistance. Cell Cycle Georget Tex 8: 158–166.

35. Curley MD, Therrien VA, Cummings CL, Sergent PA, Koulouris CR, et al. (2009) CD133 expression defines a tumor initiating cell population in primary human ovarian cancer. Stem Cells Dayt Ohio 27: 2875–2883.

36. Shi MF, Jiao J, Lu WG, Ye F, Ma D, et al. Identification of cancer stem cell-like cells from human epithelial ovarian carcinoma cell line. Cell Mol Life Sci CMLS 67: 3915–3925.

37. Silva IA, Bai S, McLean K, Yang K, Griffith K, et al. (2011) Aldehyde dehydrogenase in combination with CD133 defines angiogenic ovarian cancer stem cells that portend poor patient survival. Cancer Res 71: 3991–4001.

38. Suman S, Das TP, Damodaran C (2013) Silencing NOTCH signaling causes growth arrest in both breast cancer stem cells and breast cancer cells. Br J Cancer 109: 2587–2596.

39. Zhang Z, Dong Z, Lauxen IS, Filho MS, Nör JE (2014) Endothelial cell-secreted EGF induces epithelial to mesenchymal transition and endows head and neck cancer cells with stem-like phenotype. Cancer Res 74: 2869–2881.

40. Liu S, Cong Y, Wang D, Sun Y, Deng L, et al. (2014) Breast Cancer Stem Cells Transition between Epithelial and Mesenchymal States Reflective of their Normal Counterparts. Stem Cell Rep 2: 78–91.

41. Zhou W, Lv R, Qi W, Wu D, Xu Y, et al. (2014) Snail contributes to the maintenance of stem cell-like phenotype cells in human pancreatic cancer. PloS One 9: e87409.

42. Rowland BD, Peeper DS (2006) KLF4, p21 and context-dependent opposing forces in cancer. Nat Rev Cancer 6: 11–23.

43. Ghaleb AM, Katz JP, Kaestner KH, Du JX, Yang VW (2007) Krüppel-like factor 4 exhibits antiapoptotic activity following gamma-radiation-induced DNA damage. Oncogene 26: 2365–2373.

44. Zhou Q, Hong Y, Zhan Q, Shen Y, Liu Z (2009) Role for Kruppel-like factor 4 in determining the outcome of p53 response to DNA damage. Cancer Res 69: 8284–8292.

45. Harper JW, Adami GR, Wei N, Keyomarsi K, Elledge SJ (1993) The p21 Cdk-interacting protein Cip1 is a potent inhibitor of G1 cyclin-dependent kinases. Cell 75: 805–816.

12

MRE11-Deficiency Associated with Improved Long-Term Disease Free Survival and Overall Survival in a Subset of Stage III Colon Cancer Patients in Randomized CALGB 89803 Trial

Thomas Pavelitz[1,15], Lindsay Renfro[2,15], Nathan R. Foster[2], Amber Caracol[1,3], Piri Welsch[4], Victoria Valinluck Lao[5,6], William B. Grady[5,7], Donna Niedzwiecki[8], Leonard B. Saltz[9], Monica M. Bertagnolli[10], Richard M. Goldberg[11], Peter S. Rabinovitch[12], Mary Emond[13], Raymond J. Monnat Jr.[4,12], Nancy Maizels[1,3,12,14]*

1 Department of Immunology, University of Washington, Seattle, Washington, United States of America, 2 Division of Biomedical Statistics and Informatics, Mayo Clinic, Rochester, Minnesota, United States of America, 3 Molecular and Cellular Biology Graduate Program, University of Washington, Seattle, Washington, United States of America, 4 Department of Genome Sciences, University of Washington Medical School, Seattle, Washington, United States of America, 5 Clinical Research Division, Fred Hutchinson Cancer Research Center, Seattle, Washington, United States of America, 6 Department of Surgery, University of Washington Medical School, Seattle, Washington, United States of America, 7 Department of Medicine, University of Washington Medical School, Seattle, Washington, United States of America, 8 Cancer and Leukemia Group B Statistical Center, Duke University Medical Center, Durham, North Carolina, United States of America, 9 Memorial Sloan-Kettering Cancer Center, New York, New York, United States of America, 10 Dana-Farber Cancer Institute and Brigham and Women's Hospital, Boston, Massachusetts, United States of America, 11 The Ohio State University, Columbus, Ohio, United States of America, 12 Department of Pathology, University of Washington Medical School, Seattle, Washington, United States of America, 13 Department of Biostatistics, University of Washington, Seattle, Washington, United States of America, 14 Department of Biochemistry, University of Washington, Seattle, Washington, United States of America, 15 Department of Chemistry, University of Washington, Seattle, Washington, United States of America

Abstract

Purpose: Colon cancers deficient in mismatch repair (MMR) may exhibit diminished expression of the DNA repair gene, *MRE11*, as a consequence of contraction of a T_{11} mononucleotide tract. This study investigated MRE11 status and its association with prognosis, survival and drug response in patients with stage III colon cancer.

Patients and Methods: Cancer and Leukemia Group B 89803 (Alliance) randomly assigned 1,264 patients with stage III colon cancer to postoperative weekly adjuvant bolus 5-fluorouracil/leucovorin (FU/LV) or irinotecan+FU/LV (IFL), with 8 year follow-up. Tumors from these patients were analyzed to determine stability of a T_{11} tract in the *MRE11* gene. The primary endpoint was overall survival (OS), and a secondary endpoint was disease-free survival (DFS). Non-proportional hazards were addressed using time-dependent covariates in Cox analyses.

Results: Of 625 tumor cases examined, 70 (11.2%) exhibited contraction at the T_{11} tract in one or both *MRE11* alleles and were thus predicted to be deficient in MRE11 (dMRE11). In pooled treatment analyses, dMRE11 patients showed initially reduced DFS and OS but improved long-term DFS and OS compared with patients with an intact MRE11 T_{11} tract. In the subgroup of dMRE11 patients treated with IFL, an unexplained early increase in mortality but better long-term DFS than IFL-treated pMRE11 patients was observed.

Conclusions: Analysis of this relatively small number of patients and events showed that the dMRE11 marker predicts better prognosis independent of treatment in the long-term. In subgroup analyses, dMRE11 patients treated with irinotecan exhibited unexplained short-term mortality. MRE11 status is readily assayed and may therefore prove to be a useful prognostic marker, provided that the results reported here for a relatively small number of patients can be generalized in independent analyses of larger numbers of samples.

Trial Registration: ClinicalTrials.gov NCT00003835

Editor: Pierlorenzo Pallante, Institute of Experimental Endocrinology and Oncology G. Salvatore' (IEOS), Italy

Funding: Research reported here was supported by National Institutes of Health National Cancer Institute P01 CA077852 (WBG, PSR, RJM, NM); and NIH F31 GM073318 and HHMI MedIntoGrad Scholar Awards (AC). The funders had no role in study design, data collection and analysis, decision to publish, or preparation of the manuscript.

Competing Interests: The authors have declared that no competing interests exist.

* Email: maizels@u.washington.edu

Introduction

Colorectal cancer (CRC) is the third most common cancer, and the second most common cause of cancer-related death in the US, after lung cancer [1]. There will be an estimated 143,000 new cases in the US in 2013, and more than 51,000 deaths due to this cancer. It is important to identify markers that report on disease prognosis.

Like many other types of cancer, CRC is characterized by deficiencies in DNA repair pathways that can affect evolution of the tumor, its response to chemotherapy, and survival in the short and long term [2]. Approximately 15% of sporadic CRC and most hereditary CRC are characterized by deficient mismatch repair (MMR-D), which is also common in other cancers, including endometrial and gastric tumors [3–5]. MMR-D CRC are recognized as a distinct pathological and clinical subclass, with better long-term prognosis but possibly limited response to standard adjuvant chemotherapy consisting of 5-fluorouracil (FU) and leucovorin (LV) [2,6,7].

Deficient MMR elevates the somatic mutation rate and destabilizes simple sequence repeats, or microsatellites, which in turn can affect gene sequence and gene functions [8]. Deficient MMR could affect prognosis directly or indirectly, by altering function of another gene or genes. One consequence of deficient MMR is contraction of a T_{11} tract in intron 4 of the *MRE11* gene, which is evident in over 60% of MMR-D CRC [9–11]. The T_{11} polypyrimidine tract promotes lariat formation in splicing of exon 4 to exon 5 of the MRE11 transcript. Contraction of that tract impairs splicing, resulting in exon skipping and synthesis of a mRNA carrying an out-of-frame stop codon. This mRNA encodes a truncated MRE11 polypeptide, with potentially dominant negative effect on function of the normal protein [12]. The status of the *MRE11* T_{11} tract can be readily determined by the standard clinical assay used to determine MMR status based on instability of neutral microsatellite markers [13].

MRE11-deficiency may affect both clonal evolution within a tumor as well as therapeutic response. MRE11 forms one component of the highly conserved MRE11/RAD50 complex, which is essential for DNA double-strand break repair mediated by both homologous recombination and non-homologous end-joining, for telomere maintenance, and for signaling in response to DNA damage [14–18]. MRE11 may in particular influence the response to topoisomerase 1 poisons, which function by trapping the normally transient covalent bond that topoisomerase 1 forms with DNA in order to relax supercoiling. This class of drugs includes the naturally occurring compound camptothecin, and its derivatives irinotecan and topotecan. MRE11 is highly conserved, and genetic analysis in the yeast, *S. cerevisiae*, has shown that MRE11-deficiency causes extreme sensitivity to camptothecin [19]. In vitro, purified recombinant MRE11/RAD50 can cleave the covalent tyrosyl-DNA bond formed by topoisomerase 1 and resect the DNA end for repair [20]. In addition, a limited study of five CRC cell lines found that those that were MRE11/RAD50-deficient were more sensitive to irinotecan [21], but did not determine whether irinotecan resistance could be restored by complementing the MRE11/RAD50-deficiency/.

The observations summarized above lead to two hypotheses. First, MRE11-deficiency might be a useful marker for tumor prognosis; and second, that MRE11-deficient (dMRE11) tumors might respond better to treatment with topoisomerase 1 poisons than MRE11-proficient (pMRE11) tumors. These possibilities were of particular interest because of the readiness with which MRE11 status can be assayed during standard clinical molecular profiling [13].

The utility of irinotecan has been assessed for adjuvant treatment of stage III CRC in a two arm Cancer and Leukemia Group B (CALGB) 89803 clinical trial, which compared DFS and OS in patients treated with FU/LV alone or in combination with irinotecan. No difference in OS or DFS was reported overall, but patients with MMR-D tumors exhibited somewhat improved and extended DFS if treatment included irinotecan [22]. This trial therefore provided informative samples for addressing the question of whether MRE11 status correlated with DFS, OS, or with response to irinotecan. In order to determine whether MRE11 status predicts DFS, OS, or response to IFL, we analyzed MRE11 status in 625 tumor samples from patients in the CALGB 89803 clinical trial, both overall and by treatment with FU/LV therapy with or without irinotecan, while accounting for potential relationships with other patient characteristics including MMR.

Materials and Methods

The protocol for this trial and supporting CONSORT checklist are available as supporting information; see Protocol S1 and Checklist S1.

Study population

Patients in this study were participants in the NCI-sponsored Cancer and Leukemia Group B (CALGB) adjuvant therapy trial for stage III colon cancer comparing therapy with the weekly Roswell Park regimen of 5-fluorouracil (FU) and leucovorin (FU/LV) with the weekly bolus regimen of irinotecan, FU, and leucovorin (CALGB 89803; [23]). A total of 1264 patients were recruited between April, 1999, and April, 2001. All patients underwent complete surgical resection and started chemotherapy between postoperative days 21 to 56. Patients were randomly assigned by computer to two treatment arms, 629 patients to FU plus LV and 635 patients to irinotecan plus FU plus LV (Figure 1). The primary study endpoint was overall survival (OS). Disease-free survival (DFS) was a secondary endpoint. Follow-up was captured as of March, 2008.

Consort Diagram

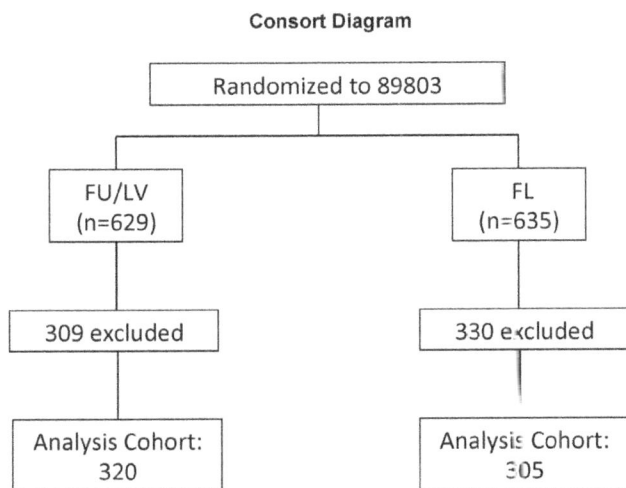

Figure 1. Consort diagram. Outline of CALGB 89803 randomized trial which generated the 625 samples tested.

Table 1. Demographics of Study Population by MRE11 Status.

	Ineligible MRE11 Analyses (N = 639)	Eligible MRE11 Analyses (N = 625)	Total (N = 1264)	p value
Treatment arm				0.3121[1]
5FU/LV	309 (48.4%)	320 (51.2%)	629 (49.8%)	
CPT-11/5FU/LV	330 (51.6%)	305 (48.8%)	635 (50.2%)	
Age at study entry				0.0144[2]
Mean (SD)	59.2 (11.5)	60.5 (11.4)	59.9 (11.5)	
Median	59.0	63.0	61.0	
Range	(21.0–85.0)	(24.0–85.0)	(21.0–85.0)	
Gender				0.6415[1]
Male	359 (56.2%)	343 (54.9%)	702 (55.5%)	
Female	280 (43.8%)	282 (45.1%)	562 (44.5%)	
Tumor Site				0.5030[1]
Missing	17	11	28	
Distal	268 (43.1%)	253 (41.2%)	521 (42.2%)	
Proximal	354 (56.9%)	361 (58.8%)	715 (57.8%)	
Performance status				0.4169[1]
Missing	18	9	27	
0	458 (73.8%)	467 (75.8%)	925 (74.8%)	
1	158 (25.4%)	147 (23.9%)	305 (24.7%)	
2	5 (0.8%)	2 (0.3%)	7 (0.6%)	
Positive Nodes				0.1703[2]
N	624	616	1240	
Mean (SD)	3.4 (3.3)	3.7 (3.6)	3.6 (3.4)	
Median	2.0	3.0	2.0	
Range	(0.0–29.0)	(1.0–24.0)	(0.0–29.0)	
Histologic Grade				0.2419[1]
Missing	17	10	27	
Grade 1/2	478 (76.8%)	455 (74.0%)	933 (75.4%)	
Grade 3/4	144 (23.2%)	160 (26.0%)	304 (24.6%)	
T-Stage				0.7941[1]
Missing	18	13	31	
T12	83 (13.4%)	74 (12.1%)	157 (12.7%)	
T3	486 (78.3%)	487 (79.6%)	973 (78.9%)	
T4	52 (8.4%)	51 (8.3%)	103 (8.4%)	
MMR Status				0.7890[1]
Missing	310	44	354	
MMR-I	283 (86.0%)	496 (85.4%)	779 (85.6%)	
MMR-D	46 (14.0%)	85 (14.6%)	131 (14.4%)	
BRAF600				0.8919[1]
Missing	567	40	607	
Wild-Type	61 (84.7%)	492 (84.1%)	553 (84.2%)	
Mutant	11 (15.3%)	93 (15.9%)	104 (15.8%)	
KRAS				0.8518[1]
Missing	569	41	610	
Wild-Type	45 (64.3%)	382 (65.4%)	427 (65.3%)	
Mutant	25 (35.7%)	202 (34.6%)	227 (34.7%)	
P53				0.2703
Missing	439	216	655	

Table 1. Cont.

	Ineligible MRE11 Analyses (N = 639)	Eligible MRE11 Analyses (N = 625)	Total (N = 1264)	p value
Wild-Type	103 (51.5%)	230 (56.2%)	333 (54.7%)	
Mutant	97 (48.5%)	179 (43.8%)	276 (45.3%)	

[1]chi-squared tests, for difference between MRE11-eligible and MRE11-ineligible patients.
according to relevant factors.
[2]Wilcoxon test for difference between MRE11-eligible and MRE11-ineligible patients according to relevant factors.

Ethics statement

The study was approved by the Mayo Clinic Institutional Review Board and the North Central Cancer Treatment Group (now part of Alliance for Clinical Trials in Oncology). CALGB protocol 89803 was reviewed by the institutional review board of each participating center. All patients gave written informed consent before participation.

Trial structure and organization

This trial was conducted by CALGB with participation by the North Central Cancer Treatment Group, National Cancer Institute of Canada Clinical Trials Group, Eastern Cooperative Oncology Group, Southwest Oncology Group, and the National Cancer Institute Cancer Trials Support Unit. The protocol and list of participating sites are available as Supporting Information. The

CALGB data safety monitoring board reviewed safety data twice yearly and efficacy data at protocol-specified intervals in accordance with CALGB policies. The CALGB Statistical Center at Duke University in Durham, NC, maintained the clinical and laboratory database.

Treatment

After central registration, eligible patients were randomly assigned (by computer, using a randomized fixed block design) to receive FU/LV or FU/LV in combination with irinotecan (IFL). Treatment has previously been described in detail [24]. In brief, the FU/LV group received the Roswell Park regimen, consisting of weekly LV 500 mg/m^2 intravenously over 2 hours, with a bolus of FU 500 mg/m^2 by intravenous injection 1 hour after initiation of LV, for 6 consecutive weeks followed by a 2-week rest, for four cycles (32 weeks). The IFL group received weekly

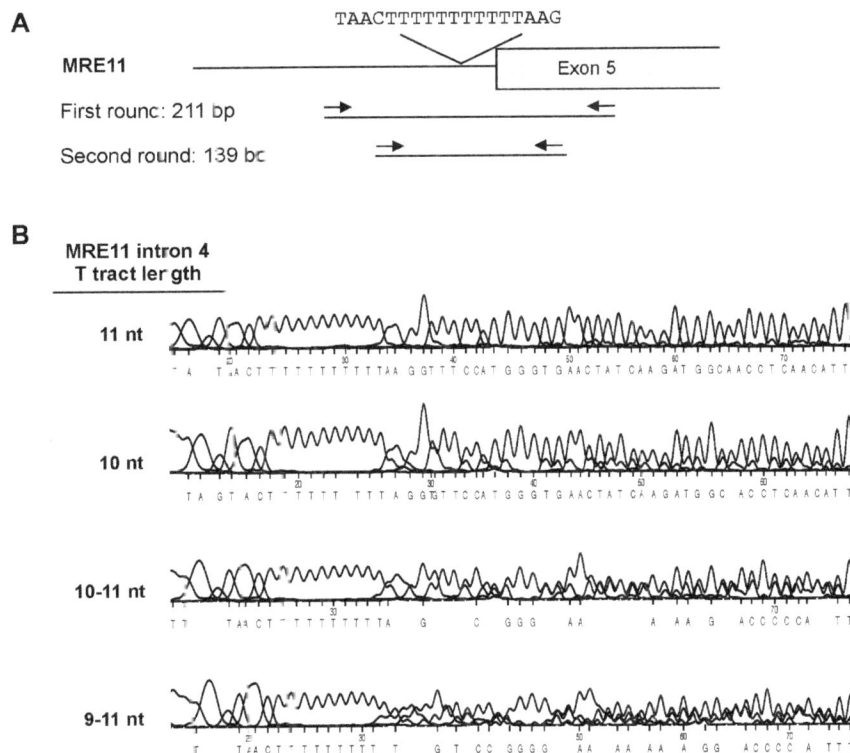

Figure 2. Genomic PCR assay of *MRE11* intron 4 T$_{11}$ tract. (A) Diagram of the *MRE11* intron 4/exon 5 junction, showing the T$_{11}$ tract in intron 4, flanking sequence and primers. Contraction of the T$_{11}$ tract impairs the lariat formation step in mRNA splicing and leads to skipping of exon 5. The resulting mutant mRNA encodes a truncated MRE11 polypeptide with potentially dominant negative effect on protein function [12]. MRE11 is essential for cell viability, and the *MRE11* mutations that occur in MMR-D CRC are not null alleles but reduce expression and activity of the MRE11 protein. (B) Sequence traces of the region of *MRE11* intron 4 that carries the T$_{11}$ tract in four tumor samples. Lengths of tracts in nt shown at left.

Table 2. Demographics by MRE11 Status (dMRE11 vs. pMRE11).

	dMRE11 (N = 70)	pMRE11 (N = 555)	Total (N = 625)	p value
Treatment arm				0.2194[1]
5FU/LV	31 (44.3%)	289 (52.1%)	320 (51.2%)	
CPT-11/5FU/LV	39 (55.7%)	266 (47.9%)	305 (48.8%)	
Age at study entry				0.2133[2]
Mean (SD)	60.8 (14.0)	60.5 (11.1)	60.5 (11.4)	
Median	66.0	62.0	63.0	
Range	(24.0–81.0)	(24.0–85.0)	(24.0–85.0)	
Gender				0.2603[1]
Male	34 (48.6%)	309 (55.7%)	343 (54.9%)	
Female	36 (51.4%)	246 (44.3%)	282 (45.1%)	
Tumor site				<0.0001[1]
Missing	2	9	11	
Distal	10 (14.7%)	243 (44.5%)	253 (41.2%)	
Proximal	58 (85.3%)	303 (55.5%)	361 (58.8%)	
Performance status				0.8624[1]
Missing	2	7	9	
0	51 (75.0%)	416 (75.9%)	467 (75.8%)	
1	17 (25.0%)	130 (23.7%)	147 (23.9%)	
2	0 (0.0%)	2 (0.4%)	2 (0.3%)	
Positive nodes				0.4688[2]
N	68	548	616	
Mean (SD)	4.2 (4.1)	3.7 (3.5)	3.7 (3.6)	
Median	3.0	3.0	3.0	
Range	(1.0–22.0)	(1.0–24.0)	(1.0–24.0)	
Histologic Grade				0.0001[1]
Missing	2	8	10	
Grade 1/2	37 (54.4%)	418 (76.4%)	455 (74.0%)	
Grade 3/4	31 (45.6%)	129 (23.6%)	160 (26.0%)	
T-Stage				0.1056[1]
Missing	2	11	13	
T12	6 (8.8%)	68 (12.5%)	74 (12.1%)	
T3	52 (76.5%)	435 (80.0%)	487 (79.6%)	
T4	10 (14.7%)	41 (7.5%)	51 (8.3%)	
MMR Status				<0.0001[1]
Missing	3	41	44	
MMR-I	14 (20.9%)	482 (93.8%)	496 (85.4%)	
MMR-D	53 (79.1%)	32 (6.2%)	85 (14.6%)	
BRAF600				<0.0001[1]
Missing	4	36	40	
Wild-Type	33 (50.0%)	459 (88.4%)	492 (84.1%)	
Mutant	33 (50.0%)	60 (11.6%)	93 (15.9%)	
KRAS				<0.0001[1]
Missing	3	38	41	
Wild-Type	59 (88.1%)	323 (62.5%)	382 (65.4%)	
Mutant	8 (11.9%)	194 (37.5%)	202 (34.6%)	
P53				0.0300[1]
Missing	22	194	216	
Wild-Type	34 (70.8%)	196 (54.3%)	230 (56.2%)	
Mutant	14 (29.2%)	165 (45.7%)	179 (43.8%)	

Table 2. Cont.

	dMRE11 (N = 70)	pMRE11 (N = 555)	Total (N = 625)	p value
RAD50				0.8062[1]
Missing	36	544	580	
Wild-Type	23 (67.6%)	7 (63.6%)	30 (66.7%)	
Mutant	11 (32.4%)	4 (36.4%)	15 (33.3%)	

[1]chi-squared test.
[2]Wilcoxon Rank-Sum test.

irinotecan 125 mg/m^2 over 90 minutes followed immediately by intravenous bolus injections of LV 20 mg/m^2, then FU 500 mg/m^2, for 4 consecutive weeks followed by a 2-week rest, for five cycles (30 weeks).

DNA extraction

DNA was extracted from archived formalin-fixed paraffin-embedded tumor tissue by incubating the paraffin-extracted, rehydrated tissue in 50 mM Tris HCl (pH 8.5) with 0.5% Tween 20 and 20 mg/ml proteinase K for 3 hr at 55°C; or by incubating the tissue in Instagene (BioRad, Hercules, CA) and 30 mg/ml proteinase K for 3 hr at 55°C. After the incubation, the sample was then incubated at 95°C for 9 minutes, vortexed briefly, and then subjected to centrifugation to pellet any undigested material or the Instagene, respectively. The extracted DNA was then aliquoted and stored at −20°C until needed for the PCR based assays.

Determination of MRE11 and RAD50 mononucleotide tract lengths

Mononucleotide tract length was determined by PCR amplification and DNA sequencing, using a well-established approach widely used to characterize the heterogeneity in mononucleotide tracts characteristic of MMR-deficient colorectal, gastric and endometrial tumors, and not evident in normal tissue or MMR-proficient tumor samples (e.g. [9–11,25]). The assay involves PCR amplification of the region carrying mononucleotide tract, followed by DNA sequence analysis. This same simple procedure is used to assess microsatellite instability diagnostic of mismatch repair deficiency.

A total of 625 samples generated DNA suitable for analysis of the region of *MRE11* intron 4 containing the T$_{11}$ tract, 320 from the FU/LV study arm and 305 from the IFL arm (Figure 1).

Nested PCR primers were used to amplify a region containing the mononucleotide tract of interest in MRE11 intron 4. MRE11 amplification was with first round primers, MRE11×1F, 5′-GTGGTCATATGCCAATGTAGATTATGC-3′, and MRE11×1R, 5′-CCCTGTGGGATCGTCATGATTGCC-3′, produced a 211 bp product. and with second round primers, MRE11×2F, 5′-GGAGGAGAATCTTAGGGAAAACAGC-3′, and MRE11×2R, 5′-GATTGCCATGAATACTAAACACTGG-3′, produced a 139 bp product MRE11 was sequenced in both forward and reverse directions with the second round PCR primers.

RAD50 status was determined for 34 CRCs with contractions in *MRE11*. Amplification was with first round primers R50×1F, 5′-CTCCCAGTTCATTACTCAGC-3′, and R50×1R, 5′-GACAGGGCATACCACCT-3′, produced a 326 bp product; and with second round primers R50×2F, 5′-GCTAACAGACGAAAAC-CAG-3′, and R50×2R, 5′-CATACCAGCTCAGAGTCC-3′, produced a 301 bp product. RAD50 was sequenced in reverse orientation with primer 5′-CATACCAGCTCAGAGTCC-3′.

MRE11 status and RAD50 status were determined by visual inspection of tracings from automated sequencing in both the forward and reverse direction by investigators blinded to MMR status, which had been determined independently [22,26]. Results are presented in Tables 1 and 2.

Determination of MMR status

MMR status of tumor samples had been previously determined by IHC, supplemented in some cases by analysis of microsatellite stability using the Bethesda panel markers [22,25]. MMR status of

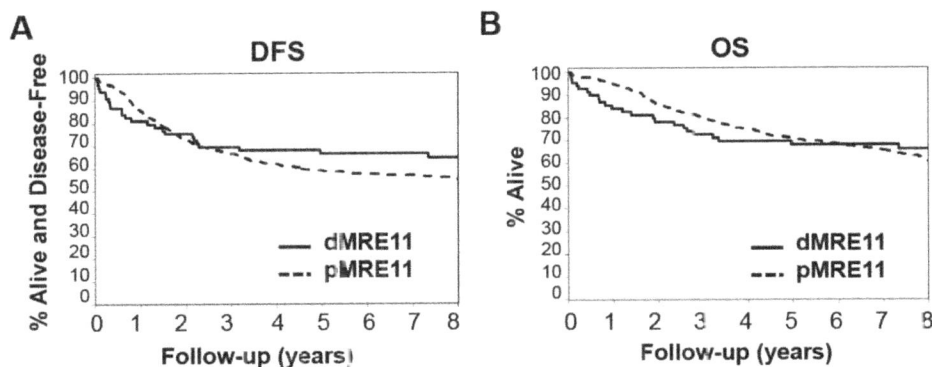

Figure 3. Tumor MRE11 status is significantly prognostic for DFS and OS. (A) Disease free survival for dMRE11 (n = 70; events = 24); 5-yr rate: 67% (95% CI: 56–79%) vs. pMRE11 (n = 555; events = 240); 5-yr rate: 59% (95% CI: 55–63%). (B) Overall survival for dMRE11 (n = = 70; events = 23); 5-yr rate: 68% (95% CI: 58–80%) vs. pMRE11 (n = 555; events = 154); 5-yr rate: 71% (95% CI: 67–75%).

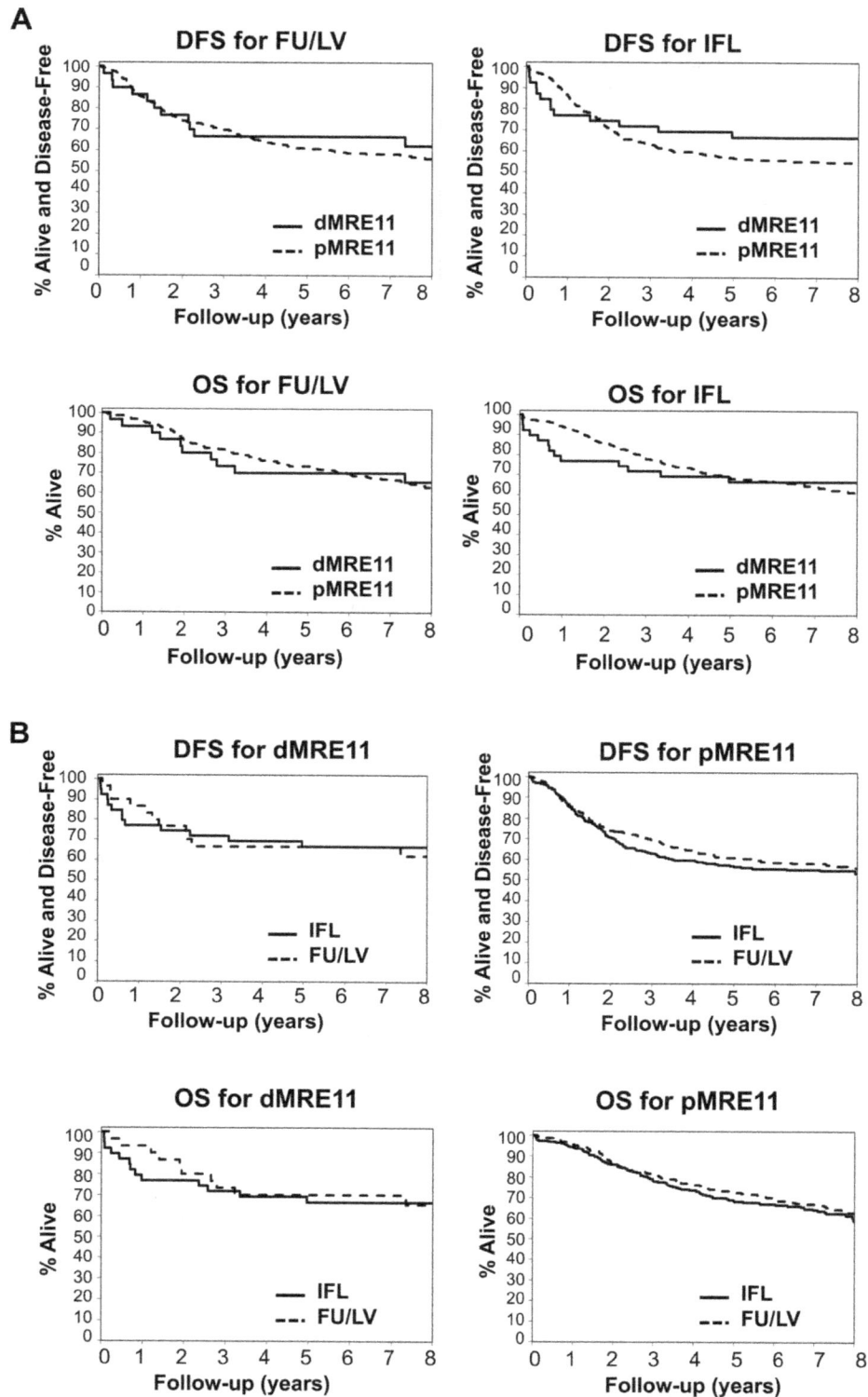

Figure 4. Assessment of tumor MRE11 status as predictive of benefit from FU/LV and IFL. (A) Top: Disease free survival for dMRE11 vs. pMRE11 treated with FU/LV [n = 320; dMRE11 n = 31; events = 11; 5-yr rate: 67% (95% CI: 52–86%); pMRE11 n = 289; events = 122; 5-yr rate: 61% (95% CI: 56–67%)] or with IFL [n = 305; dMRE11 n = 39; events = 13; 5-yr rate: 67% (95% CI: 53–83%); pMRE11 n = 266; events = 118; 5-yr rate: 57% (95% CI: 51–63%)]. Bottom: Overall survival for dMRE11 vs. pMRE11, treated with FU/LV [n = 320; dMRE11 n = 31; events = 10; 5-yr rate: 70% (95% CI: 55–89%); pMRE11 n = 289; events = 98; 5-yr rate: 73% (95% CI: 68–79%)] or with IFL [n = 305; dMRE11 n = 39; events = 13; 5-yr rate: 67% (95% CI: 53–83%); pMRE11 n = 266; events = 96; 5-yr rate: 69% (95% CI: 63–75%)]. (B) Top: Disease-free survival for IFL vs. FU/LV treated dMRE11 [n = 70; IFL N = 39; events = 13; 5-yr rate: 67% (95% CI: 53–83%); FU/LV n = 31; events = 11; 5-yr rate: 67% (95% CI: 52–86%)] or pMRE11 (n = 555; IFL n = 266; events = 118; 5-yr rate: 57% (95% CI: 51–63%; FU/LV n = 289; events = 122; 5-yr rate: 61% (95% CI: 56–67%)]. Bottom: Overall survival for IFL vs. FU/LV-treated

dMRE11 [n = 70; IFL n = 39; events = 13; 5-yr rate: 67% (95% CI: 53–83%); FU/LV n = 31; events = 10; 5-yr rate: 70% (95% CI: 55–89%) or pMRE11 [(n = 555; IFL n = 266; events = 96; 5-yr rate: 59% (95% CI: 63–75%); FU/LV n = 289; events = 98; 5-yr rate: 73% (95% CI: 68–79%)].

a subset of samples was independently confirmed in a blinded analysis by PCR amplification and sequencing 5 microsatellite markers (Promega, Madison, WI). Samples were classified as MMR-D if 3 or more markers exhibited instability.

Statistical methods

The goal of this study was to determine whether tumor MRE11 status was associated with outcome for patients with stage III colon cancer treated either with FU/LV alone or in combination with irinotecan. The joint primary endpoints were OS, measured from entry onto the clinical trial until death from any cause; and DFS, measured from study entry until documented progression of disease or death from any cause. OS and DFS distributions were estimated overall and within categories defined by MRE11 and treatment, using Kaplan-Meier methodology. Differences in OS and DFS between groups were tested using the log-rank test. The effects of MRE11 on OS and DFS were analyzed using Cox proportional hazards models. Where the Cox proportional hazards assumption was significantly violated according to the method of Grambsch and Therneau [27], time-varying coefficients were introduced through automated selection of one or more cutpoints on the time axis, which in turn optimally satisfied the proportional hazards assumption in a piecewise fashion [28]. The potential predictive ability of MRE11 was explored through two-way interactions with treatment arm, and through partial interactions when the effect of MRE11 was modeled as time-dependent. Interactions that were both statistically significant (p< 0.01) and of interpretable clinical relevance were required to conclude meaningful predictive ability of MRE11. Multivariable Cox models were used to study the MRE11 effect while controlling for treatment and clinicopathologic factors including age, sex, tumor location, performance status, number of positive lymph nodes, tumor stage, and tumor grade. Potential MRE11 interactions with and adjustments by MMR, KRAS, and BRAF were also explored. For the purposes of this analysis, follow-up was limited to 8 years. All statistical analyses were performed by Alliance statisticians.

Results

Determination of MRE11 status

Tumor DNA suitable for PCR amplification was extracted from a total of 625 CRC specimens, 320 from the FU/LV group and 305 from the ILV group (Consort Diagram, Figure 1). The 625 specimens represent 49% of the 1264 patients enrolled on CALGB 89803 [23]. The region of MRE11 intron 4 containing the T_{11} tract was amplified and sequenced (Figure 2A), using a well-established assay (e.g. [9–11,25]). Examples show sequences of a control sample with uniform T_{11} tracts on both alleles, and of samples in which both alleles carried 10 nt tracts, or tracts ranging from 10–11 or 9–11 nt (Figure 2B). Tract length heterogeneity was not a PCR or sequencing artefact, as length heterogeneity was not evident in DNA from normal cells, and identical tract lengths were deduced from sequencing a single sample in both directions (not shown). Heterogeneity could reflect the presence of multiple sub-clonal populations within the tumor.

Cases were scored based on the number of nucleotides lost by contraction: an 11 nt tract was scored as 0; a 10–11 nt tract as 1; tracts of 9–11 nt as 2; and tracts of 10 nt (due to loss of 1 nt on each allele) as 2. A total of 555 cases (89%) carried an intact T_{11} tract (score 0); while 70 cases (11%) had contractions of 1–6 nt in length (1 nt, n = 36; 2 nt, n = 26; 3 nt, n = 6; 4 nt, n = 1; and 6 nt, n = 1). The overall frequency of MRE11 T_{11} contractions was 11%, comparable to that reported in other analyses of CRC specimens [9–11,25]. Approximately equal numbers of cases exhibited contractions of 1 nt (36 cases, 5.8%) or 2 or more nt (34 cases, 5.8%). Due to an imbalance of cases with no contractions versus any contraction, and the small number of cases in each contraction category, we defined a dichotomous MRE11 T_{11} tract variable: no contractions or MRE11 proficient (pMRE11, 555 cases) versus any contraction or MRE11 deficient (dMRE11, 70 cases). Using this dichotomized classification, MRE11 T_{11} tract contraction status was found to be significantly associated with tumor site, histological grade, MMR status, and BRAF, KRAS, and P53 mutation status (Table 2).

Determination of RAD50 status

In some MMR-D CRC, an exonic A_9 tract in the RAD50 gene is destabilized, causing a frameshift mutation and synthesis of a truncated protein [29]. In an exploratory analysis, we determined this frequency among tumor DNAs extracted from 34 CRCs with contractions in MRE11 (18 cases with MRE11 scores of 1, and 16 with scores of 2). The RAD50 A_9 tract was unstable in 11/34 cases (3 with MRE11 scores of 1, and 8 with scores of 2) or 32% of CRCs analyzed, similar to the frequency of 40% previously reported [11].

Determination of MMR status

MMR status of all CALGB 89803 samples had previously been determined by IHC, genomic sequencing with the Bethesda panel markers, or both [26]. That analysis classified MMR as intact (MMR-I) in 86% of the samples, and deficient (MMR-D) in 14% (Table 1). Instability of the MRE11 T_{11} tract was strongly associated with MMR deficiency thus determined: 79% of dMRE11 CRCs were MMR-D, and 21% MMR-I (chi-squared test, p<0.0001; Table 2).

In an exploratory analysis, MMR status was separately determined by PCR and sequencing at the University of Washington (UW) clinical diagnostic facility, exclusively using commercial primers (Promega) that interrogate different neutral and non-polymorphic markers than the Bethesda panel markers. A total of 83 CRCs were analyzed, including 63 of the 70 dMRE11 samples. Of these, 50 CRC were classified as MMR-D by CALGB and 56 by the UW (chi-squared test, p<0.0001).

Instability at the MRE11 T_{11} tract and the RAD50 A_9 tract is predicted to correlate with MMR-D. To get a sense of whether the different assays used by CALGB and UW might over-count or under-count MMR-D tumors, we asked if the 9 CRC classified as MMR-I by the CALGB assays but as MMR-D by the UW assay were dMRE11 or pMRE11. All of these were dMRE11, and two of them were also dRAD50. This raises the possibility that the MRE11 T_{11} tract might be usefully included among markers for determination of MMR status.

Tumor MRE11 status is significantly prognostic for DFS and OS

The relationship between MRE11 status and DFS and OS was determined using data captured as of March 10, 2008, representing a median follow-up of >6.0 years. Univariate analyses of OS and DFS based solely on MRE11 status of the 625 CRCs assayed, independent of chemotherapeutic regimen, showed that dMRE11 patients exhibited no significant improvement in OS (HR 0.98; 95% CI, 0.64 to 1.51) or DFS (HR 0.80; 95% CI, 0.52 to 1.21) relative to pMRE11 patients. However, Kaplan-Meier plots of OS and DFS by MRE11 status (Figure 3) revealed a possible violation of the proportional hazards assumption, with the two curves crossing during the follow-up period for each endpoint. Non-proportionality was statistically confirmed, with the null hypothesis of proportional hazards rejected for both DFS (p = 0.0038) and OS (p = 0.0005).

To resolve this violation of the Cox modeling assumptions, a piecewise proportional hazard model was constructed for each endpoint (DFS and OS), resulting in time dependent coefficients (HRs) for MRE11 status, as follows. First, an automated searching algorithm over a grid of time points $\{t_1 = 0.1$ years, $t_2 = 0.2$ years, ..., $t_{79} = 7.9$ years$\}$ was used to identify the cutpoint t^* for which the proportional hazards assumption was optimally satisfied on either side of the cutpoint; specifically, t^* is defined as the value of t yielding the largest maximized log partial likelihood among Cox models containing separate MRE11 effects (HRs) for the two time intervals defined by t. Piecewise proportionality was then tested and confirmed in the final models for OS and DFS, producing the final (univariate) models for MRE11. The same cutpoints and time-dependent coefficients were used in subsequent interaction and multivariable Cox models.

The optimal cut-point identified for OS was 3.4 years. Prior to 3.4 years, dMRE11 patients experience significantly worse OS relative to pMRE11 patients (HR = 10.95, 95% CI: 6.83 to 17.55, p<0.0001), while after 3.4 years dMRE11 is associated with improved OS (HR = 0.09, 95% CI: 0.02 to 0.37, p = 0.0008), independent of treatment arm. The cut-point identified for DFS was 3.3 years. Prior to 3.3 years, dMRE11 was associated with worse outcomes (HR = 7.02, 95% CI: 4.49 to 10.99, p<0.0001), while after 3.3 years DFS is improved relative to pMRE11 patients (HR = 0.07, 95% CI: 0.02 to 0.30, p = 0.0002). MRE11 status remained significant overall when adjusted for clinical/tumor variables (age, sex, number of positive nodes, tumor stage, grade, and site of primary tumor).

In relation to other patient biomarkers, MRE11 is jointly significant in multivariable models with KRAS (OS and DFS), BRAF (OS and DFS), and P53 mutation status (OS only). Furthermore, MRE11 remains a significant predictor for both OS (p<0.0001) and DFS (p<0.0001) after adjustment for MMR, while MMR is not significant in these models (DFS p = 0.799; OS p = 0.647). No significant interactions between MRE11 and biomarkers were observed.

Univariate analyses for RAD50 status showed no significant relationship with OS or DFS. Covariate-adjusted models for RAD50 were not performed due to the limited sample size (n = 34) and small number of events.

Assessment of tumor MRE11 status as predictive of benefit from IFL and FU/LV

MRE11 status was assessed as a potential predictor benefit from IFL through partial interactions with treatment in piecewise Cox (non-proportional hazards) models for DFS and OS. Kaplan-Meier plots for the MRE11 effect are presented by treatment arm in Figure 4A, while plots for the corresponding treatment effect are presented by MRE11 status in Figure 4B. While some differences in the treatment effect by MRE11 status are visually apparent, the treatment-by-MRE11 interaction was not significant for either endpoint. Among irinotecan-treated patients (Figure 4A, right), however, dMRE11 patients exhibited worse DFS than

pMRE11 patients during the first year of follow-up (based on a subset-selected cut-point; p<0.0001), but improved outcomes thereafter (p = 0.004). Similarly, dMRE11 patients were at increased risk of death for the first 3.5 years of follow-up relative to pMRE11 patients (p<0.0001), and decreased risk thereafter (p = 0.011). These relationships remained significant when adjusted for age, sex, nodal status, tumor stage, grade, and site of primary tumor, but this subgroup analysis among IFL-treated patients should be considered as exploratory given the small sample size and non-significance of the treatment-by-MRE11 interaction.

Discussion

This analysis of treated outcomes in a cohort of stage III CRC patients treated with FU/LV or IFL showed that, after controlling for unexpected non-proportional hazards, MRE11 status is significantly prognostic for both DFS and OS, and remains significant when adjusted for clinicopathologic variables and published significant markers such as MMR, KRAS, BRAF, and p53. Furthermore, after adjusting for MMR, MRE11 remains a significant prognostic marker, while the converse is not true. In an exploratory subgroup analysis, MRE11 status was associated with differences in OS and DFS among patients treated with IFL. The latter finding is clinically interesting, but based on a relatively small number of patients, and could be further investigated in studies enrolling larger numbers of patients. The impact on response might best be assessed in a study of stage IV patients with measurable metastatic disease, although it has been shown on many occasions that the effects of anti-tumor therapies differ between stage III and stage IV disease.

MMR status had previously been shown to be both a prognostic marker [2,6,7] and predictor of response to IFL relative to FU/LV [22]. In light of the strong correlation between dMRE11 and MMR-D status noted here, it is not surprising that the prognostic and predictive patterns for the two markers parallel one another. However, in multivariable prognostic models for DFS or OS containing both markers, MRE11 but not MMR status remained highly statistically significant during both early and late time periods. Thus, the significance of MRE11 status does not reflect its dependence on MMR status.

It should be noted that dMRE11 patients treated with IFL exhibited better long-term DFS than pMRE11 patients in the same treatment arm, although dMRE11 patients had an unexplained increased mortality in the first 2 years post-treatment. There was no relationship between poor initial response and clinical factors such as age, sex or nodal status. Therapy with irinotecan extended over only 30 weeks, while the difference in response did not become evident until later (Figure 4), so early treatment-associated toxicity alone is unlikely to explain this difference.

The analysis of MRE11 function in the response to irinotecan was undertaken based on results of basic mechanistic studies showing that MRE11/RAD50 contributes to repair of DNA damage induced by topoisomerase 1 poisons [19,20]. Topoisomerase 1 poisons (like irinotecan) and topoisomerase 2 poisons (like etoposide) both promote formation of protein-DNA adducts, which are cytotoxic if not repaired. Some insight into the considerable short-term mortality among dMRE11 patients treated with irinotecan may be provided by studies of mice deficient in the enzyme TDP2, which repairs damage induced by topoisomerase 2 poisons [30]. These mice are hypersensitive to etoposide, and respond to treatment by dramatic weight loss accompanied by villous atrophy in the small intestine and lymphoid toxicity [31]. Analogously, dMRE11 tumor cells may be hypersensitive to irinotecan, but at the single dose tested the cytotoxic response may create a local milieu conducive to tumor cell proliferation, for example by promoting expression of growth factors or by limiting the immune response to the tumor during the early stages of tumor development. If so, drug hypersensitivity could cause poor outcomes in early but not in later years post-treatment.

MRE11 T_{11} tract instability can be measured using an easy and reliable standard clinical assay like that already used to interrogate microsatellite instability. Analysis of the relatively small number of patients and events reported here showed that the dMRE11 marker predicts better prognosis independent of treatment in the long-term, suggesting that MRE11 may be a useful prognostic marker. Generalizability will require that these findings can be independently validated in another dataset that examines larger numbers of patients.

Deficiency in MRE11 occurs not only in colon cancer but also other solid tumors with deficient mismatch repair. Analysis of independent relevant datasets will be necessary to establish whether the results reported here extend to these other cancers.

Supporting Information

Protocol S1 Cancer and Leukemia Group B, CALBG 89803. Protocol for phase III intergroup trial of irinotecan (CPT-11) plus fluorouracil/leucovorin (5-FU/LV) versus fluorouracil/leucovorin alone after curative resection for patients with stage III colon cancer.

Checklist S1 CONSORT 2010 checklist. Checklist of information to include when reporting a randomised trial.

Institutions S1 CALBG 89803 Institutions. Institutions and investigators that participated in the initial CALGB 89803 study.

Acknowledgments

We are grateful to our Program Project Colleagues at the UW (P01 CA077852) for their valuable insights and support.

Author Contributions

Contributed to the writing of the manuscript: TP LR NRF AC PW VVL WBG DN LBS MMB PSR ME RJM NM. Conceived and designed the experiments: TP AC PW PSR ME RJM NM. Performed the experiments: TP AC NRF PW VVW. Analyzed the data: TP LR NRF AC PW PSR ME RJM NM. Contributed reagents/materials/analysis tools: DN LBS MMB VVL WBG RMG.

References

1. Meyerhardt JA, Mayer RJ (2005) Systemic therapy for colorectal cancer. N Engl J Med 352: 476–487.
2. Hewish M, Lord CJ, Martin SA, Cunningham D, Ashworth A (2010) Mismatch repair deficient colorectal cancer in the era of personalized treatment. Nat Rev Clin Oncol 7: 197–208.
3. Peltomaki P (2001) DNA mismatch repair and cancer. Mutat Res 488: 77–85.
4. Peltomaki P (2001) Deficient DNA mismatch repair: a common etiologic factor for colon cancer. Hum Mol Genet 10: 735–740.
5. Rustgi AK (2007) The genetics of hereditary colon cancer. Genes Dev 21: 2525–2538.
6. Popat S, Hubner R, Houlston RS (2005) Systematic review of microsatellite instability and colorectal cancer prognosis. J Clin Oncol 23: 609–618.
7. Sinicrope FA, Foster NR, Thibodeau SN, Marsoni S, Monges G, et al. (2011) DNA mismatch repair status and colon cancer recurrence and survival in clinical trials of 5-fluorouracil-based adjuvant therapy. J Natl Cancer Inst 103: 863–875.
8. Kunkel TA, Erie DA (2005) DNA mismatch repair. Annu Rev Biochem 74: 681–710.
9. Ottini L, Falchetti M, Saieva C, De Marco M, Masala G, et al. (2004) MRE11 expression is impaired in gastric cancer with microsatellite instability. Carcinogenesis 25: 2337–2343.
10. Giannini G, Rinaldi C, Ristori E, Ambrosini MI, Cerignoli F, et al. (2004) Mutations of an intronic repeat induce impaired MRE11 expression in primary human cancer with microsatellite instability. Oncogene 23: 2640–2647.
11. Miquel C, Jacob S, Grandjouan S, Aime A, Viguier J, et al. (2007) Frequent alteration of DNA damage signalling and repair pathways in human colorectal cancers with microsatellite instability. Oncogene 26: 5919–5926.
12. Wen Q, Scorah J, Phear G, Rodgers G, Rodgers S, et al. (2008) A mutant allele of MRE11 found in mismatch repair-deficient tumor cells suppresses the cellular response to DNA replication fork stress in a dominant negative manner. Mol Biol Cell 19: 1693–1705.
13. Boland CR, Thibodeau SN, Hamilton SR, Sidransky D, Eshleman JR, et al. (1998) A National Cancer Institute Workshop on Microsatellite Instability for cancer detection and familial predisposition: development of international criteria for the determination of microsatellite instability in colorectal cancer. Cancer Res 58: 5248–5257.
14. Williams RS, Moncalian G, Williams JS, Yamada Y, Limbo O, et al. (2008) Mre11 dimers coordinate DNA and bridging and nuclease processing in double-strand-break repair. Cell 135: 97–109.
15. Adelman CA, Petrini JH (2009) Division of labor: DNA repair and the cell cycle specific functions of the Mre11 complex. Cell Cycle 8: 1510–1514.
16. Attwooll CL, Akpinar M, Petrini JH (2009) The Mre11 Complex and the Response to Dysfunctional Telomeres. Mol Cell Biol.
17. Truong LN, Li Y, Shi LZ, Hwang PY, He J, et al. (2013) Microhomology-mediated end joining and homologous recombination share the initial end resection step to repair DNA double-strand breaks in mammalian cells. Proc Natl Acad Sci U S A 110: 7720–7725.
18. Stracker TH, Roig I, Knobel PA, Marjanovic M (2013) The ATM signaling network in development and disease. Front Genet 4: 37.
19. Hamilton NK, Maizels N (2010) MRE11 function in response to topoisomerase poisons is independent of its function in double-strand break repair in Saccharomyces cerevisiae. PLoS One 5: e15387.
20. Sacho EJ, Maizels N (2011) DNA repair factor MRE11/RAD50 cleaves 3'-phosphotyrosyl bonds and resects DNA to repair damage caused by topoisomerase 1 poisons. J Biol Chem 286: 44945–44951.
21. Vilar E, Scaltriti M, Balmana J, Saura C, Guzman M, et al. (2008) Microsatellite instability due to hMLH1 deficiency is associated with increased cytotoxicity to irinotecan in human colorectal cancer cell lines. Br J Cancer 99: 1607–1612.
22. Bertagnolli MM, Niedzwiecki D, Compton CC, Hahn HP, Hall M, et al. (2009) Microsatellite instability predicts improved response to adjuvant therapy with irinotecan, fluorouracil, and leucovorin in stage III colon cancer: Cancer and Leukemia Group B Protocol 89803. J Clin Oncol 27: 1814–1821.
23. Saltz LB, Niedzwiecki D, Hollis D, Goldberg RM, Hantel A, et al. (2007) Irinotecan fluorouracil plus leucovorin is not superior to fluorouracil plus leucovorin alone as adjuvant treatment for stage III colon cancer: results of CALGB 89803. J Clin Oncol 25: 3456–3461.
24. Kakar S, Aksoy S, Burgart LJ, Smyrk TC (2004) Mucinous carcinoma of the colon: correlation of loss of mismatch repair enzymes with clinicopathologic features and survival. Mod Pathol 17: 696–700.
25. Giannini G, Ristori E, Cerignoli F, Rinaldi C, Zani M, et al. (2002) Human MRE11 is inactivated in mismatch repair-deficient cancers. EMBO Rep 3: 248–254.
26. Bertagnolli MM, Redston M, Compton CC, Niedzwiecki D, Mayer RJ, et al. (2011) Microsatellite instability and loss of heterozygosity at chromosomal location 18q: prospective evaluation of biomarkers for stages II and III colon cancer–a study of CALGB 9581 and 89803. J Clin Oncol 29: 3153–3162.
27. Grambsch P, Therneau T (1994) Proportional hazards tests and diagnostics based on weighted residuals. Biometrika 81: 515–526
28. Klein JP, Moeschberger ML (2003) Survival Analysis: Techniques for Censored and Truncated Data. New York, NY: Springer.
29. Kim NG, Choi YR, Baek MJ, Kim YH, Kang H, et al. (2001) Frameshift mutations at coding mononucleotide repeats of the hRAD50 gene in gastrointestinal carcinomas with microsatellite instability. Cancer Res 61: 36–38.
30. Zeng Z, Cortes-Ledesma F, El Khamisy SF, Caldecott KW (2011) TDP2/TTRAP is the major 5'-tyrosyl DNA phosphodiesterase activity in vertebrate cells and is critical for cellular resistance to topoisomerase II-induced DNA damage. J Biol Chem 286: 403–409.
31. Gomez-Herreros F, Romero-Granados R, Zeng Z, Alvarez-Quilon A, Quintero C, et al. (2012) TDP2-dependent non-homologous end-joining protects against topoisomerase II-induced DNA breaks and genome instability in cells and in vivo. PLoS Genet 9: e1003226.

13

Impact of Age-Associated Cyclopurine Lesions on DNA Repair Helicases

Irfan Khan[1][◑], Avvaru N. Suhasini[1][◑][¤], Taraswi Banerjee[1], Joshua A. Sommers[1], Daniel L. Kaplan[2], Jochen Kuper[3], Caroline Kisker[3], Robert M. Brosh, Jr.[1]*

1 Laboratory of Molecular Gerontology, National Institute on Aging, National Institutes of Health, NIH Biomedical Research Center, Baltimore, Maryland, United States of America, 2 Department of Biomedical Sciences, Florida State University College of Medicine, Tallahassee, Florida, United States of America, 3 Rudolf Virchow Center for Experimental Biomedicine, Institute for Structural Biology, University of Würzburg, Würzburg, Germany

Abstract

8,5′ cyclopurine deoxynucleosides (cPu) are locally distorting DNA base lesions corrected by nucleotide excision repair (NER) and proposed to play a role in neurodegeneration prevalent in genetically defined Xeroderma pigmentosum (XP) patients. In the current study, purified recombinant helicases from different classifications based on sequence homology were examined for their ability to unwind partial duplex DNA substrates harboring a single site-specific cPu adduct. Superfamily (SF) 2 RecQ helicases (RECQ1, BLM, WRN, RecQ) were inhibited by cPu in the helicase translocating strand, whereas helicases from SF1 (UvrD) and SF4 (DnaB) tolerated cPu in either strand. SF2 Fe-S helicases (FANCJ, DDX11 (ChlR1), DinG, XPD) displayed marked differences in their ability to unwind the cPu DNA substrates. Archaeal *Thermoplasma acidophilum* XPD (taXPD), homologue to the human XPD helicase involved in NER DNA damage verification, was impeded by cPu in the non-translocating strand, while FANCJ was uniquely inhibited by the cPu in the translocating strand. Sequestration experiments demonstrated that FANCJ became trapped by the translocating strand cPu whereas RECQ1 was not, suggesting the two SF2 helicases interact with the cPu lesion by distinct mechanisms despite strand-specific inhibition for both. Using a protein trap to simulate single-turnover conditions, the rate of FANCJ or RECQ1 helicase activity was reduced 10-fold and 4.5-fold, respectively, by cPu in the translocating strand. In contrast, single-turnover rates of DNA unwinding by DDX11 and UvrD helicases were only modestly affected by the cPu lesion in the translocating strand. The marked difference in effect of the translocating strand cPu on rate of DNA unwinding between DDX11 and FANCJ helicase suggests the two Fe-S cluster helicases unwind damaged DNA by distinct mechanisms. The apparent complexity of helicase encounters with an unusual form of oxidative damage is likely to have important consequences in the cellular response to DNA damage and DNA repair.

Editor: Sergey Korolev, Saint Louis University, United States of America

Funding: This work was supported by the Intramural Research program of the National Institutes of Health, National Institute on Aging and by the Fanconi Anemia Research Fund (to R.M.B.) and through the Deutsche Forschungsgemeinschaft (Forschungszentrum FZ82 and KI-562/2 to C.K.). The funders had no role in study design, data collection and analysis, decision to publish, or preparation of the manuscript.

Competing Interests: The authors have declared that no competing interests exist.

* Email: broshr@mail.nih.gov

¤ Current address: Department of Medicine, Division of Hematology & Medical Oncology, Unversity of Texas Health Science Center, San Antonio, Texas, United States of America

◑ These authors contributed equally to this work.

Introduction

Oxidative DNA damage represented by a spectrum of bases or sugar modifications is incurred by reactive oxygen species that arise from endogenous biochemical processes and can also be induced exogenously by environmental agents such as chemical compounds (e.g., aldehydes, peroxides) or ionizing radiation. Oxidative DNA lesions in nuclear and/or mitochondrial genomes result in perturbations to cellular DNA replication and transcription; furthermore, their accumulation predisposes individuals to accelerated tissue aging, neurodegeneration, and cancer. A variety of oxidative DNA lesions exist, and recent efforts have focused on establishing meaningful relationships between the accumulation of a particular oxidative lesion and aberrant cellular and organismal phenotypes as well as the pathways for repairing and tolerating the spectrum of oxidative DNA lesions [1].

A class of endogenous oxidative DNA lesions that has attracted considerable attention for potential roles in human disease and mutagenesis is 8,5′-cyclopurine-2′-deoxynucleoside (cPu) [2]. The occurrence of cyclopurines in affected tissues may serve as a biomarker for disease or cancer risk, and effectiveness of therapeutic drugs [3,4]. The cPu DNA lesion arises from hydroxyl radical attack of the H5-atom of the sugar moiety leading to a carbon centered radical that reacts with the C8 position of the purine (guanine (G) or adenine (A)), ultimately creating a very stable glycosidic covalent bond in the cyclization reaction (**Fig. 1**). Structural studies indicate that the presence of the cyclopurine lesion in double-stranded DNA perturbs helix twist and base pair stacking [5,6]. Consistent with the structural results, cPu lesions are corrected by nucleotide excision repair (NER) [7,8], which is unusual because the vast majority of oxidative DNA base lesions are repaired by base excision repair (BER) [9]; however, the mechanistic steps involved in recognition and verification of a cPu lesion by the NER machinery are not well understood. Biochemical and cellular studies demonstrate that cPu lesions can interfere with replication [10], inhibit gene expression [7], perturb transcription factor binding to cognate recognition sequences [11], and induce transcriptional mutagenesis [12], leading researchers to investigate their role in disease pathology. Xeroderma pigmentosum (XP) Group C and Cockayne syndrome (CS) Group A patient keratinocytes [13,14] and tissues of CSB knockout mice [15] contained cPu lesions after exposure to low dose ionizing radiation and tissues from CSB knockout mice. It is hypothesized that cPu lesions are involved in XP neurological disease [16]. Furthermore, the stability of cPu base damage *in vivo* is supported by observations that under controlled environmental conditions, cPu lesions accumulate with age in wild-type mice compared to young mice, and also in congenic progeroid Ercc1−/Δ mice deficient in the XPF-ERCC1 endonuclease implicated in NER [17].

While the effects of cPu lesions on the functions of DNA polymerases [18–22], DNA nucleases [19,23,24], and RNA polymerase II [7] have been determined, there have been no studies on the impact of cPu damage on DNA unwinding enzymes known as helicases. Helicases represent a prominent class of proteins in cellular nucleic acid metabolism that are important in not only DNA replication and transcription, but also DNA repair, recombination, and chromosome segregation; moreover, a number of genetic disorders characterized by age-related symptoms and cancer are linked to mutations in helicase genes [25]. Covalent or noncovalent DNA modifications that alter helicase function are thought to play a role in processes involving replication stress, DNA damage signaling, and DNA repair [26]. In terms of eukaryotic NER, the XPD helicase is believed to play

an instrumental role in DNA damage verification that is necessary for subsequent steps to process and replace the damaged DNA with correct nucleotides [27,28]. Because helicases are now widely recognized as key enzymes in processes that are either directly affected by DNA damage or are themselves implicated in the DNA damage response, we have carefully examined the potential effects of cPu lesions on the DNA unwinding function of helicases which play a role in human disease. Our findings from biochemical studies with purified recombinant DNA helicases and defined DNA substrates harboring a site- and strand-specific cPu lesion provide the first evidence for their unique and wide ranging effects on DNA helicases that are highly likely to encounter the abundant and stable oxidized base damage.

Materials and Methods

Recombinant DNA helicase proteins

Recombinant human FANCJ [29], DDX11 (ChlR1) [30], RECQ1 [31], WRN [32], *E. coli* (Ec) EcDnaB [33], EcDinG [34], and *Thermoplasma acidophilum* (ta) XPD [35] were purified as previously described. EcRecQ was purchased from Abcam. Human recombinant BLM protein was kindly provided by Dr. Ian Hickson (University of Copenhagen). EcUvrD protein was kindly provided by Drs. Ting Xu and Wei Yang (NIDDK, National Institutes of Health). Superfamily designation and polarity for each helicase utilized in this study is provided in **Table 1**.

DNA substrates

Cyclo dA and Cyclo dG phosphoramidites were purchased from Berry & Associates (Dexter, MI). Synthesis and purification by polyacrylamide gel electrophoresis (PAGE) of oligonucleotides including those which used cyclo dA or cyclo dG phosphorami-

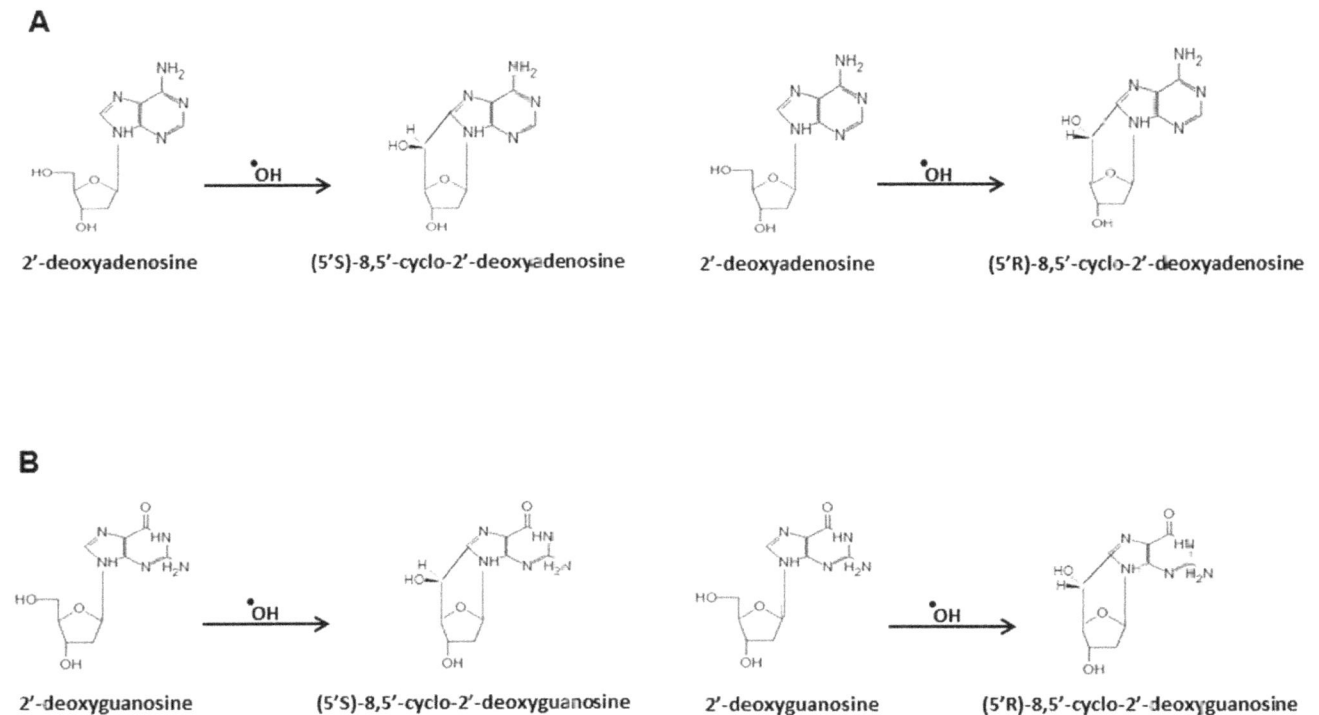

Figure 1. Conversion of adenine and guanine bases to cyclo dA and cyclo dG bases. A, Formation of 2'-deoxyadenosine to (5'S) 8,5'-cyclo-2'-dA and (5'R) 8,5'-cyclo-2'-dA. B, Formation of 2'-deoxyguanosine to (5'S) 8,5'-cyclo-2'-dG and (5'R) 8,5'-cyclo-2'-dG.

Table 1. DNA Helicases used in this study.

Superfamily	Helicases	Polarity
1	EcUvrD	3' to 5'
2	BLM, RECQ1, WRN, EcRecQ	3' to 5'
	EcDinG, DDX11, FANCJ, taXPD	5' to 3'
4	EcDnaB	5' to 3'

dites for synthesis was performed by Loftstrand Labs (Rockville, MD). The DNA substrates used were 5'-^{32}P-end-labeled partial duplex forked substrates labeled and annealed as described previously [36]. The forked substrates contained 5' and 3' single-stranded tails of 41 nucleotide (nt) and a 25 base pair (bp) duplex region. The sequences of the DNA substrates are provided in **Table S1**.

Standard helicase assays

Helicase reactions were carried out in 20 µl volumes which contained 10 fmol of the forked duplex DNA substrate carrying the cyclopurine lesion either in the top, bottom, or neither strand. The reactions were performed using previously described conditions (FANCJ [37], DDX11 (ChlR1) [30], taXPD [35,38], RECQ1 [31], WRN [32] EcRecQ [31], BLM [39], EcDnaB [33], EcDinG [34], and EcUvrD [40]). Unless stated otherwise, each of the helicase reactions were carried out by adding the indicated concentration of helicase protein to the reaction mixture followed by incubation at the appropriate temperature for the specified period of time. FANCJ, DDX11, taXPD, RECQ1, WRN, Ec RecQ, EcDnaB, EcDinG and EcUvrD were incubated for 15 min, while BLM was incubated for 30 min. Reactions were quenched with 20 µl of 2X Stop Buffer, containing 17.5 mM EDTA, 0.6% SDS, 0.02% bromophenol blue, 0.02% xylene cyanol and 10-fold excess of unlabeled oligonucleotide which contained the same sequence as the labeled strand. The unlabeled oligonucleotide was added to prevent reannealing. The quenched helicase reaction mixture samples were electrophoresed on non-denaturing 12% polyacrylamide (19:1 acrylamide-bisacrylamide) gels, visualized using a PhosphorImager, and quantified with ImageQuant Sofware.

Sequestration helicase assays

For helicase sequestration experiments, FANCJ (9.6 nM) or RECQ1 (8.8 nM) was preincubated for 3 min at 30°C or 37°C, respectively, with ATP (2 mM) and the indicated amounts of unlabeled forked duplex competitor DNA substrates containing the cdA lesion in the top strand, bottom strand, or neither strand. Subsequently, 10 fmol of radiolabeled 19 bp forked duplex, also known as the tracker substrate [41], was added to the mixture and incubated for an additional 10 min at 30°C (FANCJ) or 37°C (RECQ1). The helicase reactions were then quenched and resolved on 12% polyacrylamide gels and visualized as described under "Standard helicase assays".

Protein trap kinetic helicase assays

For protein trap kinetic helicase assays, FANCJ (0.6 nM), DDX11 (1 nM), EcUvrD (1 nM), and RECQ1 (7 nM) were preincubated for 3 min at 24°C with 5 nM of the radiolabeled forked duplex DNA substrate carrying the cyclo dA lesion in the top, bottom, or neither strand. After 3 min, ATP (2 mM) and

500 nM oligo dT$_{200}$ (to serve as protein trap) was added simultaneously to the reaction mixture and incubated at 30°C or 37°C. Aliquots (20 µl) of the reaction mixture were quenched at 10-sec intervals with 2X Stop Buffer containing a 10-fold excess of unlabeled oligonucleotide with the same sequence as the labeled strand. Products of helicase reaction mixtures were then resolved on 12% polyacrylamide gels and visualized as described under "Standard helicase assays".

Results

Up to this point, there has been no assessment of the effect of cPu base damage on DNA unwinding by any helicase. Given that cPu lesions arising from oxidative stress are believed to be fairly abundant [2,16,17,42,43], interfere with DNA replication and transcription, and play a prominent role in mutagenesis and human disease, we undertook a systematic investigation of the effect of cPu on DNA unwinding by purified recombinant DNA helicases from different classifications based on sequence homology (**Table 1**). The DNA substrates used for this study are composed of partially complementary single-stranded oligonucleotides containing a single cPu (dA or dG) in either the top or bottom strand within the double-stranded region of a forked duplex. Nine bp reside between the 41-nucleotide single-stranded tails and the site of the cPu adduct and 15 bp reside between the lesion and blunt duplex end on the opposite side of the DNA substrate (**Table S1**). The control substrate consisted of the same oligonucleotides except there was no cPu lesion present in either strand.

Effects of a cyclopurine lesion on DNA unwinding by RecQ helicases under multi-turnover conditions

We began with the human RecQ DNA helicase BLM implicated in the hereditary chromosomal instability disorder Bloom Syndrome, and also the human RECQ1 DNA helicase which is not yet reported to be genetically linked to a human disease but thought to play a role in cancer suppression [44]. BLM unwound the control DNA substrate and the substrate with the cyclo dA (**Fig. 2A**) or cyclo dG (**Fig. 2C**) lesion in the top (non-translocating) strand similarly and in a protein concentration dependent manner. The substrate with the cyclo dA (**Fig. 2A, B**) or cyclo dG (**Fig. 2C, D**) lesion in the bottom (translocating) strand was poorly unwound, especially for the cyclo dG adduct in which only 2% substrate was unwound compared to nearly 40% of the control substrate or substrate with the non-translocating strand cyclo dG lesion.

RECQ1 was inhibited by the cyclo dA in the translocating strand, showing nearly a four-fold reduced level of helicase activity at the 9 nM RECQ1 concentration where 80% of the control substrate as well as the substrate with the lesion in the non-translocating strand was unwound, compared to only 20%

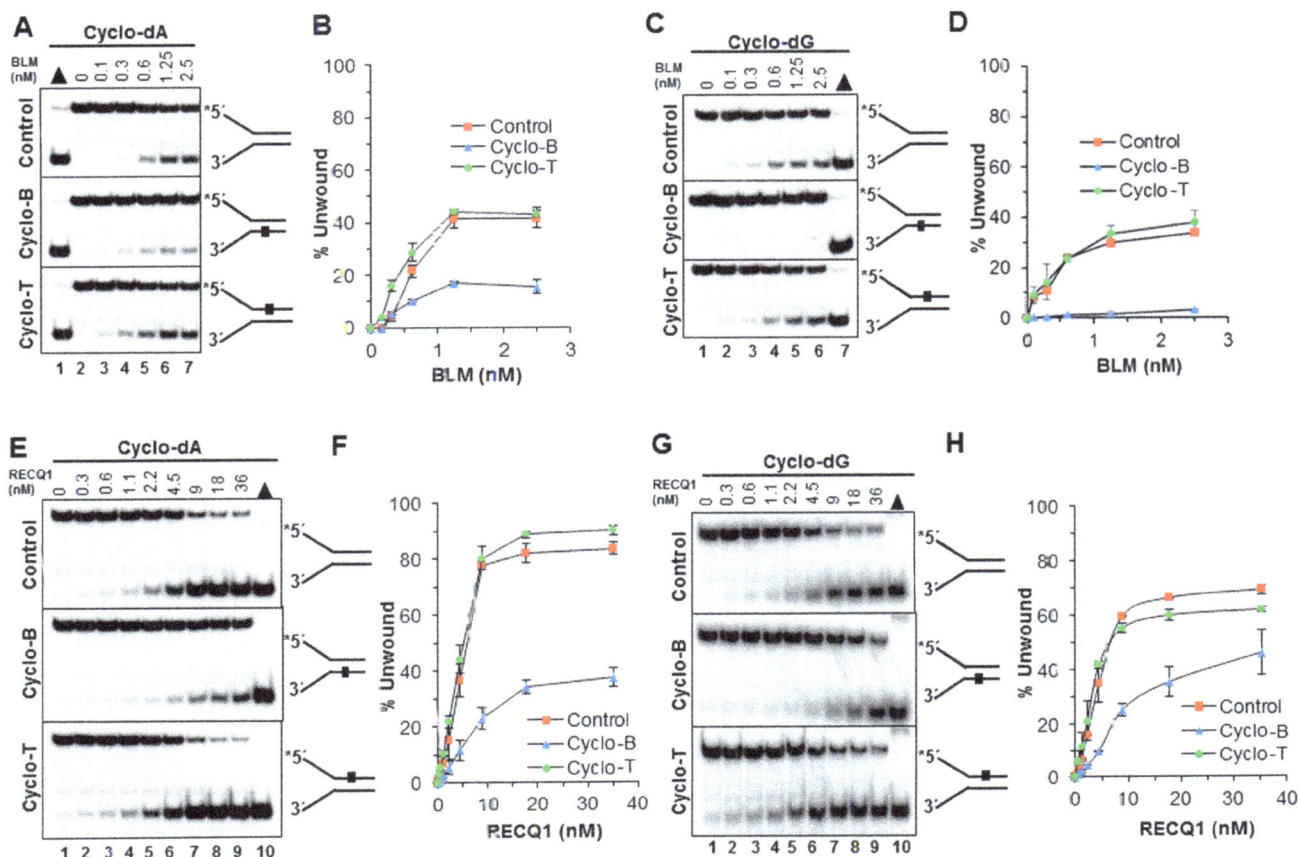

Figure 2. Effect of a site- and strand-specific cyclopurine lesion on BLM or RECQ1 helicase activity. Helicase reactions were carried out by incubating the indicated BLM or RECQ1 concentrations with 0.5 nM forked duplex DNA that contained a cyclopurine lesion in the top strand (nontranslocating-Cyclo T), bottom strand (translocating-Cyclo B), or neither strand (Control) at 37°C for 15 min (RECQ1) or 30 min (BLM) under standard helicase assay conditions described in the Materials and Methods. A, BLM unwinding of undamaged and cyclo dA damaged DNA substrates. Lane 1, heat-denatured DNA substrate control; lane 2, no enzyme control; lanes 3–7, indicated concentrations of BLM. B, Quantification of BLM helicase activity on cdA substrates with error bars. C, BLM unwinding of undamaged and cyclo dG damaged DNA substrates. Lane 1, no enzyme control; lanes 2–6, indicated concentrations of BLM, lane 7 heat-denatured DNA substrate control. D, Quantification of BLM helicase activity on cdG substrates with error bars. E, RECQ1 unwinding of undamaged and cyclo dA damaged DNA substrates. Lane 1, no enzyme control; lanes 2–9, indicated concentrations of RECQ1; lane 10, heat-denatured DNA substrate control. F, Quantification of RECQ1 helicase activity on cdA substrates with error bars. G, RECQ1 unwinding of undamaged and cyclo dG damaged DNA substrates. Lane 1, no enzyme control; lanes 2–9, indicated concentrations of RECQ1; lane 10, heat-denatured DNA substrate control. H, Quantification of RECQ1 helicase activity on cdG substrates with error bars.

of the substrate with the cyclo dA in the translocating strand (**Fig. 2E, F**). RECQ1 was also similarly inhibited by the cyclo dG substrates, although the differences were less dramatic compared to cyclo dA (**Fig. 2G, H**). We also tested another human RecQ helicase, WRN which is implicated in Werner Syndrome [45]. Analysis of reaction products from ATP-dependent WRN helicase assays revealed partial inhibition by the cyclo dA in the translocating strand (**Fig. 3A, B**), but not to the extent as observed for BLM or RECQ1 helicase. EcRecQ helicase was also affected by the cyclo dA in a strand-specific manner, showing inhibition only when the adduct was positioned in the translocating strand (**Fig. 3C, D**). Collectively, the results from DNA unwinding assays with human BLM, WRN, RECQ1, and EcRecQ demonstrated that the RecQ helicases were inhibited by the cPu to different extents when the lesion resided in the helicase translocating strand of the forked duplex DNA molecule.

A cyclopurine lesion does not inhibit DNA unwinding by Superfamily 1 or 4 DNA helicases under multi-turnover conditions

Our observations that a single cyclopurine residing in the duplex was able to inhibit unwinding by all the RecQ helicases tested led us to ask what the effect of a cyclopurine would be on DNA unwinding by EcUvrD, a SF1 bacterial helicase implicated in NER and mismatch repair [46]. Here it is relevant that the major contacts between SF1 helicases and DNA are believed to be with the bases via hydrophobic interactions in contrast to SF2 helicase in which electrostatic interactions between the ionic side chains of amino acids in the helicase protein and the negatively charged sugar-phosphate backbone prevail [47]. Surprisingly, EcUvrD was resistant to any detectable inhibition by the cyclopurine adduct residing in either the translocating or non-translocating strands of the DNA substrate (**Fig. 4A, B**).

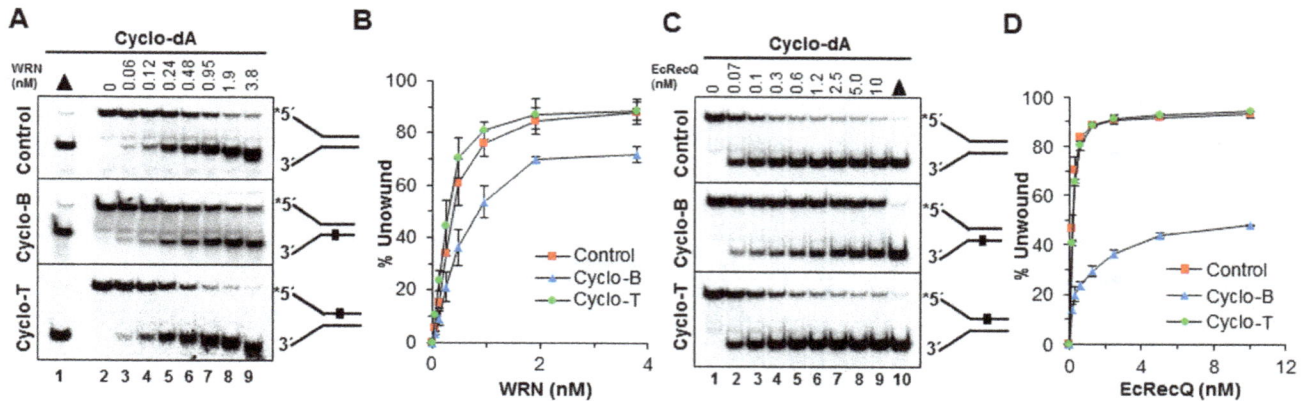

Figure 3. Effect of a site- and strand-specific cyclopurine lesion on WRN or EcRecQ helicase activity. Helicase reactions of 20 μl were carried out by incubating the appropriate WRN or EcRecQ concentrations with 0.5 nM forked duplex DNA that contained a cyclopurine lesion in the top strand (nontranslocating-Cyclo T), bottom strand (translocating-Cyclo B), or neither strand (Control) at 37°C for 15 min under standard helicase assay conditions described in the Materials and Methods. A, WRN unwinding of undamaged and cyclo dA damaged DNA substrates. lane 1, heat denatured DNA substrate control, lane 2 no enzyme control, lane 3–9, indicated concentrations of WRN. B, Quantification of WRN helicase activity on cdA substrates with error bars. C, EcRecQ unwinding of undamaged and cyclo dA damaged DNA substrates. Lane 1, no enzyme control; lanes 2–9, indicated concentrations of EcRecQ; lane 10, heat-denatured DNA substrate control. D, Quantification of EcRecQ helicase activity on cdA substrates with error bars.

We next tested the SF4 DNA helicase EcDnaB, a hexameric ring-like helicase that is responsible for unwinding complementary strands at the replication fork in *E. coli*. EcDnaB unwinds forked duplex DNA by inserting one strand within the donut hole of the hexamer and extruding the other strand outside the central channel [48]. Therefore, it is believed that the replicative helicase unwinds duplex DNA by a fundamentally different mechanism from a number of DNA repair helicases that operate as monomers or dimers. Experimental studies with EcDnaB and the forked duplex substrates containing the cyclo dA lesion demonstrated that EcDnaB, like the SF1 helicase EcUvrD, was unaffected by the cyclopurine residing in either the translocating or non-translocating strands (**Fig. 4C, D**). Based on these results, we conclude that the sensitivity of SF2 RecQ helicases to a single cyclopurine lesion residing in the duplex is not generally observed by representative DNA helicases from SF1 or SF4.

Effects of a cyclopurine lesion on DNA unwinding by Fe-S cluster helicases under multi-turnover conditons

We next tested the *E. coli* Fe-S cluster helicase, DinG. EcDinG was resistant to the cyclo dA lesion in either strand (**Fig. 4E, F**). Also tested were three Fe-S cluster DNA helicases important for chromosomal stability and implicated in genetic diseases: DDX11 (ChlR1) linked to Warsaw Breakage syndrome [49], archaeal *Thermoplasma acidophilum* XPD (taXPD), whose human homologue is linked to Xeroderma Pigmentosum [50], and FANCJ linked to Fanconi Anemia and associated with breast cancer [51]. The control undamaged DNA substrate was unwound by DDX11 in a protein concentration–dependent manner, achieving 60–80% substrate unwound at the highest protein concentrations (**Fig. 5A, C**). The presence of a cyclo dA lesion in either the top or bottom strand did not inhibit DDX11 helicase activity throughout the protein titration. In fact, DDX11 unwinding of the substrate with cyclo dA in the bottom (non-translocating) strand was slightly better than the control substrate or the substrate with the lesion in the top strand (**Fig. 5B**). Similar observations were made for DDX11 helicase activity on the forked duplex substrate series with the cyclo dG lesion (**Fig. 5D**).

The modest effects of a cyclopurine seen with EcDinG and DDX11 led us to investigate how taXPD might behave when it encounters the cycloadduct damage. This question was particularly interesting to us because taXPD is believed to play a critical role in DNA damage verification during a relatively early step of NER [50]. Given the biochemical evidence that cPu is a substrate for the NER pathway [7,52], we investigated the ability of taXPD to unwind forked duplex substrates with cyclo dA in the top (translocating) or bottom (non-translocating) strands. As shown in **Fig. 5E, F**, taXPD was strongly inhibited by the cyclo dA in the non-translocating strand. Similar behavior with taXPD was also seen with the cyclo dG substrates (**Fig. 5G, D**). At 40 nM taXPD, less than 10% of the forked duplex with cyclo dA in the non-translocating strand was unwound compared to 60% of the control forked duplex or the substrate with cyclo dA in the translocating strand.

A series of experiments were also performed with FANCJ helicase. FANCJ unwound the DNA substrates in a protein concentration-dependent manner in the 15-min incubation. However, in this case there was markedly less unwinding by FANCJ of the DNA substrate harboring the cyclo dA (**Fig. 6A, B**) or cyclo dG (**Fig. 6C, D**) in the top (translocating) strand. Throughout the FANCJ protein titration range of 0.15–2.4 nM, there was consistently a 2- to 3-fold better unwinding of the control undamaged DNA substrate compared to the substrate with either cyclo dA or cyclo dG in the helicase translocating strand. Based on these results, we conclude that the Fe-S cluster helicases are differentially affected by the cyclopurine lesions, with taXPD being impeded by either cyclo dA or cyclo dG in the non-translocating strand, inhibition of FANCJ helicase activity by the translocating strand cyclo dA or cyclo dG lesion, and no effect of the cyclopurine lesion on DDX11 or EcDinG.

Sequestration studies with SF2 helicases and forked duplex competitor DNA harboring a cyclopurine lesion

Previously, we observed that certain forms of DNA damage to the base (*e.g.*, thymine glycol) [53] or sugar-phosphate backbone [41] resulted in helicase sequestration by the lesion. To address if this is the case for a cyclopurine, helicase sequestration experi-

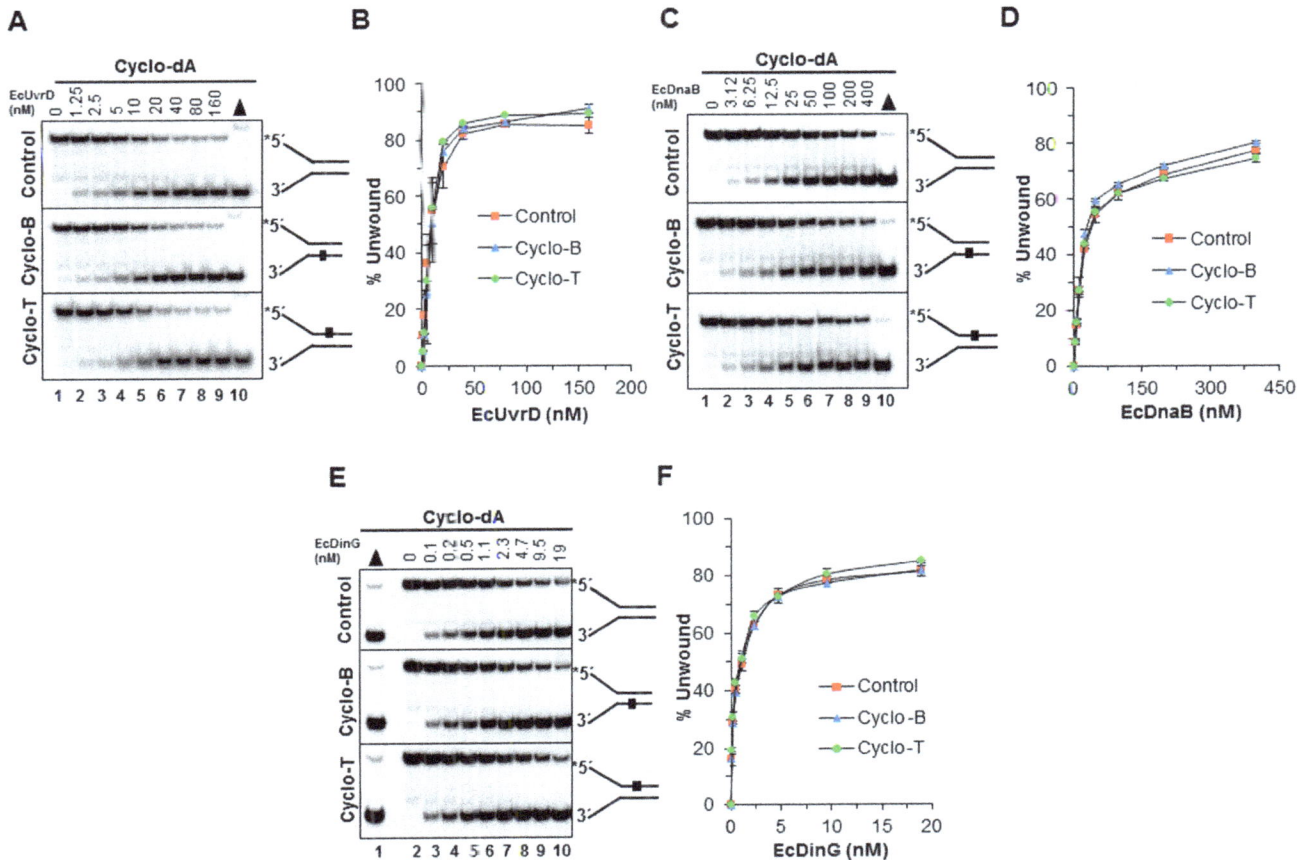

Figure 4. Effect of a site- and strand-specific cyclopurine lesion on EcUvrD, EcDnaB or EcDinG helicase activity. Helicase reactions were carried out by incubating the appropriate EcUvrD, EcDnaB or EcDinG concentrations with 0.5 nM forked duplex DNA that contained a cyclopurine lesion in the top strand (nontranslocating-Cyclo T), bottom strand (translocating-Cyclo B), or neither strand (Control) at 37°C for 15 min under standard helicase assay conditions described in the Materials and Methods. A, EcUvrD unwinding of undamaged and cyclo dA damaged DNA substrates. Lane 1, no enzyme control; lanes 2–9, indicated concentrations of EcUvrD; lane 10, heat-denatured DNA substrate control. B, Quantification of EcUvrD helicase activity on cdA substrates with error bars. C, EcDnaB unwinding of undamaged and cyclo dA damaged DNA substrates. Lane 1, no enzyme control; lanes 2–9, indicated concentrations of EcDnaB; lane 10, heat-denatured DNA substrate control. D, Quantification of EcDnaB helicase activity on cdA substrates with error bars. E, EcDinG unwinding of undamaged and cyclo dA damaged DNA substrates. Lane 1, heat-denatured DNA substrate control; lane 2, no enzyme control; lanes 3–10, indicated concentrations of EcDinG. F, Quantification of EcDinG helicase activity on cdA substrates with error bars.

ments were performed to evaluate if FANCJ (5' to 3' helicase) or RECQ1 (3' to 5' helicase) was differentially trapped during unwinding of DNA substrate molecules containing the cyclo dA lesion in the translocating versus non-translocating strand. If the helicase is sequestered when it encounters the cyclo dA in the strand it is predominantly translocating, then the enzyme would be less available to unwind a forked duplex tracker substrate added subsequently to the reaction mixture. A schematic for the experimental procedure is shown in **Fig. 7A**. Throughout the competitor DNA titration range, FANCJ helicase activity on the tracker substrate was inhibited to a significantly greater extent when the helicase was preincubated with the unlabeled forked duplex harboring a cyclo dA lesion in the top (translocating) strand compared to the control undamaged forked substrate (**Fig. 7B, D**). For example, FANCJ was able to only unwind 44% of the tracker substrate when the helicase was preincubated with 2.5 fmol of the forked duplex containing the cyclo dA adduct in the translocating strand whereas 98% of the tracker substrate was unwound when FANCJ was preincubated with the undamaged forked duplex. At this same amount of competitor DNA

containing cyclo dA in the non-translocating strand, FANCJ was able to unwind 82% of the tracker substrate. Using 5 fmol of competitor DNA containing the cdA lesion in the translocating strand, only 15% of the tracker substrate was unwound by FANCJ. At this same level of competitor DNA with no damage, FANCJ unwound 53% of the tracker substrate. An intermediate level of FANCJ helicase activity on the tracker substrate was observed when FANCJ was preincubated with the competitor DNA containing the cdA in the non-translocating strand.

In contrast to the experimental results for FANCJ, sequestration experiments performed with RECQ1 demonstrated that the cyclo dA adduct positioned in either the bottom (translocating) or top (non-translocating) strand had no discernible effect on the ability of RECQ1 to unwind the tracker substrate compared to preincubation with the control undamaged forked duplex (**Fig. 7C, E**). Thus, despite the finding that RECQ1 helicase activity is inhibited by the cyclo dA in the translocating strand, RECQ1 is not trapped by the lesion. This would suggest that when RECQ1 becomes blocked by the lesion, it may dissociate from the

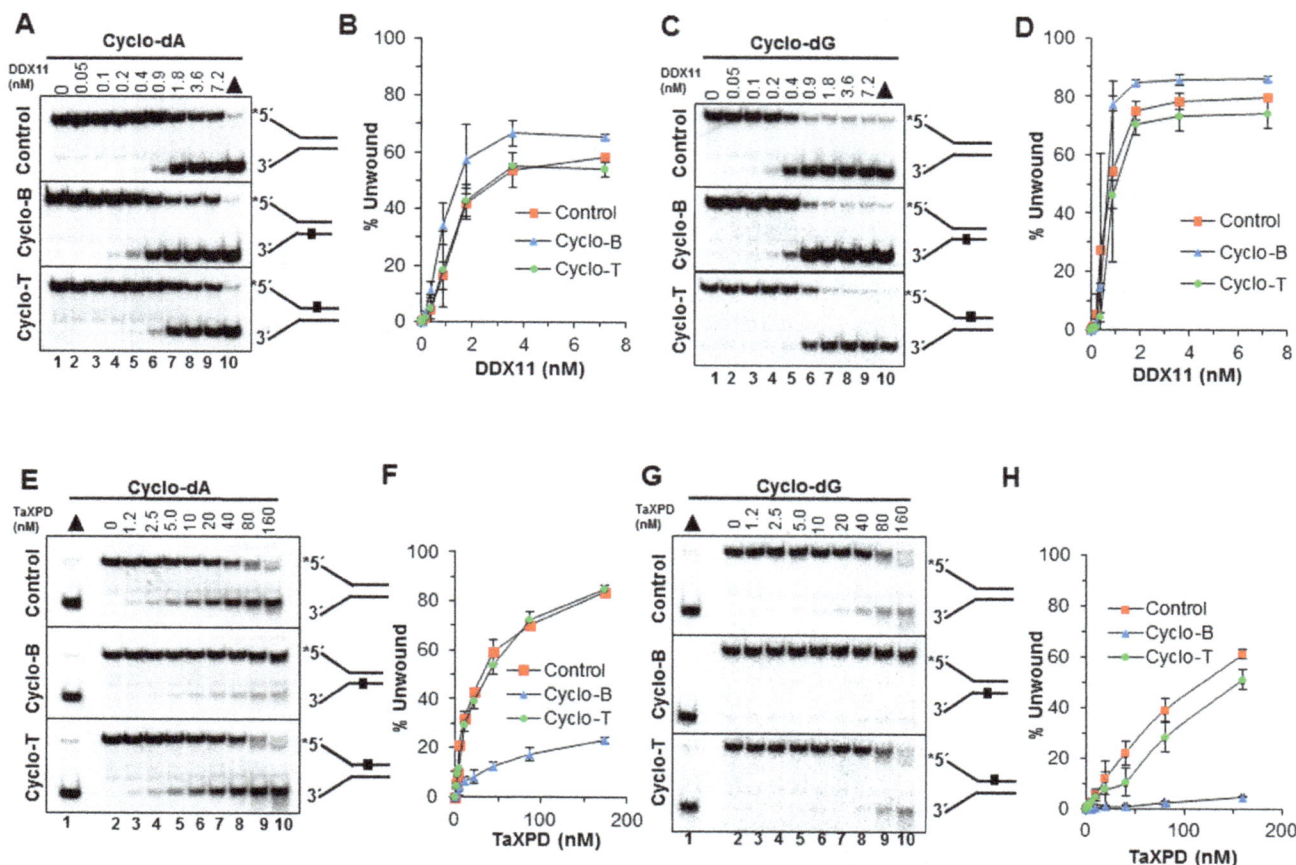

Figure 5. Effect of a site- and strand-specific cyclopurine lesion on DDX11 or taXPD helicase activity. Helicase reactions of 20 µl were carried out by incubating the appropriate DDX11 or taXPD concentrations with 0.5 nM forked duplex DNA that contained a cyclopurine lesion in the top strand (translocating-Cyclo T), bottom strand (nontranslocating-Cyclo B), or neither strand (Control) at 37°C, for 15 min under standard helicase assay conditions described in the Materials and Methods. A, DDX11 unwinding of undamaged and cyclo dA damaged DNA substrates. Lane 1, no enzyme control; lanes 2–9, indicated concentrations of DDX11; lane 10, heat-denatured DNA substrate control. B, Quantification of DDX11 helicase activity on cdA substrates with error bars. C, DDX11 unwinding of undamaged and cyclo dG damaged DNA substrates. Lane 1, no enzyme control; lanes 2–9, indicated concentrations of DnaB; lane 10, heat-denatured DNA substrate control. D, Quantification of DDX11 helicase activity on cdG substrates with error bars. E, taXPD unwinding of undamaged and cyclo dA damaged DNA substrates. Lane 1, heat-denatured DNA substrate control; lane 2, no enzyme control; lanes 3–10, indicated concentrations of taXPD. F, Quantification of taXPD helicase activity on cdA substrates with error bars. G, taXPD unwinding of undamaged and cyclo dG damaged DNA substrates. Lane 1, heat-denatured DNA substrate control; lane 2, no enzyme control, lanes 3–10, indicated concentrations of taXPD. H, Quantification of taXPD helicase activity on cdG substrates with error bars.

DNA and become available to bind and unwind the tracker substrate.

Protein trap kinetic helicase assays with cyclopurine substrate to simulate single-turnover conditions

To further reexamine the effect of a cyclopurine lesion on helicase activity, we performed kinetic assays with a protein trap to stimulate single turnover conditions (**Fig. 8A**). FANCJ (0.6 nM), DDX11 (1 nM), RECQ1 (7 nM), or EcUvrD (1 nM) were allowed to bind the 5 nM forked duplex substrate containing the cyclo dA lesion in the top, bottom, or neither strand. Helicase reactions were initiated by the simultaneous addition of ATP and 500 nM oligo dT_{200} which served as a protein trap to bind helicases free in solution, helicases that dissociated from the DNA substrate, or helicases that completed unwinding of the forked duplex and dissociated from the single-stranded unwound products during the reaction incubation phase. Reaction mixture samples were removed at 10-sec intervals to establish initial linear rates of DNA unwinding by FANCJ, DDX11, RECQ1, and EcUvrD

(**Fig. 8B, 8C, 8D, 8E**). Under these conditions, we determined that FANCJ unwound the control undamaged forked duplex substrate at a rate of 0.12 bp sec^{-1} FANCJ $monomer^{-1}$ (**Fig. 9**). The forked duplex substrate with cyclo dA in the top, translocating strand was unwound at a rate of 0.012 bp sec^{-1} FANCJ $monomer^{-1}$, a 10-fold slower kinetics compared to the control substrate. In contrast to these results for FANCJ, the rate of DDX11 helicase activity was only reduced 1.4-fold by the translocating strand cyclo dA (**Fig. 9**). The forked duplex with cyclo dA in the bottom, non-translocating strand was unwound relatively efficiently compared to the control substrate for both FANCJ and DDX11. Like the Fe-S cluster helicases, the rates of DNA unwinding under single-turnover conditions for the 3′ to 5′ helicases EcUvrD and RECQ1 were only affected by cyclo dA in the translocating strand, (which in these cases would be the bottom strand) (**Fig. 9**); however, the inhibition by cyclo dA was greater for RECQ1 (4.5-fold) compared to EcUvrD (2.5-fold). Based on these results, we conclude that a single cyclo dA lesion in the helicase translocating strand of the 25-bp forked duplex substrate significantly slowed down FANCJ and RECQ1 unwinding but only modestly affected DDX11 and EcUvrD.

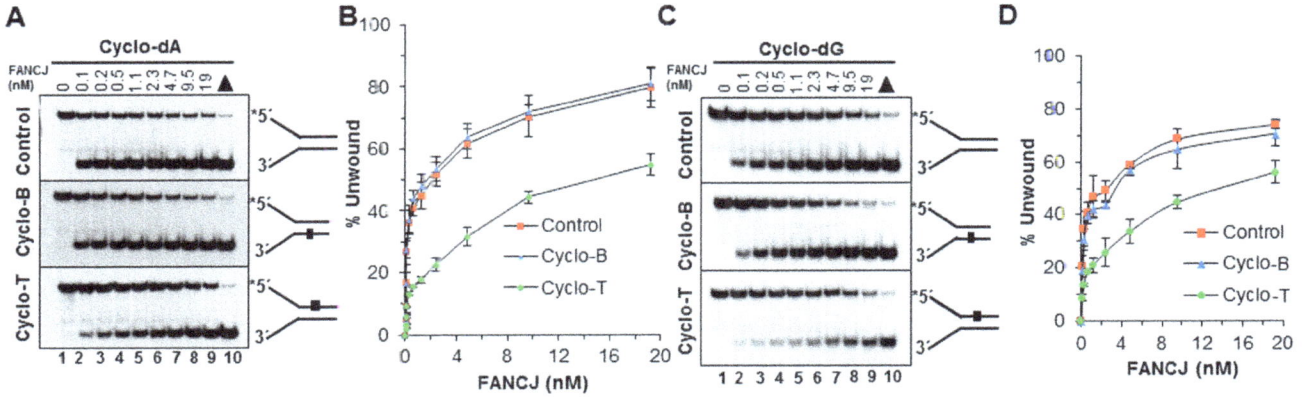

Figure 6. Effect of a site- and strand-specific cyclopurine lesion on FANCJ helicase activity. Helicase reactions were carried out by incubating the appropriate FANCJ concentrations with 0.5 nM forked duplex DNA that contained a cyclopurine lesion in the top strand (translocating-Cyclo T), bottom strand (nontranslocating-Cyclo B), or neither strand (Control) at 30°C for 15 min under standard helicase assay conditions described in the Materials and Methods. *E*, FANCJ unwinding of undamaged and cyclo dA damaged DNA substrates. Lane 1, no enzyme control; lanes 2–9 indicated concentrations of FANCJ; lane 10, heat- denatured DNA substrate control. *F*, Quantification of FANCJ helicase activity on cdA substrates with error bars. *G*, FANCJ unwinding of undamaged and cyclo dG damaged DNA substrates. lane 1, no enzyme control; lanes 2–9, indicated concentrations of FANCJ; lane 10, heat- denatured DNA substrate control. *H*, Quantification of FANCJ helicase activity on cdG substrates with error bars.

Discussion

The strong ability of cPu lesions to block replication and transcription, coupled with their accumulation with aging or progeria in mice, has compelled researchers to understand how

cPu lesions exert their cytotoxic effects and how efficiently they are detected and corrected by the cellular DNA repair machinery. Their structural perturbation to the DNA double helix is similar to that of the UV-induced photoproduct cyclobutane pyrimidine dimer (CPD) [54,55], which may help to explain why the

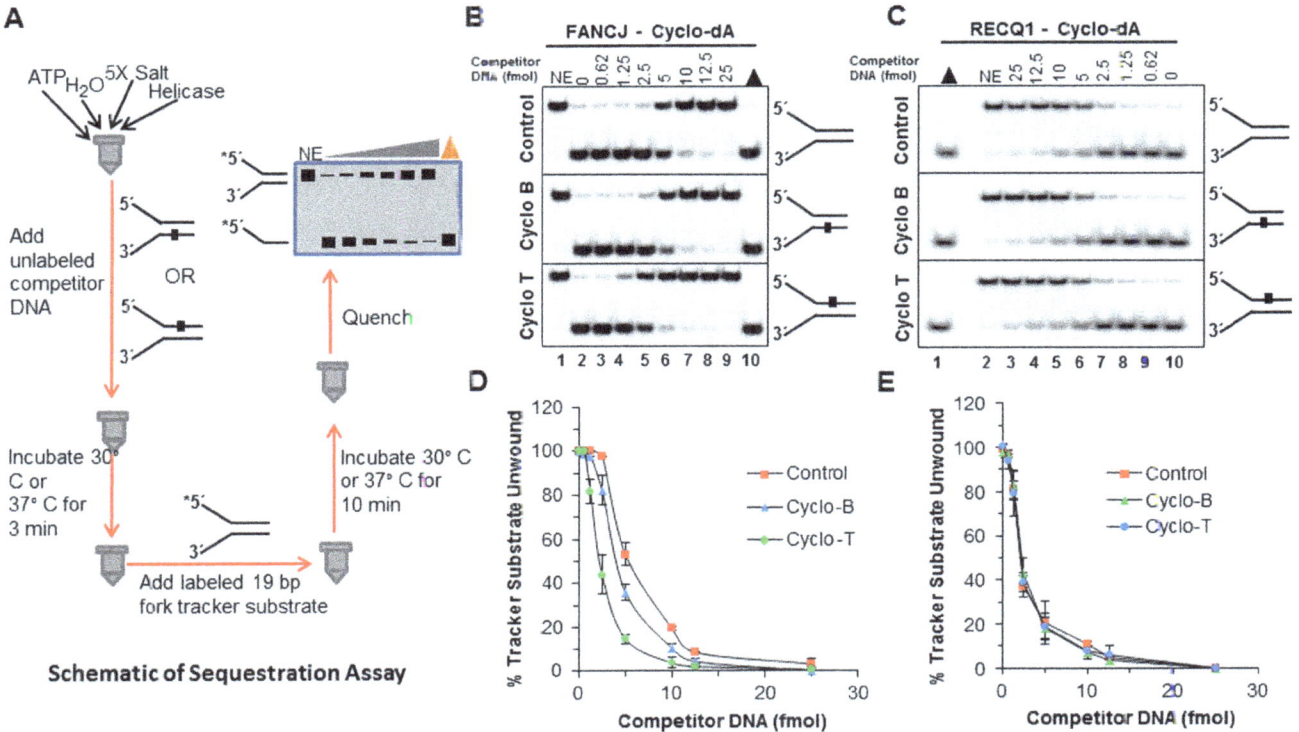

Figure 7. Sequestration of FANCJ, but not RECQ1, by cyclo dA. *A*, Schematic of sequestration assay. Sequestration assays were performed with 9.6 nM FANCJ or 8.8 nM RECQ1 and the indicated concentrations of the competitor DNA forked duplex at 30°C (FANCJ) or 37°C (RECQ1) under sequestration assay conditions described in the Materials and Methods. *B* and *C*, FANCJ (*B*) or RECQ1 (*C*) unwinding of undamaged 19 bp tracker DNA substrate after incubation with unlabeled forked duplex DNA molecules that contained cyclo dA in the top, bottom, or neither strand. *D and E*, Quantification of FANCJ and RECQ1 helicase activity from representative sequestration experiments shown in panels *B* and *C*, respectively.

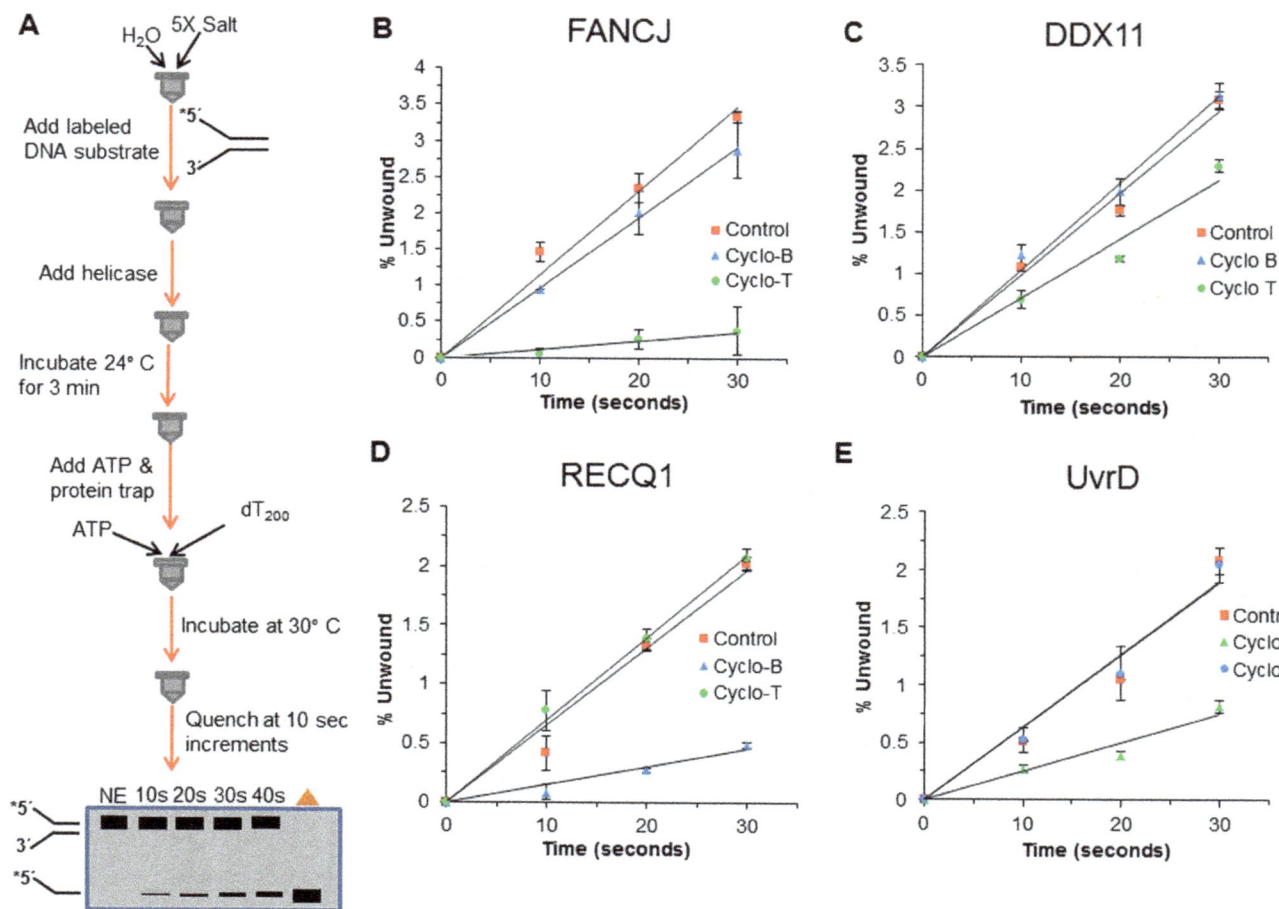

Figure 8. Protein trap kinetics assay to measure FANCJ, DDX11, RECQ1, and EcUvrD rates of unwinding DNA substrates with cyclo dA. Reactions were performed under protein trap kinetic assay kinetics conditions described in the Materials and Methods. *A*, Schematic of protein trap kinetics helicase assay. *B*, Quantification of FANCJ helicase activity on cdA DNA substrates. *C*, Quantification of DDX11 helicase activity on cdA DNA substrates. *D*, Quantification of RECQ1 helicase activity on cdA DNA substrates. *E*, Quantification of EcUvrD helicase activity on cdA DNA substrates.

oxidatively induced cPu is a substrate of NER [7,52]. In addition, a recent study suggests that cdA adducts found at 3′ termini of double-strand breaks can be removed by human Apurinic Endonuclease 1 (APE1), suggesting an alternative pathway for cleansing genomic cPu lesions [24]. Due to their distinctive biological effects as well as their impressive chemical stability and distorting effects on the DNA helix, we set out to assess in a systematic manner the effects of cyclo dA or cyclo dG adducts on DNA unwinding catalyzed by a panel of helicases, a number of which are defective in hereditary disorders and are implicated in pathways required to preserve genomic stability. These efforts have led us to conclude that the effects of cyclopurine lesions on helicase-catalyzed DNA unwinding are of quite a broad range, and to some extent not easily classified according to helicase family or even within the same species of conserved helicase proteins. The RecQ helicases (human BLM, RECQ1, WRN, and EcRecQ) behaved in the most predictable manner in which the cPu lesion residing in the translocating strand was found to be inhibitory to DNA unwinding, whereas there was little to no effect of the cPu in the non-translocating strand on helicase function. In contrast, the cPu lesion exerted non-uniform effects on DNA unwinding by Fe-S cluster helicases that varied widely in terms of strand-specificity and damage recognition among those helicases tested (FANCJ,

ChlR1 (DDX11), taXPD, and EcDinG). Finally, under multi-turnover conditions DNA unwinding by the classic *E. coli* DNA repair helicase UvrD (which is believed to unwind double-stranded DNA as a homo-dimer [56]) or the replicative hexameric ring-like helicase EcDnaB [57] was not affected in any significant manner by the cPu lesion irrespective of strand residence.

In order to further examine the effect that cPu had on helicase activity, rates of unwinding for select helicases were conducted under single-turnover conditions. The SF2 Fe-S cluster helicase FANCJ is strongly inhibited by the cyclopurine lesion, a result that is consistent with the strand-specific inhibition observed under the multi-turnover conditions. In contrast, the rate of DNA unwinding by the Fe-S cluster helicase DDX11 is only modestly affected by the cyclopurine damage, a result that is also consistent with what was observed under multi-turnover conditions. Thus, DDX11 possesses an intrinsic ability to unwind and bypass the cyclopurine, even in the translocating strand, without invoking the requirement for additional helicase molecules to load on the same substrate and help stalled DDX11 helicase molecule translocate forward. In the case of 3′ to 5′ helicases, SF1 helicase EcUvrD is detectably affected by the translocating strand cyclopurine under single-turnover conditions, whereas the enzyme fully tolerated the lesion under multi-turnover conditions. These results suggest that the

Helicase	Directionality	Control Rate of Unwinding*	Cyclo B Rate of Unwinding*	Cyclo T Rate of Unwinding*
FANCJ		0.12±0.004	0.10±0.004	0.012±0.010
DDX11		0.062±0.002	0.066±0.004	0.045±0.002
UvrD		0.040±0.002	0.016±0.001	0.040±0.005
RECQ1		0.0058±0.0003	0.0013±0.0001	0.0062±0.0004

*Rate expressed as bp unwound sec^{-1} helicase monomer $^{-1}$

Figure 9. Protein trap kinetic rates for FANCJ, DDX11, RECQ1, and EcUvrD. Rates of unwinding were calculated for each helicase on undamaged DNA substrates and DNA substrates containing a cyclo dA damage in the translocating or non-translocating strand. Rates were determined based on experimental data from Figure 8.

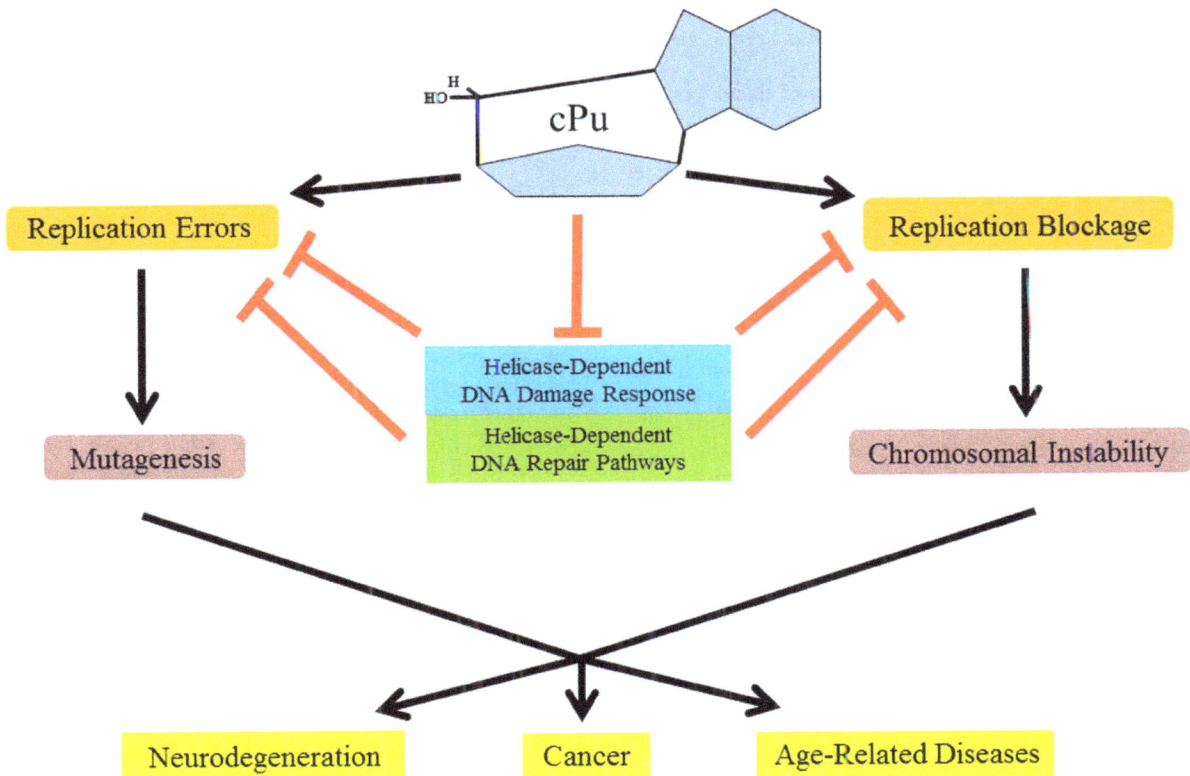

Figure 10. The accumulation of cyclopurine lesions in genomic DNA can cause replication errors or blockage leading to deleterious effects on the fidelity of DNA synthesis and maintenance of genomic stability which have negative outcomes for human health. The functions of certain DNA helicases can be adversely affected by cyclopurines and other forms of DNA damage which potentially impair helicase-dependent DNA damage response and repair pathways. See text for details.

ability of EcUvrD to efficiently unwind the DNA substrate with the translocating strand cyclopurine lesion in a protein concentration manner under multi-turnover conditions may be in part due to the loading of more than a single functional helicase molecule on the DNA substrate during the reaction incubation period. In contrast, the 3′ to 5′ helicase RECQ1 is more negatively affected in its ability to unwind the DNA substrate with the translocating strand cyclopurine lesion under either single-turnover or multi-turnover conditions. Thus, inhibition of both RECQ1 and FANCJ stalling by the cyclopurine lesion in the translocating strand is not efficiently overcome by increasing the number of helicase molecules in solution.

The selective deterrence of DNA unwinding by the RecQ helicases when the cPu lesion resided in the translocating strand is interesting in light of recent experimental findings that BLM [58] and Arabidopsis RecQ homologs [59] have the ability to switch strands upon encountering undamaged double-stranded DNA and effectively translocate on the opposite strand away from the duplex. Based on the strand-switching model, it could be suggested that when RecQ helicase molecules encounter a helix-distorting lesion such as cPu, a population of helicase molecules may switch strands and translocate on the opposite strand away from the lesion, enabling the unwound strands to reanneal behind it. Although it is unknown if a DNA lesion causes the acceleration of RecQ strand-switching, it seems probable that strand-specific inhibition of DNA unwinding by a RecQ helicase caused by an adduct such as cPu would increase the probability of the helicase to undergo a strand-switching event. From a biological perspective, cPu lesions are likely to modulate the functional roles of RecQ helicases which are generally believed to involve sensing DNA damage at the replication fork or facilitating the processing of DNA ends or recombinant DNA molecules that arise in early or later steps of double-strand break repair [25].

FANCJ was the sole Fe-S cluster helicase tested that displayed a sensitivity similar to that of the RecQ helicases in which inhibition was observed only when the cPu adduct resided in the helicase translocating strand. To our knowledge, strand-switching by FANCJ or any Fe-S helicase for that matter has not been examined, leaving in question the mechanistic basis for inhibition of FANCJ helicase by the cPu lesion. Unlike most, if not all RecQ helicases, FANCJ does not efficiently catalyze strand annealing of pre-existing complementary single-stranded DNA molecules [37]. If helicase-catalyzed strand annealing is a signature event of strand-switching by a RecQ helicase, FANCJ is likely to behave differently when it encounters helicase roadblocks. Consistent with this notion, FANCJ, but not RECQ1, was partially sequestered by the cPu. Protein trap kinetic assays demonstrated that the rate of FANCJ helicase activity was reduced 10-fold by the translocating strand cyclo dA. In contrast, the sequence-related ChlR1 and EcDinG helicases fully tolerated the cPu lesion in either the translocating or non-translocating strands. Therefore, the Fe-S cluster helicases ChlR1 and EcDinG are likely to unwind damaged DNA by a mechanism that is distinguishable from FANCJ.

Previously, the effects of more classic NER lesions such as the UV photoproduct CPD have been examined for their effects on DNA binding and unwinding by various archaeal XPD helicases [50,55,60,61]. In the current study, we analyzed the effect of a cPu lesion on taXPD helicase activity. taXPD was inhibited by the cPu lesion residing in the helicase non-translocating strand, but unaffected by the cPu in the helicase translocating strand. Recently, it was shown that *Ferroplasma acidarmanus XPD* (faXPD) utilizes its conserved Fe-S cluster domain as a damage sensor pocket, which scans for lesions when translocating on a DNA substrate [50]. Biophysical studies suggest that taXPD utilizes its damage sensor function in order to recognize distinct NER-type lesions at different positions when translocating on a DNA bubble substrate [55]. taXPD preferentially recognized a bulky fluorescein lesion residing in the translocating strand, whereas it detected a CPD lesion located in the non-translocating strand more readily. It was proposed that the fluorescein adduct may distort the helix in a manner that directly impedes passage of single-stranded DNA through the central hole of the helicase protein. In contrast, the CPD lesion may pass through the central hole, but likely comes into contact with the damage sensor when present on the non-translocating strand and thus inhibits taXPD [55]. Based on our results, it is plausible that the cPu lesion is recognized by taXPD in a similar fashion to a CPD lesion.

It is also possible that the differences in sensitivity of Fe-S cluster helicases to DNA damage such as a cPu adduct could be due to other mechanisms. Recent experimental evidence from the Barton lab suggested that DNA repair proteins (*Sulfolobus acidocaldarius* XPD and Endonuclease III) with redox active Fe-S clusters can utilize charge transport along the DNA double helical molecules as a means for detecting DNA lesions and recruiting other repair proteins [62]. It remains to be seen to what extent the cPu lesion affects electron transport along the axis of the DNA double helix, and what role this may play in helicase function or recruitment of other DNA damage repair proteins. Interestingly, the aforementioned APE1 has redox capability which is thought to be important for cell growth and differentiation [63], but it is not well understood if the redox function plays a role in the recognition or excision of oxidized bases.

The noted effects of cPu lesions on DNA helicases has implications for how these adducts may have an impact on replication and other areas of DNA metabolism. In a recent study, it was found that cPu adducts inhibit DNA replication and lead to increased mutation frequencies at the lesion sites through base pair transversions [22]. Certain translesion synthesis (TLS) polymerases can promote efficient bypass of the cPu adduct, but can cause mutations at the lesion sites [21,22]. Interestingly, FANCJ was reported to promote TLS pol eta-dependent bypass of UV-induced DNA damage [64], raising the possibility that the helicase may facilitate TLS past cPu adducts. It is plausible that a helicase like FANCJ which was inhibited by a cPu lesion may help to recruit a TLS polymerase to facilitate DNA synthesis. The ability of cellular DNA replication and repair machinery, including DNA damage response and repair pathways dependent on DNA helicases, to suppress replication errors induced by cyclopurines and other oxidative DNA lesions has important consequences for aging and age-related diseases (**Fig. 10**). It is believed that stem cell function is impaired by age-dependent accumulation of damaged DNA [65]. Extrinsic and intrinsic factors can induce molecular effectors such as reactive oxygen species to cause genomic and epigenomic changes in stem cells that debilitate function, leading to abnormal differentiated cells which in turn contribute to tissue dysfunction and aging [66]. Because cPu adducts have been shown to accumulate in an age-dependent manner [17], it is reasonable to speculate that their metabolism will have important consequences for stem cell dysfunction with aging.

Supporting Information

Table S1 DNA substrates used in this study. Lower case red font "a" or "g" denotes cyclo dA or cyclo dG, respectively.

Acknowledgments

This work was supported by the Intramural Research program of the National Institutes of Health, National Institute on Aging and by the Fanconi Anemia Research Fund (to R.M.B; and through the Deutsche Forschungsgemeinschaft (Forschungszentrum Fz82 and KI-562/2; to C.K.).

Author Contributions

Conceived and designed the experiments: IK ANS RMB. Performed the experiments: IK ANS TB JAS. Analyzed the data: IK ANS TB JAS RMB. Contributed reagents/materials/analysis tools: IK ANS TB JAS DLK JK CK RMB. Contributed to the writing of the manuscript: IK ANS RMB.

References

1. Berquist BR, Wilson DM, III (2012) Pathways for repairing and tolerating the spectrum of oxidative DNA lesions. Cancer Lett 327: 61–72. doi: 10.1016/j.canlet.2012.02.001.

2. Jaruga P, Dizdaroglu M (2008) 8,5′-Cyclopurine-2′-deoxynucleosides in DNA: mechanisms of formation, measurement, repair and biological effects. DNA Repair (Amst) 7: 1413–1425. doi: 10.1015/j.dnarep.2008.06.005.

3. Anderson KM, Jaruga P, Ramsey CR, Gilman NK, Green VM, et al. (2006) Structural alterations in breast stromal and epithelial DNA: the influence of 8,5′-cyclo-2′-deoxyadenosine. Cell Cycle 5: 1240–1244. doi 10.4161/cc.5.11.2816.

4. Jaruga P, Rozalski R, Jawien A, Migdalski A, Olinski R, et al. (2012) DNA damage products (5′R)- and (5′S)-8,5′-cyclo-2′-deoxyadenosines as potential biomarkers in human urine for atherosclerosis. Biochemistry 51: 1822–1824. doi: 10.1021/bi201912c.

5. Huang H, Das RS, Basu AK, Stone MP (2011) Structure of (5′S)-8,5′-cyclo-2′-deoxyguanosine in DNA. J Am Chem Soc 133: 20357–20368. doi: 10.1021/ja207407n.

6. Zaliznyak T, Lukin M, de los Santos C (2012) Structure and stability of duplex DNA containing (5′S)-5′,8-cyclo-2′-deoxyadenosine: an oxidatively generated lesion repaired by NER. Chem Res Toxicol 25: 2103–2111. doi: 10.1021/tx300193k.

7. Brooks PJ, Wise DS, Berry DA, Kosmoski JV, Smerdon MJ, et al. (2000) The oxidative DNA lesion 8,5′-(S)-cyclo-2′-deoxyadenosine is repaired by the nucleotide excision repair pathway and blocks gene expression in mammalian cells. J Biol Chem 275: 22355–22362. doi: 10.1074/jbc.M002259200.

8. Kuraoka I, Bender C, Romieu A, Cadet J, Wood RD, et al. (2000) Removal of oxygen free-radical-induced 5′,8-purine cyclodeoxynucleosides from DNA by the nucleotide excision-repair pathway in human cells. Proc Natl Acad Sci U S A 97: 3832–3837. doi: 10.1073/pnas.070471597.

9. Svilar D, Goellner EM, Almeida KH, Sobol RW (2011) Base excision repair and lesion-dependent subpathways for repair of oxidative DNA damage. Antioxid Redox Signal 14: 2491–2507. doi: 10.1089/ars.2010.3466.

10. Jasti VP, Das RS, Hilton BA, Weerasooriya S, Zou Y, et al. (2011) (5′S)-8,5′-cyclo-2′-deoxyguanosine is a strong block to replication, a potent pol V-dependent mutagenic lesion, and is inefficiently repaired in Escherichia coli. Biochemistry 50: 3862–3865. doi: 10.1021/bi2004944.

11. Marietta C, Gulam H, Brooks PJ (2002) A single 8,5′-cyclo-2′-deoxyadenosine lesion in a TATA box prevents binding of the TATA binding protein and strongly reduces transcription in vivo. DNA Repair (Amst) 1: 967–975. doi: 10.1015/S1568-7864(02)00148-9.

12. Marietta C, Brooks PJ (2007) Transcriptional bypass of bulky DNA lesions causes new mutant RNA transcripts in human cells. EMBO Rep 8: 388–393. doi: 10.1038/sj.embor.7400932.

13. D'Errico M, Parlanti E, Teson M, de Jesus BM, Degan P, et al. (2006) New functions of XPC in the protection of human skin cells from oxidative damage. EMBO J 25: 4305–4315. doi: 10.1038/sj.emboj.7601277.

14. D'Errico M, Parlanti E, Teson M, Degan P, Lemma T, et al. (2007) The role of CSA in the response to oxidative DNA damage in human cells. Oncogene 26: 4336–4343. doi: 10.1038/sj.onc.1210232.

15. Kirkali G, de Souza-Pinto NC, Jaruga P, Bohr VA, Dizdaroglu M (2009) Accumulation of (5′S)-8,5′-cyclo-2′-deoxyadenosine in organs of Cockayne syndrome complementation group B gene knockout mice. DNA Repair (Amst) 8: 274–278. doi: 10.1016/j.dnarep.2008.09.009.

16. Brooks PJ (2008) The 8,5′-cyclopurine-2′-deoxynucleosides: candidate neuro-degenerative DNA lesions in xeroderma pigmentosum, and unique probes of transcription and nucleotide excision repair. DNA Repair (Amst) 7: 1168–1179. doi: 10.1016/j.dnarep.2008.03.016.

17. Wang J, Clauson CL, Robbins PD, Niedernhofer LJ, Wang Y (2012) The oxidative DNA lesions 8,5′-cyclopurines accumulate with aging in a tissue-specific manner. Aging Cell 11: 714–716. doi: 10.1111/j.1474-9726.2012.00828.x.

18. Kamakura N, Yamamoto J, Brooks PJ, Iwai S, Kuraoka I (2012) Effects of 5′,8-cyclodeoxyadenosine triphosphates on DNA synthesis. Chem Res Toxicol 25: 2718–2724. doi: 10.1021/tx300351p.

19. Kuraoka I, Robins P, Masutani C, Hanaoka F, Gasparutto D, et al. (2001) Oxygen free radical damage to DNA. Translesion synthesis by human DNA polymerase eta and resistance to exonuclease action at cyclopurine deoxynucleoside residues. J Biol Chem 276: 49283–49288. doi: 10.1074/jbc.M107779200.

20. Pednekar V, Weerasooriya S, Jasti VP, Basu AK (2014) Mutagenicity and Genotoxicity of (5′S)-8,5′-Cyclo-2′-Cyclo-2′-deoxyadenosine in Escherichia coli and replication of (5′S)-8,5′-cyclopurine-2′-deoxynucleosides in vitro by DNA Polymerase IV, Exo-Free Klenow Fragment, and Dpo4. Chem Res Toxicol 27: 200–10. doi: 10.1021/tx4002786.

21. Swanson AL, Wang J, Wang Y (2012) Accurate and efficient bypass of 8,5′-cyclopurine-2′-deoxynucleosides by human and yeast DNA polymerase eta. Chem Res Toxicol 25: 1682–1691. doi: 10.1021/tx3001576.

22. You C, Swanson AL, Dai X, Yuan B, Wang J, et al. (2013) Translesion synthesis of 8,5′-cyclopurine-2′-deoxynucleosides by DNA polymerases eta, iota, and zeta. J Biol Chem 288: 28548–28556. doi: 10.1074/jbc.M113.480459.

23. Jaruga P, Theruvathu J, Dizdaroglu M, Brooks PJ (2004) Complete release of (5′S)-8,5′-cyclo-2′-deoxyadenosine from dinucleotides, oligodeoxynucleotides and DNA, and direct comparison of its levels in cellular DNA with other oxidatively induced DNA lesions. Nucleic Acids Res 32: e87. doi: 10.1093/nar/gnh087.

24. Mazouzi A, Vigouroux A, Aikeshev B, Brooks PJ, Saparbaev MK, et al. (2013) Insight into mechanisms of 3′-5′ exonuclease activity and removal of bulky 8,5′-cyclopurine adducts by apurinic/apyrimidinic endonucleases. Proc Natl Acad Sci U S A 110: E3071-E3080. doi: 10.1073/pnas.1305281110.

25. Brosh RM Jr (2013) DNA helicases involved in DNA repair and their roles in cancer. Nature Reviews Cancer 13: 542–53. doi: 10.1038/nrc3560.

26. Suhasini AN, Brosh RM Jr (2010) Mechanistic and biological aspects of helicase action on damaged DNA. Cell Cycle 9: 2317–2329. doi: 10.4161/cc.9.12.11902.

27. Egly JM, Coin F (2011) A history of TFIIH: Two decades of molecular biology on a pivotal transcription/repair factor. DNA Repair (Amst) 10: 714–21. doi: 10.1016/j.dnarep.2011.04.021.

28. Fuss JO, Tainer JA (2011) XPB and XPD helicases in TFIIH orchestrate DNA duplex opening and damage verification to coordinate repair with transcription and cell cycle via CAK kinase. DNA Repair (Amst) 10: 697–713. doi: 10.1016/j.dnarep.2011.04.028.

29. Cantor S, Drapkin R, Zhang F, Lin Y, Han J, et al. (2004) The BRCA1-associated protein BACH1 is a DNA helicase targeted by clinically relevant inactivating mutations. Proc Natl Acad Sci U S A 101: 2357–2362. doi: 10.1073/pnas.0308717101.

30. Wu Y, Sommers JA, Khan I, De Winter JP, Brosh RM Jr (2012) Biochemical characterization of Warsaw breakage syndrome helicase. J Biol Chem 287: 1007–1021. doi: 10.1074/jbc.M111.276022.

31. Sharma S, Sommers JA, Choudhary S, Faulkner JK, Cui S et al. (2005) Biochemical analysis of the DNA unwinding and strand annealing activities catalyzed by human RECQ1. J Biol Chem 280: 28072–84. doi: 10.1074/jbc.M500264200.

32. Sharma S, Otterlei M, Sommers JA, Driscoll HC, Dianov GL, et al. (2004) WRN helicase and FEN-1 form a complex upon replication arrest and together process branch-migrating DNA structures associated with the replication fork. Mol Biol Cell 15: 734–750. doi: 10.10.91/mbc.E03-08-0567.

33. Kaplan DL, O'Donnell M (2002) DnaB drives DNA branch migration and dislodges proteins while encircling two DNA strands. Mol Cell 10: 647–657. doi: 10.1016/S1097-2765(02)00642-1.

34. Bharti SK, Sommers JA, George F, Kuper J, Hamon F, et al. (2013) Specialization among iron-sulfur cluster helicases to resolve G-Quadruplex DNA structures that threaten genomic stability. J Biol Chem 288: 28217–29. doi: 10.1074/jbc.M113.496463.

35. Wolski SC, Kuper J, Hanzelmann P, Truglio JJ, Croteau DL, et al. (2008) Crystal structure of the FeS cluster-containing nucleotide excision repair helicase XPD. PLoS Biol 6: e149. doi: 10.1371/journal.pbio.0060149.

36. Brosh RM, Waheed J, Sommers JA (2002) Biochemical characterization of the DNA substrate specificity of Werner syndrome helicase. J Biol Chem 277: 23236–45. doi: 10.1074/jbc.M111446200.

37. Gupta R, Sharma S, Sommers JA, Jin Z, Cantor SB, et al. (2005) Analysis of the DNA substrate specificity of the human BACH1 helicase associated with breast cancer. J Biol Chem 280: 25450–25460. doi: 10.1074/jbc.M501995200.

38. Rudolf J, Makrantoni V, Ingledew WJ, Stark MJ, White MF (2006) The DNA Repair Helicases XPD and FancJ have essential iron-sulfur domains. Mol Cell 23: 801–808. doi: 10.1016/j.molcel.2006.07.019.

39. Suhasini AN, Rawtani NA, Wu Y, Sommers JA, Sharma S, et al. (2011) Interaction between the helicases genetically linked to Fanconi anemia group J and Bloom's syndrome. EMBO J 30: 692–705. doi: 10.1038/emboj.2010.362.

40. Cadman CJ, Matson SW, McGlynn P (2006) Unwinding of forked DNA structures by UvrD. J Mol Biol 362: 18–25. doi: 10.1016/j.jmb.2006.06.032.

41. Suhasini AN, Sommers JA, Yu S, Wu Y, Xu T, et al. (2012) DNA repair and replication fork helicases are differentially affected by alkyl phosphotriester lesion. J Biol Chem 287: 19188–19198. doi: 10.1074/jbc.M112.352757.

42. Mitra D, Luo X, Morgan A, Wang J, Hoang MP, et al. (2012) An ultraviolet-radiation-independent pathway to melanoma carcinogenesis in the red hair/fair skin background. Nature 491: 449–453. doi: 10.1038/nature11624.

43. Wang J, Yuan B, Guerrero C, Bahde R, Gupta S, et al. (2011) Quantification of oxidative DNA lesions in tissues of Long-Evans Cinnamon rats by capillary high-

performance liquid chromatography-tandem mass spectrometry coupled with stable isotope-dilution method. Anal Chem 83: 2201–2209. doi: 10.1021/ac103099s.

44. Sharma S, Doherty KM, Brosh RM Jr (2006) Mechanisms of RecQ helicases in pathways of DNA metabolism and maintenance of genomic stability. Biochem J 398: 319–337. doi:10.1042/BJ0060450.

45. Monnat RJ Jr (2010) Human RECQ helicases: roles in DNA metabolism, mutagenesis and cancer biology. Semin Cancer Biol 20: 329–339. doi: 10.1016/j.semcancer.2010.10.002.

46. Kuper J, Kisker C (2013) DNA helicases in NER, BER, and MMR. Adv Exp Med Biol 767: 203–224. doi: 10.1007/978-1-4614-5037-5_10.

47. Singleton MR, Dillingham MS, Wigley DB (2007) Structure and mechanism of helicases and nucleic acid translocases. Annu Rev Biochem 76: 23–50. doi: 10.1146/annurev.biochem.76.052305.115300.

48. Kaplan DL (2000) The 3′-tail of a forked-duplex sterically determines whether one or two DNA strands pass through the central channel of a replication-fork helicase. J Mol Biol 301: 285–299. doi: 10.1006/jmbi.2000.3965.

49. Bharti SK, Khan I, Banerjee T, Sommers JA, Wu Y, et al. (2014) Molecular functions and cellular roles of the ChlR1 (DDX11) helicase defective in the rare cohesinopathy Warsaw breakage syndrome. Cell Mol Life Sci 71: 2625–39. doi: 10.1007/s00018-014-1569-4.

50. Mathieu N, Kaczmarek N, Ruthemann P, Luch A, Naegeli H (2013) DNA quality control by a lesion sensor pocket of the Xeroderma pigmentosum group D helicase subunit of TFIIH. Current Biology 23: 204–12. doi: 10.1016/j.cub.2012.12.032.

51. Cantor SB, Guillemette S (2011) Hereditary breast cancer and the BRCA1-associated FANCJ/BACH1/BRIP1. Future Oncol 7: 253–261. doi: 10.2217/fon.10.191.

52. Menoni H, Hoeijmakers JH, Vermeulen W (2012) Nucleotide excision repair-initiating proteins bind to oxidative DNA lesions in vivo. J Cell Biol 199: 1037–1046. doi: 10.1083/jcb.201205149.

53. Suhasini AN, Sommers JA, Mason AC, Voloshin ON, Camerini-Otero RD, et al. (2009) FANCJ helicase uniquely senses oxidative base damage in either strand of duplex DNA and is stimulated by Replication Protein A to unwind the damaged DNA substrate in a strand-specific manner. J Biol Chem 284: 18458–18470. doi: 10.1074/jbc.M109.012229.

54. Brooks PJ (2007) The case for 8,5′-cyclopurine-2′-deoxynucleosides as endogenous DNA lesions that cause neurodegeneration in xeroderma pigmentosum. Neuroscience 145: 1407–1417. doi: 10.1016/j.neuroscience.2006.10.025.

55. Buechner CN, Heil K, Michels G, Carell T, Kisker C, et al. (2014) Strand-specific recognition of DNA Damages by XPD provides insights into nucleotide excision repair substrate versatility. J Biol Chem 289: 3613–3624. doi: 10.1074/jbc.M113.523001.

56. Maluf NK, Fischer CJ, Lohman TM (2003) A dimer of Escherichia coli UvrD is the active form of the helicase in vitro. J Mol Biol 325: 913–935. doi: 10.1016/S0022-2836(02)01277-9.

57. Patel SS, Picha KM (2000) Structure and function of hexameric helicases. Annu Rev Biochem 2000 69: 651–97. doi: 10.1146/annurev.biochem.69.1.651.

58. Yodh JG, Stevens BC, Kanagaraj R, Janscak P, Ha T (2009) BLM helicase measures DNA unwound before switching strands and hRPA promotes unwinding reinitiation. EMBO J 28: 405–416. doi: 10.1038/emboj.2008.298.

59. Klaue D, Kobbe D, Kemmerich F, Kozikowska A, Puchta H, et al. (2013) Fork sensing and strand switching control antagonistic activities of RecQ helicases. Nat Commun 4: 2024. doi: 10.1038/ncomms3024.

60. Mathieu N, Kaczmarek N, Naegeli H (2010) Strand- and site-specific DNA lesion demarcation by the xeroderma pigmentosum group D helicase. Proc Natl Acad Sci U S A 107: 17545–17550. doi: 10.1073/pnas.1004339107.

61. Rudolf J, Rouillon C, Schwarz-Linek U, White MF (2009) The helicase XPD unwinds bubble structures and is not stalled by DNA lesions removed by the nucleotide excision repair pathway. Nucleic Acids Res 38: 931–41. doi: 10.1093/nar/gkp1058.

62. Sontz PA, Mui TP, Fuss JO, Tainer JA, Barton JK (2012) DNA charge transport as a first step in coordinating the detection of lesions by repair proteins. Proc Natl Acad Sci U S A 109: 1856–1861. doi: 10.1073/pnas.1120063109.

63. Li M, Wilson DM, III (2014) Human apurinic/apyrimidinic endonuclease 1. Antioxid Redox Signal 20: 678–707. doi: 10.1089/ars.2013.5492.

64. Xie J, Litman R, Wang S, Peng M, Guillemette S, et al. (2010) Targeting the FANCJ-BRCA1 interaction promotes a switch from recombination to poleta-dependent bypass. Oncogene 29: 2499–2508. doi: 10.1038/onc.2010.18.

65. Behrens A, van Deursen JM, Rudolph KL, Schumacher B (2014) Impact of genomic damage and ageing on stem cell function. Nat Cell Biol 16: 201–207. doi: 10.1038/ncb2928.

66. Liu L, Rando TA (2011) Manifestations and mechanisms of stem cell aging. J Cell Biol 193: 257–266. doi: 10.1083/jcb.201010131.

14

Analysis of Tumor Suppressor Genes Based on Gene Ontology and the KEGG Pathway

Jing Yang[1⑨], **Lei Chen**[2⑨], **Xiangyin Kong**[1]*, **Tao Huang**[3]*, **Yu-Dong Cai**[4]*

1 The Key Laboratory of Stem Cell Biology, Institute of Health Sciences, Shanghai Jiao Tong University School of Medicine (SJTUSM) and Shanghai Institutes for Biological Sciences (SIBS), Chinese Academy of Sciences (CAS), Shanghai, People's Republic of China, **2** College of Information Engineering, Shanghai Maritime University, Shanghai, People's Republic of China, **3** Department of Genetics and Genomic Sciences, Mount Sinai School of Medicine, New York, New York, United States of America, **4** Institute of Systems Biology, Shanghai University, Shanghai, People's Republic of China

Abstract

Cancer is a serious disease that causes many deaths every year. We urgently need to design effective treatments to cure this disease. Tumor suppressor genes (TSGs) are a type of gene that can protect cells from becoming cancerous. In view of this, correct identification of TSGs is an alternative method for identifying effective cancer therapies. In this study, we performed gene ontology (GO) and pathway enrichment analysis of the TSGs and non-TSGs. Some popular feature selection methods, including minimum redundancy maximum relevance (mRMR) and incremental feature selection (IFS), were employed to analyze the enrichment features. Accordingly, some GO terms and KEGG pathways, such as biological adhesion, cell cycle control, genomic stability maintenance and cell death regulation, were extracted, which are important factors for identifying TSGs. We hope these findings can help in building effective prediction methods for identifying TSGs and thereby, promoting the discovery of effective cancer treatments.

Editor: William B. Coleman, University of North Carolina School of Medicine, United States of America

Funding: This work was supported by the National Basic Research Program of China (2011CB510102, 2011CB510101), the National Natural Science Foundation of China (31371335, 61202021, 61373028, 11371008, 81030015), Innovation Program of Shanghai Municipal Education Commission (12ZZ087, 12YZ120), the Shanghai Educational Development Foundation (12CG55) and the grant from "The First-class Discipline of Universities in Shanghai." The funders had no role in study design, data collection and analysis, decision to publish, or preparation of the manuscript.

Competing Interests: The authors have declared that no competing interests exist.

* Email: xykong@sibs.ac.cn (XK); tohuangtao@126.com (TH); cai_yud@126.com (YDC)

⑨ These authors contributed equally to this work.

Introduction

Currently, cancer is the second most common cause of death, following cardiovascular disease. Cancer that originates from the epithelial cells or mesenchymal cells is characterized by uncontrolled cell proliferation. In malignancy, cancer cells invade adjacent normal tissues and metastasize through blood circulation, lymphokinesis or body cavity transfer. In this process, proteins that are coded by tumor suppressor genes (TSGs) play vital roles in the mechanisms associated with cellular growth, DNA damage, apoptosis and metabolic regulation [1].

It has been reported that tumor suppressor inactivation and haploinsufficiency occur at several different levels in tumor patients. In the past decades, many classic TSGs have been widely identified, which are silenced by recurrent LOH (loss of heterozygosity) and physical deletion in the tumor genome. Increasing evidence has shown the abnormal DNA methylation or histone modifications, and non-coding RNA affect the expression of TSGs at the epigenetic level and post-transcriptional level, respectively [2,3].

The first identified TSG was retinoblastoma protein (Rb), which was identified by studies of familial retinoblastoma in early childhood. Based on this, the "two-hit" hypothesis was introduced by Knudson in 1971 [4,5]. As a guardian to the normal cell cycle, the Rb protein is responsible for the G1/S checkpoint and maintains regular cell growth. In addition to loss of heterozygosity, the high frequent mutations or partial deletions are mainly located in exon13~exon17 of Rb and have been found in various cancer types, especially in lung cancer, breast cancer, osteosarcoma and bladder cancer, with a frequency ranging from 15% to 50% [6–10]. Like Rb, the p53 protein family as a key element of the tumor suppression network, exerts much of its growth arrest in the cell cycle and induces apoptosis. Changes to p53 are involved in various cancers. Genetic variation mainly missense mutations, in p53 are often regarded as the driver mutations that confer apoptosis evasion and abnormal cell growth of tumor cells, especially those that originate from the epithelial tissue. More than 86% of point mutations occur in the evolutionary conservative regions, especially four mutation hotspots [11,12]. In addition, p53 is silenced via LOH in the genome and hypermethylation at the epigenetic level in cancer patients [13,14].

Like Rb and p53, some tumor suppressor proteins control cell behaviors directly by arresting cell proliferation, disturbing the cell cycle and inducing apoptosis, and these are called the gatekeepers. The destiny of a cell is also affected indirectly by some tumor suppressor proteins that are associated with mutation accumulation and genome stability maintenance such as BRCA1 and BRCA2, which are also referred to as caretakers [15,16].

Additionally inherited mutations of BRCA1 and BRCA2 (breast cancer 1/2) are associated with patients who have hereditary breast cancer, accounting for 5–10% of all breast cancer patients [17]. Loss function of their products causes abnormal homologous recombination and genome instability, which increases the susceptibility to breast and ovarian cancer [18].

Unlike the activated oncogene, suppression of TSGs occurs more frequently, providing evidence for understanding the initiation and progress of various cancers. The identification and subsequent activation of TSGs can facilitate controlling cell proliferation, restraining the biological activity of cancer. In this study, we attempted to investigate the characteristics of TSGs. The TSGs retrieved from the web-based database, TSGene (tumor suppressor gene database), facilitated our investigation of TSGs. These genes were called 'positive genes' and all of the remaining genes in the STRING were selected as 'negative genes'. Gene Ontology (GO) is an acknowledged bioinformatics tool for representing gene product properties across all species by defined GO terms, the function of the genes and their products were represented by the GO terms and predicted by the GO annotation effectively [19,20]. In contrast, the Kyoto Encyclopedia of Genes and Genomes (KEGG) is a comprehensive database based on known molecular interaction networks and is usually used to understand biological pathways and systems [21]. In view of this, the enrichment scores of the GO terms and KEGG pathways were used to encode all genes investigated in this study. Minimum redundancy maximum relevance (mRMR) and incremental feature selection (IFS) [22] combined with a prediction engine were employed to analyze these features. The analysis of the extracted GO terms and KEGG pathways suggests that they are related to TSGs. In addition, the extracted GO terms and KEGG pathways were used to predict the novel TSGs, indicating that they may help build effective computational methods for identifying TSGs.

Materials and Methods

Dataset

We compiled 716 human TSGs in the TSGene database (http://bioinfo.mc.vanderbilt.edu/TSGene/download.cgi), which were collected from two resources: public databases and literature reports. In detail, 187 (human) and 170 (human) known TSGs were retrieved from UniProtKB (28 January, 2012) and the TAG database (http://www.binfo.ncku.edu.tw/TAG/GeneDoc.php) (29 March, 2012), respectively, with only 41 overlapped genes by mapping to the Entrez gene symbols. By combining two exhaustive searches, PubMed and Gene Reference Into Function (GeneRIF) [23,24], and after overlapping and synonymous genes with same the Entrez gene ID were filtered, 637 protein-coding TSGs and 79 non-coding TSGs were identified [25]. Because the

encoding method described in Section "Encoding method" employed the neighbors of each investigated TSG in the STRING, we obtained 615 genes with their ensembl protein IDs in the STRING. These genes were termed 'positive genes' and are given in Table S1. The remaining 17,985 ensembl protein IDs in the STRING were considered 'negative genes'.

The number of negative genes was much larger than that of the positive genes. This is an imbalanced dataset. Inspired by some studies dealing with this type of data [26,27], we divided the 17,985 negative genes into six datasets, $A_1, A_2, \ldots, A_6$, where $A_1, A_2, \ldots, A_5$ contained 3,075 negative genes and, A_6 contained 2,610 negative genes. The 615 positive genes were put into each of these datasets, comprising six new datasets, $S_1, S_2, \ldots, S_6$, i.e., S_i ($i = 1,2,3,4,5,6$) consisting of genes in A_i ($i = 1,2,3,4,5,6$) and 615 positive genes.

Encoding method

To analyze the characteristics of the TSGs, it is very important to encode each gene with its essential properties. GO is an acknowledged bioinformatics tool for representing gene product properties across all species by defined GO terms, while KEGG is a comprehensive database based on known molecular interaction networks and usually includes the biological pathway and system information [21]. Therefore, we selected GO terms and KEGG pathways to code each gene. TSGs have a strong relationship with some GO terms and KEGG pathways. On the other hand, the enrichment method of GO can reflect the relationship between the genes and GO terms [28]. It is reasonable to use this method to encode genes and analyze the relationship of the TSGs and GO terms. Furthermore, this method can also be extended to KEGG pathways [29] to find the relationship between the genes and KEGG pathways.

GO enrichment. For one gene g and one GO term GO_j, the GO enrichment score is defined as the $-\log_{10}$ of the hypergeometric test P value [28–30] of a gene set G containing g's direct neighbors in the protein-protein interaction network of STRING and GO term GO_j, which can be calculated by:

$$S_{GO}(g, GO_j) = -\log_{10}\left(\sum_{k=m}^{n} \frac{\binom{M}{m}\binom{N-M}{n-m}}{\binom{N}{n}} \right) \quad (1)$$

where N is the number of overall proteins in human, M is the number of proteins annotated to the GO term GO_j, n is the number of proteins in G, and m is the number of proteins in G, which are annotated to the GO term GO_j. The high score for one gene and one GO term implies that the gene and GO term have a

Table 1. The number of remaining features after using Cramer's coefficient to exclude non-essential features.

Dataset	Number of remaining features
S_1	3,347
S_2	3,837
S_3	4,632
S_4	4,270
S_5	4,956
S_6	6,661

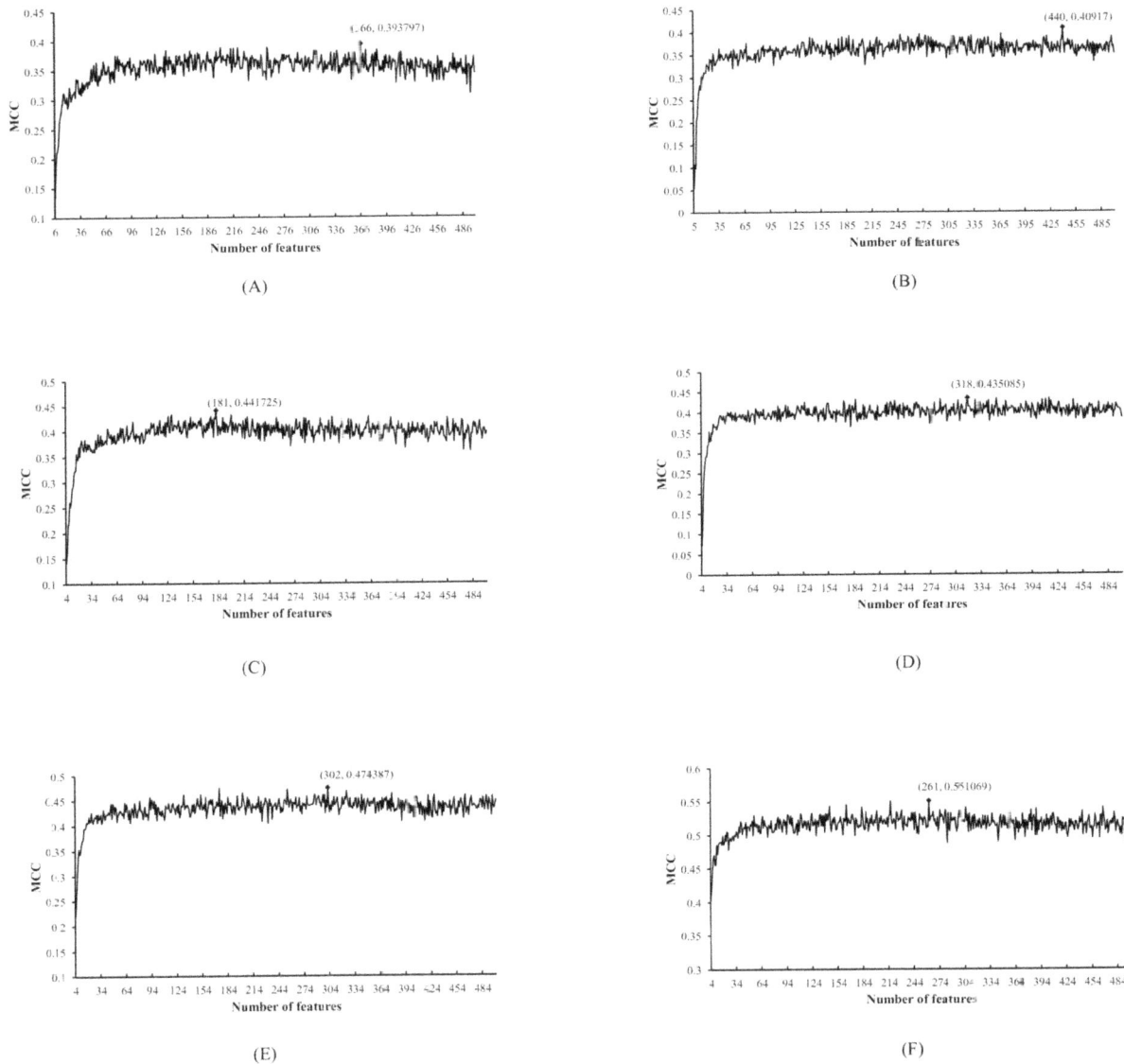

Figure 1. Six IFS-curves for six datasets. In detail, (A) shows the IFS-curve for the dataset S_1; (B) shows the IFS-curve for the dataset S_2; (C) shows the IFS-curve for the dataset S_3; (D) shows the IFS-curve for the dataset S_4; (E) shows the IFS-curve for the dataset S_5; (F) shows the IFS-curve for the dataset S_6. The Y-axis represents the Matthews's correlation coefficient (MCC) and the X-axis represents the number of features participating in the classification model.

Table 2. The number of features in the optimal feature set for each dataset and the MCC values obtained by using these features.

Dataset	Number of features in the optimal feature set	Maximum MCC value
S_1	366	0.3938
S_2	440	0.4092
S_3	181	0.4417
S_4	318	0.4351
S_5	302	0.4744
S_6	261	0.5511
Mean		0.4509

special relationship. The 12,877 GO terms induced 12,877 GO enrichment scores.

KEGG enrichment. For one gene g and one KEGG pathway P_j, the KEGG enrichment score is defined as the $-\log_{10}$ of the hypergeometric test P value [29] of a gene set G containing g's direct neighbors in the protein-protein interaction network of STRING and KEGG pathway P_j, which can be computed as follows:

$$S_{KEGG}(g,P_j) = -\log_{10}\left(\sum_{k=m}^{n} \frac{\binom{M}{m}\binom{N-M}{n-m}}{\binom{N}{n}}\right) \quad (2)$$

where N is the number of overall proteins in human, M is the number of proteins in the KEGG pathway P_j, n is the number of proteins in G, m is the number of proteins in both G and P_j. Additionally, the higher the KEGG enrichment score for g and P_j, the stronger the relationship between them. The 239 KEGG pathways induced 239 features of KEGG enrichment scores.

Each of the 12,877 GO enrichment scores or each of the 239 KEGG enrichment scores can be considered a dimension. Accordingly, each gene g can be represented by a vector in $12,877+239 = 13,116$-D space, which is formulated as:

$$v_g = (S_{GO}(g,GO_1),\ldots,S_{GO}(g,GO_{12877}),$$
$$S_{KEGG}(g,P_1),\ldots,S_{KEGG}(g,P_{239}))^T \quad (3)$$

Prediction method

Dagging is a well-known meta classifier. The main idea of this classifier is to integrate multiple classifiers derived from a single learning algorithm that is trained by disjoint samples of the original dataset [31]. The brief description of this method is as follows. For a training dataset $\Im$ with samples $s_1, s_2, \ldots, s_n$, construct k disjoint subsets by randomly taking n' samples in $\Im$, without replacement, such that $kn' \leq n$. These subsets were used to train a basic classifier (*e.g.*, support vector machine) and derive k classification models, $M_1, M_2, \ldots, M_k$. For a query sample, each of these models M_i ($1 \leq i \leq k$) provides a predicted result. The predicted result of dagging integrated these results by majority voting.

In Weka 3.6.4 [32], the classifier "Dagging" implements the dagging classifier mentioned above. Here, it was adopted as the prediction engine. For convenience, it was run with its default parameters. In detail, the SMO (Sequential Minimal Optimization), which implements John Platt's sequential minimal optimization algorithm for solving the optimization problem during the training of a support vector classifier using polynomial or Gaussian kernels [33,34], is set as the basic classifier, and k is set to 10.

Evaluation method

Ten-fold cross-validation is a widely used cross-validation method for evaluating the performance of different classification models [35−38]. Compared to the Jackknife test [39,40], the 10-fold cross-validation test requires less computing time and provides similar results for a given dataset. Therefore, the current study adopted this cross-validation method to evaluate the performance of the prediction method.

To represent the predicted results of a two-class classification problem, a confusion matrix was often employed, which contained the following four entries: true positives (TP), true negative (TN), false positives (FP), and false negative (FN) [41,42]. Based on these values, the prediction accuracy (ACC), specificity (SP), sensitivity (SN) [42] and Matthews's correlation coefficient (MCC) [43] were often used to evaluate the predicted results, which can be computed by

$$\begin{cases} ACC = \dfrac{TP+TN}{TP+TN+FP+FN} \\ SP = \dfrac{TN}{TN+FP} \\ SN = \dfrac{TP}{TP+FN} \\ MCC = \dfrac{TP \cdot TN - FP \cdot FN}{\sqrt{(TN+FN) \cdot (TN+FP) \cdot (TP+FN) \cdot (TP+FP)}} \end{cases} \quad (4)$$

As mentioned in Section "Dataset", five datasets were constructed in this study to reduce the size difference of the 'positive genes' and 'negative genes'. However, each dataset still had very different class sizes. In detail, the number of 'negative genes' was at least 4 times as many as that of 'positive genes'. Thus, the ACC is not appropriate for evaluating the predicted results on the whole. MCC, as a balanced measure even if the classes are of very different sizes, was employed as the key measurement.

Feature selection method

As mentioned in Section "Encoding method", each gene was represented by 13,116 features of the enrichment scores, which indicated the relationship between the genes and GO terms or KEGG pathways. TSGs are related to some GO terms and KEGG pathways. To identify key GO terms and KEGG pathways, some feature selection methods were employed in this study. The procedure of the feature selection method included two stages: (I) Cramer's coefficient [44,45], which used to discard non-essential features and (II) minimum redundancy maximum relevance (mRMR), incremental feature selection (IFS) [22] and Dagging [31] for further selection.

The Cramer's coefficient [44,45], derived from the Pearson Chi-square test [46], is a statistical measure of two variables. Its value is between 0 and 1. According to the fact that a high Cramer's coefficient of two variables indicates a strong association of two variables, features with low Cramer's coefficients to samples' class labels were deemed non-essential features. Here, we used 0.1 as the threshold and features with Cramer's coefficients lower than 0.1 were excluded.

The second stage of the feature selection involved the mRMR, IFS and Dagging. In detail, the mRMR method sorted the remaining features in two lists, while the IFS and Dagging were used to extract key features based on the feature lists obtained by the mRMR method. The mRMR method, proposed by *Peng et al.* [22], has two criteria: Max-Relevance and Min-Redundancy, producing the following two feature lists: (I) MaxRel feature list and (II) mRMR feature list. The MaxRel feature list sort features only based on the Max-Relevance criterion, while the mRMR feature list sort features based on both the Max-Relevance and Min-Redundancy. In this study, these two lists were formulated as follows:

$$\begin{cases} \text{MaxRel features list}: F_{MaxRel} = [f_1^M, f_2^M, \cdots f_N^M] \\ \text{mRMR features list}: F_{mRMR} = [f_1^m, f_2^m, \cdots f_N^m] \end{cases} \quad (5)$$

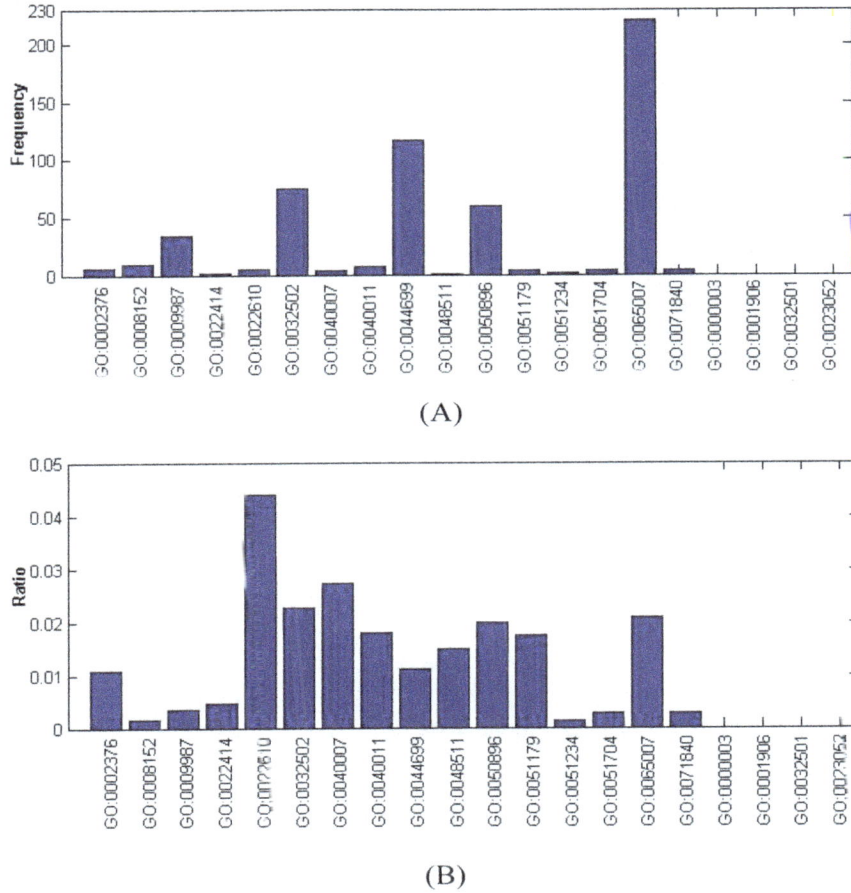

Figure 2. Frequency and ratio of GO terms of biological process in OS. (A) Frequency of GO terms of biological process in OS. (B) Ratio of GO terms of biological process in OS.

where N is the total number of features. The mRMR method has been widely used in recent years to analyze complicated biological problems [36,47−52]. Since the mRMR feature list was built with both the Max-Relevance and Min-Redundancy criteria in mind, it was used to extract important features by combining the IFS and Dagging. This procedure was as follows:

(I) Construct N feature set from the mRMR features list F_{mRMR}, say $F^1_{mRMR}, F^2_{mRMR}, \ldots, F^N_{mRMR}$, such that $F^i_{mRMR} = [f^m_1, f^m_2, \cdots, f^m_i](1 \le i \le N)$, i.e. F^i_{mRMR} consisted of the first i features in F_{mRMR}.

(II) For each F^i_{mRMR}, Dagging was conducted on samples represented by features in F^i_{mRMR}, evaluated by 10-fold cross-validation, thereby obtaining ACC, SP, SN and MCC (cf. **Eq. 4**).

(III) The feature set that can produce the maximum MCC is the optimal feature set. Additionally, an IFS-curve was plotted with the MCC value as its Y-axis and the superscript i of F^i_{mRMR} (the number of features that participate in the classification) as its X-axis.

Results and Discussion

Results of the feature selection

As mentioned in Section "Dataset", 6 datasets, $S_1, S_2, \ldots, S_6$, were constructed. For each, we calculated the Cramer's coeffi-

cients of the features and the samples' class labels. Then, the features with Cramer's coefficients lower than 0.1 were excluded. The remaining features were kept for the further selection. The number of remaining features for each dataset is shown in **Table 1**.

The mRMR method, IFS method and Dagging were used to analyze the remaining features for each dataset S_i. The mRMR program, downloaded from http://research.janelia.org/peng/proj/mRMR/, was executed on each dataset S_i, in which each sample was represented by the remaining features. For convenience, the mRMR method was conducted with its default parameters. As mentioned in Section "Feature selection method", the MaxRel features list and mRMR features list were obtained for each dataset S_i. However, to reduce the computation time, we only obtained the first 500 features in each of the two feature lists, which are summarized in Table S2.

The IFS method and classifier Dagging were executed according to the mRMR features list for each dataset S_i, which was evaluated by 10-fold cross-validation. The SNs, SPs, ACCs and MCCs obtained for each dataset S_i are given in Table S3. For easy observation, we plotted an IFS-curve for each dataset S_i. The six IFS-curves are shown in **Figure 1**; the maximum MCCs for datasets $S_1, S_2, \ldots, S_6$ were 0.3938, 0.4092, 0.4417, 0.4351, 0.4744, and 0.5511, respectively. These values are listed in **Table 2**, in which the numbers of the features used to obtain these maximum MCCs are also listed. In detail, by using the first

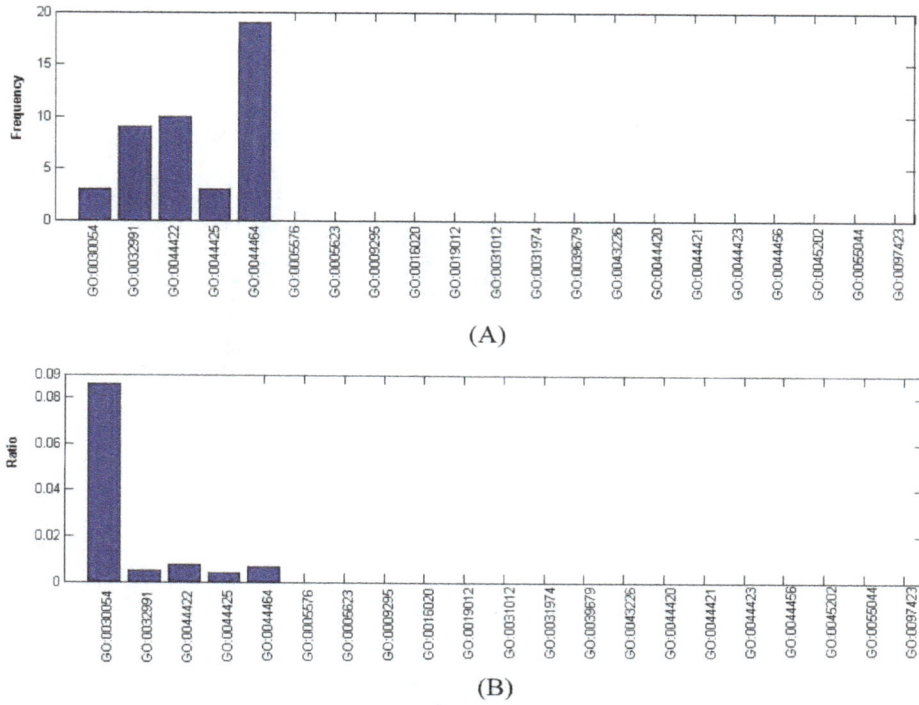

Figure 3. Frequency and ratio of GO terms of cellular component in *OS.* (A) Frequency of GO terms of cellular component in *OS.* (B) Ratio of GO terms of cellular component in *OS.*

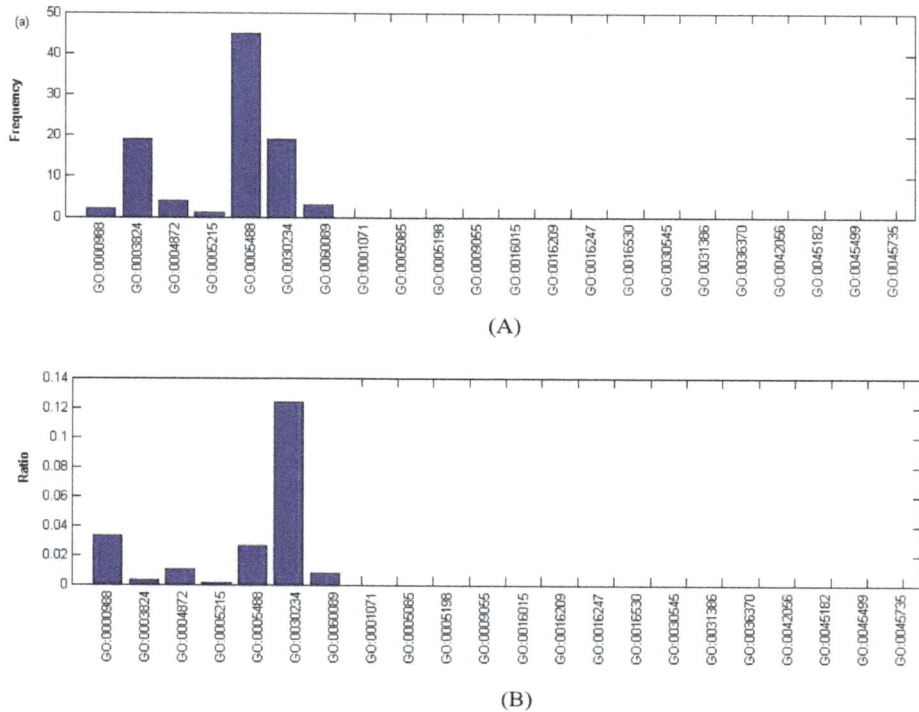

Figure 4. Frequency and ratio of GO terms of molecular function in *OS.* (A) Frequency of GO terms of molecular function in *OS.* (B) Ratio of GO terms of molecular function in *OS.*

Table 3. Top forty putative tumor suppressors based on features in the total optimal feature set.

Ensembl ID	Number of key tumor suppressor functions[a]	Gene symbol
ENSP00000297261	353	SHH
ENSP00000324806	353	GSK3B
ENSP00000389184	345	MARK2
ENSP00000264657	338	STAT3
ENSP00000355069	338	PAX2
ENSP00000293549	337	WNT1
ENSP00000353483	331	MAPK8
ENSP00000263253	331	EP300
ENSP00000218894	327	SUPT20H
ENSP00000328181	327	NOG
ENSP00000228872	327	CDKN1B
ENSP00000338548	325	FGF1
ENSP00000250003	322	MYOD1
ENSP00000206249	322	ESR1
ENSP00000245451	321	BMP4
ENSP00000352514	317	RUNX2
ENSP00000348986	316	INS-IGF2
ENSP00000263025	315	MAPK3
ENSP00000354558	313	MTOR
ENSP00000363822	311	AR
ENSP00000361066	310	NCOA3
ENSP00000339004	309	FOXG1
ENSP00000320604	309	FAXDC2
ENSP00000338018	308	HIF1A
ENSP00000278385	308	CD44
ENSP00000216797	306	NFKBIA
ENSP00000222330	304	GSK3A
ENSP00000255465	304	CCNA1
ENSP00000222726	303	HOXA5
ENSP00000334458	303	GATA4
ENSP00000264498	303	FGF2
ENSP00000323588	302	SOX2
ENSP00000392858	299	TNF
ENSP00000302665	299	IGF1
ENSP00000338297	298	-
ENSP00000362649	297	HDAC1
ENSP00000318977	297	GEN1
ENSP00000343745	296	DICER1
ENSP00000265165	294	LEF1
ENSP00000415481	293	PROM1

[a]The value in this column is the number of features in the total optimal feature set whose values are greater than $-\log_{10}(0.05)$.

366, 440, 181, 318, 302, and 261 features in the mRMR features lists of the six datasets (see Table S3), respectively, the MCCs calculated by **Eq. 4** were 0.3938, 0.4092, 0.4417, 0.4351, 0.4744, and 0.5511, respectively. Accordingly, six optimal feature sets, OS_1, OS_2, ..., OS_6 can be obtained by selecting the first 366, 440, 181, 318, 302, and 261 features in six mRMR feature lists of six datasets, respectively.

Analysis of the GO terms in the total optimal feature set

As mentioned in Section "Results of the feature selection", six optimal feature sets were obtained. We took the union operation of these sets and obtained a new dataset denoted by OS $(OS = OS_1 \cup \cdots \cup OS_6)$ and termed the total optimal feature set, consisting of 708 enrichment features of the GO terms and 9 enrichment features of the KEGG pathways, which are available in Table S4. The analysis of 708 GO terms is described below.

Seven hundred and eight GO terms can be divided into the following three parts: (1) Biological Process (BF); (2) Cellular Component (CC); and (3) Molecular Function (MF). We mapped the 708 GO terms to the children terms of three GO domains. As we can see in **Figures 2–4**, the GO terms in the *OS* were significantly enriched in some specific children terms with a high frequency and high ratio, which is defined as "the number of each GO term"/"the scale of the number of its children terms".

Biological process GO terms. The top five biological process GO terms of the frequency shown in **Figure 2(A)** are GO: 0065007: biological regulation (221), GO: 0044699: single-organism process (117), GO: 0032502: developmental process (75), GO: 0050896: response to stimulus (60) and GO: 0009987: cellular process (35). The top five biological process terms with large base numbers that perform fundamental functions in organisms and tumor suppressor proteins may be functional disturbance in health maintenance of cancer patients.

For the ratio of the biological process GO terms shown in **Figure 2(B)**, the top five are GO: 0022610: biological adhesion (4.39%, 5/114), GO: 0040007: growth (2.72%, 4/147), GO: 0032502: developmental process (2.28%, 75/3294), GO:0065007: biological regulation (2.09%, 221/10551) and GO:0050896: response to stimulus (2.0%, 60/3001). The GO terms biological adhesion and response to stimulus should be noted and relevant TS proteins act in the alarm reaction and have protective roles in tumorigenesis and the metastasis process. The GO term single-organism process involved in death and cell proliferation is highlighted too, although its percentage is not high. The destiny of an organism is critically regulated by the cell cycle and apoptosis in which TSGs play an important part. TSGs act like brakes on a car and are involved in maintenance of the cell cycle checkpoints and apoptosis induction [53].

Cells are under constant attack by various agents and oncogenic DNA variants form because of endogenous (normal cell metabolite) and exogenous agents (chemical species and physical mutagens). To maintain genome stability, TSGs participated in multiple mechanisms to repair DNA damage and arrest cell proliferation. In DNA double-strand break repair (DSBR), several TS genes, including ATM, NBS1, BRCA1 and BRCA2, are activated by DNA damage to induce cell cycle checkpoint arrest and DSB repair complex formation [54]. The highly conserved DNA mismatch repair (MMR) proteins composed of MSH2, MLH1, PMS1 and PMS2 tumor suppressor proteins in people, are required to correct base mismatches that are formed in response to exogenous or endogenous substances. If the expression of MLH1 or MSH2 is suppressed, cells lose the ability to perform mismatch repair and have resistance to alkylation mutagens that would normally activate G2/M checkpoint or apoptosis [55]. In nucleotide excision repair (NER), the DNA repair genes are regulated by p53 to remove bulky DNA adducts including pyrimidine dimmers induced by UV [56]. Normal, unrepaired DNA variants promote cells apoptosis.

Normally, cell proliferation is tightly regulated in different periods of the cell cycle. The pRb (retinoblastoma protein), known as the first TSG, maintains the G1/S checkpoint through its regulation of the E2F family. Inactivation of pRb, which caused by mutations, promoter methylation or interaction with oncoproteins, results in loss of control of the checkpoint R, allowing for uncontrolled cell proliferation [57,58]. In addition, cancer cells inhibit the expression of many other tumor suppressor proteins to gain malignant proliferation ability. For example, with mutations or the low expression of TGF-βR II (transforming growth factor

βreceptor II) and its downstream proteins Smad2/3/4 (SMAD family member 2/3/4), cancer cells will be insensitive to the proliferation inhibition of TGF [59,60]. Similar to pRb, the INK4 (cyclin -dependent kinase inhibitor, *e.g.,* p16INK4A) family, which is regulated by TGF-β, can block CDK, causing cell growth arrest in a different period of the cell cycle. The dysfunction of INK4 or TGF-βR II will allow cells to pass through the checkpoint abnormally and accumulate variations [61,62].

Apoptosis, known as programmed cell death, can be initiated by two distinct signaling pathways, BCL2 induced and death receptor induced, which ultimately converge in the caspase cascade. The most famous TSG, p53, is mutated in ~50% of human cancers and related to some tumor suppression network [14]. p53 is a transcriptional regulator that can be activated by DNA damage, certain oncogenes and other cytotoxic stress signals, triggering cell cycle arrest (G1/S checkpoint), DNA repair and apoptosis. Dysfunction of p53 caused by mutations or methylation prevents the damage-induced cell cycle arrest and apoptosis [63,64]. As a TSG, PTEN (phosphatase with tensin homology) negatively regulates the PI3K (the phosphatidylinositol 3-kinase) pathway, preventing inappropriate metabolism via effects on TOR and promoting cell proliferation via effects on proapoptotic proteins [65]. CYLD(cylindromatosis), first identified as a TSG in the familial cylindromatosis, is a DUB (deubiquitinase) of the USP subfamily. Multiple myeloma patients with dysfunction of CYLD have abnormal activation of NF-kB and cell cycle and apoptosis dysfunction [66,67]. The insufficient activation of caspase 8 (apoptosis-related cysteine peptidase), a key TS gene in the caspase cascade, leads to the interruption of signal transduction from death receptors, inducing normal apoptosis [68,69].

Many tumor cell types acquire the capacity to invade and metastasize though loss of cell-cell adhesion or cell-ECM (extracellular matrix) junctions. The silencing or suppression of E-cadherin, which is regulated by promoter methylation, histone methylation, transcriptional repression or frequent mutations cause EMT (epithelial-mesenchymal transition), disruption of cell contacts, tumor cell detachment and invasion [70,71]. Integrins, a family of heterodimeric transmembrane proteins, mediate cell–ECM (extracellular matrix) interactions. Aberrant integrin can induce the activation of proteolytic enzymes and cause degradation of the extracellular matrix and basement membrane, promoting tumor cells metastasis [72]. MMPs (matrix metalloproteinase) are endopeptidases that are involved in the breakdown of the extracellular matrix; they are regulated by inhibitors, TIMPs (Tissue Inhibitor of Metalloproteinases). Loss of function of TIMPs, which are TSGs, may cause a MMP/TIMP equilibrium shift into a malignant status [73,74].

Except the features above, which help us comprehend the relevance between tumor suppressors and specific GO terms or pathways, some rare investigated terms were highlighted such as metabolic process (GO:0008152), reproductive process (GO:0022414), locomotion (GO:0040011), localization (GO:0051179)/establishment of localization (GO:0051234) and multi-organism process (GO:0051704). These features remind us tumor suppressors participate in protein localization intracellular, various cells migration and locomotion intercellular, complex metabolic process and multi-organism process in the whole organism. Particularly, in some tumor types, tumor suppressors play key roles in reproductive process, usually related to hormone and hormone receptors. These features are not studies deeply as others, but need more attention to mine novel tumor suppressors.

Cellular component GO terms. It can be seen from **Figure 3(A)** that the top five CC GO terms with regard to frequency are GO:0044464: cell part (19), GO:0044422: organelle part (10), GO:0032991: macromolecular complex (9), GO:0030054: cell junction (3), and GO:0044425: membrane part (3), which also have a corresponding high percentage. Their ratios (cf. **Figure 3(B)**) are GO: 0030054: cell junction (8.57%, 3/35), GO: 0044422: organelle part (0.73%, 10/1361), GO: 0044464: cell part (0.67%, 19/2823), GO: 0032991: macromolecular complex (0.49%, 9/1824), and GO:0044425: membrane part (0.41%, 3/724). Cell junction is a cellular component that forms connections between two cells or between a cell and the extracellular matrix. As discussed above, TSGs such as E-cadherin and integrin play critical roles in tumor cell adhesion and metastasis. Additionally, organelles, including the mitochondria, ribosomes and UPS (ubiquitin-proteasome system), participate in the biological process involved in carcinogenesis. Many macromolecular complexes consist of tumor suppressor protein inside cells, such as TSgene SMAD2/3(SMAD family member 2/3) in the SMAD protein complex [75] and SMARCB1(SWI/SNF related, matrix associated, actin dependent regulator of chromatin, subfamily b, member 1) in the Swi/Snf complex [76].

Molecular function the GO terms. It can be observed from **Figure 4(A)** that the five highest frequency of MF GO terms are GO: 0005488: binding (45), GO: 0003824: catalytic activity (19), GO: 0030234: enzyme regulator activity (19), GO:0004872: receptor activity (4), and GO:0060089: molecular transducer activity (3). On one hand, these high frequency MF GO terms consist of a huge number of proteins that perform basic biological functions; on the other hand, the catalytic activity and enzyme regulator are involved in most vital biological processes, including cell proliferation, DNA damage repair and apoptosis. The cell junction requires protein binding and enzymes catalyze, which can involve biological processes such as phosphorylation, acetylation, the cell-extracellular matrix link and cell cycle control. The transcription factor Dp (DPDP-polypeptide) forms a complex with E2F1 to regulate its binding to DNA and the expression of certain genes (such as myc) catalyzed by enzymes [77]. Genomic instability is essential in almost all tumor factors, and mutations in ATM (ataxia telangiectasia mutated) which belongs to the PI3/PI4-kinase family, leave DSBs (DNA double-strand breaks) unrepaired [78]. The receptor proteins transduce extracellular or intracellular messenger to the biological effectors, triggering a serial biochemical reaction. The typical receptor protein and tumor suppressors in the TGF-β signaling pathway are TGF-βR II and BMPR2 (bone morphogenetic protein receptor, type II (serine/threonine kinase)) [79]. The five most common MF GO terms (cf. **Figure 4(B)**) are GO: 0030234: enzyme regulator (12.33%, 19/154), GO: 0000988: protein binding transcription factor activity (3.28%, 2/61), GO: 0005488: binding (2.64%, 45/1703), GO:0004872: receptor activity (1.02%, 4/391), and GO:0060089: molecular transducer activity (0.74%, 3/405). The corresponding percentages of the top five MF terms are similar to the top MF frequency, which are associated with the BP percentage and CC percentage and participate in tumorigenesis at different level.

Directed acyclic graph (DAG) analysis of the GO children terms. To further understand the function of the selected GO terms, we analyzed the directed acyclic graph of the GO children terms. We found that the GO children terms clustered in several particular modules under the primary GO terms discussed above. In addition to cell adhesion, the cellular response to UV-induced DNA damage and subsequent activated apoptotic signaling pathway and cell cycle regulation, phosphate metabolism, signal transduction and some molecular complex were highlighted in the biological modules.

The phosphorus utilization including phosphorylation and dephosphorylation catalyzed by kinases and phosphatases, respectively, is a key mechanism in a number of vital cellular pathways such as the cell cycle, cell proliferation and apoptosis. Mutations or low expression in certain TSGs, such as PTP (protein tyrosine phosphatase), should bring the phosphorylation/dephosphorylation ratio out of balance [80,81].

Cancer is a disease of aberrant signal transduction. In the functioning biological system, tumor suppressors keep the signaling cascades in balance, such as for the TGF-βR II and Smad2/3/4 in TGFβ signaling pathways [59,60] and ptch1 protein (patched 1) in hedgehog pathway [82].

In addition, some molecular complex and enzyme activity should be noticed. The SWI/SNF complex, which contains a subunit from the BAF family, mediated chromatin remodeling in cell differentiation, proliferation and DNA repair. Several components of the SWI/SNF complex, such as BAF47, function as tumor suppressors, and BRM and BRG1 act as putative tumor suppressors, which is evidenced by frequently loss of heterozygosity [83].

Analysis of the KEGG pathways in the total optimal feature set

Nine KEGG pathway terms in the *OS*, were hsa04115 (p53 signaling pathway), hsa00100 (steroid biosynthesis), hsa05213 (endometrial cancer), hsa05216 (thyroid cancer), hsa05218 (melanoma), hsa05219 (bladder cancer), hsa05220 (chronic myeloid leukemia), hsa05221 (acute myeloid leukemia) and hsa05223 (non-small cell lung cancer). As discussed above, p53 participates in cell death regulation and cell cycle control as a key central element. Aberrant genetic inactivation or diminished expression of p53 was found in the most of KEGG cancers terms. In addition to Rb in bladder cancer and chronic myeloid leukemia [7,84−86], abnormal PTEN was also found in thyroid cancer and endometrial cancer [7,84−86]. In melanoma, chronic myeloid leukemia and non-small cell lung cancer patients, there is reported silence or suppression of ink4a/arf leading to cell cycle disorder and sustained cellular proliferation [7,84−86]. Steroids and steroid metabolism have markedly influenced in some cancer types, such as breast cancer and prostate cancer, which may mediate the apoptosis network [87,88].

Unlike oncogenes, TSGs act as guardians regulating the network of cell cycle and apoptosis factors involved in controlling cell fate. Furthermore, maintaining genomic stability and balanced cell adhesion demand that the TSGs perform normal physiological functions.

Analysis of candidate tumor suppressors predicted based on optimal features

We try to predict the novel TSGs based on features in the total optimal feature set, *i.e.*, the key functions that defines tumor suppressor. For each 'negative gene', we counted the number of key tumor suppressor functions that it was annotated onto. The genes with great number of key tumor suppressor functions were considered as candidate tumor suppressors, since they shared similar functions with the known tumor suppressors. Since oncogene and tumor suppressor are two sides of a coin, their functions are difficult to distinguish. To better prioritize candidate tumor suppressor, we removed the 330 oncogenes from oncogene family of GSEA MSigDB (Molecular Signatures DATAbase, http://www.broadinstitute.org/gsea/msigdb/gene_families.jsp) and 251 oncogenes from HGNC (HUGO Gene Nomenclature Committee, http://www.genenames.org/) with the oncogene as the keyword. MSigDB is an online database, which collected annotated genes sets for GSEA analyze and categorize genes into gene family to provide a functional overview. HGNC is a collection of unique symbols and names for genes, ncRNA genes and pseudogenes. Subsequently, the overlap genes between these genes and the 'negative genes' were filtered out, 17,553 ensembl protein IDs remain in the end, which are available in Table S5.

Our study performs the gene enrichment and pathway enrichment analysis, providing a support to identify novel tumor suppressor in these features and pathways. In **Table 3**, we revealed a list of novel tumor suppressor genes, which shared at least 293 key annotations with known tumor suppressors. It has been demonstrated part of them play suppressive roles in tumorigenesis and more genes need verification by functional evidence and a larger clinical pathological characteristics data set. There are many tumor suppress genes proved partly, such as EP300 [89−91], GATA4 [92], ESR1 [93] and NFKBIA [94,95], which still need a large clinic data validation and functional research.

Glycogen synthase kinase 3 beta (GSK3β) belongs to the glycogen synthase kinase subfamily. GSK2β regulated Wnt signaling and PI3K/Akt pathway negatively, which play key roles in cell cycle, anti-apoptosis and invasion [96,97]. It has been identified suppression of GSK3β in many tumor types including, oral squamous cell carcinoma (OSCC), lung cancer, cutaneous squamous cell carcinoma and esophageal carcinoma [98−101]. Inhibition of constitutively active GSK3β leads to epithelial-mesenchymal transition (EMT) transition during tumorigenesis [102]. In vitro, GSK3β play a negative regulator of myeloid cell leukemia-1(Mcl-1), which has anti-apoptotic function and is correlated to the poor prognosis of breast cancer patients [98,103,104]. Although there are some controversial reports, GSK3β is a putative tumor suppressor and need more studies [105,106].

Homeobox A5 (HOXA5) is belonging to a DNA-binding transcription factor family, homeobox genes cluster A, and regulates organism gene expression, adult differentiation and embryonic development in organism. It has been observed a frequently increased methylation of the HOXA5 promoter region in various tumor tissues [107−109] and is related to decreased expression [107,110]. In addition, HOXA5 up-regulates p53 transcription through binding to a target element in its promoter [111]. These evidences document that HOXA5 is a putative tumor suppressor for tumorigenesis. But it still warrants further functional studies that how HOXA5 suppress tumorigenesis in animal model and in clinic.

Holliday Junction 5′ Flap Endonuclease, previous named gen endonuclease homolog 1 (GEN1) is an enzyme, evolved in Holliday junctions (HJs) formation during homologous recombination and DNA repair. The activity of Yen1, the ortholog of GEN1, is inhibited by phosphorylation events in the G1/S transition, keep inactive through S-phase and G2, and activated by dephosphorylation at the later stages of mitosis [112,113]. Similarly, in the early stages of the cell cycle, GEN1 is excluded

from the nucleus, and access chromatin and HJs [113]. GEN1 participates in some specific features: cell cycle, DNA repair and phosphorylation/dephosphorylation, which involved in many tumor suppressors. In Bloom's syndrome cells, depletion of GEN1 results in severe chromosome abnormalities [114]. It has been identified rare recessive at-risk alleles of GEN1 in breast cancer by Ekaterina Sh [115−117], and two somatic frameshift mutations in breast cancer cell lines and primary tumors through exome sequencing [114]. Above all, GEN1 is a novel tumor suppressor akin to some other DNA repair genes, BRCA1 and BRCA2 in breast cancer, although there is rare study prove GEN1 make a high-appreciable contribution to breast cancer. In future study, it would be focus on the methylation or LOH level and anti-tumorigenesis mechanism to explore function of GEN1.

Besides these genes discussed above, our study reveals more novel candidate tumor suppressors including SHH, STAT3, SUPT20H and GSK3A, which are highlighted and need more focus and research in future cancer research.

Conclusions

This study summarizes the enrichment analysis of TSGs. The features of the GO and KEGG pathway enrichment scores were used to encode the investigated genes and some feature selection methods were employed to analyze these features. The analysis of the 708 GO terms and 9 KEGG pathways implies that they are strongly related to the determination of TSGs. We hope that effective methods based on these GO terms and KEGG pathways can be built to identify TSGs.

Supporting Information

Table S1 List of 615 tumor suppressor genes.

Table S2 List of the MaxRel features lists and mRMR features lists obtained by mRMR method for each dataset.

Table S3 List of the SNs, SPs, ACCs and MCCs obtained by IFS and Dagging for each dataset S_i.

Table S4 List of 717 Features in the final optimal feature set.

Table S5 List of the novel tumor suppressors predicted based on features in the total optimal feature set.

Author Contributions

Conceived and designed the experiments: TH YDC. Performed the experiments: LC YDC. Analyzed the data: JY LC XK TH. Contributed reagents/materials/analysis tools: JY TH. Contributed to the writing of the manuscript: JY LC.

References

1. Hanahan D, Weinberg RA (2011) Hallmarks of cancer: the next generation. Cell 144: 646−674.
2. Sherr CJ (2004) Principles of tumor suppression. Cell 116: 235−246.
3. Shlien A, Malkin D (2010) Copy number variations and cancer susceptibility. Curr Opin Oncol 22: 55−63.
4. Knudson AG, Jr. (1971) Mutation and cancer: statistical study of retinoblastoma. Proc Natl Acad Sci U S A 68: 820−823.
5. Lee WH, Bookstein R, Hong F, Young LJ, Shew JY, et al. (1987) Human retinoblastoma susceptibility gene: cloning, identification, and sequence. Science 235: 1394−1399.

6. Brandau S, Bohle A (2001) Bladder cancer. I. Molecular and genetic basis of carcinogenesis. Eur Urol 39: 491−497.
7. Giacinti C, Giordano A (2006) RB and cell cycle progression. Oncogene 25: 5220−5227.
8. Pietilainen T, Lipponen P, Aaltomaa S, Eskelinen M, Kosma VM, et al. (1995) Expression of retinoblastoma gene protein (Rb) in breast cancer as related to established prognostic factors and survival. Eur J Cancer 31A: 329−333.
9. Wadayama B, Toguchida J, Shimizu T, Ishizaki K, Sasaki MS, et al. (1994) Mutation spectrum of the retinoblastoma gene in osteosarcomas. Cancer Res 54: 3042−3048.

10. Burkhart DL, Sage J (2008) Cellular mechanisms of tumour suppression by the retinoblastoma gene. Nat Rev Cancer 8: 671–682.

11. Volkenandt M, Schlegel U, Nanus DM, Albino AP (1991) Mutational analysis of the human p53 gene in malignant melanoma. Pigment Cell Res 4: 35–40.

12. Nigro JM, Baker SJ, Preisinger AC, Jessup JM, Hostetter R, et al. (1989) Mutations in the p53 gene occur in diverse human tumour types. Nature 342: 705–708.

13. Muller PA, Vousden KH (2013) p53 mutations in cancer. Nat Cell Biol 15: 2–8.

14. Chuikov S, Kurash JK, Wilson JR, Xiao B, Justin N, et al. (2004) Regulation of p53 activity through lysine methylation. Nature 432: 353–360.

15. Levitt NC, Hickson ID (2002) Caretaker tumour suppressor genes that defend genome integrity. Trends Mol Med 8: 179–186.

16. Levine AJ (1997) p53, the cellular gatekeeper for growth and division. Cell 88: 323–331.

17. Nicoletto MO, Donach M, De Nicolo A, Artioli G, Banna G, et al. (2001) BRCA-1 and BRCA-2 mutations as prognostic factors in clinical practice and genetic counselling. Cancer Treat Rev 27: 295–304.

18. Scully R, Livingston DM (2000) In search of the tumour-suppressor functions of BRCA1 and BRCA2. Nature 408: 429–432.

19. Ashburner M, Ball CA, Blake JA, Botstein D, Butler H, et al. (2000) Gene ontology: tool for the unification of biology. The Gene Ontology Consortium. Nat Genet 25: 25–29.

20. Altshuler D, Daly MJ, Lander ES (2008) Genetic mapping in human disease. Science 322: 881–888.

21. Kanehisa M, Goto S, Sato Y, Furumichi M, Tanabe M (2012) KEGG for integration and interpretation of large-scale molecular data sets. Nucleic Acids Res 40: D109–114.

22. Peng H, Long F, Ding C (2005) Feature selection based on mutual information: criteria of max-dependency, max-relevance, and min-redundancy. IEEE Transactions on Pattern Analysis and Machine Intelligence 27: 1226–1238.

23. Lu Z, Cohen KB, Hunter L (2007) GeneRIF quality assurance as summary revision. Pac Symp Biocomput: 269–80.

24. Acland A, Agarwala R, Barrett T, Beck J, Benson DA, et al. (2014) Database resources of the National Center for Biotechnology Information. Nucleic Acids Res 42(D1): D7–D17.

25. Zhao M, Sun J, Zhao Z (2013) TSGene: a web resource for tumor suppressor genes. Nucleic acids research 41: D970-D976.

26. He Z, Huang T, Shi X, Hu L, Chen L, et al. (2011) Computational Analysis of Protein Tyrosine Nitration; 2010. pp. 35–42.

27. Chen L, Qian ZL, Fen KY, Cai YD (2010) Prediction of Interactiveness Between Small Molecules and Enzymes by Combining Gene Ontology and Compound Similarity. Journal of Computational Chemistry 31: 1766–1776.

28. Carmona-Saez P, Chagoyen M, Tirado F, Carazo JM, Pascual-Montano A (2007) GENECODIS: a web-based tool for finding significant concurrent annotations in gene lists. Genome Biol 8: R3.

29. Huang T, Zhang J, Xu ZP, Hu LL, Chen L, et al. (2012) Deciphering the effects of gene deletion on yeast longevity using network and machine learning approaches. Biochimie 94: 1017–1025.

30. Chen L, Li B-Q, Feng K-Y (2013) Predicting Biological Functions of Protein Complexes Using Graphic and Functional Features. Current Bioinformatics 8: 545–551.

31. Ting KM, Witten IH (1997) Stacking bagged and dagged models; San Francisco, CA. pp. 367–375.

32. Witten IH, Frank E (2005) Data Mining: Practical machine learning tools and techniques: Morgan Kaufmann Pub.

33. Platt J, editor (1998) Fast training of support vector machines using sequential minimal optimization. Cambridge, MA: MIT Press.

34. Keerthi SS, Shevade SK, Bhattacharyya C, Murthy KRK (2001) Improvements to Platt's SMO algorithm for SVM classifier design. Neural Computation 13: 637–649.

35. Kohavi R. (1995) A Study of Cross-Validation and Bootstrap for Accuracy Estimation and Model Selection; San Mateo. pp. 1137–1143.

36. Li B-Q, Feng K-Y, Chen L, Huang T, Cai Y-D (2012) Prediction of Protein-Protein Interaction Sites by Random Forest Algorithm with mRMR and IFS. PLoS ONE 7: e43927.

37. Ding C, Dubchak I (2001) Multi-class protein fold recognition using support vector machines and neural networks. Bioinformatics 17: 349–358.

38. Martin S, Roe D, Faulon J-L (2005) Predicting protein–protein interactions using signature products. Bioinformatics 21: 218–226.

39. Chen L, Zeng WM, Cai YD, Feng KY, Chou KC (2012) Predicting Anatomical Therapeutic Chemical (ATC) Classification of Drugs by Integrating Chemical-Chemical Interactions and Similarities. PLoS ONE 7: e35254.

40. Chen L, Lu J, Zhang N, Huang T, Cai Y-D (2014) A hybrid method for prediction and repositioning of drug Anatomical Therapeutic Chemical classes. Molecular BioSystems 10: 868–877.

41. Baldi P, Brunak S, Chauvin Y, Andersen C, Nielsen H (2000) Assessing the accuracy of prediction algorithms for classification: an overview. Bioinformatics 16: 412–424.

42. Chen L, Feng KY, Cai YD, Chou KC, Li HP (2010) Predicting the network of substrate-enzyme-product triads by combining compound similarity and functional domain composition. BMC bioinformatics 11: 293.

43. Matthews B (1975) Comparison of the predicted and observed secondary structure of T4 phage lysozyme. Biochimica et Biophysica Acta (BBA)-Protein Structure 405: 442–451.

44. Cramér H (1946) Mathematical Methods of Statistics: Princeton university press.

45. Kendall M, Stuart A (1979) The Advanced Theory of Statistics, vol. 2, Inference and Relationship. New York: Macmillan.

46. Harrison KM, Kajese T, Hall HI, Song R (2008) Risk factor redistribution of the national HIV/AIDS surveillance data: an alternative approach. Public health reports 123: 618–627.

47. Zhang Y, Ding C, Li T (2008) Gene selection algorithm by combining reliefF and mRMR. BMC genomics 9: S27.

48. Chen L, Zeng W-M, Cai Y-D, Huang T (2013) Prediction of Metabolic Pathway Using Graph Property, Chemical Functional Group and Chemical Structural Set. Current Bioinformatics 8: 200–207.

49. Li Z, Zhou X, Dai Z, Zou X (2010) Classification of G-protein coupled receptors based on support vector machine with maximum relevance minimum redundancy and genetic algorithm. BMC bioinformatics 11: 325.

50. Ding C, Peng H (2005) Minimum redundancy feature selection from microarray gene expression data. J Bioinform Comput Biol 3: 185–205.

51. Mohabatkar H, Mohammad Beigi M, Esmaeili A (2011) Prediction of GABAA receptor proteins using the concept of Chou's pseudo-amino acid composition and support vector machine. Journal of Theoretical Biology 281: 18–23.

52. Mohabatkar H, Mohammad Beigi M, Abdolahi K, Mohsenzadeh S (2013) Prediction of Allergenic Proteins by Means of the Concept of Chous Pseudo Amino Acid Composition and a Machine Learning Approach. Medicinal Chemistry 9: 133–137.

53. Delbridge AR, Valente LJ, Strasser A (2012) The role of the apoptotic machinery in tumor suppression. Cold Spring Harb Perspect Biol 4: a008789.

54. Dasika GK, Lin SC, Zhao S, Sung P, Tomkinson A, et al. (1999) DNA damage-induced cell cycle checkpoints and DNA strand break repair in development and tumorigenesis. Oncogene 18: 7883–7899.

55. Young LC, Hays JB, Tron VA, Andrew SE (2003) DNA mismatch repair proteins: potential guardians against genomic instability and tumorigenesis induced by ultraviolet photoproducts. J Invest Dermatol 121: 435–440.

56. Smith ML, Ford JM, Hollander MC, Bortnick RA, Amundson SA, et al. (2000) p53-mediated DNA repair responses to UV radiation: studies of mouse cells lacking p53, p21, and/or gadd45 genes. Mol Cell Biol 20: 3705–3714.

57. Dannenberg JH, van Rossum A, Schuijff L, te Riele H (2000) Ablation of the retinoblastoma gene family deregulates G(1) control causing immortalization and increased cell turnover under growth-restricting conditions. Genes Dev 14: 3051–3064.

58. Sage J, Mulligan GJ, Attardi LD, Miller A, Chen S, et al. (2000) Targeted disruption of the three Rb-related genes leads to loss of G(1) control and immortalization. Genes Dev 14: 3037–3050.

59. Derynck R, Zhang Y, Feng XH (1998) Smads: transcriptional activators of TGF-beta responses. Cell 95: 737–740.

60. Yang J, Song K, Krebs TL, Jackson MW, Danielpour D (2008) Rb/E2F4 and Smad2/3 link survivin to TGF-beta-induced apoptosis and tumor progression. Oncogene 27: 5326–5338.

61. Beausejour CM, Krtolica A, Galimi F, Narita M, Lowe SW, et al. (2003) Reversal of human cellular senescence: roles of the p53 and p16 pathways. EMBO J 22: 4212–4222.

62. Mitrea DM, Yoon MK, Ou L, Kriwacki RW (2012) Disorder-function relationships for the cell cycle regulatory proteins p21 and p27. Biol Chem 393: 259–274.

63. Vousden KH, Lane DP (2007) p53 in health and disease. Nat Rev Mol Cell Biol 8: 275–283.

64. Vazquez A, Bond EE, Levine AJ, Bond GL (2008) The genetics of the p53 pathway, apoptosis and cancer therapy. Nat Rev Drug Discov 7: 979–987.

65. Slomovitz BM, Coleman RL (2012) The PI3K/AKT/mTOR pathway as a therapeutic target in endometrial cancer. Clin Cancer Res 18: 5856–5864.

66. Annunziata CM, Davis RE, Demchenko Y, Bellamy W, Gabrea A, et al. (2007) Frequent engagement of the classical and alternative NF-kappaB pathways by diverse genetic abnormalities in multiple myeloma. Cancer Cell 12: 115–130.

67. Zhang XJ, Liang YH, He PP, Yang S, Wang HY, et al. (2004) Identification of the cylindromatosis tumor-suppressor gene responsible for multiple familial trichoepithelioma. J Invest Dermatol 122: 658–664.

68. Mandruzzato S, Brasseur F, Andry G, Boon T, van der Bruggen P (1997) A CASP-8 mutation recognized by cytolytic T lymphocytes on a human head and neck carcinoma. J Exp Med 186: 785–793.

69. Kim HS, Lee JW, Soung YH, Park WS, Kim SY, et al. (2003) Inactivating mutations of caspase-8 gene in colorectal carcinomas. Gastroenterology 125: 708–715.

70. Espada J, Peinado H, Lopez-Serra L, Setien F, Lopez-Serra P, et al. (2011) Regulation of SNAIL1 and E-cadherin function by DNMT1 in a DNA methylation-independent context. Nucleic Acids Res 39: 9194–9205.

71. van Roy F, Berx G (2008) The cell-cell adhesion molecule E-cadherin. Cell Mol Life Sci 65: 3756–3788.

72. Hood JD, Cheresh DA (2002) Role of integrins in cell invasion and migration. Nat Rev Cancer 2: 91–100.

73. Bourboulia D, Stetler-Stevenson WG (2010) Matrix metalloproteinases (MMPs) and tissue inhibitors of metalloproteinases (TIMPs): Positive and negative regulators in tumor cell adhesion. Semin Cancer Biol 20: 161–168.

74. Roy R, Yang J, Moses MA (2009) Matrix metalloproteinases as novel biomarkers and potential therapeutic targets in human cancer. J Clin Oncol 27: 5287–5297.

75. Fleming NI, Jorissen RN, Mouradov D, Christie M, Sakthianandeswaren A, et al. (2013) SMAD2, SMAD3 and SMAD4 mutations in colorectal cancer. Cancer Res 73: 725–735.

76. Lee RS, Roberts CW (2013) Linking the SWI/SNF complex to prostate cancer. Nat Genet 45: 1268–1269.

77. Milton A, Luoto K, Ingram L, Munro S, Logan N, et al. (2006) A functionally distinct member of the DP family of E2F subunits. Oncogene 25: 3212–3218.

78. Shiloh Y, Ziv Y (2013) The ATM protein kinase: regulating the cellular response to genotoxic stress, and more. Nat Rev Mol Cell Biol 14: 197–210.

79. Piccirillo SG, Reynolds BA, Zanetti N, Lamorte G, Binda E, et al. (2006) Bone morphogenetic proteins inhibit the tumorigenic potential of human brain tumour-initiating cells. Nature 444: 761–765.

80. Julien SG, Dube N, Hardy S, Tremblay ML (2011) Inside the human cancer tyrosine phosphatome. Nat Rev Cancer 11: 35–49.

81. Jacob ST, Motiwala T (2005) Epigenetic regulation of protein tyrosine phosphatases: potential molecular targets for cancer therapy. Cancer Gene Ther 12: 665–672.

82. Merchant AA, Matsui W (2010) Targeting Hedgehog–a cancer stem cell pathway. Clin Cancer Res 16: 3130–3140.

83. Reisman D, Glaros S, Thompson EA (2009) The SWI/SNF complex and cancer. Oncogene 28: 1653–1668.

84. Singhal S, Vachani A, Antin-Ozerkis D, Kaiser LR, Albelda SM (2005) Prognostic implications of cell cycle, apoptosis, and angiogenesis biomarkers in non-small cell lung cancer: a review. Clin Cancer Res 11: 3974–3986.

85. Knowles MA (2006) Molecular subtypes of bladder cancer: Jekyll and Hyde or chalk and cheese? Carcinogenesis 27: 361–373.

86. Renneville A, Roumier C, Biggio V, Nibourel O, Boissel N, et al. (2008) Cooperating gene mutations in acute myeloid leukemia: a review of the literature. Leukemia 22: 915–931.

87. Sharifi N, Auchus RJ (2012) Steroid biosynthesis and prostate cancer. Steroids 77: 719–726.

88. Risbridger GP, Davis ID, Birrell SN, Tilley WD (2010) Breast and prostate cancer: more similar than different. Nat Rev Cancer 10: 205–212.

89. Kim MS, Lee SH, Yoo NJ, Lee SH (2013) Frameshift mutations of tumor suppressor gene EP300 in gastric and colorectal cancers with high microsatellite instability. Hum Pathol 44: 2064–2070.

90. Gayther SA, Batley SJ, Linger L, Bannister A, Thorpe K, et al. (2000) Mutations truncating the EP300 acetylase in human cancers. Nat Genet 24: 300–303.

91. Tamura G (2006) Alterations of tumor suppressor and tumor-related genes in the development and progression of gastric cancer. World J Gastroenterol 12: 192–198.

92. Hellebrekers DM, Lentjes MH, van den Bosch SM, Melotte V, Wouters KA, et al. (2009) GATA4 and GATA5 are potential tumor suppressors and biomarkers in colorectal cancer. Clin Cancer Res 15: 3990–3997.

93. Hishida M, Nomoto S, Inokawa Y, Hayashi M, Kanda M, et al. (2013) Estrogen receptor 1 gene as a tumor suppressor gene in hepatocellular carcinoma detected by triple-combination array analysis. Int J Oncol 43: 88–94.

94. Bredel M, Scholtens DM, Yadav AK, Alvarez AA, Renfrow JJ, et al. (2011) NFKBIA deletion in glioblastomas. N Engl J Med 364: 627–637.

95. Sigglekow ND, Pangon L, Brummer T, Molloy M, Hawkins NJ, et al. (2012) Mutated in colorectal cancer protein modulates the NFkappaB pathway. Anticancer Res 32: 73–79.

96. Katoh M (2007) Networking of WNT, FGF, Notch, BMP, and Hedgehog signaling pathways during carcinogenesis. Stem Cell Rev 3: 30–38.

97. Thornton TM, Pedraza-Alva G, Deng B, Wood CD, Aronshtam A, et al. (2008) Phosphorylation by p38 MAPK as an alternative pathway for GSK3beta inactivation. Science 320: 667–670.

98. Ma C, Wang J, Gao Y, Gao TW, Chen G, et al. (2007) The role of glycogen synthase kinase 3beta in the transformation of epidermal cells. Cancer Res 67: 7756–7764.

99. Suzuki M, Shinohara F, Endo M, Sugazaki M, Echigo S, et al. (2009) Zebularine suppresses the apoptotic potential of 5-fluorouracil via cAMP/PKA/CREB pathway against human oral squamous cell carcinoma cells. Cancer Chemother Pharmacol 64: 223–232.

100. Zheng H, Saito H, Masuda S, Yang X, Takano Y (2007) Phosphorylated GSK3beta-ser9 and EGFR are good prognostic factors for lung carcinomas. Anticancer Res 27: 3561–3569.

101. Lu Z, Liu H, Xue L, Xu P, Gong T, et al. (2008) An activated Notch1 signaling pathway inhibits cell proliferation and induces apoptosis in human esophageal squamous cell carcinoma cell line EC9706. Int J Oncol 32: 643–651.

102. Yan D, Avtanski D, Saxena NK, Sharma D (2012) Leptin-induced epithelial-mesenchymal transition in breast cancer cells requires beta-catenin activation via Akt/GSK3- and MTA1/Wnt1 protein-dependent pathways. J Biol Chem 287: 8598–8612.

103. Ding Q, He X, Xia W, Hsu JM, Chen CT, et al. (2007) Myeloid cell leukemia-1 inversely correlates with glycogen synthase kinase-3beta activity and associates with poor prognosis in human breast cancer. Cancer Res 67: 4564–4571.

104. Farago M, Dominguez I, Landesman-Bollag E, Xu X, Rosner A, et al. (2005) Kinase-inactive glycogen synthase kinase 3beta promotes Wnt signaling and mammary tumorigenesis. Cancer Res 65: 5792–5801.

105. Cao Q, Lu X, Feng YJ (2006) Glycogen synthase kinase-3beta positively regulates the proliferation of human ovarian cancer cells. Cell Res 16: 671–677.

106. Yang J, Takahashi Y, Cheng E, Liu J, Terranova PF, et al. (2010) GSK-3beta promotes cell survival by modulating Bif-1-dependent autophagy and cell death. J Cell Sci 123: 861–870.

107. Strathdee G, Sim A, Soutar R, Holyoake TL, Brown R (2007) HOXA5 is targeted by cell-type-specific CpG island methylation in normal cells and during the development of acute myeloid leukaemia. Carcinogenesis 28: 299–309.

108. Shiraishi M, Sekiguchi A, Oates AJ, Terry MJ, Miyamoto Y (2002) HOX gene clusters are hotspots of de novo methylation in CpG islands of human lung adenocarcinomas. Oncogene 21: 3659–3662.

109. Maroulakou IG, Spyropoulos DD (2003) The study of HOX gene function in hematopoietic, breast and lung carcinogenesis. Anticancer Res 23: 2101–2110.

110. Houghton J, Stoicov C, Nomura S, Rogers AB, Carlson J, et al. (2004) Gastric cancer originating from bone marrow-derived cells. Science 306: 1568–1571.

111. Raman V, Martensen SA, Reisman D, Evron E, Odenwald WF, et al. (2000) Compromised HOXA5 function can limit p53 expression in human breast tumours. Nature 405: 974–978.

112. Matos J, West SC (2014) Holliday junction resolution: Regulation in space and time. DNA Repair (Amst) 19: 176–181.

113. Matos J, Blanco MG, Maslen S, Skehel JM, West SC (2011) Regulatory control of the resolution of DNA recombination intermediates during meiosis and mitosis. Cell 147: 158–172.

114. Wechsler T, Newman S, West SC (2011) Aberrant chromosome morphology in human cells defective for Holliday junction resolution. Nature 471: 642–646.

115. Kuligina E, Sokolenko AP, Mitiushkina NV, Abysheva SN, Preobrazhenskaya EV, et al. (2013) Value of bilateral breast cancer for identification of rare recessive at-risk alleles: evidence for the role of homozygous GEN1 c.2515_2519delAAGTT mutation. Fam Cancer 12: 129–132.

116. Forbes SA, Bhamra G, Bamford S, Dawson E, Kok C, et al. (2008) The Catalogue of Somatic Mutations in Cancer (COSMIC). Curr Protoc Hum Genet Chapter 10: Unit 10 11.

117. Wood LD, Parsons DW, Jones S, Lin J, Sjoblom T, et al. (2007) The genomic landscapes of human breast and colorectal cancers. Science 318: 1108–1113.

15

The Role of BRCA Status on the Prognosis of Patients with Epithelial Ovarian Cancer

Chaoyang Sun[9], **Na Li**[9], **Dong Ding**[9], **Danhui Weng, Li Meng, Gang Chen***, **Ding Ma***

Department of Obstetrics and Gynaecology, Tongji Hospital, Tongji Medical College, Huazhong University of Science and Technology, Wuhan, Hubei, China

Abstract

Objective: The role of BRCA dysfunction on the prognosis of patients with epithelial ovarian cancer (EOCs) remains controversial. This systematic review tried to assess the role of BRCA dysfunction, including BRCA1/2 germline, somatic mutations, low BRCA1 protein/mRNA expression or BRCA1 promoter methylation, as prognostic factor in EOCs.

Methods: Studies were selected for analysis if they provided an independent assessment of BRCA status and prognosis in EOC. To make it possible to aggregate survival results of the published studies, their methodology was assessed using a modified quality scale.

Results: Of 35 evaluable studies, 23 identified BRCA dysfucntion status as a favourable prognostic factor. No significant differences were detected in the global score of quality assessment. The aggregated hazard ratio (HR) of overall survival (OS) of 34 evaluable studies suggested that BRCA dysfunction status had a favourable impact on OS (HR = 0.69, 95% CI 0.61–0.79), and when these studies were categorised into BRCA1/2 mutation and low protein/mRNA expression of BRCA1 subgroups, all of them demonstrated positive results (HR = 0.67, 95% CI: 0.57–0.78; HR = 0.62, 95% CI: 0.51–0.75; and HR = 0.51, 95% CI: 0.33–0.78, respectively), except for the subgroup of BRCA1 promoter methylation (HR = 1.59, 95% CI: 0.72–3.50). The meta-analysis of progression-free survival (PFS), which included 18 evaluable studies, demonstrated that BRCA dysfunction status was associated with a longer PFS in EOC (HR = 0.69, 95% CI: 0.63–0.76).

Conclusions: Patients with BRCA dysfunction status tend to have a better outcome, but further prospective clinical studies comparing the different BRCA statuses in EOC is urgently needed to specifically define the most effective treatment for the separate patient groups.

Editor: Alexander James Roy Bishop, University of Texas Health Science Center at San Antonio, United States of America

Funding: The authors have no support or funding to report.

Competing Interests: The authors have declared that no competing interests exist.

* E-mail: gumpc@126.com (GC); dma@tjh.tjmu.edu.cn (DM)

[9] These authors contributed equally to this work.

Introduction

Epithelial ovarian carcinoma (EOC) is the fifth leading cause of cancer death in women [1], and the five-year relative survival rates for the late stage of EOC were less than 10% between 2004 and 2008 [2]. Despite advances in surgery and the wide use of platinum-based chemotherapy, the long-term outcome remains poor as a result of recurrences and the emergence of drug resistance, necessitating the discovery of biomarkers for predicting which patients will benefit or not benefit from systemic chemotherapy. Moreover, the lack of active therapeutic agents for patients with platinum-resistant cancers impels researchers to discover novel molecular targets helping define subsets of patients who may benefit the most from specific treatment.

In 1996, a detailed case-control analysis reported that BRCA1/2 germline mutations were beneficial prognostic factors for patients with EOC [3]. Since then, many scientists have tried to discover the real association between BRCA1/2 germline

mutation status and the prognosis of EOC in subsequent studies, generating conflicting results [3–8]. Although, the mechanism underlying the association between BRCA1/2 germline mutations and survival is not fully understood, *in vitro* experiments have shown that BRCA1/2 deficient cells display a deficiency in repairing double-strand DNA breaks by homologous recombination [9–11]. This biological mechanism may be responsible for increased chemo-sensitivity, which results in a longer progression-free survival (PFS) and overall survival (OS) [12]. More inspiringly, BRCA1/2 mutation carries can obtain an excellent response from targeted therapies, such as the poly (ADP) ribose polymerase (PARP) inhibitor (Olaparib) [13,14]. However, BRCA1/2 germline mutation carriers only account for 10% to 15% of EOCs. Fortunately, recent data suggest that many sporadic EOCs display "BRCAness", or dysfunction of BRCA1/2. Additionally, in sporadic EOCs, low BRCA1 expression detected by immunohistochemistry (IHC) or RT-PCR or BRCA1 promoter methylation had also been reported as a clinically useful tool to provide important information on prognosis [15].

The aim of this study was to assess the role of BRCA dysfunction status, including BRCA1/2 germline/somatic mutations, low BRCA1 protein/mRNA expression or BRCA1 promoter methylation in sporadic EOCs, on prognosis in EOCs by carrying out a systematic review of the literature followed by a meta-analysis, and to estimate to what extent do these BRCA statuses influence patients' prognosis.

Methods

Publication Selection

This study has been registered at the International Prospective Register of Systematic Reviews (PROSPERO, http://www.crd.york.ac.uk/prospero/display_record.asp?ID = CRD42011001747) in 2011. An electronic search of Medline, Embase, and CNKI (China National Knowledge Infrastructure) was used to select articles with the following keywords: 'ovarian neoplasm', 'ovarian tumour', 'ovarian carcinoma', 'ovarian malignance' or 'ovarian cancer' and 'BRCA1', 'BRCA2' or 'BRCA*' and 'prognos*', 'surviv*', 'outcome' or 'marker'. This search strategy was complemented by examining the personal bibliography of the authors. To avoid overlap between patient populations, when authors reported results obtained on the same patient cohorts in several publications, only the most recent report or the most complete one was included in the analysis. The search was updated in September 2013. A study must have been published as a full paper in the English or Chinese language. To be eligible for inclusion, studies had to meet the following criteria: addressed epithelial ovarian cancer and analysed patients' prognosis according to BRCA statuses (assessed BRCA1/2 mutations, assessed BRCA1/2 protein expression through IHC or assessed mRNA level through RT-PCR, and/or assessed BRCA1 promoter methylation in the primary tumour (not in metastatic tissue or in tissue adjacent to the tumour)). The primary outcome was overall survival (OS) and the secondary outcome was progression-free survival (PFS).

Data Extraction and Methodological Assessment

The data retrieved from the reports included authors, years of studies and publications, patients' resources, population size, methods, histology, stage and treatment. To avoid bias in the data abstraction process, three reviewers (Chaoyang Sun, Na Li, Dong Ding) abstracted the data independently and subsequently compared the results. All of the data were checked for internal consistency, and disagreements were resolved by discussion.

To assess methodology, three investigators (Chaoyang Sun, Na Li, Dong Ding) read each publication independently and scored them according to the European Lung Cancer Working Party (ELCWP) scoring scale, with some modification (Method S1 in File S1) [16]. The scores were compared, and a consensus value for each item was reached in meetings attended by at least two investigators. The score evaluates a number of aspects of methodology, which were grouped into four main categories: design, laboratory methods, generalisability of results and the analysis of the study data. Each category had a maximum score of 10 points, giving a theoretical total maximum score of 40 points. The final scores were expressed as percentages ranging from 0 to 100%, with higher values reflecting better methodological quality.

Statistical Methods

A study was considered to be significant if the P-value for the statistical test comparing the survival distributions between the

groups of BRCA dysfunction and normal BRCA status was < 0.05. The study was called 'positive' when BRCA dysfunction status was found as a favourable prognostic factor for survival. Other situations were called 'negative', including when a significant survival difference was found, but the group of patients with BRCA dysfunction status fared worse.

Non-parametric tests were used to compare the distribution of the quality scores according to the value of a discrete variable (Mann-Whitney tests).

For the quantitative aggregation of the survival results, we measured the impact of BRCA dysfunction status on prognosis by the hazard ratio (HR) between the survival distributions of the two BRCA status groups. For each study, the HR was extracted or estimated by a method that depended on the results provided in the publication. The most accurate method was to retrieve the HR estimate and its variance from the reported results or to calculate it directly using parameters provided by the authors for univariate analysis: the confidence interval (CI) for the HR, the log-rank statistic, its P-value or the O-E statistic (difference between numbers of observed and expected events). If these parameters were not available, we evaluated the total number of events, the number of patients at risk in each group and the log-rank statistic or it's P-value, allowing for the calculation of an approximation of the HR estimate. Finally, if the only useful data were in the form of graphical representations of the survival distributions, we extracted survival rates at specified times to reconstruct the HR estimate and its variance, with the assumption that during the study follow-up, the rate of patients censored was constant [17]. If this latter method was used, three independent persons read the curves to reduce imprecision in the reading variations.

If survival was reported separately for particular subgroups, these results were included in the meta-analysis of the corresponding subgroups. The same patients were never considered more than once in each analysis. The individual HR estimates were combined into an overall HR using the method published by Yusuf S and Peto R et al [18]. If the assumption of homogeneity had to be rejected, we used a random-effects model as a second step. By convention, an observed HR <1 implied better survival for the group with BRCA dysfunction status. This impact of BRCA status on survival was considered to be statistically significant if the 95% CI for the overall HR did not include 1.

Horizontal lines indicate the 95% CI, and each box represents the HR point estimate; the box size is proportional to the number of patients included in the study. A funnel plot and Begg's linear regression test were used to investigate any possible publication bias [19].

For all analyses, a two-sided P value of <0.05 was considered to be statistically significant. All analyses were performed using SPSS version 13.0 (SPSS, Chicago, IL) and STATA version 10.0 software (Stata Corporation, College Station, TX).

Studies that were eligible for the systematic review were called 'eligible', and those providing data for the meta-analysis were called 'evaluable'.

Results

Study Selection and Characteristics

The primary search yielded a total of 1,231 publications, 1030 of which were excluded by title screening. Abstracts of the remaining 201 papers were reviewed, resulting in 162 being excluded and leaving 39 as candidate articles [3–8,15,20–51]. To reach a final decision on which articles were to be included in the meta-analysis, we examined all 39 papers in detail, which resulted in the further exclusion of 4 papers because survival information was not available for three papers [29,35,46] and one study's [42] subjects overlapped with a subsequent study that the authors published six years later [26] (Figure 1). All eligible articles were reviewed by three independent investigators. The main features of the 39 studies eligible for the systematic review, which were published between 1996 and 2013, are shown in Table S1 in File S1. All of the eligible literatures were case-control studies. A total of 26 studies investigated BRCA1/2 germline and/or somatic mutations, while low BRCA1 protein/mRNA expressions and BRCA1 promoter methylation statuses in sporadic EOCs were studied in nine, two, and two studies, respectively.

As shown in Table 1, 26 studies were performed on BRCA1/2 germline and/or somatic mutions. Twenty-one (21/26, 80.8%) studies investigated the germline BRCA1/2 mutation alone, four (4/26, 15.4%) studies investigated BRCA mutation status including germline and somatic BRCA1/2 mutation together, and the one (1/26, 3.8%) study left investigated BRCA1 dysfunction secondary to germline, somatic BRCA1 mutation or BRCA1 promoter methylation. The detailed information of these 26 studies was listed in Table 1. Eighteen (18/26, 69.2%) papers identified BRCA1/2 mutation as a good prognostic factor for survival, while the remaining eight (8/26, 30.8%) concluded that BRCA1/2 mutation was not a prognostic factor for survival.

Immunohistochemistry (IHC) was used in 9 studies to detect the low expression of BRCA1 protein in sporadic EOCs. The MS110 clone antibody was used in 88.9% (8/9) of the studies. Various experimental procedures were performed with the same cut-off value (<10% positive cells) except for one study [49], and the summary proportion of low expression of BRCA1 (with cut-off value as <10% positive cells) in sporadic ovarian cancer was 55.2% (Table 2).

BRCA1 mRNA expression and BRCA1 promoter methylation in sporadic EOCs were studied in two papers each. Both articles identified the low expression of BRCA1 mRNA as a significantly better predictor of prognosis, while the other two papers on BRCA1 promoter methylation showed negative results (Table 3).

Quality Assessment

Overall, the global quality assessment score, expressed as a percentage, ranged between 36.7% and 89.4%, with a median of 70.6% (Table S2A in File S1, mean ± SD values are shown).

No statistically significant difference of scores were found between the 35 evaluable and 4 non-evaluable studies. There was also no statistically significant difference between the scores of the 26 positive studies and 13 negative studies, except the positive ones had better sub-scores for laboratory methodology (P = 0.016). The difference in the global and four subgroup scores between the studies classified according to the types of BRCA dysfunction statuses was not significant.

Table S2B in File S1 shows the scores for the 35 studies classified as evaluable for the meta-analysis. There was no significant difference between significant and not significant studies in the global score, except for the sub-score of generalisability (P = 0.013). Moreover, the different types of BRCA dysfunction status did not affect the overall quality assessment or the four subgroup scores.

Meta-analysis of BRCA Status and OS of Ovarian Cancer

The absence of significant qualitative differences between positive and negative trials allowed us to perform a quantitative aggregation of the survival data. Subgroup analysis was performed because the heterogeneity of the trials was obvious: the studies had reported on patients with different BRCA dysfunction statuses (BRCA1/2 germline/somatic mutations, low BRCA1 expression tested by IHC or RT-PCR, and BRCA1 promoter methylation in sporadic EOCs). In this study, we combined studies of germline, somatic BRCA1/2 mutations together as one intervention called the BRCA1/2 mutations in subgroup meta-analysis.

The overall meta-analysis of OS included 34 aggregable studies with 7,986 patients (one studies only provided PFS). The test of overall heterogeneity was significant ($I^2 = 61.7\%$, P = 0.000), which primarily came from the BRCA1/2 mutation subgroup ($I^2 = 64.4\%$, P = 0.000), while the heterogeneity of the remaining three subgroups (low BRCA1 expression by IHC or RT-PCR and BRCA1 promoter methylation in sporadic EOCs) was not significant. BRCA dysfunction status was associated with a better OS, with HR = 0.69, 95% CI: 0.61–0.79 in random-effects model (HR = 0.72, 95% CI: 0.61–0.79 in fixed-effects model). In the subgroup analyses according to different BRCA statuses, BRCA1/2 mutations (1,686 cases and 4,941 controls) and low BRCA1 expression by IHC (500 cases and 362 controls) or RT-PCR (72 cases and 49 controls) were statistically significantly better prognostic factors for survival (HR = 0.69, 95% CI: 0.59–0.80; HR = 0.62, 95% CI: 0.51–0.75; and HR = 0.51, 95% CI: 0.33–0.78 in the random-effects model, respectively; and HR = 0.72, 95% CI: 0.67–0.78; HR = 0.62, 95% CI: 0.51–0.75; and HR = 0.51, 95% CI: 0.33–0.78 in the fixed-effects model, respectively). However, BRCA1 promoter methylation (62 cases and 196 controls) was not associated with better prognosis (HR = 1.59, 95% CI: 0.72–3.50 in the random-effects model and HR = 1.40, 95% CI: 0.94–2.09 in the fixed-effects model) (Figure 2).

When BRCA mutation was subdivided into BRCA1 or BRCA2 subgroups, the meta-analysis showed that both BRCA1 and BRCA2 mutations predicted better OS (HR = 0.78, 95% CI: 0.69–0.87 and HR = 0.65, 95% CI: 0.50–0.86 in a fixed and random-effects model, respectively) (Figure 3A, 3B).

Meta-analysis of BRCA Status and PFS of Ovarian Cancer

The overall meta-analysis of PFS included 13 evaluable studies with 3,394 patients. The overall heterogeneity and the heteroge-

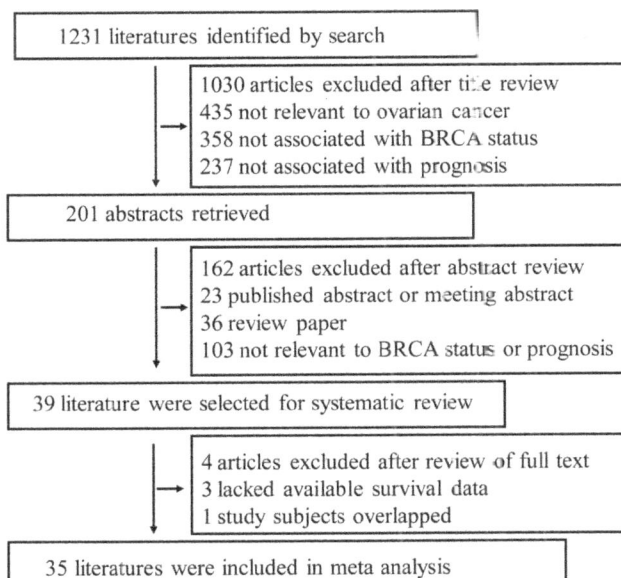

```
┌─────────────────────────────────────┐
│ 1231 literatures identified by search │
└─────────────────────────────────────┘
              │
              │   ┌──────────────────────────────────────────┐
              ├──▶│ 1030 articles excluded after title review  │
              │   │ 435 not relevant to ovarian cancer         │
              │   │ 358 not associated with BRCA status        │
              │   │ 237 not associated with prognosis          │
              │   └──────────────────────────────────────────┘
              ▼
┌─────────────────────────────────────┐
│ 201 abstracts retrieved              │
└─────────────────────────────────────┘
              │
              │   ┌──────────────────────────────────────────┐
              ├──▶│ 162 articles excluded after abstract review│
              │   │ 23 published abstract or meeting abstract  │
              │   │ 36 review paper                            │
              │   │ 103 not relevant to BRCA status or prognosis│
              │   └──────────────────────────────────────────┘
              ▼
┌─────────────────────────────────────┐
│ 39 literature were selected for systematic review │
└─────────────────────────────────────┘
              │
              │   ┌──────────────────────────────────────────┐
              ├──▶│ 4 articles excluded after review of full text│
              │   │ 3 lacked available survival data           │
              │   │ 1 study subjects overlapped                │
              │   └──────────────────────────────────────────┘
              ▼
┌─────────────────────────────────────┐
│ 35 literatures were included in meta analysis │
└─────────────────────────────────────┘
```

Figure 1. Flow chart of publication selection.

Table 1. Characteristics of studies of patients with BRCA1/2 mutated ovarian cancer.

First author	Study year, published year	Country	Histology	Stage	No. of cases/controls	Laboratory methods	BRCA status	Germline/somatic	Mutation Types	Treatment	Survival result
Aida	1984–1996,1998	Japan	se	I-III	13/29	SCCP,PCR,seq	BRCA1	Germ	Deleterious	2	positive
Alsop	2002–2006,2012	Austrilia	se	I-IV	118/536	PCR,seq, MLPA	BRCA1/2	Germ	Deleterious	2	positive
Artioli	,2010	Italian	all	I-IV	48/40	PCR,seq	BRCA1/2	Germ	Deleterious	1+2	positive
Boyd	1986–1998,2000	U.S.A	all	I-IV	88/100	PCR,seq	BRCA1/2	Germ	Deleterious	2	positive
Brozek	1995–2004,2008	Poland	se+CCC	I-IV	21/130	DHPLC,RFLP,seq	BRCA1/2	Germ	Deleterious+ VUS	2	positive
Buller	1990–2000,2002	U.S.A	all	I-IV	59/59	PTT,SSCP,seq	BRCA1	Mixed	Deleterious+ VUS	2	negative
Cass	1990–2001,2003	U.S.A	all	III-IV	29/25	SSCR,seq	BRCA1/2	Germ	Deleterious	2	positive
Chetrit	1994–1999,2008	Israel	all	I-IV	213/392	PCR,seq	BRCA1/2	Germ	Deleterious	2	positive
David	1994–1999,2002	Israel	all	I-IV	229/549	SCCP,seq	BRCA1/2	Germ+Somatic	Deleterious	2	positive
Dann	1999–2007,2012	U.S.A	all	II-IV	15/38	PCR,seq	BRCA1/2	Germ+Somatic	Deleterious	2	negative
Gallagher	1996–2006,2011	U.S.A	all	III-IV	36/74	PCR,seq	BRCA1/2	Germ	Deleterious	2	positive
Hennessy	1990–2006,2010	U.S.A	all	I-IV	43/192	PCR,seq	BRCA1/2	Germ+Somatic	Deleterious	2	positive
Hyman	2001–2010,2012	U.S.A	se	III-IV	69/298	PCR,seq	BRCA1/2	Germ	Deleterious	2	positive
Johannsson	1958–1995,1998	Swedish	all	I-IV	38/97	PTT,SSCP,seq	BRCA1	Germ	Deleterious	2+3	negative
Lacour	1996–2007,2011	U.S.A	all	III-IV	95/183	PCR,seq	BRCA1/2	Germ	Deleterious	–	positive
Majdak	1997–2002,2005	Poland	se+Mu	I-IV	18/171	F-CSGE,seq	BRCA1	Germ	Deleterious	2	positive
McLaughlin	1995–1995,2002–2004,2012	Canada	all	I-IV	218/1408	PTT, seq,DGGE, DHPLC	BRCA1/2	Germ	Deleterious	2	negative
Pal	2000–2003,2007	West central Florida	all	III-IV	32/177	PCR,seq	BRCA1/2	Germ	Deleterious+ VUS	–	negative
Pharoah	,1999	U.K	all	I-IV	151/119	PTT,SSCP	BRCA1/2	Germ	Deleterious	–	negative
Ramus	1992–1997,2001	Israel	all	I-IV	27/71	SSCP,PCR,seq	BRCA1/2	Germ	Deleterious	–	negative
Rubin	,1996	U.S.A	all	III-IV	43/43	SSCP,PCR,seq	BRCA1	Germ	Deleterious+ VUS	–	positive
Tan	1991–2006,2008	U.K	all	III-IV	22/44	SCCP,seq	BRCA1/2	Germ	Deleterious+ VUS	2	positive
Vencken	1980–2009,2011	Netherlands	all	I-IV	112/222	PCR,seq	BRCA1/2	Germ	unknown	2	positive
Yang	,2011	multi-country	all	III-IV	59/251	exom seq	BRCA1/2	Germ+Somatic	Deleterious+ VUS	2	positive
Zweemer	,1999	Netherlands	–	–	42/84	PTT,PCR	BRCA1/2	Germ	Deleterious	–	positive
Zweemer	,2001	Netherlands	All	I-IV	23/17	PTT,PCR,seq	BRCA1/2	Germ	Deleterious	–	negative

Histology: pathological histology of ovarian cancer, se=serous ovarian cancer, CCC=clear cell cancer of, Mu=mucinous ovarian cancer. all=almost all of the epithelial ovarian cancer types, including serous, mucinous, clear cell cancer, etc.

Laboratory methods: laboratory methods used to detect BRCA1/2 mutation, PTT=Protein truncation test, SSCP=Single-Strand Conformation Polymorphism, seq=sequencing, DGGE=fluorescent multiplex denaturing gradient gel electrophoresis, MLPA=multiplex ligation-dependent probe amplification, DHPLC=Denaturing high performance liquid chromatography, RFLP=Restriction fragment length polymorphisms, F-CSGE=Fluorescence-based Conformation Sensitive Gel Electrophoresis.

Germline/somatic: Germ=germline mutation, Mixed=BRCA1 germline/somatic mutation or BRCA1 promoter methylation.

Mutation types: VUS=variants of unknown significance.

Treatment: chemotherapy used, 1=only Platinum was used, 2=Platinum-based chemotherapy, 3=other agents without Platinum, like Paclitaxel, etc.

Table 2. Characteristics of studies of patients of ovarian cancer with low BRCA1 expression measured by IHC.

First author	Study year, published year	Country	stage	Histology	No. of cases/controls	Clone	dilution	Retrieval	readers	Double blind	Cut off	Low%	treatment	Survival result
Weberpals	2008,2011	Canada	II-IV	all	75/41	MS110	1:100	-	2	Yes	10%	65%	1	positive
Carser	1998-2004,2011	U.K	I-IV	all	120/172	MS110	-	steam heat	2	Yes	10%	41%	1	positive
Gan	1991-2007,2013	U.K	I-IV	se	112/19	MS110	1:80	microwave	1	Yes	≤70*	84.4%	2	positive
Kaern	1990-1992,2005	Norway	III	all	30/16	MS110	1:200	microwave	2	No	10%	65.20%	2	negative
Sirisabya	1996-1999,2007	Thailand	I-III	all	87/12	-	-	microwave	1	No	10%	87.80%	1	negative
Thrall	,2006	U.S.A	I-III	all	97/55	MS110	1:50	steam heat	2	Yes	10%	63.8%	1	positive
Swisher	,2009	U.S.A	I-IV	all	39/76	MS110	1:250	steam heat		No	10%	34%	?	positive
Radosa	2000-2005,2011	Germany	III-IV	all	12/15	MS110	1:200	heat	2	Yes	10%	44.40%	1	positive
Yu	1996-1998,2005	China	I-IV	all	35/15	MS110	1:100	-			10%	70%	2	negative

Histology: pathological histology of ovarian cancer, all = almost all of the epithelial ovarian cancer types, including serous, mucinous, clear cell cancer, etc, se = serous ovarian cancer.
Treatment: chemotherapy used, 1 = only Platinum was used, 2 = Platinum-based chemotherapy.
*BRCA1 (H-score≤70) defined as the BRCA1-deficient group.

Table 3. Characteristics of studies of patients of ovarian cancer with low BRCA1 mRNA expression or BRCA1 promoter methylation.

	First author	Study year, published year	Country	Histology	stage	No. of cases/controls	Methods of methylation detecting	Treatment	significance
RT-PCR	Quinn	,2007	U.K	all	I-IV	47/23		2	positive
	Weberpals	1997-2005,2009	Canada	all	II-IV	25/26		2	positive
methylation	Wiley	1991-2000,2006	Italy	all	I-IV	44/171	MSP	2	negative
	Chiang	1986-2001,2006	USA	-	I-IV	10/25	MSRE+ Southern blot+ MSP	2	negative

Histology: pathological histology of ovarian cancer, all = almost all of the epithelial ovarian cancer types, including serous, mucinous, clear cell cancer, etc.
Methods of methylation detecting: methods of methylation detecting, MSP = methylation-specific polymerase chain reaction (PCR) analysis, MSRE = methylation-sensitive restriction enzyme digestion.
Treatment: chemotherapy used, 2 = Platinum-based chemotherapy.

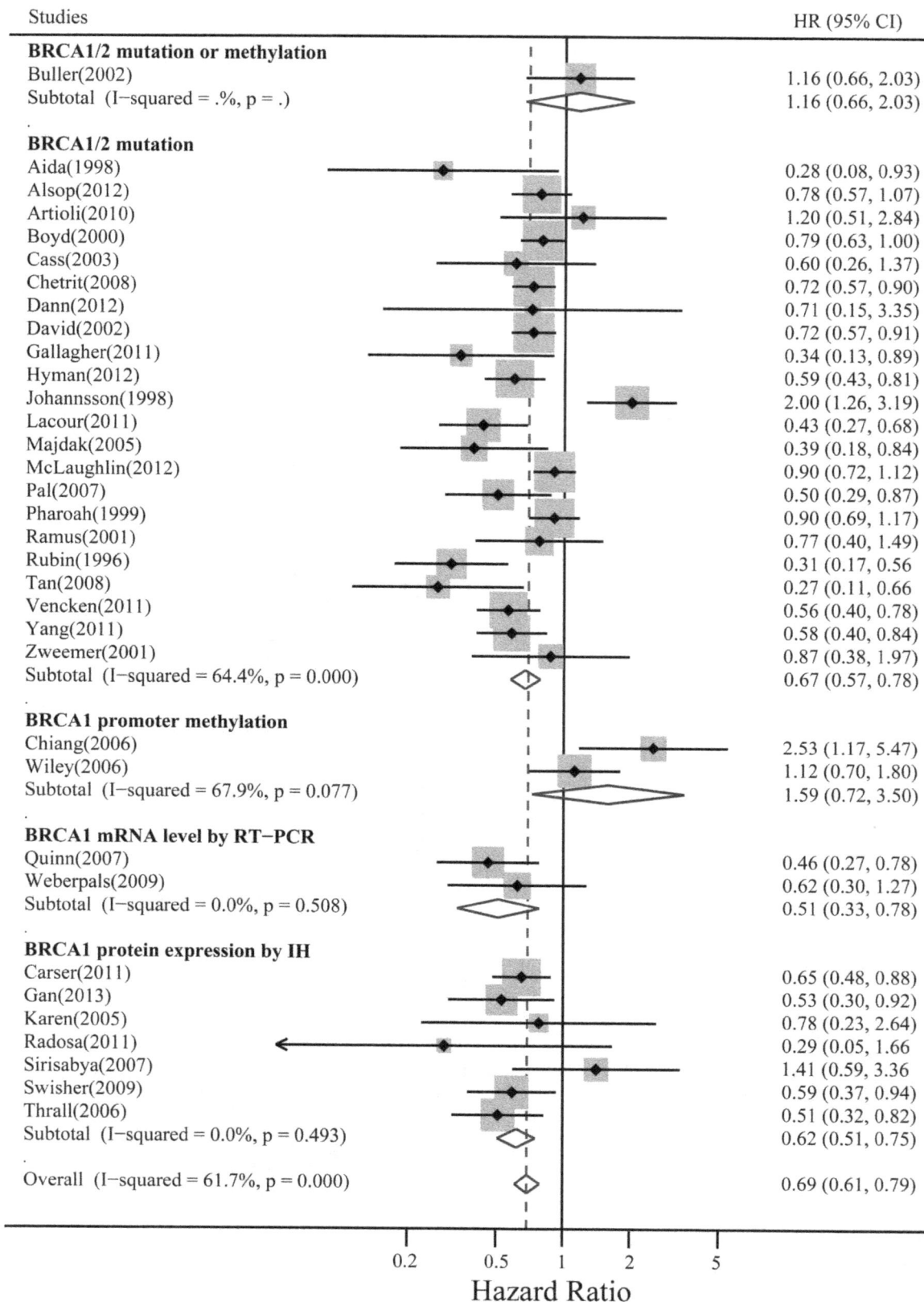

Figure 2. Summary hazard ratios (HRs) and 95% confidence intervals (CIs) of epithelial ovarian cancer OS for BRCA dysfunction status. Horizontal lines represent 95% CIs; diamonds represent summary estimates with corresponding 95% CIs. Test for heterogeneity: $P = .000$, $I^2 = 61.7\%$. A random-effects model was used for analysis.

A

Studies	HR (95% CI)
Aida(1998)	0.28 (0.08, 0.93)
Alsop(2012)	0.87 (0.59, 1.27)
Boyd(2000)	0.65 (0.42, 0.99)
Buller(2002)	1.13 (0.43, 2.99)
Chetrit(2008)	0.82 (0.64, 1.06)
McLaughlin(2012)	0.89 (0.67, 1.18)
Pal(2007)	0.59 (0.28, 1.25)
Pharoah(1999)	0.95 (0.72, 1.25)
Ramus(2001)	0.71 (0.27, 1.84)
Vencken(2011)	0.56 (0.41, 0.76)
Yang(2011)	0.70 (0.45, 1.10)
Overall (I−squared = 20.2%, p = 0.251)	0.78 (0.69, 0.87)

Hazard Rates

B

Studies	HR (95% CI)
Alsop(2012)	0.95 (0.60, 1.50)
Boyd(2000)	0.62 (0.32, 1.19)
Chetrit(2008)	0.54 (0.36, 0.80)
McLaughlin(2012)	0.94 (0.68, 1.29)
Pal(2007)	0.43 (0.20, 0.90)
Pharoah(1999)	0.94 (0.56, 1.58)
Ramus(2001)	0.88 (0.44, 1.74)
Vencken(2011)	0.29 (0.12, 0.71)
Yang(2011)	0.33 (0.16, 0.69)
Overall (I−squared = 55.1%, p = 0.023)	0.65 (0.50, 0.86)

Hazard Rates

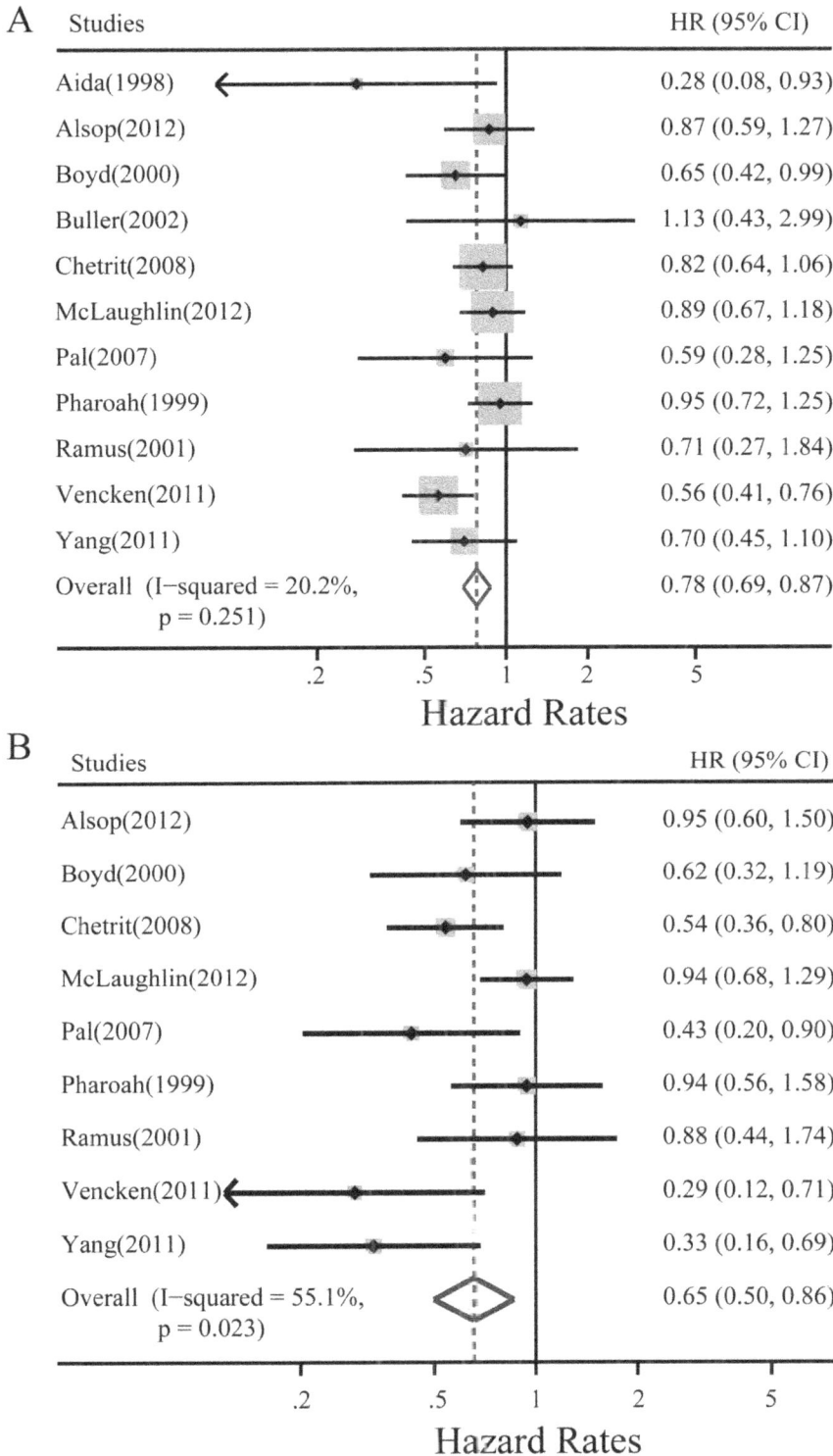

Figure 3. Subgroup meta-analysis of summary hazard ratios (HRs) and 95% confidence intervals (CIs) of ovarian cancer OS for different BRCA mutation statuses. A: BRCA1 mutation. B: BRCA2 mutation. Horizontal lines represent 95% CIs; diamonds represent summary estimates with corresponding 95% CIs. Test for heterogeneity: A: P =.251, I^2 = 20.2%, a fixed-effects model was used; B: P = .023, I^2 = 55.1%, a random-effects model was used.

neity of all subgroups were not significant. BRCA dysfunction status was associated with a better PFS in ovarian cancer, with HR = 0.69 (95% CI: 0.63–0.76, fixed-effect model). In the subgroup analyses according to different BRCA statuses, BRCA1/2 mutation and low BRCA1 expression by IHC were statistically significant predictors for longer PFS (HR = 0.65, 95%

Studies   HR (95% CI)

BRCA1/2 mutation

Aida(1998)   0.75 (0.08, 6.90)

Alsop(2012)   0.75 (0.60, 0.94)

Boyd(2000)   0.50 (0.36, 0.69)

Cass(2003)   0.58 (0.30, 1.14)

Dann(2012)   0.62 (0.29, 1.32)

Hennessy(2010)   0.65 (0.44, 0.96)

Lacour(2011)   0.61 (0.43, 0.86)

Majdak(2005)   0.58 (0.31, 1.09)

Vencken(2011)   0.67 (0.52, 0.87)

Yang(2011)   0.65 (0.47, 0.90)

Subtotal (I–squared = 0.0%, p = 0.878)   0.65 (0.57, 0.73)

BRCA1 protein expression by IHC

Carser(2011)   0.74 (0.55, 0.99)

Gan(2013)   0.60 (0.35, 1.04)

Radosa(2011)   0.44 (0.13, 1.44)

Sirisabya(2007)   1.42 (0.65, 3.11)

Thrall(2006)   0.64 (0.42, 0.97)

Weberpals(2011)   0.56 (0.35, 0.89)

Subtotal (I–squared = 3.4%, p = 0.395)   0.69 (0.57, 0.83)

BRCA1 promoter methylation

Chiang(2006)   1.55 (0.81, 2.98)

Wiley(2006)   1.32 (0.82, 2.12)

Subtotal (I–squared = 0.0%, p = 0.696)   1.40 (0.95, 2.05)

Heterogeneity between groups: p = 0.001

Overall (I–squared = 29.3%, p = 0.118)   0.69 (0.63, 0.76)

```
        0.2       0.5      1      2      5
```

Hazard Ratio

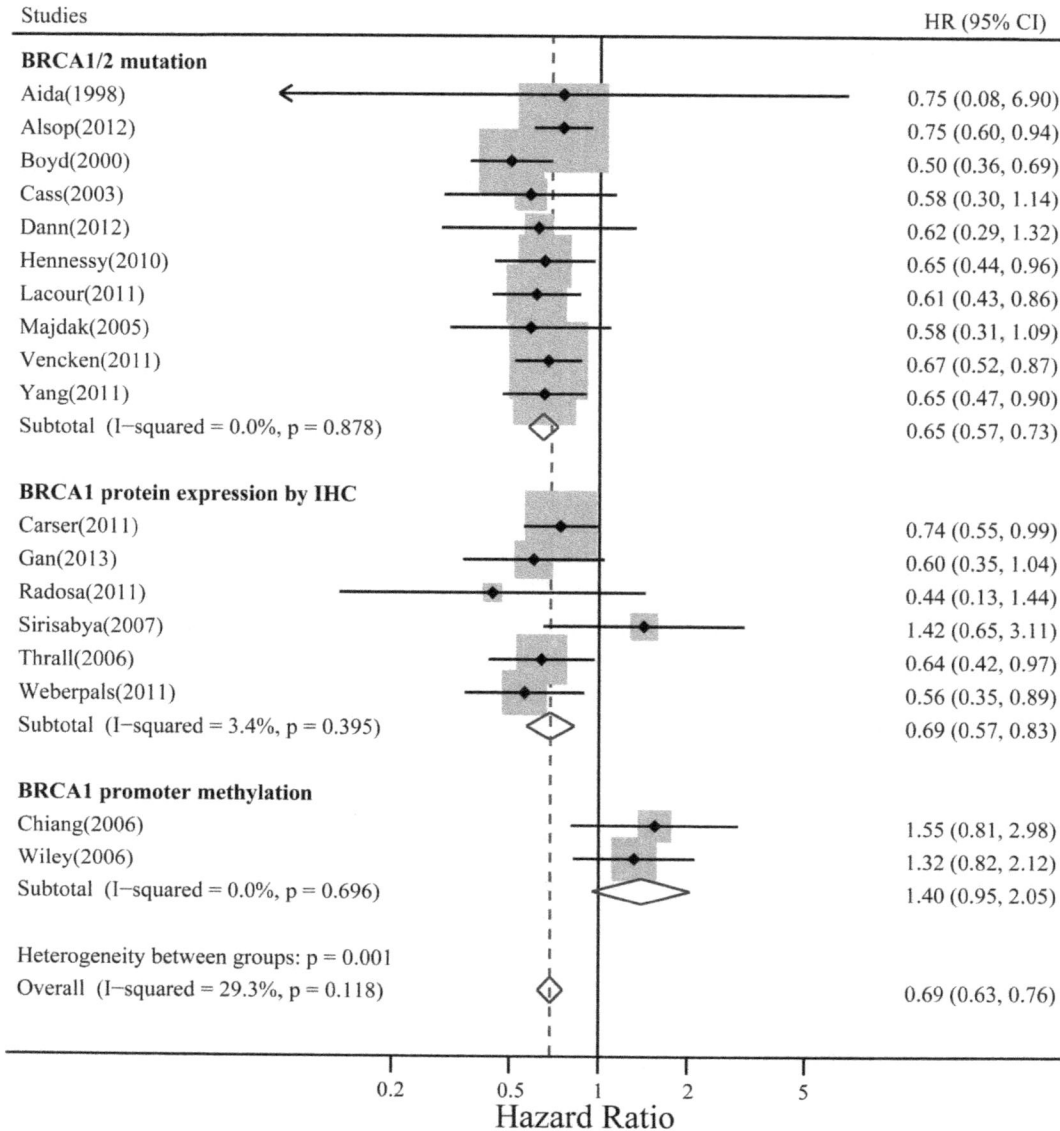

Figure 4. Summary hazard ratios (HRs) and 95% confidence intervals (CIs) of ovarian cancer PFS for BRCA dysfunction status. Horizontal lines represent 95% CIs; diamonds represent summary estimates with corresponding 95% CIs. Test for heterogeneity: $P = .118$, $I^2 = 29.3\%$. A fixed-effects model was used.

CI: 0.57–0.73 and HR = 0.69, 95% CI: 0.57–0.83 in a fixed-effect model, respectively). However, BRCA1 promoter methylation was not associated with better PFS (HR = 1.40, 95% CI: 0.95–2.05) (Figure 4).

Publication Bias

Publication bias statistics were determined using Begg's linear regression test. No publication bias was found for the studies used for the meta-analysis for overall survival (Begg's test, $P = 0.221$) (Figure 5A); moreover, there is no publication bias was found for the studies used for the meta-analysis for PFS (Begg's test, $P = 0.880$) (Figure 5B).

Discussion

Our systematic review of the literature and meta-analysis demonstrate an improved prognosis in patients whose EOC

display BRCA1/2 dysfunction, relative to those whose EOC display normal BRCA1/2 function. Although the comparison of prognostic benefit between BRCA1 and BRCA2 mutation was not feasible, the aggregated HRs indicated that patients with a BRCA2 mutation (HR = 0.65) may have a better prognosis than patients with a BRCA1 mutation (HR = 0.78). During the preparation of this manuscript, Bolton et al also reported BRCA1/2 germline mutation was associated with improved survival and BRCA2 carriers had the best prognosis, these findings are consistent with our results [52].

Although BRCA1/2 germline mutation carriers only account for small proportions of EOCs, fortunately, it has been estimated that approximately 50% sporadic EOCs show dysfunction of BRCA1/2 through different mechanisms. Our study is the first meta-analysis, to our knowledge, to assess if low BRCA1/2 expression status of sporadic EOCs could show similar effects on

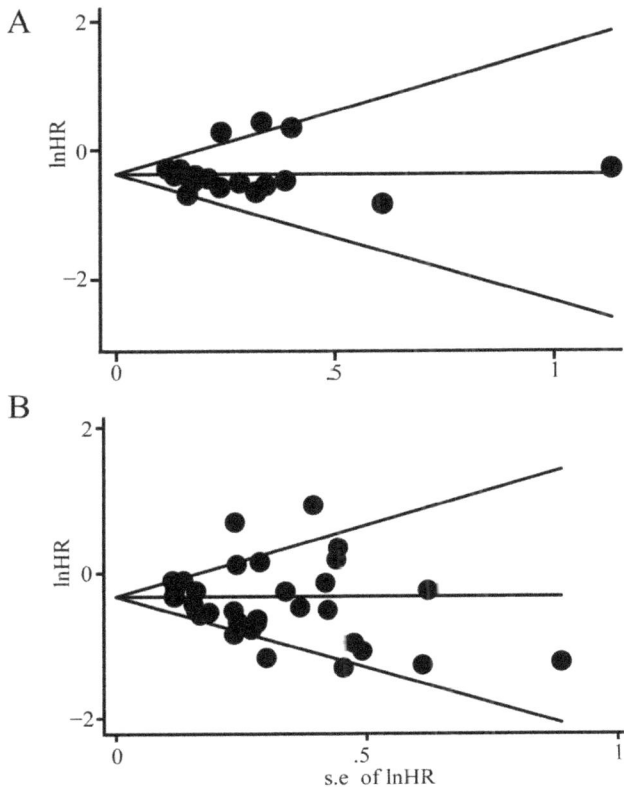

Figure 5. Begg's funnel plots of the natural logarithm of the hazard ratios (HRs) and the SE of the natural logarithm of the HRs for all of the included studies reported with OS and PFS. A: Begg's funnel plots for all of the included studies reported with OS, the dashed line represents 95% confidence intervals (CIs). Circles represent individual studies. Begg's test: $P = 0.221$. B: Begg's funnel plots for all of the included studies reported with PFS, the dashed line represents 95% confidence intervals (CIs). Circles represent individual studies. Begg's test: $P = 0.880$.

prognosis to BRCA1/2 mutation carriers. Our results showed that low BRCA1 expression measured by IHC or RT-PCR but not BRCA1 promoter methylation is a good prognostic factor for both OS and PFS in patients of sporadic EOCs, indicating that low BRCA1 expression status in sporadic EOCs show similar clinical effects on prognosis to germline mutations carriers. However, it is still difficult to draw a definite conclusion because these results were based on small numbers and require confirmation in larger studies, especially for low BRCA1 expression measured by RT-PCR and BRCA1 promoter methylation status. Swisher et al had stated that BRCA1 promoter methylation only occurs in a small proportion of sporadic ovarian cancer with low BRCA1 expression [33], therefore, other mechanisms that could cause low BRCA1 expression need to be further investigated.

In our study, patients whose EOC displays BRCA dysfunction had a favourable prognosis. BRCA1/2 gene products play a pivotal role in DNA repair mechanisms. The better prognosis of patients with BRCA dysfunction may be explained by their inability to repair double-strand DNA breaks caused by platinum-based chemotherapy. As we mentioned above, although the comparison of prognostic benefit between the BRCA1 and BRCA2 mutation was not feasible, the aggregated HR for OS

for BRCA2 mutants was lower than that for BRCA1 mutants. It has been established by several research groups that BRCA2-mutated cells are recombination deficient and undergo significantly reduced homologous recombination repair of DNA double-strand breaks [13,53]. Functionally, the primary function of BRCA2 appears to be regulation of the RAD51 protein, which is required for double-strand break repair by homologous recombination [10], indicating that BRCA2 lesions cause more substantial homologous recombination defects than BRCA1 lesions, because BRCA1 is more versatile. However, to date, there are no reports regarding the association between low BRCA2 expression and the prognosis of patients with sporadic EOCs. So, large population-based studies are urgently needed to discover the proportion of low BRCA2 expression patients among sporadic EOCs and the real role of low BRCA2 expression status on survival.

Our results may have important implications for the clinical management of EOCs. Ovarian carcinoma is clinically highly heterogeneous. Our study revealed that both BRCA1/2 mutations and low BRCA1 expression are associated with favourable survival in EOC, so, these BRCA statuses can guide choice of post-operative treatment decisions. Additionally, it has been demonstrated that a deficiency of the BRCA gene confers substantial sensitivity to a new class of agents, namely poly-ADP-ribose polymerase-1 (PARP1) inhibitors [13,14]. A number of phase I and II studies have reported the successful applications of PARP inhibitors in BRCA1/2 mutation carries of ovarian and breast cancer, and phase III studies are underway [13,14,54]. So, routine testing BRCA1/2 germline mutation status of EOCs may now be warranted. A large proportion of sporadic EOCs demonstrate BRCA deficiency, whether these patients could also benefit from PARP1 inhibitor are still unclear. Moreover, a reliable assay to detect these patients is required. Our meta-analysis supports the IHC technique as a promising assay to detect a portion of sporadic ovarian cancer displaying BRCAness. Although RT-PCR may also be a potential assay to discover the BRCAness, the supporting positive literature was limited and without standard experimental protocols and uniform cut-off values. Large prospective clinical trials are expected for further validation.

In conclusion, EOCs patients with BRCA dysfunction status have better outcomes, but more fundamental studies and further prospective clinical studies are urgently needed. Furthermore, EOCs should be stratified by different BRCA statuses to specifically define the most effective treatment for the separate patient groups in further clinical studies.

Supporting Information

File S1 Contains the following files: **Method S1:** The quality score for methodology modified according to the European Lung Cancer Working Party (ELCWP) scoring scale [1]. **Table S1:** Main characteristics and results of eligible studies. **Table S2:** Methodological assessment.

Checklist S1 PRISMA checklist.

Author Contributions

Conceived and designed the experiments: GC DM. Performed the experiments: NL. Analyzed the data: CYS DHW. Contributed reagents/materials/analysis tools: DD LM. Wrote the paper: CYS.

References

1. Jemal A, Siegel R, Xu J, Ward E (2010) Cancer statistics, 2010. CA Cancer J Clin 60: 277–300.
2. (2011) Ovarian cancer, five-year stage-specific relative survival rates (2004–2008). J Natl Cancer Inst 103: 1287.
3. Rubin SC, Benjamin I, Behbakht K, Takahashi H, Morgan MA, et al. (1996) Clinical and pathological features of ovarian cancer in women with germ- line mutations of BRCA1. New England Journal of Medicine 335: 1413–1416.
4. Gallagher DJ, Konner JA, Bell-McGuinn KM, Bhatia J, Sabbatini P, et al. (2011) Survival in epithelial ovarian cancer: a multivariate analysis incorporating BRCA mutation status and platinum sensitivity. Ann Oncol 22: 1127–1132.
5. Vencken PM, Kriege M, Hoogwerf D, Beugelink S, van der Burg ME, et al. (2011) Chemosensitivity and outcome of BRCA1- and BRCA2-associated ovarian cancer patients after first-line chemotherapy compared with sporadic ovarian cancer patients. Ann Oncol 22: 1346–1352.
6. Johannsson OT, Ranstam J, Borg A, Olsson H (1998) Survival of BRCA1 breast and ovarian cancer patients: a population-based study from southern Sweden. J Clin Oncol 16: 397–404.
7. Tan DS, Rothermundt C, Thomas K, Bancroft E, Eeles R, et al. (2008) "BRCAness" syndrome in ovarian cancer: a case-control study describing the clinical features and outcome of patients with epithelial ovarian cancer associated with BRCA1 and BRCA2 mutations. J Clin Oncol 26: 5530–5536.
8. Yang D, Khan S, Sun Y, Hess K, Shmulevich I, et al. (2011) Association of BRCA1 and BRCA2 mutations with survival, chemotherapy sensitivity, and gene mutator phenotype in patients with ovarian cancer. JAMA 306: 1557–1565.
9. Bhattacharyya A, Ear US, Koller BH, Weichselbaum RR, Bishop DK (2000) The breast cancer susceptibility gene BRCA1 is required for subnuclear assembly of Rad51 and survival following treatment with the DNA cross-linking agent cisplatin. J Biol Chem 275: 23899–23903.
10. Davies AA, Masson JY, McIlwraith MJ, Stasiak AZ, Stasiak A, et al. (2001) Role of BRCA2 in control of the RAD51 recombination and DNA repair protein. Mol Cell 7: 273–282.
11. Kowalczykowski SC (2002) Molecular mimicry connects BRCA2 to Rad51 and recombinational DNA repair. Nat Struct Biol 9: 897–899.
12. Cooke SL, Brenton JD (2011) Evolution of platinum resistance in high-grade serous ovarian cancer. Lancet Oncol 12: 1169–1174.
13. Audeh MW, Carmichael J, Penson RT, Friedlander M, Powell B, et al. (2010) Oral poly(ADP-ribose) polymerase inhibitor olaparib in patients with BRCA1 or BRCA2 mutations and recurrent ovarian cancer: a proof-of-concept trial. Lancet 376: 245–251.
14. Fong PC, Boss DS, Yap TA, Tutt A, Wu P, et al. (2009) Inhibition of poly(ADP-ribose) polymerase in tumors from BRCA mutation carriers. N Engl J Med 361: 123–134.
15. Weberpals JI, Tu D, Squire JA, Amin MS, Islam S, et al. (2011) Breast cancer 1 (BRCA1) protein expression as a prognostic marker in sporadic epithelial ovarian carcinoma: an NCIC CTG OV.16 correlative study. Ann Oncol.
16. Steels E, Paesmans M, Berghmans T, Branle F, Lemaitre F, et al. (2001) Role of p53 as a prognostic factor for survival in lung cancer: a systematic review of the literature with a meta-analysis. Eur Respir J 18: 705–719.
17. Parmar MK, Torri V, Stewart L (1998) Extracting summary statistics to perform meta-analyses of the published literature for survival endpoints. Stat Med 17: 2815–2834.
18. Yusuf S, Peto R, Lewis J, Collins R, Sleight P (1985) Beta blockade during and after myocardial infarction: an overview of the randomized trials. Prog Cardiovasc Dis 27: 335–371.
19. Sterne JA, Egger M (2001) Funnel plots for detecting bias in meta-analysis: guidelines on choice of axis. J Clin Epidemiol 54: 1046–1055.
20. Carser JE, Quinn JE, Michie CO, O'Brien EJ, McCluggage WG, et al. (2011) BRCA1 is both a prognostic and predictive biomarker of response to chemotherapy in sporadic epithelial ovarian cancer. Gynecol Oncol.
21. Kaern J, Aghmesheh M, Nesland JM, Danielsen HE, Sandstad B, et al. (2005) Prognostic factors in ovarian carcinoma stage III patients. Can biomarkers improve the prediction of short- and long-term survivors? International Journal of Gynecological Cancer 15: 1014–1022.
22. Buller RE, Shahin MS, Geisler JP, Zogg M, De Young BR, et al. (2002) Failure of BRCA1 dysfunction to alter ovarian cancer survival. Clinical Cancer Research 8: 1196–1202.
23. Boyd J, Sonoda Y, Federici MG, Bogomolniy F, Rhei E, et al. (2000) Clinicopatholic features of BRCA-linked and sporadic ovarian cancer. Journal of the American Medical Association 283: 2260–2265.
24. Aida H, Takakuwa K, Nagata H, Tsuneki I, Takano M, et al. (1998) Clinical features of ovarian cancer in Japanese women with germ-line mutations of BRCA1. Clinical Cancer Research 4: 235–240.
25. Cass I, Baldwin RL, Varkey T, Moslehi R, Narod SA, et al. (2003) Improved survival in women with BRCA-associated ovarian carcinoma. Cancer 97: 2187–2195.
26. Chetrit A, Hirsh-Yechezkel G, Ben-David Y, Lubin F, Friedman E, et al. (2008) Effect of BRCA1/2 mutations on long-term survival of patients with invasive ovarian cancer: The National Israeli Study of Ovarian Cancer. Journal of Clinical Oncology 26: 20–25.
27. Wiley A, Katsaros D, Chen H, Rigault de la Longrais IA, Beeghly A, et al. (2006) Aberrant promoter methylation of multiple genes in malignant ovarian tumors and in ovarian tumors with low malignant potential. Cancer 107: 299–308.
28. Weberpals J, Garbuio K, O'Brien A, Clark-Knowles K, Doucette S, et al. (2009) The DNA repair proteins BRCA1 and ERCC1 as predictive markers in sporadic ovarian cancer. Int J Cancer 124: 806–815.
29. Zweemer RP, Verheijen RH, Menko FH, Gille JJ, van Diest PJ, et al. (1999) Differences between hereditary and sporadic ovarian cancer. Eur J Obstet Gynecol Reprod Biol 82: 151–153.
30. Chiang JW, Karlan BY, Cass l, Baldwin RL (2006) BRCA1 promoter methylation predicts adverse ovarian cancer prognosis. Gynecologic Oncology 101: 403–410.
31. Quinn JE, James CR, Stewart GE, Mulligan JM, White P, et al. (2007) BRCA1 mRNA expression levels predict for overall survival in ovarian cancer after chemotherapy. Clin Cancer Res 13: 7413–7420.
32. Thrall M, Gallion HH, Kryscio R, Kapali M, Armstrong DK, et al. (2006) BRCA1 expression in a large series of sporadic ovarian carcinomas: a Gynecologic Oncology Group study. Int J Gynecol Cancer 16 Suppl 1: 166–171.
33. Swisher EM, Gonzalez RM, Taniguchi T, Garcia RL, Walsh T, et al. (2009) Methylation and protein expression of DNA repair genes: association with chemotherapy exposure and survival in sporadic ovarian and peritoneal carcinomas. Mol Cancer 8: 48.
34. Pharoah PD, Easton DF, Stockton DL, Gayther S, Ponder BA (1999) Survival in familial, BRCA1-associated, and BRCA2-associated epithelial ovarian cancer. United Kingdom Coordinating Committee for Cancer Research (UKCCCR) Familial Ovarian Cancer Study Group. Cancer Res 59: 868–871.
35. Brozek I, Ochman K, Debniak J, Morzuch L, Ratajska M, et al. (2008) High frequency of BRCA1/2 germline mutations in consecutive ovarian cancer patients in Poland. Gynecologic Oncology 108: 433–437.
36. Zweemer RP, Verheijen RH, Coebergh JW, Jacobs IJ, van Diest PJ, et al. (2001) Survival analysis in familial ovarian cancer, a case control study. European journal of obstetrics, gynecology, and reproductive biology 98: 219–223.
37. Ramus SJ, Fishman A, Pharoah PD, Yarkoni S, Altaras M, et al. (2001) Ovarian cancer survival in Ashkenazi Jewish patients with BRCA1 and BRCA2 mutations. Eur J Surg Oncol 27: 278–281.
38. Radosa MP, Hafner N, Camara O, Diebolder H, Mothes A, et al. (2011) Loss of BRCA1 Protein Expression as Indicator of the BRCAness Phenotype Is Associated With Favorable Overall Survival After Complete Resection of Sporadic Ovarian Cancer. Int J Gynecol Cancer.
39. Artioli G, Borgato L, Cappetta A, Wabersich J, Mocellin S, et al. (2010) Overall survival in BRCA-associated ovarian cancer: Case-control study of an Italian series. European Journal of Gynaecological Oncology 31: 658–661.
40. Lacour RA, Westin SN, Meyer LA, Wingo SN, Schorge JO, et al. (2011) Improved survival in non-Ashkenazi Jewish ovarian cancer patients with BRCA1 and BRCA2 gene mutations. Gynecologic Oncology 121: 358–363.
41. Majdak EJ, Debniak J, Milczek T, Cornelisse CJ, Devilee P, et al. (2005) Prognostic impact of BRCA1 pathogenic and BRCA1/BRCA2 unclassified variant mutations in patients with ovarian carcinoma. Cancer 104: 1004–1012.
42. David YB, Chetrit A, Hirsh-Yechezkel G, Friedman E, Beck BD, et al. (2002) Effect of BRCA mutations on the length of survival in epithelial ovarian tumors. Journal of Clinical Oncology 20: 463–466.
43. Hennessy BTJ, Timms KM, Carey MS, Gutin A, Meyer LA, et al. (2010) Somatic mutations in BRCA1 and BRCA2 could expand the number of patients that benefit from poly (ADP ribose) polymerase inhibitors in ovarian cancer. Journal of Clinical Oncology 28: 3570–3576.
44. Pal T, Permuth-Wey J, Kapoor R, Cantor A, Sutphen R (2007) Improved survival in BRCA2 carriers with ovarian cancer. Familial Cancer 6: 113–119.
45. Sirisabya N, Manchana T, Termrungreunglert W, Triratanachat S, Charuruks N, et al. (2007) Prevalence of BRCA1 expression in epithelial ovarian cancer: Immunohistochemical study. Journal of the Medical Association of Thailand 90: 9–14.
46. Yu M, Hao J, Jiao Z (2005) A study on the expression of BRCA1 & P53 and their correlation in epithelial ovarian cancer. Chinese Journal of Clinical Oncology 32: 18–20.
47. Alsop K, Fereday S, Meldrum C, deFazio A, Emmanuel C, et al. (2012) BRCA mutation frequency and patterns of treatment response in BRCA mutation-positive women with ovarian cancer: a report from the Australian Ovarian Cancer Study Group. J Clin Oncol 30: 2654–2663.
48. Dann RB, DeLoia JA, Timms KM, Zorn KK, Potter J, et al. (2012) BRCA1/2 mutations and expression: response to platinum chemotherapy in patients with advanced stage epithelial ovarian cancer. Gynecol Oncol 125: 677–682.
49. Gan A, Green AR, Nolan CC, Martin S, Deen S (2013) Poly(adenosine diphosphate-ribose) polymerase expression in BRCA-proficient ovarian high-grade serous carcinoma; association with patient survival. Hum Pathol 44: 1638–1647.
50. Hyman DM, Long KC, Tanner EJ, Grisham RN, Arnold AG, et al. (2012) Outcomes of primary surgical cytoreduction in patients with BRCA-associated high-grade serous ovarian carcinoma. Gynecol Oncol 126: 224–228.

51. McLaughlin JR, Rosen B, Moody J, Pal T, Fan I, et al. (2013) Long-term ovarian cancer survival associated with mutation in BRCA1 or BRCA2. J Natl Cancer Inst 105: 141–148.

52. Bolton KL, Chenevix-Trench G, Goh C, Sadetzki S, Ramus SJ, et al. (2012) Association between BRCA1 and BRCA2 mutations and survival in women with invasive epithelial ovarian cancer. JAMA 307: 382–390.

53. Kortmann U, McAlpine JN, Xue H, Guan J, Ha G, et al. (2011) Tumor growth inhibition by olaparib in BRCA2 germline-mutated patient-derived ovarian cancer tissue xenografts. Clin Cancer Res 17: 783–791.

54. Kummar S, Chen A, Ji J, Zhang Y, Reid JM et al. (2011) Phase I study of PARP inhibitor ABT-888 in combination with topotecan in adults with refractory solid tumors and lymphomas. Cancer Res 71: 5626–5634.

16

Exome-Wide Somatic Microsatellite Variation Is Altered in Cells with DNA Repair Deficiencies

Zalman Vaksman[1], Natalie C. Fonville[1], Hongseok Tae[1¤], Harold R. Garner[1,2*]

1 Virginia Bioinformatics Institute, Virginia Tech, Blacksburg, Virginia, 24061, United States of America, 2 Genomeon LLC, Floyd, Virginia, 24091, United States of America

Abstract

Microsatellites (MST), tandem repeats of 1–6 nucleotide motifs, are mutational hot-spots with a bias for insertions and deletions (INDELs) rather than single nucleotide polymorphisms (SNPs). The majority of MST instability studies are limited to a small number of loci, the Bethesda markers, which are only informative for a subset of colorectal cancers. In this paper we evaluate non-haplotype alleles present within next-gen sequencing data to evaluate somatic MST variation (SMV) within DNA repair proficient and DNA repair defective cell lines. We confirm that alleles present within next-gen data that do not contribute to the haplotype can be reliably quantified and utilized to evaluate the SMV without requiring comparisons of matched samples. We observed that SMV patterns found in DNA repair proficient cell lines without DNA repair defects, MCF10A, HEK293 and PD20 RV:D2, had consistent patterns among samples. Further, we were able to confirm that changes in SMV patterns in cell lines lacking functional BRCA2, FANCD2 and mismatch repair were consistent with the different pathways perturbed. Using this new exome sequencing analysis approach we show that DNA instability can be identified in a sample and that patterns of instability vary depending on the impaired DNA repair mechanism, and that genes harboring minor alleles are strongly associated with cancer pathways. The MST Minor Allele Caller used for this study is available at https://github.com/zalmanv/MST_minor_allele_caller.

Editor: Michael Shing-Yan Huen, The University of Hong Kong, Hong Kong

Funding: This work was funded by the Virginia Bioinformatics Institute Medical Informatics Systems Division director's funds, Virginia Bioinformatics Institute Genomics Research Lab Small Grant (CLF-1172), high performance computing was supported by a grant from the National Science Foundation (OCI-1124123) and NSF S-STEM grant (DUE-0850198). This work was supported by these 4 funds. The first two funds were internal university funds (Virginia Tech), and the latter two were from the National Science Foundation (NSF). None had a role in the study design, data collection and analysis, decision to publish, or preparation of the manuscript. These funds supported portions of author salaries and benefits, computer costs, laboratory supplies, sequencing services, publication costs, and overhead (indirect expenses to the university).

Competing Interests: HT currently works at Caris Life Sciences; the work for this paper was done when he was employed at Virginia Tech and is in no way connected to his current employment. Harold Garner is owner and founder of Genomeon, however Genomeon was not involved in funding or directing this work.

* Email: garner@vbi.vt.edu

¤ Current address: Bioinformatics group, Caris Life Sciences, Phoenix, Arizona, 85040, United States of America.

Introduction

Microsatellites (MSTs) are regions of repetitive DNA at which 1–6 nucleotides are tandemly repeated; and are present ubiquitously throughout the genome, both in gene and intergenic regions. Observations of somatic variation in MSTs have demonstrated that MST mutation rates are between 10 and 1000 time higher than that of surrounding DNA [1,2], rendering microsatellites mutational "hot-spots" [3,4]. The increased mutational rate of MSTs is thought to be primarily due DNA polymerase slippage and mis-alignment of the slipped structure due to local homology [5–7]. This difference in primary mutational mechanism suggests that, unlike non-repetitive DNA whose mutational spectrum is primarily SNPs, microsatellites are more prone to INDELs [4,7,8]. Specifically MSTs are prone to INDELs that are 'in-phase' or result in expansion or contraction by complete repeat units. For example, a dimer microsatellite will typically expand or contract by 2N nucleotides while a trimer will expand or contract by 3N [1].

MSTs are found in and around a significant number of coding and promoter regions and specific microsatellite variations have been linked to over 40 disorders, such as the CAG microsatellite whose expansion is associated with Huntington's disease and the CGG repeat whose expansion is associated with Fragile X [1,9]. In addition, a more general increase in MST instability has been associated with colon cancer, which, if detected, results in better prognosis and can influence treatment [10,11]. Currently, MST instability is clinically defined based on the results of a kit that tests somatic variation of 18–21 "susceptible" loci (PowerPlex 21, Promega). Although the test has been shown to be effective for identifying MST unstable colon cancer [12], it is significantly less effective for most other disorders including other cancers [13–15]. The ability to capture and discern variation patterns exome-wide would provide a more accurate and useful clinical data for a broader range of disorders. In recent reports next-gen sequencing has been used to uncover MST instability in intestinal and endometrial cancers by observing genotype changes in MSTs between tumor and healthy tissue [14,15].

The goal of this research was to identify patterns of somatic variation in MSTs as a possible marker for genomic instability. We hypothesize that the variable nature of MSTs and the quantification of minor allele content makes them ideal candidates for in-depth next-gen analysis and that somatic variation of microsatellite loci can be quantified using high-depth sequencing. A broadening of the definition of MST instability to include changes in somatic variability and using an exome/genome-wide approach may enable a more accurate diagnosis of patients then what is currently provided by PowerPlex 21.

Somatic variability, novel genomic polymorphisms that arise within a cell population not found in the progenitors, plays a critical role in cellular reprogramming leading to the development and progression of cancer [16]. Suppression of mutations is essential for genomic stability, therefore cells have evolved multiple mechanisms to repair damaged or unpaired nucleotides [17,18]. Currently the only established DNA repair defect that that has been directly linked to MST instability is mismatch repair (MMR). MMR impairments have been shown to increase somatic variation at MSTs in both cell lines and tumors [19–21]. Although the role other DNA repair mechanisms such as inter-strand crosslink repair (as seen in Fanconi anemia genes) and homologous recombination (HR) play in MST instability is less clear, both are important for genomic and chromosomal stability (reviewed by [22,23]).

In this study we first show that we can robustly detect signatures of MST mutation bias and somatic variation occurring in cell lines in next-gen data including a high frequency of in-phase INDELs. We are then able to construct a pattern of somatic MST variation (SMV) by using DNA repair proficient cell lines. Our results indicate that ~5% of microsatellite loci show somatic variation, i.e. have at least one additional non-haplotype allele present. Finally, we are able to differentiate between cell lines with known defects in various DNA repair mechanisms (mismatch repair, DNA crosslink repair, homologous recombination), which correlate with an altered distribution of loci with non-haplotype alleles. These findings suggest that signatures that distinctly define specific defective DNA repair mechanisms can be gleaned from next-gen sequencing data and that this information has the potential to be utilized for detection of individuals with altered levels of somatic variation that are at increased risk of disease or the evaluation of patient's tumor that may yield clinically actionable information.

Methods

Cells, DNA prep and sequencing

HEK (human embryonic kidney) and MCF10A (immortalized breast epithelial) and HEK293 (human embryonic kidney) cells were obtained from ATCC. PD20 and PD20 RV:D2 (FANCD2 and FANCD2 retrovirally corrected) cell lines were obtained from the Fanconi Anemia Foundation (Eugene OR). Sequencing data for Capan-1 cells was previously published by Barber and coworkers [12].

PD20, PD20 RV:D2 and HEK293 cells were grown at 37°C with 5% CO_2, in DMEM supplemented with 10% FBS (Invitrogen) and 1X pen/strep (Invitrogen) to 80% confluence. MCF10A cells were grown to confluence in DMEM/F12 medium (Invitrogen, Carlsbad, CA), supplemented with 5% horse serum (Invitrogen), antibiotics- 1X Pen/Strep (Invitrogen), 20 ng/mL EGF (Peprotech, Rocky Hill, NJ), 0.5 mg/mL hydrocortisone (Sigma), 100 ng/mL cholera toxin (Sigma), and 10 µg/mL insulin (Sigma) at 37°C with 5% CO_2. All cell lines were collected by trypsinazation and prepared for DNA extraction. DNA was extracted using the Qiagen DNAeasy kit (Qiagen) as per manufacturers instructions.

Since PD20 RV:D2 were derived from PD20 cells by retroviral insertion of the corrected FANCD2 gene we confirmed the maintenance of the corrected version using the sequencing data. Further, a comparison of growth-curves showed an order of magnitude more cells 48 hours after exposure to the DNA interstrand cross-linker Cisplatin, confirming a partial rescue phenotype.

Sequencing and analysis pipeline

Exome paired-end libraries were prepared using the Agilent (Chicago, IL) SureSelectXT Human All Exon V4 capture library. 2×100 bp reads were obtained using an Illumina (San Diego, CA) HiSeq 2500 instrument in Rapid Run mode on a HiSeq Rapid v1 flowcell. Indexed reads were de-multiplexed with CASAVA v1.8.2.

Paired-end sequencing reads were trimmed using fastX_Toolkit and aligned to HG19/GRCh37 human reference genome (http://www.genome.ucsc.edu) using BWA-mem. The output was then sorted, indexed and PCR duplicates were removed using SAMTOOLS [24]. Bam files were then locally realigned and target loci marked using GATK IndelRealigner and TargetIntervals. MST alleles were retrieved and analyzed using software described in the next section.

Microsatellite minor-allele software

A catalogue of MST loci was generated from the HG19/GRCh37 reference genome using Tandem Repeats Finder [25] (with the following parameters: 2.7.7.80.10.18.6). The list was filtered to remove any loci that were shorter than 8 nucleotides, had less than 3 copies of a given motif unit or were below 85% sequence purity. Duplicated loci were identified based on sequence purity and sequence length and were removed.

MSTs were analyzed using a custom MST minor-allele caller based on GenoTan and ReviSTER software [26,27], which were developed by this group to improve MST haplotype predictions (https://github.com/zalmanv/MST_minor_allele_caller). The minor-allele caller extracts marked MSTs from bam files using SAMTOOLs. MST loci are called based on predicted alignments and an adjustable length flanking sequence (this study used either 5 or 7 nucleotide sequence). Reads with low base call scores (below a base score of 28) for nucleotides within the repeats and those with mapping quality score below 10% were eliminated. Alleles are initially called only when two or more reads, verified in both directions of a paired-end run, have the same sequence. All alleles for a given locus are binned with the number of supporting paired-end reads. The final number of alleles is computed based on a user specified minimal requirement of substantiating reads (for this study the minimum number of substantiating reads is either 2 or 3 reads per allele). If more than one allele per locus was found, zygosity and the sequence length difference from the most common allele were recorded. Heterozygotic loci were called using the following criteria as described and confirmed in the GenoTan and ReviSTER manuscripts [26,27]: 1) it is the second most common allele, 2) The number of confirming reads is greater than 25% of the total reads for the locus or greater than 50% of the depth for the most common allele, if the total is below 25% of the total depth.

In addition to MST loci, we also generated a somatic variability profile for non-MST loci. To make the data comparable we randomly selected 3 million loci, each consisting of 15 nucleotides segments, from the HG19 genome. We then filtered out any loci that intersected with our MST and were left with over 2 million loci. The same pipeline as for MSTs was used to generate the data for non-MST loci. This data yielded information on the number of loci with minor alleles and type of mutation (SNPs and INDELs).

Sequence validation and allele calls validated by independent Sanger sequencing method

The MST minor-allele caller we use in this paper is a modified version of a published and experimentally verified code, however to further validate the multi-allele capability of the modified code 30 loci, including 17 showing multiple alleles, were verified using Sanger sequencing. Figure S1A in file S1 shows the data from the minor-allele caller output at one of these loci, chr10:72639137-72639161, at which we would predict at least 3 alleles to be present in this sample (MCF10A) with lengths of 21, 23, and 25 nucleotides. Sanger sequencing confirmed that multiple alleles were present, with the alleles being greater than 21 nucleotides long (figure S1B in file S1). Of the 30 loci 28 loci verified the genotype and 14 of 17 loci with minor alleles also had visible minor alleles by Sanger sequencing.

Modeling error rates to establish rules that differentiate errors from high confidence minor alleles

Two methods were used to generate models of NGS runs for chromosomes 17 and 21; 1) Wgsim (https://github.com/lh3/wgsim) a commonly used paired-end read generator and 2) in-house designed generator. Both methods were set to have a per nucleotide error rate between 0.5% and 5%. The major difference between the two methods was that wgsim was used to obtain modeling data with fairly similar coverage (read depth) across the reference chromosome while the lab-designed algorithm allowed for a more variable coverage as is observed in a typical next-gen sequencing run. The generated fastq files were run through the same pipeline as actual real sequencing data. The accuracy of the pipeline was analyzed by the verification of the predicted alignment. Predicted error rates ranged between 1.3% and 1.9%, with the majority of errors due to misalignments.

Results

We modified a previously published and verified MST genotyper [26] to enumerate all possible alleles present within next-gen data, as opposed to only capturing the most common (haplotype) alleles. We first characterized the error which may cause false positive allele calls via a parametric sensitivity study conducted on *in-silico* generated data, and showed that our measure can then be used to accurately quantify minor alleles and thus be used to distinguish between mutational mechanisms that are exhibited in different cell lines. To accomplish this, we establish a baseline SMV profile from DNA repair proficient cell lines, and compared this to what is seen in cell lines with various DNA repair defects.

Characterizing the effect of sequencing error on minority allele calling

This analysis evaluates each MST locus to establish the one or two alleles that define the genotype, then it robustly calls additional non-haplotype or 'minor' alleles that are present at lower frequency within next-gen data. However, the accuracy of such minority allele calls can be significantly affected by sequencing errors found within the raw reads that map to each locus. To minimize the number of false positive 'alleles', we first established the minimal number of reads necessary for confirming

an allele in the presence of typical next-gen errors. It has been established by a number of studies that 3 reads mapped to a loci is sufficient to properly call major alleles [28–30]. To corroborate this, we created an *in-silico* sequencing data set for chromosomes 21 and 17, with randomly generated errors ranging from 0.5% to 5% which mimicked next-gen sequencing data in both the error types that were created and read coverage per locus (results depicted in figure 1).

We first determined the parameters required to optimize the measurement of the fraction of loci *without* minor alleles in sequencing data with the above-mentioned error rates. Alignment and zygosity calling accuracy is displayed in table S1 in file S1. The sequencing data generator produced between 8 and 10.5 million reads that contained over 58,000 targeted MSTs. Over 98.5% of the reads mapped correctly with an accuracy of over 99.8% in coding regions (regions captured by exome sequencing). The accuracy of zygosity calls was over 99.98% for all error rates. Next we varied the minimum number of reads covering a locus required to call an allele. Changing the threshold from 2 confirming reads (figure 1A) to 3 confirming reads (figure 1B) statistically and significantly decreased the fraction of loci with more alleles than the haplotype number (1 if homozygotic or 2 if heterozygotic). Using a threshold of 2 confirming reads per allele, the fraction of loci without minor alleles identified (due to sequencing errors being interpreted as alleles) was 19–62% for simulated data sets with error rates ranging between 5%–0.5% respectively (figure 1A), indicating that requiring only 2 reads to identify an allele leads to a high level of false alleles. By increasing the threshold to 3 confirming reads the percent of loci without minor alleles increases to 73–99% for the same data set (figure 1B). By increasing to 4 confirming reads per allele we further increase the number of loci without minor alleles 87%–99% (figure S2A in file S1). However, at error rates close to the actual HiSeq rates (of ~1%), we only saw a modest increase in the number of loci without minor alleles, a change from 97% (3 reads per allele) to 99% (4 reads per allele). This is in contrast to an increase from 61% with 2 reads per allele to 97% with 3 confirming reads per allele.

We next examined how sequencing error might affect the number of alleles present in our data. To do this we used modeling data with error rates similar to the actual HiSeq error rate (1%) and 2.5% error (figure 2), and determined the average read depth per locus with increasing alleles. For the *in-silico* generated data, we found a linear increase in the total read depth as the number of alleles increased (using 2–4 confirming reads per allele) up to 8 alleles (figures 2 and Figure S2 in File S1). A comparison of these results to actual sequencing data from our cell lines (discussed in more detail later) shows that when 3 or more reads are required to confirm an allele, the number of alleles called for a given read depth is greater than what would be expected from error, even at a rate of 2.5% which is substantially more than the observed next-gen error rate of 1% (figure 2B and Figure S2B in File S1), i.e. more alleles are called at a lower read depth in the actual data than would be present due to error. Based on these results, requiring a minimum of 3 reads covering a locus to confirm an allele minimizes the number of 'false' alleles being identified due to sequencing error.

Polymerase slippage vs. nucleotide misincorporation

Another potential source of error in calling alleles from sequencing data is amplification errors induced during the library preparation process [31]. These errors would likely be present at higher frequency than errors generated during sequencing [31,32]; therefore cannot be minimized by solely increasing the minimum

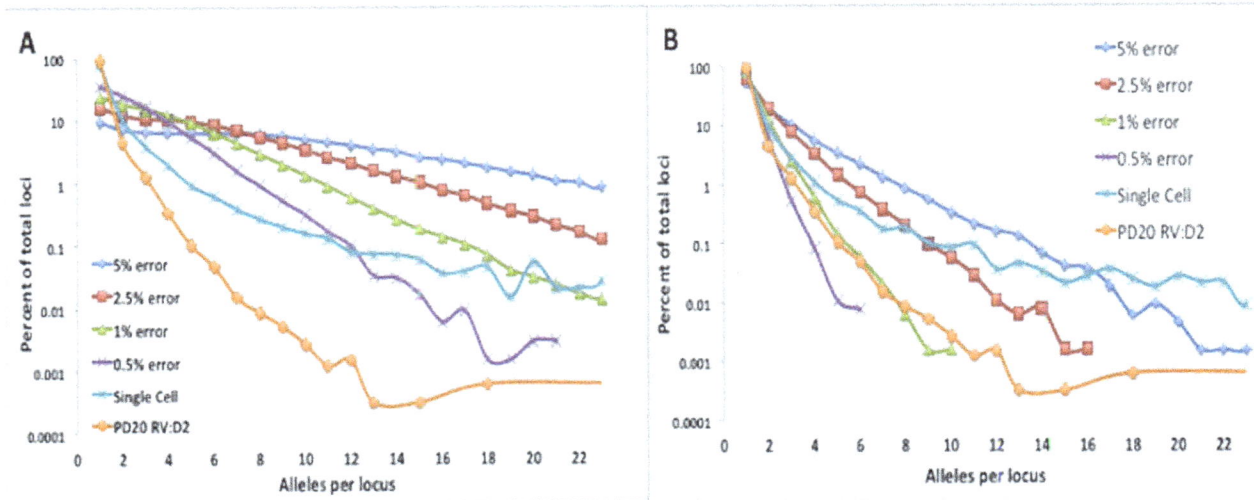

Figure 1. Effects of sequencing error and the minimum number of reads required to call an allele on the number of alleles called in sequencing data. Modeling data with different error frequencies (0.5%–5%) showed an increase in loci with multiple alleles as error increased when both 2 (A) and 3 (B) reads were minimally required to call an allele. In contrast, standard exome sequencing data from DNA repair proficient cells (PD20 RV:D2 cells) and exome sequencing after whole genome amplification from a single cell were insensitive to the cut-off used.

read coverage (as above). Somatic mutation of MSTs is primarily associated with polymerase slippage [33,34], which is thought to cause the characteristic INDEL bias [31,35,36]. In contrast, nucleotide mis-incorporation errors during in-vitro amplification would be predicted to lead primarily to SNPs in sequencing data [37]. Both of the mentioned DNA synthesis methods would lead to an increase in the number of loci with non-haplotype alleles, however with a predicted variation pattern that is distinctly different. To differentiate between the two predicted SMV patterns including minority alleles, and to assess the influence of nucleotide mis-incorporation/amplification error on our results, we compared a standard exome sequence from cells which are proficient for DNA repair (described later) that did not undergo whole genome amplification (WGA) with data from the sequencing of a single cell [38] which would be expected to have no somatic variation within the sample, but has necessarily undergone WGA to generate the quantity of DNA necessary for sequencing. Therefore, for the WGA sample, presumably all non-haplotype alleles present are due to amplification error. As expected, genome amplification increases the number of loci with non-haplotype alleles (figure 1) to 11.3% and 7% of the total with a threshold of 2 and 3 reads, respectively. The DNA repair proficient cells, which did not undergo extensive amplification, were only decreased by 1.7%, from 7% to 5.3%, by altering the minimum read cutoff. From this it can be concluded that neither errors during library prep nor during the sequencing run account for more than 4 percent of the total non-haplotype alleles detected.

Approximately 85% of mutations found within microsatellite loci in the WGA single-cell data were SNPs, which is expected as a consequence of polymerase errors during amplification. These results were comparable to those predicted by our model, which showed that ~88% of the total minor alleles were composed of alleles carrying SNPs rather than INDELs (Figure 3). In contrast, SNPs account for only 36% (±3.4%) of the total minor alleles in DNA repair proficient cell lines. In addition, although for all the DNA repair proficient cell lines the most common MST motifs with minor alleles observed were mono-nucleotide repeats found within 56%–66% of loci, loci containing tri-nucleotide motifs

accounted for over 55% of the total loci with minor alleles in the WGA data (table S2 in file S1). These results further support the hypothesis that this approach can differentiate between distinct MST mutational profiles: INDELs, particularly at mono-nucleotide runs predominantly reflect DNA repair proficient biological SMV whereas SNPs in MSTs, particularly at tri-nucleotide motif containing loci are predominantly amplification-induced errors or potentially due to altered DNA maintenance capacity. This is further supported by a similar study that has found that the majority of MSTs that are variable within the normal population (individuals sequenced as part of the 1,000 Genomes Project) are predominantly INDELs at mono-nucleotide runs [30].

MST vs non-MST regions

MSTs are considered to be more susceptible to mutations than the surrounding non-repetitive DNA regions [3,14,39]. Because of this, one could expect that non-MST regions would have less somatic variability (non-MST equivalent of SMV) than MST regions. In order to perform a fair comparison with the MST data, 2 million segments consisting of 15 nucleotides each were randomly selected throughout the genome. The same analysis as was performed on loci containing MSTs was also applied to these non-MST regions. It was found that for these non-MST loci the average fraction of loci that were homozygotic was 98.9% with a standard deviation of 0.2, while only 96.7% of the MST containing loci was homozygotic. Even more significant, only 2% (standard deviation of 0.2) of the non-MST loci (homozygotic and heterozygotic) had minor alleles, while 5.1% of the MST loci harbored minor alleles (table 1). Further, a comparison of SNP and INDEL distributions indicated that, unlike MST regions where INDEL variations prevail (64%), SNPs account for the majority (96.9%) of the differences in minor alleles at non-MST loci (table 2). Taken together, these results confirm that, consistent with the literature, MSTs are more susceptible to mutation [2–4,34].

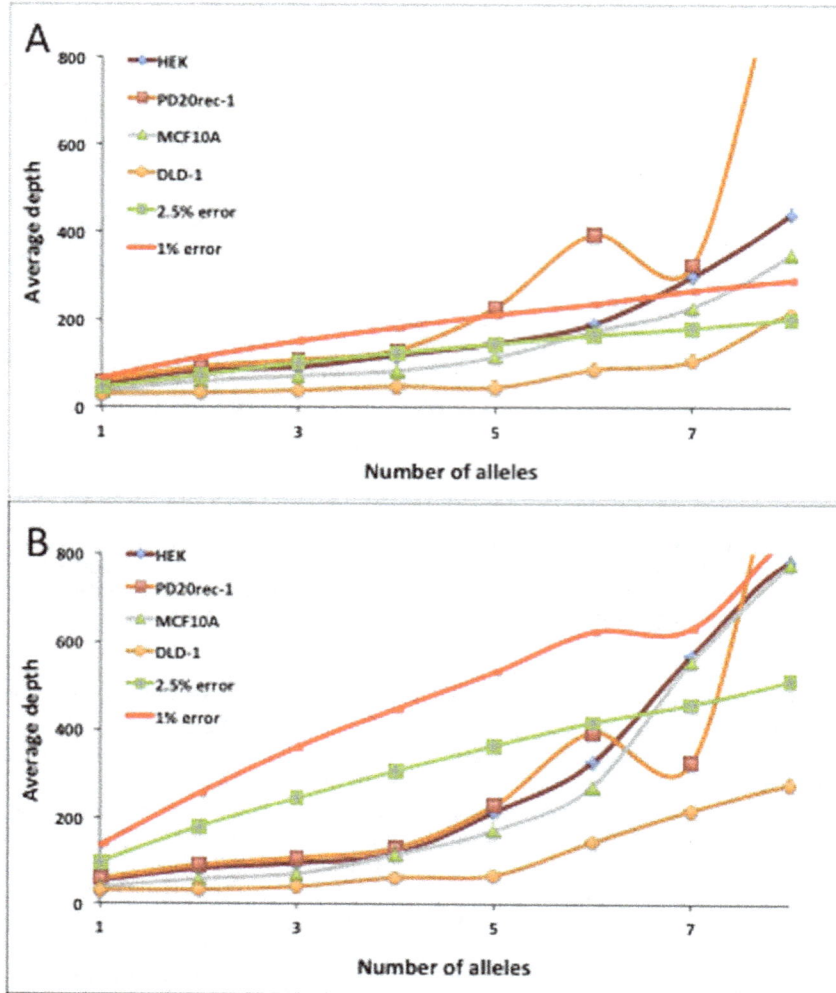

Figure 2. Variation in average depth per locus cannot explain the number of loci with minor alleles. The average read depth at loci with increasing numbers of alleles using A) 2 and B) 3 confirming reads per allele for in-silico generated data using 1% and 2.5% induced error rate for 4 different cell lines.

Reproducibility within a cell line

The objective of this study is to characterize the pattern of SMV from DNA repair proficient cells and then compare to cell populations in which DNA repair is compromised. SMV changes associated with disease will likely be subtle and require highly reproducible control data. To test the reproducibility of SMV measurements within a cell line, two biological replicate cultures of PD20 RV:D2 (PD20 RV:D2-1 and PD20 RV:D2-2) cells were grown separately and sequenced. PD20 RV:D2 are fibroblasts derived from an individual with Fanconi Anemia subgroup D2, retroviraly complimented with a functional copy of FANCD2 [40]. Using a minimum read depth cutoff of 15 to genotype a given loci, we successfully called over 280 K and 250 K loci (at an average depth of 52 and 45 reads per locus) for PD20 RV:D2-1 and 2 respectively. Both samples showed a similar SNP to INDEL ratio, with INDELs making up over ~67% of the minor alleles (table 2). A genotype analysis showed that approximately 96.8% of called loci were homozygous while heterozygosity was observed in ~3.2% of the loci called (table 1). Comparison of those loci that were called in both samples shows that haplotype discordance (i.e. homo- or heterozygotic using standard genotyping) was 1.1%

(table 3), of which 92% were due the fraction of reads supporting a second allele being below the haplotype threshold (see method) and was therefore counted as a minor allele instead of a second haplotype allele, as is the convention in established genotype callers. Only 173 discordant loci were due to sequence differences between the two samples.

For the purpose of this study SMV is defined by the presence of variant MST alleles that are supported by a minimum of 3 confirming reads but do not contribute to haplotype. An analysis of variant MST alleles found a total of 5.4% and 5.3% of MST loci in the PD20 RV:D2-1 and 2 samples, respectively, had 1 or more minor alleles (table 1). The concordance of loci without minor alleles in either sample is 93.9% while 3.4% of loci have at least one minor allele in both samples. By concordance we mean a locus has minor alleles or the same haplotype in multiple samples. Conversely, discordance, where a locus in only one of the compared samples had minor alleles, was 2.7% (table 3). To confirm the significance of these values, we calculated the probabilities of concordance and discordance based on a cohort of randomly selected loci (5.4% and 5.3% of a total samples), which was <0.25% concordant, and compared with our results.

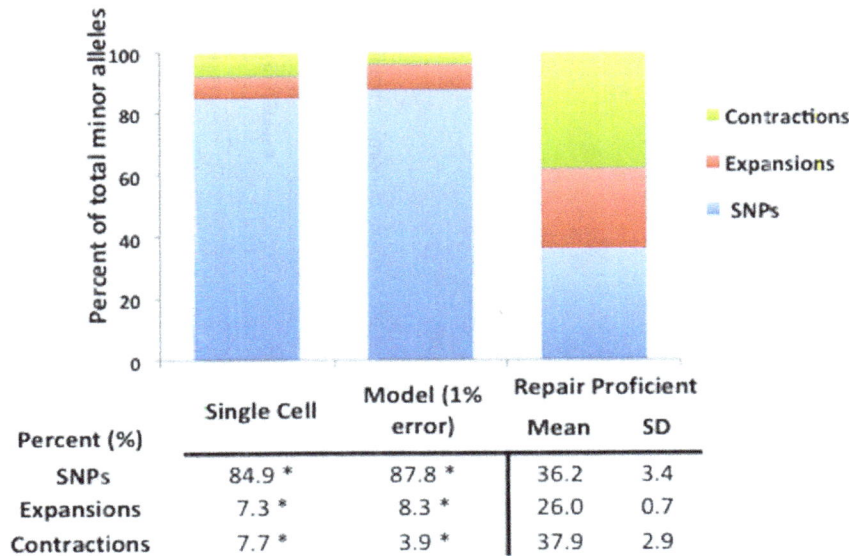

Percent (%)	Single Cell	Model (1% error)	Repair Proficient	
			Mean	SD
SNPs	84.9 *	87.8 *	36.2	3.4
Expansions	7.3 *	8.3 *	26.0	0.7
Contractions	7.7 *	3.9 *	37.9	2.9

Figure 3. DNA repair proficient cells vary significantly from the *in-silico* modeling and single cell sequencing analysis with respect to SNPs and INDELs. The percent of SNPs, expansion and contractions for single cell sequencing and the *in-silico* model as well as the mean and standard deviation for the control cell lines. * significant difference p<0.01.

Using a Pearson's goodness of fit X^2, we verified that the concordant loci are not randomly distributed (p<0.0001). To determine within cell line reproducibility we compared the percent of loci having minor alleles by chromosome as a whole and binned into a million base regions. A linear regression model comparing the percent of loci with minor alleles for each chromosome (as depicted in figure S3 in file S1) shows a significant correlation ($R^2 = 0.85$ and p<0.001) between two independently cultured samples (Figure 4A). Similarly, a comparison of the binned chromosome also shows a significant correlation ($R^2 = 0.60$ and p<0.001, figure 4B). Visualization of the distribution of fraction of MST loci showing somatic variation in a representative chromosome (chr1), depicted in figure 5, indicates specific chromosomal regions that may harbor SMV "hot-spots". An evaluation of MST loci in translated (exon) regions found over 820 genes containing MSTs with a minimum of 2 minor alleles in both PD20 RV:D2 samples, with some of genes found within segments of chromosome 1 with increased SMV depicted in figure 5 (a complete list of exonal MSTs with the minor alleles called, for all cell lines discussed in this paper are available in File S2).

Taken together these results support our hypothesis that this method truly reflects SMV rather than error generated during sequencing and that the results are highly reproducible. The data further suggests that within an individual or cell line, specific genomic regions may contain MSTs that are more susceptible to somatic variability.

Reproducibility between cell lines

To begin to establish a SMV baseline for DNA repair proficient cells, we compared the haplotype, minor allele and SNP/INDEL distributions for two DNA repair proficient cell lines and the PD20 RV:D2 cells discussed above. MCF10A cells are immortalized breast epithelial cells derived from a healthy human female and HEK293 cells are a human embryonic kidney cell line derived from a healthy male fetus. Sequencing produced over 45 million reads with over 170 K microsatellite loci called at an average depth of 42 reads per locus for HEK293 cells and over 190 K

microsatellite loci called at an average depth of 39 reads per locus for MCF10A cells. Considering major alleles only, 96.4% and 97.0% of all MST loci, respectively, are homozygotic (table 1). The average fraction of loci with minor alleles for all three cell lines was 5.1% with a standard deviation of 0.4%. Although MCF10A cells had fewer loci with minor alleles than the PD20 RV:D2 and HEK293 cells (4.5% compared with 5.3% and 5.4% respectively, table 1), and showed a difference in the fraction of secondary alleles with SNPs compare to INDELS (table 2), MCF10A was not considered an outlier (using Grubb's test for outliers). When we compared the haplotype and minor allele concordance between two non-related cell lines, MCF10A and PD20 RV:D2, we found that 3.8% of loci have different genotypes with only 60% due to haplotype differences. For those loci with minor alleles, discordance is 4.0% and concordance is only 2.0%, the result is significantly above what would be anticipated by chance with Pearson's X^2 (i.e. <0.3%,). Interestingly, a full factorial comparison of the fraction of loci with minor alleles for each chromosome (as depicted in figure S4 in file S1), using a linear regression model, found a non-significant correlation ($R^2 = 0.061$ and p<0.23, figure 4C). However, a correlation using the 1 million base bins is significant with an R^2 value of 0.33 and a p<0.0001 (figure 4D), supporting the concept that certain regions contain minor allele susceptibility hot spots. These results demonstrate substantial reproducibility between unrelated independently grown DNA repair proficient cell lines even when the samples are derived from different tissues of origin. These results also suggest that a baseline profile of SMV can be established for DNA repair proficient cells to compare to cell lines with DNA repair defects.

SMV in cells with compromised DNA repair capacity

Thus far we have established that (1) three DNA repair proficient cell lines show similar SMV with low variability both within and between cell lines and that (2) we can differentiate between different SMV trends based on the ratio of INDELs to SNPs. However, the larger goal of this study is to compare SMV

Table 1. Exome sequencing data indicates that MST and non-MST haplotype and somatic polymorphism are reproducible in DNA repair proficient cell lines.

Percent (%)	Microsatellite loci				Repair Proficient		Non-Microsatellite loci				Repair Proficient	
	PD20 RV:D2-1	PD20 RV:D2-2	MCF10A	HEK293	Mean	SD	PD20 RV:D2-1	PD20 RV:D2-2	MCF10A	HEK293	Mean	SD
Homo-zyg	96.8	96.8	96.4	97.0	96.7	0.3	99.0	99.0	98.6	99.1	98.9	0.2
Hetero-zyg	3.2	3.2	3.6	3.0	3.3	0.3	1.0	1.0	1.4	0.9	1.1	0.2
Multi-alleles	5.4	5.3	4.5	5.3	5.1	0.4	1.7	2.0	2.1	2.1	2.0	0.2

Table 2. MST and non-MST containing loci from exome sequencing of DNA repair proficient cells, but not from sequencing of a single cell after whole genome amplification, show the expected high ratio of INDELs (expansions and contractions) to SNPs.

Percent (%)	Microsatellite loci				Repair Proficient		Non-microsatellite loci				Repair Proficient	
	PD20 RV:D2-1	PD20 RV:D2-2	MCF10A	HEK293	Mean	SD	PD20 RV:D2-1	PD20 RV:D2-2	MCF10A	HEK293	Mean	SD
SNPs	33.6	32.7	41.4	36.9	36.2	3.4	96.9	96.6	96.8	97.2	96.9	0.2
Expansions	26.2	27.0	25.3	25.5	26.0	0.7	1.3	1.6	1.6	1.4	1.5	0.1
Contractions	40.3	40.3	33.3	37.5	37.9	2.9	1.8	1.8	1.6	1.3	1.6	0.2

Table 3. Percent concordance/discordance of haplotype and loci with minor alleles for cell lines.

	Genotype	More then haplotype alleles		Haplotype Allele number
	Discordance	Concordance	Discordance	Concordance
PD20 RV:D2-1 & -2	1.06	3.43	2.69	93.88
PD20rec-1 & PD20	1.15	2.50	3.07	94.43
PD20rec-1 & MCF10A	3.79	1.99	3.95	94.10
PD20rec-1 & Capan-1	2.68	1.92	12.68	85.40
MCF10A & Capan-1	2.19	1.24	13.62	85.10

patterns between cell lines representative of healthy individuals and those that may have altered DNA repair capacity. To test this, we evaluated 3 cell lines commonly used to study DNA repair and stability. DLD-1 cells are MST instability (MSI) high colon cancer cell line, impaired in Mismatch repair (MMR), selected as positive controls for this study [41]. Capan-1 cells were sequenced previously [12] and are a BRCA2- cell line that can propagate in culture. PD20 cells are from a FANCD2(-) cell line from which the PD20 RV:D2 cells were derived [40]. Both the Capan-1 cells and the PD20 cells have mutations in genes that are involved in

normal DNA repair (homologous recombination and interstrand crosslink repair, respectively).

For DLD-1 and PD20 cells, the number of loci that passed filters ranged between 185 K and 260 K with an average depth of between of 56 and 62 reads per locus respectively. Only 124 K loci were called for Capan-1 cells, with an average depth of 71 reads per locus. To capture MST differences between the DNA repair proficient and DNA repair defective cell lines we first evaluated haplotypes and the presence of minor alleles for each cell line. Both DLD-1 and Capan-1 cells significantly differ with respect to

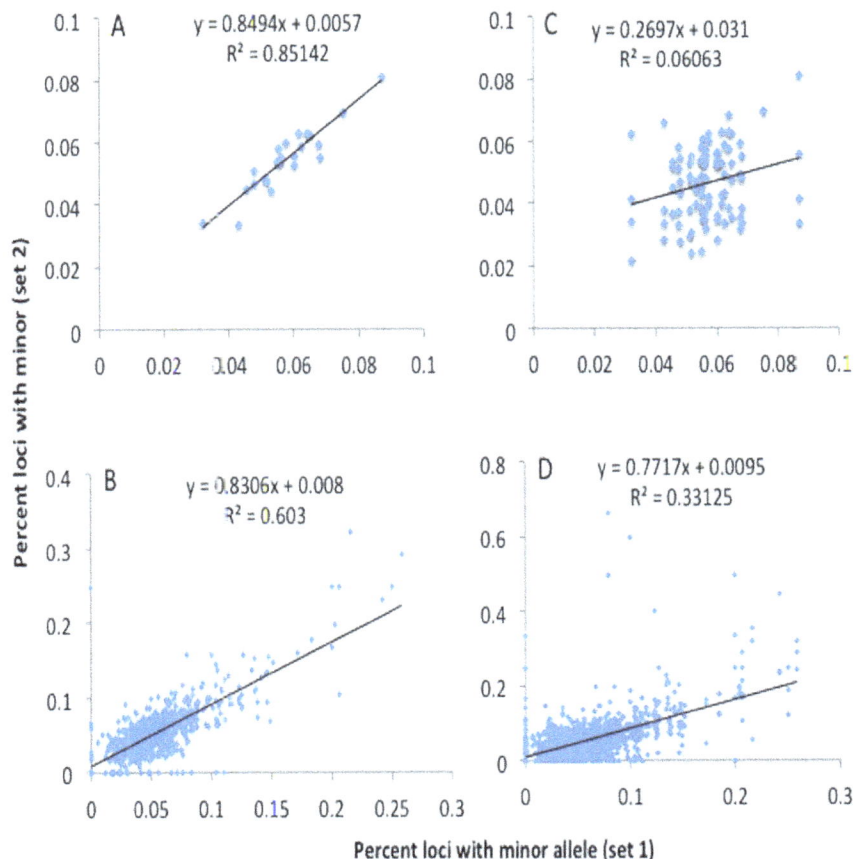

Figure 4. A regression analysis indicates a significant within and between cell line correlation in the fraction of loci with one or more minor alleles. Full factorial plots of the fraction of loci with minor alleles by chromosome, regression line and correlation coefficient for A) PD20 RV:D2-1 and 2 C) PD20 RV:D2-1, 2, MCF10A and HEK293. Also full factorial plots of the fraction of loci with minor alleles for the corresponding 1 million base segments of all the chromosomes, a regression line and the correlation coefficient for B) PD20 RV:D2-1 and 2 D) PD20 RV:D2-1, 2, MCF10A and HEK293.

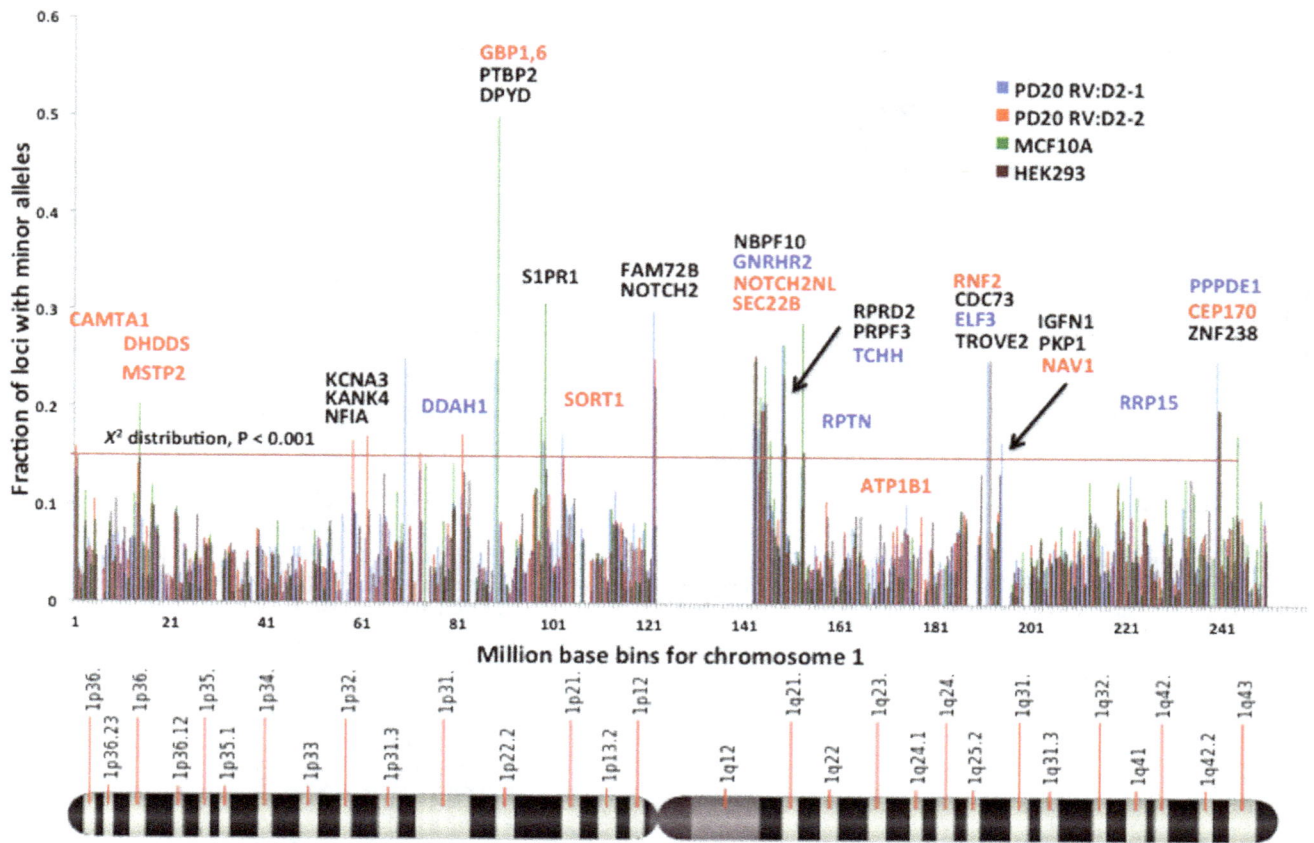

Figure 5. The distribution of MST loci showing somatic variability for chromosome 1 binned into 1 million base regions in PD20 and the derived PD20 RV:D2 cell line. The horizontal line demarcates outlier segments, based on a X^2 distribution. All genes shown were found to contain exonal MSTs that with at least 2 minor alleles in both PD20 RV:D2 samples and were found in regions that exceeded the demarcated level. Genes shown in red were found to contain exonal MSTs with at least 2 minor alleles in all 4 DNA repair proficient cell line samples and those shown in blue were found in 3 of the 4 samples. The chromosome image shown at the bottom was obtained from http://en.wikipedia.org/wiki/Chromosome_1 _(human).

haplotype distribution from DNA repair proficient cells (table 4). Capan-1 cells showed a significant decrease in heterozygotic loci, 2.1% compare to 3.3% for DNA repair proficient, which was anticipated due to the known trend for loss of heterozygosity in these cells as reported in the literature due to gene conversion in the absence of BRCA2 [42,43]. In contrast, there was an increase (5.5%) in hetereozygotic loci in DLD-1 cells, which can potentially be attributed to increased mutation due to the MMR defects responsible for the MSI in DLD-1 cells. Surprisingly, haplotype distribution analysis at non-MST loci shows that DLD-1 cells, but not Capan-1 differ significantly from DNA repair proficient (1.8% compared to 1.2% for DLD-1 and Capan-1 respectively). This was unexpected because neither mutation mechanism (homologous recombination nor MMR) would necessarily be restricted to MST vs non-MST regions. A comparison of SNPs and INDELs in the DNA repair impaired cell lines showed Capan-1 cells significantly differed from the DNA repair proficient mean in the fraction of SNPs, with 47% and 91% for MST and non-MST loci respectively (table 5). Conversely, DLD-1 and PD20 cells were not found to be different from DNA repair proficient cell lines. For the DNA repair proficient cells the mean fraction of loci with minor alleles was 5.1% with a SD of 0.4%. Capan-1 cells showed again, a greater susceptibility to mutation with a significant increase (6.2%) in the number of loci with minor alleles (table 4). In contrast, PD20 and DLD-1 cells both show a significant

decrease in loci with minor alleles, 3.1% and 3.2% respectively. This was surprising, particularly because the PD20 cells showed a decrease with respect to their corrected cell line PD20 RV:D2. Concordance of loci with minor alleles between the two related cell lines, PD20 and PD20 RV:D2, was 2.5% while discordance was 3.1%, which was significantly above chance (Pearson's X^2). However, it was greater than the concordance between PD20 RV:D2 and MCF10A, which is to be expected since PD20 and PD20 RV:D2 are related strains (Table 3).

Because Capan-1 cells displayed the highest disparity in mutation rate from DNA repair proficient cell lines, including changes in SNP:INDEL ratios, we decided to check the concordance of genotype and minor allele containing loci between them and PD20 RV:D2s (table 3). Genotype concordance for the loci that were found in both samples, was over 97.3%, even higher than when we compared PD20 RV:D2 with MCF10As. When comparing the loci with minor alleles ~2% of the total had minor alleles in both samples (were concordant) however 12% were found to have minor alleles in only one samples, meaning discordance (table 3). Although this is strikingly different, for the PD20 RV:D2 cells to MCF10A comparison, the concordance rate is still significantly greater than expected by chance. Very similar results were obtained when Capan-1 cells were compared to MCF10A cells. These results offer additional support the

Table 4. Haplotype distribution and somatic polymorphism rate differ in DNA repair defective cell lines compared to DNA repair proficient cell lines.

Percent (%)	Repair Proficient		Microsatellite loci Repair impaired cell lines			Repair Proficient		Non-microsatellite loci repair impaired cell lines		
	Mean	SD	PD20	DLD-1	Capan-1	Mean	SD	PD20	DLD-1	Capan-1
Homo-zyg	96.7	0.3	97.2 [#]	94.5 [#]	97.9 [#]	98.9	0.2	98.8	98.2 [#]	99.2
Hetero-zyg	3.3	0.3	2.8	5.5 [#]	2.1 [#]	1.1	0.2	1.2	1.8 [#]	0.8
Multi-alleles	5.1	0.4	3.1 [#]	3.2 [#]	6.2 [#]	2.0	0.2	1.2 [#]	1.2 [#]	3.7 [#]

[#] significantly different p<0.01 - z-test.

Table 5. SNP and INDEL fractions differ in DNA repair defective cell lines compared to DNA repair proficient cells.

Percent (%)	Repair Proficient		Microsatellite loci Repair impaired cell lines			Repair Proficient		Non-microsatellite loci repair impaired cell lines		
	Mean	SD	DP20	DLD-1	Capan-1	Mean	SD	PD20	DLD-1	Capan-1
SNPs	36.2	3.4	35.7	36.9	47.6 [#]	96.9	0.2	95.4 [#]	94.9 [#]	90.8 [#]
Expansions	26.0	0.7	26.3	29.7	21.2 [#]	1.5	0.1	2.1 [#]	2.2 [#]	2.8 [#]
Contractions	37.9	2.9	38.0	33.3	31.2	1.6	0.2	2.5 [#]	2.9 [#]	6.4 [#]

[#] significantly different p<0.01 - z-test.

hypothesis that some MST loci are more susceptible to mutations than others.

For DLD-1 cells, the increase in heterozygotic loci coupled with the significant reduction in the number of minor alleles is counterintuitive. This suggests the possibility of a proliferation of a small number of subpopulations. If our hypothesis is correct we would anticipate two things to occur: 1) an increase the average depth of reads that define the second allele and 2) an increase in the read depth supporting minor alleles without an increase in the number. To test our hypothesis we first compared the fraction of total reads covering the second allele regardless of haplotype and reads covering only minor alleles. As depicted in figure 6, DLD-1 cells show greater than a 4% increase with respect to the DNA repair proficient average in the fractional coverage of the second allele and more than 8% increase (figure 6A and B) for the percent coverage supporting minor alleles. Both were statistically significant. Neither Capan-1 nor PD20 were found to be different from the DNA repair proficient group for either of these parameters. These results suggest a population bottleneck where only a small number of distinct subpopulations are the predominant contributors of the reads captured by the sequencer.

SMV in exons

MSTs are present ubiquitously throughout the genome and are found in over 16% of exons [1]. Although MST expansions or contractions in promoter and interexonal regions can affect transcription, mutations in exons are the most frequently implicated in downstream effects, consistent with exons being under significant selective pressure. An analysis of heterozygotic loci found that exons had significantly less heterozygotic loci, a reduction of over 1.2% compared to untranslated regions (2.4% and 3.8% respectively, figure 7A). However the difference in the fraction of loci with minor alleles in exons and untranslated regions was not significant (5.1% and 5.6%, figure 7B). In the previous sections we showed that DLD-1 cells, a strain defective in MMR, was found, unexpectedly, to have a significant reduction in the number of MST loci with minor alleles and an increase in heterozygotic loci. Based on this comparison it appears that the results are due to the increased difference between translated and untranslated regions. As shown in figure 8A, the fraction of MST loci with minor alleles in exons is 1.1% (compared to 4.7% in untranslated regions) while the fraction of loci that are heterozygotic is 1.7%, compared to 7.9% in untranslated regions

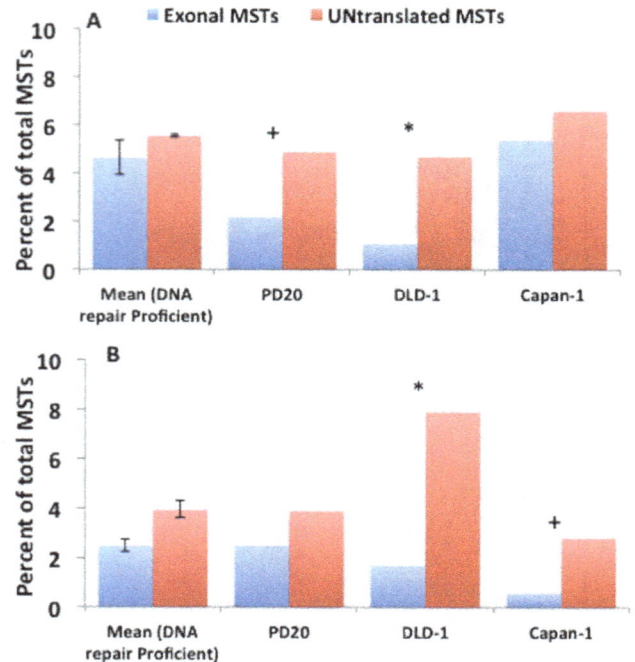

Figure 7. A comparison of the percent of heterozygotic loci and loci exhibiting SMV in exons and untranslated genomic regions in DNA repair proficient and impaired cell lines. A) The percent of MST loci that for which minor alleles were found and B) percent of heterozygotic MST loci, in exons and untranslated regions. Depicted in both figures are the means for the DNA repair proficient cell lines and the individual percentage for PD20, DLD-1 and capan-1 cell lines. (+) p<0.05 as compared to DNA proficient cells and (*) p<0.001 as compared to DNA proficient cells in measurement of the difference between exons and untranslated regions.

(figure 8B). These results further support hypothesis that DLD-1 cells have undergone a population bottleneck.

To determine the potential genetic implications of minor allele hot spots, we focused on the analysis of genes affected, specifically we inspected genes containing MST loci found in exons that with 2 or more alleles that did not contribute to the haplotype (minor alleles). This data is provided in a spreadsheet (file S2). The

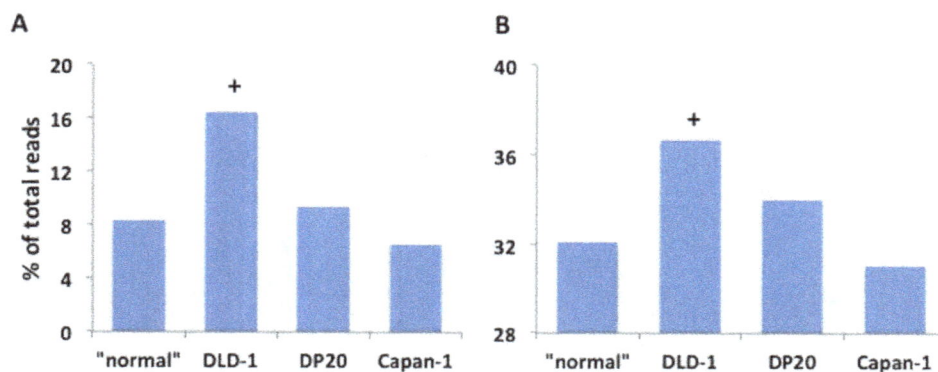

Figure 6. An increase in the fraction of reads substantiating the second alleles if present, and all minor alleles. The average fraction of reads representing A) all minor alleles (only for loci with minor alleles) and B) the second allele in both heterozygotic and homozygotic loci that have at least one minor allele, for DLD-1, PD20 and Capan-1 cells were compared to the average of the DNA repair proficient cell lines. The (+) denotes a significant difference from DNA repair proficient (p<0.01) with z-test.

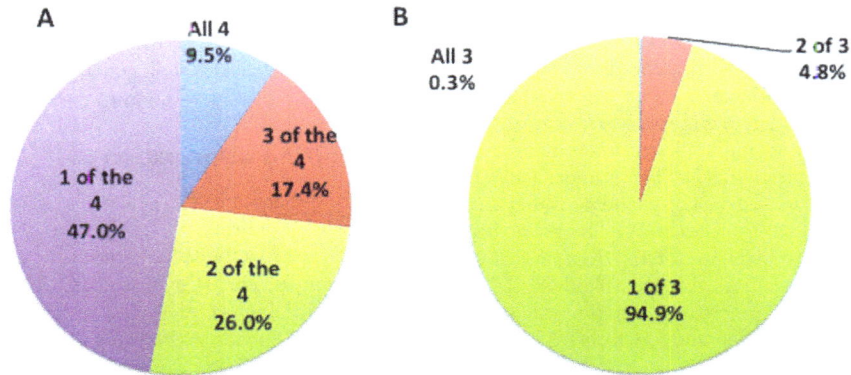

Figure 8. The distribution of genes that show SMV in DNA repair deficient cell lines appears random while those in the DNA repair proficient cell lines show significant similarity. The percent of genes with MSTs that with MSTs that have a minimum of 2 minor alleles in A) DNA repair proficient cell lines and B) DNA repair deficient cell lines that are found in all the or some of the sequenced samples. In figure B) the genes that are present in all three DNA repair deficient cell lines is 0.3% and the slice of the pie chart is not visible due to the small percentage.

spreadsheet lists the MST loci (based on the HG19 genome), gene name, cell genotype, total number of alleles, variants called and other pertinent information. Of the 2603 genes whose exons harbor minor allele containing loci found in at least one of the 4 DNA repair proficient samples sequenced 47% were found to have 2 or more minor alleles in more then one sample and 9.5% were found in all 4 samples (figure 7A). A Genome Ontology (GO) analysis of the 247 genes harboring MSTs with multiple minor alleles in all 4 samples found only a borderline (p<0.01, we use a lower p then 0.05 to compensate for the number of comparisons) significant enrichment of GOTERM categories that included transcription factors, regulators, repressors and DNA binding genes. In addition, there was no significant enrichment for any KEGG pathway categories or cataloged disorders. Conversely, of the ~1100 minor allele harboring genes found in the DNA repair impaired cell lines, only 3 (0.27%) were found in all three cell lines while 95% are in only 1 of the three cell lines (figure 7B), which suggests this concordance pattern was primarily random. Further, no genes with multiallelic MSTs were found in all of the sequenced samples and only 18 were found in 6 of the 7 cell line samples. A KEGG pathway enrichment analysis of the minor allele harboring genes found in the DNA repair impaired cell lines suggests a pattern associated with various cancer pathways. Significant KEGG terms enriched were general cancer, colorectal cancer, myeloma, cervical cancer and cell adhesion (with p<0.001). Together, these results support the hypothesis that specific MST loci in repair proficient cells are more susceptible to somatic mutations but the genes associated with them are not associated with any specific categorized pathway. In contrast, for cells that have impairments in DNA repair pathways, somatic mutations in MSTs appear in higher frequency in loci that are specific to the DNA repair deficiency, and these mutations are implicated in disease, specifically cancer.

Discussion

Somatic mutation can lead to subpopulations of cells carrying mutated alleles. These are examined in cancers, as tumors can be considered to contain subpopulations of cells, i.e. the tissues are not gnomically homogenous [44,45]. Tumors usually carry an allele or set of alleles that confirm their abnormal growth. These alleles, when detected in the tumor but not parent cells, can be the basis for important clinical treatment decisions [11,38,45]. In cell

populations with increased somatic mutation rates, like those with altered DNA repair capacity, there may be a concordant increase in subpopulation diversity. As a subpopulation propagates the mutations become more abundant, which becomes detectable in next-gen sequencing data [31,32]. A major assumption of our analysis is that an increase in the number of alleles detected in next-gen sequencing data is reflective of an increase in cell subpopulations or somatic mutation present in the sequenced sample. In this paper we evaluate allele frequencies at MSTs in various cell populations as a quantifiable indicator of variation.

The data presented here evaluate both the standard genotype and minor alleles that are present in next-gen data to establish a baseline for SMV in DNA repair proficient cells and compare this to cells with altered DNA repair capacity. The focus on cell lines with known etiologies is to establish the viability and robustness of our approach. The results show the utility in identifying the consequences of DNA repair impairments on genomic stability. There are several major objectives/findings from this analysis including (1) complimenting genomic analysis away of matched DNA samples with in-sample quantification of variation, (2) demonstrating that DNA repair proficient cells and those with different defects in DNA repair can have different SMV profiles that may be potential markers for these defects and (3) a quantitative measure of the fraction of loci that exhibit minor alleles may be reflective of subpopulations of cells with different genomic content, potentially those cells that may contribute to tumor formation. MST instability is important in the prognosis and selection of treatment for various cancers, and better, more accurate identification methods are always being sought [10,11].

These data demonstrate that the SNP:INDEL ratio at MSTs can be used to distinguish between different in-vivo mutational mechanisms and PCR amplified genomes. Both the WGA single cell sample and the Capan-1 cell line showed an increase in SNPs compared to INDELs at MST loci, however the fractions differed greatly. This is consistent with what was expected from both nucleotide mis-incorporation errors by polymerases (WGA single cell sample) and defects in DNA repair (Capan-1). Neither DLD-1 nor PD20 cells, which are defective in MMR and interstrand cross-link repair, respectively, had a significant alteration of the ratio of SNPs:INDELs at MST loci.

Capan-1 cells displayed a reduction of heterozygotic loci as compared to DNA repair proficient cell lines. This was expected since Capan-1 cells are a BRCA2- cells (impaired in homologous recombination) and have been shown to exhibit a loss of heterozygocity [43]. However, our analysis also indicates a significant increase in the fraction of loci with minor alleles. This could be due to two reasons: 1) Capan-1 cells are a hypotriploid with over 35 structural rearrangements (www.path.cam.ac.uk/%7epawefish/index.html) and with multiple chromosomal regions having more than three copies [46,47]. The minor alleles in Capan-1 cells can therefore be part of the genotype rather than somatic variation. Conversely, 2) Capan-1 cells have been reported to have an extremely high rate of INDELs and SNPs, significantly higher than expected from the hyperploidy [12]. The results shown here could be due to increased mutation rate shown with this cell line [12] and further support general genomic instability in Capan-1 cells.

Unexpectedly, although DLD-1 cells are a MST unstable cell line, they did not display either of our predicted markers for increase in MST mutation rate: 1) an increase in the number of minor alleles, as was seen with Capan-1 cells, or 2) a decrease in the number heterozygotic loci and the number of minor alleles, as we found in Capan-1 and PD20 cells (table 5). Conversely, DLD-1 cells showed both a significant increase in the number of heterozygotic loci and a reduction in the fraction of loci with more than two alleles. Further, they displayed a great reduction in both the fraction of loci with minor alleles and heterozygotic loci in exons (conserved chromosomal regions). We hypothesize that this is the result of defective MMR leading to an increase in mutations that have become fixed in the population. Alternatively, this may have resulted from a bottleneck in the growth of the cell population. If this was the case, the increase in heterozygotic loci allele may be a product of a limited set of surviving cell subpopulations. If a subpopulation with an un-repaired mutation, reached a sufficient proportion of the population due to the bottleneck it would generate sufficient reads for the locus to be mistakenly called heterozygotic. This point is reinforced by the significant increase in the portion of the total number of reads covering the second allele while the fraction of loci with minor alleles and the number of minor alleles per locus are decreased. This is important to note because it suggests that we can not only distinguish between different mutational mechanisms using the minor alleles in next-gen sequencing, but may also be able to identify cells that have experienced a growth-limiting condition as we expand this work in the future.

The work presented here is a proof-of concept of an approach to assess somatic variation in MSTs using next-gen sequencing. Using this analysis we were able to establish a SMV profile in DNA repair proficient cell lines which we can use to compare to cells with potential or known alterations in DNA repair capacity to begin to evaluate exome or whole genome sequenced samples without requiring a matched genomic sample as baseline. Based on the results presented here this approach can be used to ascertain both scientifically and clinically relevant information.

Scientifically, even with known mutations the consequences on the genome as a whole is still relatively unknown. Clinically, somatic variation is a measure of genomic stability and this approach might be used as an addition to current MST instability criteria.

Supporting Information

File S1 Contains the following files: **Figure S1.** Sanger sequencing confirms the prediction of the at least 3 different alleles, in a locus found to have minor alleles in nextGen data. A) The output produced by our caller (locus is shown in the first 5 columns in line 1) predict 3 different length alleles using a minimum of 2 reads to confirm an allele. The major allele is 23 nts with 2 minor alleles, 25 and 21 nts long. B) The sequencing chromatogram. The black arrows are showing the start point of different alleles. **Figure S2.** Effects of sequencing error and the minimum number of reads required to call an allele on of the number of alleles called in sequencing data. (A) Modeling data with different error frequencies (0.5%–5%) showed an increase in loci with multiple alleles as error increased when 4 reads were minimally required to call an allele. (B) The average read depth at loci with increasing numbers of alleles using 4 confirming reads per allele for in-silico generated data using 1% and 2.5% error rate and 4 different cell lines. **Figure S3.** The distribution of MST loci showing somatic variability by chromosome for both PD20 RV:D2 samples. **Figure S4.** The distribution of MST loci showing somatic variability by chromosome, for both PD20 RV:D2, MCF10A and HEK293 cell lines. **Table S1.** In-silico model mapping and genotyping accuracy. **Table S2.** The total minor alleles sorted by MST motif length indicate that single cell exome amplification alters the distributions observed in DNA repair proficient cell lines.

File S2 Genomic data file.

Acknowledgments

We thank the system administrators in the VBI computational core (Michael Snow, Dominik Borkowski, David Bynum, Douglas McMaster, and Vedavyas Duggirala) for technical support. We also acknowledge members of the VBI Genomics Research Lab (Saikumar Karyala, Jennifer Jenrette, Megan Friar, and Kris Lee) for the library prep, and sequencing of genomic and Sanger validation samples.

Author Contributions

Conceived and designed the experiments: ZV HRG. Performed the experiments: ZV NCF. Analyzed the data: ZV NCF HRG. Contributed reagents/materials/analysis tools: ZV HT. Wrote the paper: ZV HRG. Wrote the software: ZV HT.

References

1. Gemayel R, Vinces MD, Legendre M, Verstrepen KJ (2010) Variable tandem repeats accelerate evolution of coding and regulatory sequences. Annu Rev Genet 44: 445–477.
2. Fonville NC, Ward RM, Mittelman D (2011) Stress-induced modulators of repeat instability and genome evolution. J Mol Microbiol Biotechnol 21: 36–44.
3. Bagshaw AT, Pitt JP, Gemmell NJ (2008) High frequency of microsatellites in S. cerevisiae meiotic recombination hotspots. BMC Genomics 9: 49.
4. Payseur BA, Jing P, Haasl RJ (2011) A genomic portrait of human microsatellite variation. Mol Biol Evol 28: 303–312.
5. Delagoutte E, Goellner GM, Guo J, Baldacci G, McMurray CT (2008) Single-stranded DNA-binding protein in vitro eliminates the orientation-dependent impediment to polymerase passage on CAG/CTG repeats. J Biol Chem 283: 13341–13356.
6. Hile SE, Eckert KA (2008) DNA polymerase kappa produces interrupted mutations and displays polar pausing within mononucleotide microsatellite sequences. Nucleic Acids Res 36: 688–696.
7. Ananda G, Walsh E, Jacob KD, Krasilnikova M, Eckert KA, et al. (2013) Distinct mutational behaviors differentiate short tandem repeats from microsatellites in the human genome. Genome Biol Evol 5: 606–620.
8. Leclercq S, Rivals E, Jarne P (2010) DNA slippage occurs at microsatellite loci without minimal threshold length in humans: a comparative genomic approach. Genome Biol Evol 2: 325–335.
9. Budworth H, McMurray CT (2013) Bidirectional transcription of trinucleotide repeats: roles for excision repair. DNA Repair (Amst) 12: 672–684.
10. Xiao H, Yoon YS, Hong SM, Roh SA, Cho DH, et al. (2013) Poorly differentiated colorectal cancers: correlation of microsatellite instability with clinicopathologic features and survival. Am J Clin Pathol 140: 341–347.

11. Hong SP, Min BS, Kim TI, Cheon JH, Kim NK, et al. (2012) The differential impact of microsatellite instability as a marker of prognosis and tumour response between colon cancer and rectal cancer. Eur J Cancer 48: 1235–1243.

12. Barber LJ, Rosa Rosa JM, Kozarewa I, Fenwick K, Assiotis I, et al. (2011) Comprehensive genomic analysis of a BRCA2 deficient human pancreatic cancer. PLoS One 6: e21639.

13. Lacroix-Triki M, Lambros MB, Geyer FC, Suarez PH, Reis-Filho JS, et al. (2010) Absence of microsatellite instability in mucinous carcinomas of the breast. Int J Clin Exp Pathol 4: 22–31.

14. Yoon K, Lee S, Han TS, Moon SY, Yun SM, et al. (2013) Comprehensive genome- and transcriptome-wide analyses of mutations associated with microsatellite instability in Korean gastric cancers. Genome Res 23: 1109–1117.

15. Kim TM, Laird PW, Park PJ (2013) The landscape of microsatellite instability in colorectal and endometrial cancer genomes. Cell 155: 858–868.

16. Poduri A, Evrony GD, Cai X, Walsh CA (2013) Somatic mutation, genomic variation, and neurological disease. Science 341 1237758.

17. Harris RS, Kong Q, Maizels N (1999) Somatic hypermutation and the three R's: repair, replication and recombination. Mutat Res 436: 157–178.

18. Kunz C, Saito Y, Schar P (2009) DNA Repair in mammalian cells: Mismatched repair: variations on a theme. Cell Mol Life Sci 66: 1021–1038.

19. Baptiste BA, Ananda G, Strubczewski N, Lutzkanin A, Khoo SJ, et al. (2013) Mature microsatellites: mechanisms underlying dinucleotide microsatellite mutational biases in human cells. G3 (Bethesda) 3: 451–463.

20. Shah SN, Hile SE, Eckert KA (2010) Defective mismatch repair, microsatellite mutation bias, and variability in clinical cancer phenotypes. Cancer Res 70: 431–435.

21. Eckert KA, Mowery A, Hile SE (2002) Misalignment-mediated DNA polymerase beta mutations: comparison of microsatellite and frame-shift error rates using a forward mutation assay. Biochemistry 41: 10490–10498.

22. Roy R, Chun J, Powell SN (2012) BRCA1 and BRCA2: different roles in a common pathway of genome protection. Nat Rev Cancer 12: 68–78.

23. Kottemann MC, Smogorzewska A (2013) Fanconi anaemia and the repair of Watson and Crick DNA crosslinks. Nature 493: 356–363.

24. Li H, Handsaker B, Wysoker A, Fennell T, Ruan J, et al. (2009) The Sequence Alignment/Map format and SAMtools. Bioinformatics 25: 2078–2079.

25. Benson G (1999) Tandem repeats finder: a program to analyze DNA sequences. Nucleic Acids Res 27: 573–580.

26. Tae H, Kim DY, McCormick J, Settlage RE, Garner HR (2013) Discretized Gaussian mixture for genotyping of microsatellite loci containing homopolymer runs. Bioinformatics.

27. Tae H, McMahon KW, Settlage RE, Bavarva JH, Garner HR (2013) ReviSTER: an automated pipeline to revise misaligned reads to simple tandem repeats. Bioinformatics 29: 1734–1741.

28. McIver LJ, McCormick JF, Martin A, Fondon JW 3rd, Garner HR (2013) Population-scale analysis of human microsatellites reveals novel sources of exonic variation. Gene 516: 328–334.

29. McIver LJ NCF, Karunasena E, Garner HR (Submitted) Microsatellite genotyping reveals a signature in breast cancer exomes. Breast Cancer Research and Treatment.

30. Fonville NC LJM, Vaksman Z, Garner HR (Submitted) Microsatellites in the exome are predominantly single-allelic and invariant. Genome Biology.

31. Schmitt MW, Kennedy SR, Salk JJ, Fox EJ, Hiatt JB, et al. (2012) Detection of ultra-rare mutations by next-generation sequencing. Proc Natl Acad Sci U S A 109: 14508–14513.

32. Gundry M, Vijg J (2012) Direct mutation analysis by high-throughput sequencing: from germline to low-abundant, somatic variants. Mutat Res 729: 1–15.

33. Kruglyak S, Durrett RT, Schug MD Aquadro CF (1998) Equilibrium distributions of microsatellite repeat length resulting from a balance between slippage events and point mutations. Proc Natl Acad Sci U S A 95: 10774–10778.

34. Jarne P, Lagoda PJ (1996) Microsatellites, from molecules to populations and back. Trends Ecol Evol 11: 424–429.

35. Kanagawa T (2003) Bias and artifacts in multitemplate polymerase chain reactions (PCR). J Biosci Bioeng 96: 317–323.

36. Meyerhans A, Vartanian JP, Wain-Hobson S (1990) DNA recombination during PCR. Nucleic Acids Res 18: 1687–1691.

37. Brodin J, Mild M, Hedskog C, Sherwood E, Leitner T, et al. (2013) PCR-induced transitions are the major source of error in cleaned ultra-deep pyrosequencing data. PLoS One 8: e70388.

38. Hou Y, Song L, Zhu P, Zhang B, Tao Y, et al. (2012) Single-cell exome sequencing and monoclonal evolution of a JAK2-negative myeloproliferative neoplasm. Cell 148: 873–885.

39. Mestrovic N, Castagnone-Sereno P, Plohl M (2006) Interplay of selective pressure and stochastic events directs evolution of the MEL172 satellite DNA library in root-knot nematodes. Mol Biol Evol 23: 2316–2325.

40. Ohashi A, Zdzienicka MZ, Chen J, Couch FJ (2005) Fanconi anemia complementation group D2 (FANCD2) functions independently of BRCA2- and RAD51-associated homologous recombination in response to DNA damage. J Biol Chem 280: 14877–14883.

41. Chen TR, Hay RJ, Macy ML (1983) Intercellular karyotypic similarity in near-diploid cell lines of human tumor origins. Cancer Genet Cytogenet 10: 351–362.

42. Holt JT, Toole WP, Patel VR, Hwang H, Brown ET (2008) Restoration of CAPAN-1 cells with functional BRCA2 provides insight into the DNA repair activity of individuals who are heterozygous for BRCA2 mutations. Cancer Genet Cytogenet 186: 85–94.

43. Butz J, Wickstrom E, Edwards J (2003) Characterization of mutations and loss of heterozygosity of p53 and K-ras2 in pancreatic cancer cell lines by immobilized polymerase chain reaction. BMC Biotechnol 3: 11.

44. Tang DG (2012) Understanding cancer stem cell heterogeneity and plasticity. Cell Res 22: 457–472.

45. Schor SL (1995) Fibroblast subpopulations as accelerators of tumor progression: the role of migration stimulating factor. EXS 74: 273–296.

46. Sirivatanauksorn V, Sirivatanauksorn Y, Gorman PA, Davidson JM, Sheer D, et al. (2001) Non-random chromosomal rearrangements in pancreatic cancer cell lines identified by spectral karyotyping. Int J Cancer 91: 350–358.

47. Grigorova M, Staines JM, Ozdag H, Caldas C, Edwards PA (2004) Possible causes of chromosome instability: comparison of chromosomal abnormalities in cancer cell lines with mutations in BRCA1, BRCA2, CHK2 and BUB1. Cytogenet Genome Res 104: 333–340.

17

XRCC1 Gene Polymorphisms and Glioma Risk in Chinese Population

Li-Wen He[1,2,◑]**, Rong Shi**[1◑]**, Lei Jiang**[3◑]**, Ye Zeng**[4]**, Wen-Li Ma**[1]**, Jue-Yu Zhou**[1]*

1 Institute of Genetic Engineering, Southern Medical University, Guangzhou, China, **2** Zhujiang Hospital, Southern Medical University, Guangzhou, China, **3** Department of Neurosurgery, Changzheng Hospital, Second Military Medical University, Shanghai, China, **4** Department of Stomatology, Nanfang Hospital, Southern Medical University, Guangzhou, China

Abstract

Background: Three extensively investigated polymorphisms (Arg399Gln, Arg194Trp, and Arg280His) in the X-ray repair cross-complementing group 1 (XRCC1) gene have been implicated in risk for glioma. However, the results from different studies remain inconsistent. To clarify these conflicts, we performed a quantitative synthesis of the evidence to elucidate these associations in the Chinese population.

Methods: Data were extracted from PubMed and EMBASE, with the last search up to August 21, 2014. Meta-analysis was performed by critically reviewing 8 studies for Arg399Gln (3062 cases and 3362 controls), 8 studies for Arg194Trp (3419 cases and 3680 controls), and 5 studies for Arg280His (2234 cases and 2380 controls). All of the statistical analyses were performed using the software program, STATA (version 11.0).

Results: Our analysis suggested that both Arg399Gln and Arg194Trp polymorphisms were significantly associated with increased risk of glioma (for Arg399Gln polymorphism: Gln/Gln vs. Arg/Arg, OR = 1.82, 95% CI = 1.46–2.27, $P = 0.000$; Arg/Gln vs. Arg/Arg, OR = 1.25, 95% CI = 1.10–1.42, $P = 0.001$ and for Arg194Trp polymorphism: recessive model, OR = 1.78, 95% CI = 1.44–2.19, $P = 0.000$), whereas the Arg280His polymorphism had no influence on the susceptibility to glioma in a Chinese population.

Conclusions: This meta-analysis suggests that there may be no association between the Arg280His polymorphism and glioma risk, whereas the Arg399Gln/Arg194Trp polymorphisms may contribute to genetic susceptibility to glioma in the Chinese population. Nevertheless, large-scale, well-designed and population-based studies are needed to further evaluate gene-gene and gene–environment interactions, as well as to measure the combined effects of these XRCC1 variants on glioma risk.

Editor: Robert Lafrenie, Sudbury Regional Hospital, Canada

Funding: This work was supported by the National Natural Science Foundation of China (81201565, 81101536), Program of the Pearl River Young Talents of Science and Technology in Guangzhou, China (2013J2200042), Natural Science Foundation of Guangdong Province, China (S2012010009404, S2012010009294) and Specialized Research Fund for the Doctoral Program of Higher Education of China (20124433120001). The funders had no role in study design, data collection and analysis, decision to publish, or preparation of the manuscript.

Competing Interests: The authors have declared that no competing interests exist.

* Email: zhoujueyu@126.com

◑ These authors contributed equally to this work.

Introduction

Glioma is the most common and aggressive malignant primary brain tumor in humans, especially in adults, accounting for approximately 30% of all brain and central nervous system (CNS) tumors and 80% of all malignant brain tumors [1,2]. Currently, the therapy for glioma is a combined approach, using surgery, radiation therapy, and chemotherapy. The prognosis for glioma patients is still poor, except for pilocytic astrocytomas (WHO grade I). Fewer than 3% of glioblastoma patients are still alive at 5 years after diagnosis, with an older age being the most significant and consistent prognostic factor for poorer outcome. Despite decades of research, the etiology of glioma is poorly understood.

Many environmental and lifestyle factors including several occupations, environmental carcinogens, and diet have been reported to be associated with an elevated glioma risk, but the only factor unequivocally associated with an increased risk is high dose exposure to ionizing radiation [3,4]. However, only a minority of those exposed to ionizing radiation eventually develop glioma, suggesting that genetic factors, such as single nucleotide polymorphisms (SNPs), may be crucial to modify the risk for glioma [5,6].

DNA repair genes play a major role in the DNA mismatch repair pathway, including base excision repair (BER), nucleotide excision repair (NER), mismatch repair (MMR) and double strand break repair (DSBR), and are essential for maintaining the integrity of the genome [7,8]. The X-ray repair cross-complementing group 1 (XRCC1) gene is an important component of DNA repair and encodes a scaffolding protein that participate in the BER pathway [9–11] for repairing small base lesions derived from oxidation and alkylation damage [12]. Several nonsynonymous coding polymorphisms were identified in this gene, and the three which are most extensively studied are Arg399Gln on exon 10 (rs25487, G/A), Arg194Trp on exon 6 (rs1799782, C/T) and Arg280His on exon 9 (rs25489, G/A) [13]. These polymorphisms, which involve amino acid changes at evolutionarily conserved sequences, could alter the function of XRCC1, which may diminish repair kinetics in individuals with the variant alleles and increase the risk of glioma in humans.

To date, several epidemiologic studies have been performed to elucidate the effect of these SNPs on glioma risk. However, the results are to some extent divergent, but nevertheless intriguing. The inconsistency of these studies may be explained by differences in population background, source of controls, sample size, and also by chance. Actually differences in the allele frequencies of these three polymorphisms in Asians and Caucasians have been reported [14,15]. Since most of the previous association studies focused on Caucasians [16–25], few, if any, large-scale studies have been performed in Chinese populations. The genetic effect of XRCC1 polymorphisms on glioma risk in Chinese populations remains largely inconclusive. In addition, several new related studies of glimoa risk in Chinese populations [26–28] have since been published. Therefore, in the present study, we performed a meta-analysis to elucidate the relationship between XRCC1 polymorphisms and glioma risk in Chinese populations by combining all available studies.

Materials and Methods

Search strategy

We performed a comprehensive literature search of PubMed and EMBASE for relevant studies that tested the association between XRCC1 polymorphisms and the risk of glioma up to August 21, 2014. The following search terms and keywords were used: ("DNA repair gene" OR XRCC1 OR "X-ray repair cross-complementation group 1") AND (polymorphism OR variant OR variation OR mutation) AND (glioma OR "brain tumor"). In addition, references cited in the retrieved articles were reviewed to trace additional relevant studies missed by the search.

Inclusion criteria

Included studies were considered eligible if they met all of the following criteria: 1) studies with full text articles; 2) a case–control study evaluating at least one of these three polymorphisms in the XRCC1 gene; 3) enough data to estimate an odds ratio (OR) with 95% confidence interval (CI); 4) no overlapping data. For the studies with the same or overlapping data by the same authors, we selected the ones with the most subjects.

Data extraction

Data were extracted independently by three investigators. For conflicting evaluations, an agreement was reached following discussion. For each study, the following characteristics were collected: first author, publication year, source of controls, genotyping method, numbers of cases and controls, genotype frequency of cases and controls, and the results of the Hardy–Weinberg equilibrium test.

Quality score evaluation

The quality of the included studies was independently assessed by three investigators (LWH, RS and LJ) according to the quality assessment criteria (shown in Table S1) that was amended from previous published meta-analyses [29,30]. All disagreements were resolved by consensus after discussion. Study quality was evaluated on a numerical score ranging from 0 to 12. If the score was ≥7, the study was categorized as "high quality"; otherwise, the study was categorized as "low quality".

Statistical analysis

We assessed the deviation from HWE for the genotype distribution in controls using a chi-squared goodness-of-fit test ($P<0.05$ was considered significant). ORs with the corresponding 95% CI were used as the common measures of assessing the strength of association between XRCC1 polymorphisms (Arg399Gln, Arg194Trp, and Arg280His) and glioma risk for each study. The pooled ORs were calculated in an additive model (a allele versus A allele, a was for the minor allele and A was for the major allele), a dominant model (aa+Aa versus AA), recessive model (aa versus Aa+AA) and a codominant model (aa versus AA, Aa versus AA). If the overall gene effect was statistically significant, further comparisons of OR_1 (aa versus AA), OR_2 (Aa versus AA) and OR_3 (aa versus Aa) were explored with a designated as the risk allele. The above pairwise differences were used to determine the most appropriate genetic model. If $OR_1 = OR_3 \neq 1$ and $OR_2 = 1$, then a recessive model was indicated. If $OR_1 = OR_2 \neq 1$ and $OR_3 = 1$, then a dominant model was indicated. If $OR_2 = 1/OR_3 \neq 1$ and $OR_1 = 1$, then a complete over-dominant model was indicated. If $OR_1 > OR_2 > 1$ and $OR_1 > OR_3 > 1$, or $OR_1 < OR_2 < 1$ and $OR_1 < OR_3 < 1$, then a co-dominant model was indicated [31]. The significance of the pooled ORs was determined using a Z-test, and the level of statistical significance was established as $P<0.05$. The heterogeneity among studies was checked by the Q test [32]. The I^2 statistic, which is a quantitative measure of the proportion of the total variation across studies due to heterogeneity [33], was also calculated. If the P value for the heterogeneity test was greater than 0.05, the Mantel–Haenszel method-based fixed effects model [34] was used to calculate the pooled OR. Otherwise, the DerSimonian and Laird method-based random effects model [35] was performed. Sensitivity analysis was performed by limiting the meta-analysis to studies conforming to HWE and omitting each study in turn to assess the stability of results, respectively. Potential publication bias was evaluated by visual inspection of the Begg funnel plots in which the standard error of log (OR) of each study was plotted against its log (OR). We also performed an Egger's linear regression test ($P<0.05$ was considered a significant publication bias) [36]. All of the statistical analyses were performed using a software program, STATA version 11.0 (Stata, College Station, TX, USA).

Results

Extraction process and study characteristics

According to our search criterion, 132 articles were retrieved. Among them, the majority were excluded after the first screening based on abstracts or titles, mainly because they were overlapped citations, not relevant to the XRCC1 polymorphisms and glioma risk, reviews, conference abstracts, or not a related gene polymorphism. Afterwards, a total of 19 full-text articles [16–28,37–42] were preliminarily identified for further detailed evaluation (Figure 1). Of these, 10 studies were excluded [16–25] because the country of source was not from China. Eventually, nine case-control studies [26–28,37–42] were selected, including 8 studies for the Arg399Gln polymorphism (3062 cases and 3362 controls), 8 studies for the Arg194Trp polymorphism (3419 cases and 3680 controls), and 5 studies for the Arg280His polymorphism

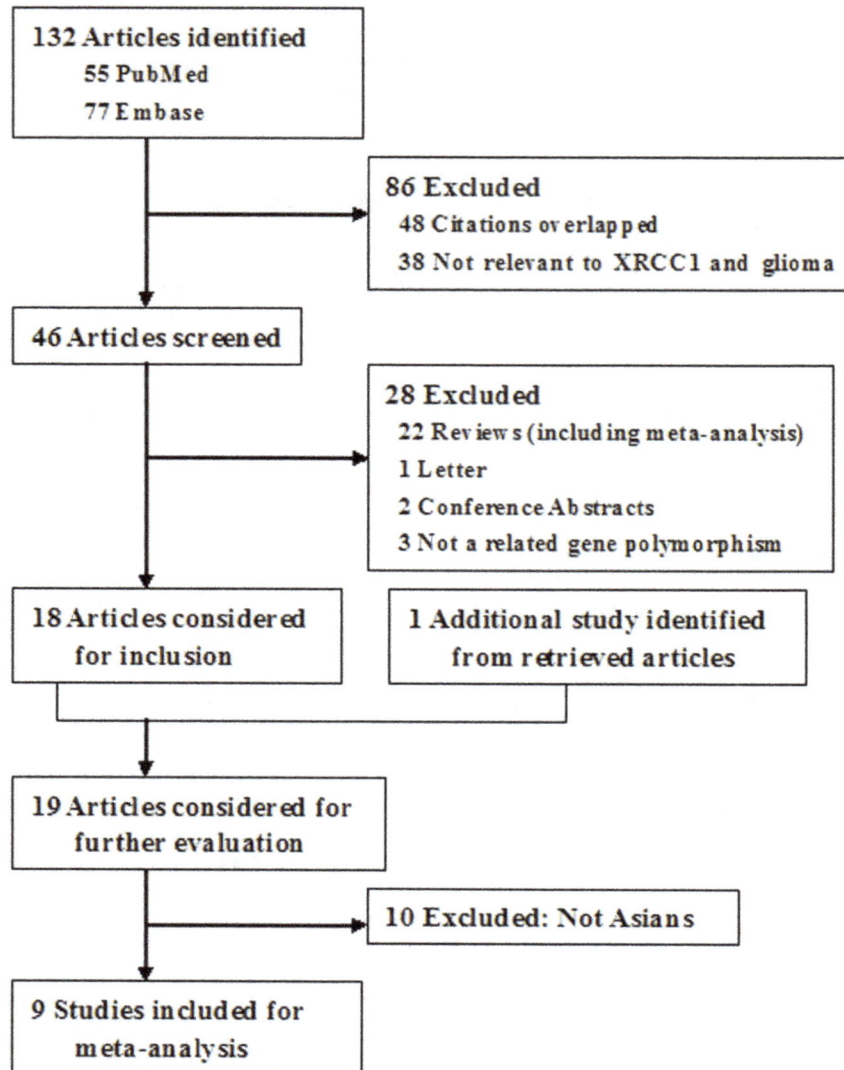

Figure 1. Flow of Included Studies.

(2234 cases and 2380 controls). With respect to the assessment of study quality, the vast majority of the included studies were high quality (shown in Table S2) except for the study by Liu *et al.* [41]. The characteristics of these included studies and the genotype distribution and allele frequency of XRCC1 polymorphisms in case and control subjects is shown in Table 1.

Meta-analysis results

The main results of the meta-analysis are shown in Table 2. According to the principle of genetic model selection by Thakkinstian *et al.* [31], the most appropriate genetic model for the Arg399Gln/Arg194Trp polymorphisms was the codominant model and the recessive model, respectively. Our results revealed that the Arg399Gln polymorphism was significantly associated with an increased risk of glioma in the Chinese population (Gln/Gln vs. Arg/Arg: OR = 1.82, 95% CI = 1.46–2.27, $P = 0.000$; Arg/Gln vs. Arg/Arg: OR = 1.25, 95% CI = 1.10–1.42, $P = 0.001$; recessive model: OR = 1.63, 95% CI = 1.32–2.01, $P = 0.000$; dominant model: OR = 1.34, 95% CI = 1.18–1.51, $P = 0.000$; additive model: OR = 1.31, 95% CI = 1.19–1.44,

$P = 0.000$; Figure 2, Table 2). For the Arg194Trp polymorphism, a significant association between this polymorphism and glioma risk was also observed (Trp/Trp vs. Arg/Arg: OR = 1.82, 95% CI = 1.48–2.25, $P = 0.000$; recessive model: OR = 1.78, 95% CI = 1.44–2.19, $P = 0.000$; dominant model: OR = 1.17, 95% CI = 1.06–1.30, $P = 0.001$; additive model: OR = 1.23, 95% CI = 1.13–1.33, $P = 0.000$; Figure 3, Table 2), with the exception of the heterozygote comparison model (OR = 1.08, 95% CI = 0.97–1.20, $P = 0.169$, Table 2). But, for the Arg280His polymorphism, we did not detect any significant association with glioma risk in any genetic model (Table 2). Since several original papers depart from the HWE which could cause unreliable results, we performed stratification analysis according to the status of HWE. Because ethnicity of all studies was Chinese and the source of controls was hospital-based, we did not carry out subgroup analysis. In addition, the subgroup analysis according to quality assessment scores is not shown because only one included study was low quality which did not materially change the corresponding pooled ORs.

Table 1. Characteristics of studies included in the meta-analysis and their genotype distributions of XRCC1 polymorphisms.

Polymorphism	First author	Year	Design	Sample size (case/control)	Case			Control			HWE in control	MAF
					AA	Aa	aa	AA	Aa	aa		
Arg399Gln	Gao	2014	HB	375	126	155	45	178	168	29	0.215	0.301
	Xu	2013	HB	886	451	365	70	469	372	45	0.008	0.261
	Pan	2013	HB	443	226	190	27	244	178	21	0.108	0.248
	Luo	2013	HB	415	111	134	51	189	181	45	0.866	0.327
	Wang	2012	HB	580	270	279	75	300	232	48	0.739	0.283
	Zhou	2011	HB	289	121	113	37	147	118	24	0.963	0.287
	Hu	2011	HB	249	58	48	21	145	75	29	<0.001	0.267
	Liu	2011	HR	89	23	37	29	28	34	27	0.026	0.494
Arg194Trp	Gao	2014	HB	376	235	73	18	279	84	13	0.041	0.146
	Xu	2013	HB	886	525	301	60	540	311	35	0.236	0.215
	Pan	2013	HB	443	301	116	27	327	101	15	0.045	0.148
	Luo	2013	HB	415	204	63	30	297	96	22	<0.001	0.169
	Liu	2012	HB	442	294	105	45	334	89	19	<0.001	0.144
	Wang	2012	HB	580	376	218	30	355	205	20	0.143	0.211
	Zhou	2011	HB	289	145	112	14	159	117	13	0.138	0.247
	Hu	2011	HB	249	71	38	18	163	64	22	<0.001	0.217
Arg280His	Gao	2014	HB	376	250	66	10	313	57	6	0.079	0.092
	Xu	2013	HB	886	618	177	91	621	178	87	<0.001	0.199
	Wang	2012	HB	580	506	115	3	473	98	9	0.140	0.100
	Zhou	2011	HB	289	218	45	8	240	44	5	0.085	0.093
	Hu	2011	HB	249	72	28	27	153	58	38	<0.001	0.269

Abbreviations: HWE, Hardy-Weinberg equilibrium; HB, hospital-based; MAF, minor allele frequency; A, the major allele; a, the minor allele.

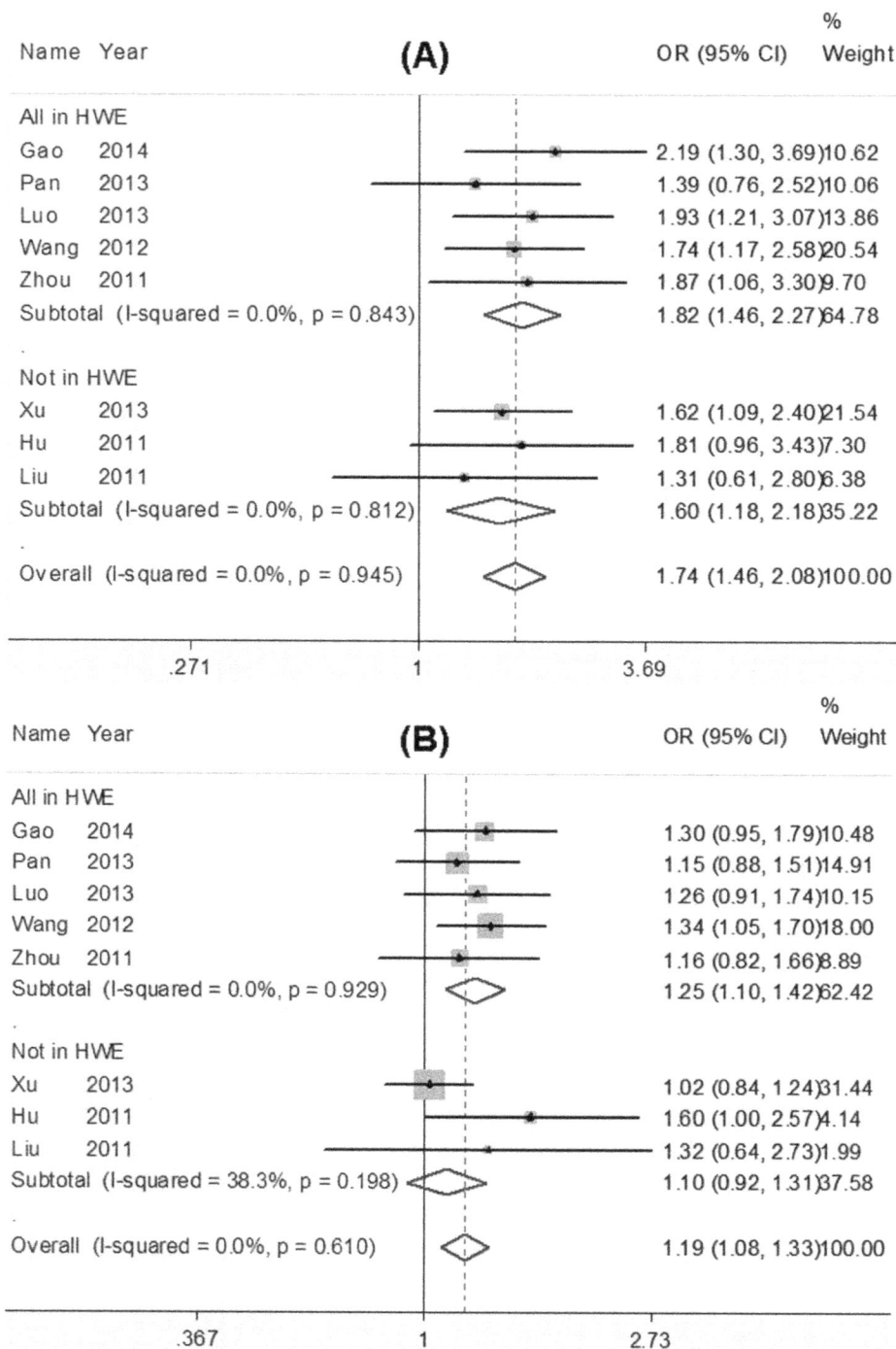

Figure 2. Forest plots of ORs with 95% CI for XRCC1 Arg399Gln polymorphism and the risk of glioma observed in Chinese population (fixed effects). The center of each square represents the OR, the area of the square is the number of sample and thus the weight used in the meta-analysis, and the horizontal line indicates the 95%CI. (A) Gln/Gln vs. Arg/Arg. (B) Arg/Gln vs. Arg/Arg.

Test of heterogeneity and sensitivity analyses

The results of heterogeneity test indicated that there was no significant heterogeneity for the Arg399Gln/Arg194Trp polymorphisms across studies. However, we found heterogeneity for the Arg280His polymorphism only in an additive model ($P_h = 0.002$, $I^2 = 77.1\%$). To explore the potential sources of heterogeneity

across studies, we determined that the study by Zhou et al. [40] could contribute to substantial heterogeneity because heterogeneity was significantly decreased, in the additive model ($P_h = 0.117$, $I^2 = 49.0\%$), after exclusion of this study. Although there were 3 and 2 studies that deviated from HWE for the Arg399Gln/Arg280His polymorphisms, respectively, the corresponding pooled

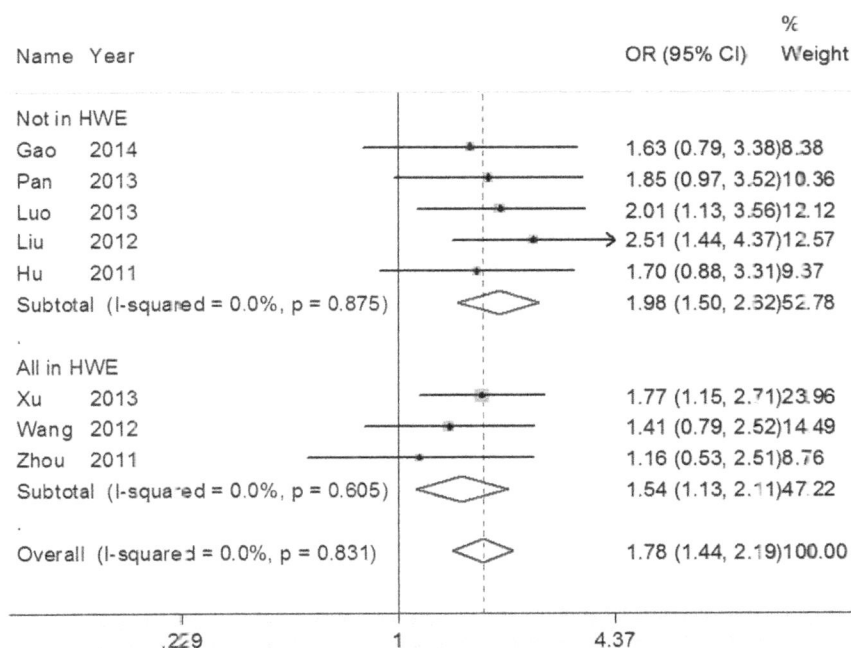

Figure 3. Forest plots of ORs with 95% CI for XRCC1 Arg194Trp polymorphism and the risk of glioma observed in recessive model among Chinese (fixed effects). The center of each square represents the OR, the area of the square is the number of sample and thus the weight used in the meta-analysis, and the horizontal line indicates the 95%CI.

ORs were not materially altered by including or not including these studies (Table 2). Similarly, the results of the Arg194Trp polymorphism remained practically unchanged in a recessive model and a codominant model when excluding the 5 studies that departed from HWE. Nevertheless, this polymorphism was no longer associated with the risk of glioma in a dominant model (OR = 1.06, 95% CI = 0.93–1.21, $P = 0.392$) and an additive model (OR = 1.10, 95% CI = 0.99–1.23, $P = 0.089$). Additionally, we also assessed the influence of each individual study on the pooled ORs by sequential omission of individual studies. The results showed the pooled ORs of these three polymorphisms were not materially altered by the contribution of any individual study, suggesting that the results of this meta-analysis are credible (data also not shown).

Publication bias

Publication bias was assessed by performing Funnel plot and Egger's regression tests under all contrast models. All of these three genetic polymorphisms showed consistent results, indicating no publication bias. Usinge the Arg399Gln polymorphism as an example; the shapes of the funnel plot did not indicate any evidence of obvious asymmetry in a codominant model (Figure 4), and the Egger's test also suggested that there was no evidence of publication bias ($P = 0.185$ for a dominant model, $P = 0.296$ for a recessive model, $P = 0.300$, or for an additive model, $P = 0.108$ for Arg/Gln vs. Arg/Arg and $P = 0.552$ for Gln/Gln vs. Arg/Arg, respectively).

Discussion

DNA damage, which leads to gene deletions, amplifications, rearrangements, and translocations occurs very frequently and results in the formation of a tumor [7,43]. Many of these mutations may lead to less effective DNA repair than normal. It is acknowledged that glioma is appreciably associated with specific mutations causing by exposure to ionizing radiation in the DNA mismatch repair pathway. XRCC1 is an essential DNA repair gene involved in BER pathway and the vast majority of previous studies have been focused on three polymorphisms (Arg399Gln, Arg194Trp, and Arg280His) in this gene. Genetic variations in this gene confers a susceptibility to tumorogeneis through the alteration of base excision repair functions [44]. At present, several systematic reviews and meta-analyses have been carried out as preliminary studies to determine the association between XRCC1 variants and glioma risk based on pervious published studies [45–54]. However, none of these studies collected sufficient data to draw a solid conclusion in a Chinese population and some results remain contradictory. Thus, Zhang et al. [52] reported that XRCC1 Arg194Trp polymorphism was not a risk factor for glioma risk in a Chinese population, which was the opposite of the conclusions made in a previous study [51]. Considering the paradoxical and underpowered conclusions of the individual studies, we conducted the most comprehensive meta-analysis using available eligible data to provide more reliable results to determine the association between the variants of the XRCC1 gene and glioma risk in the Chinese population.

Overall, our combined results based on available data from of all the studies revealed that the Arg399Gln polymorphism in XRCC1 gene was associated with increased risk of glioma among Chinese people in all genetic models, which was consistent with the conclusion of individual studies involving the Arg399Gln polymorphism [26–28,37–41]. Meanwhile, we also detected that individuals harboring the Trp/Trp genotype of the Arg194Trp polymorphism might have an increased risk of developing glioma, which was in line with the majority, but not all, previous studies [26–28,37,38,51]. As for the Arg280His polymorphism, our results did not provide any evidence of such an association with glioma risk in any genetic model, which coincided with the conclusions of

Table 2. Results of meta-analysis for Arg399Gln, Arg194Trp and Arg280His polymorphisms and the risk of glioma in Chinese population.

Genetic model	n	Recessive model				Dominant model				Homozygote				Heterozygote				Additive model			
Arg399Gln		Gln/Gln vs. Arg/Gln + Arg/Arg				Gln/Gln + Arg/Gln vs. Arg/Arg				Gln/Gln vs. Arg/Arg				Arg/Gln vs. Arg/Arg				Gln vs. Arg			
		OR(95%CI)	P_{OR}	I^2(%)	P_h	OR(95%CI)	P_{OR}	I^2(%)	P_h	OR(95%CI)	P_{OR}	I^2(%)	P_h	OR(95%CI)	P_{OR}	I^2(%)	P_h	OR(95%CI)	P_{OR}	I^2(%)	P_h
Total	8(3062/3326)	1.57(1.32–1.86)	0.000	0.0	0.926	1.27(1.15–1.41)	0.000	0.0	0.506	1.74(1.46–2.08)	0.000	0.0	0.945	1.19(1.08–1.33)	0.001	0.0	0.610	1.26(1.17–1.36)	0.000	0.0	0.567
All in HWE	5(1960/2102)	1.63(1.32–2.01)	0.000	0.0	0.877	1.34(1.18–1.51)	0.000	0.0	0.842	1.82(1.46–2.27)	0.000	0.0	0.842	1.25(1.10–1.42)	0.001	0.0	0.929	1.31(1.19–1.44)	0.000	0.0	0.750
Not in HWE	3(1102/1224)	1.46(1.10–1.96)	0.010	0.0	0.621	1.17(0.99–1.38)	0.063	39.1	0.194	1.60(1.18–2.18)	0.003	0.0	0.812	1.10(0.92–1.31)	0.281	38.3	0.198	1.18(1.04–1.35)	0.010	16.2	0.303
Arg194Trp		Trp/Trp vs. Arg/Trp + Arg/Arg				Trp/Trp + Arg/Trp vs. Arg/Arg				Trp/Trp vs. Arg/Arg				Arg/Trp vs. Arg/Arg				Trp vs. Arg			
		OR(95%CI)	P_{OR}	I^2(%)	P_h	OR(95%CI)	P_{OR}	I^2(%)	P_h	OR(95%CI)	P_{OR}	I^2(%)	P_h	OR(95%CI)	P_{OR}	I^2(%)	P_h	OR(95%CI)	P_{OR}	I^2(%)	P_h
Total	8(3419/3680)	1.78(1.44–2.19)	0.000	0.0	0.831	1.17(1.06–1.30)	0.001	15.0	0.312	1.82(1.48–2.25)	0.000	0.0	0.782	1.08(0.97–1.20)	0.169	0.0	0.666	1.23(1.13–1.33)	0.000	42.7	0.094
All in HWE	3(1781/1755)	1.54(1.13–2.11)	0.006	0.0	0.605	1.06(0.93–1.21)	0.392	0.0	0.980	1.55(1.13–2.13)	0.007	0.0	0.641	1.01(0.88–1.16)	0.920	0.0	0.966	1.10(0.99–1.23)	0.089	0.0	0.850
Not in HWE	5(1638/1925)	1.98(1.50–2.62)	0.000	0.0	0.875	1.32(1.14–1.53)	0.000	0.0	0.485	2.07(1.56–2.75)	0.000	0.0	0.852	1.17(1.00–1.38)	0.049	0.0	0.578	1.40(1.24–1.58)	0.000	1.5	0.398
Arg280His		His/His vs. Arg/His + Arg/Arg				His/His + Arg/His vs. Arg/Arg				His/His vs. Arg/Arg				Arg/His vs. Arg/Arg				His vs. Arg			
		OR(95%CI)	P_{OR}	I^2(%)	P_h	OR(95%CI)	P_{OR}	I^2(%)	P_h	OR(95%CI)	P_{OR}	I^2(%)	P_h	OR(95%CI)	P_{OR}	I^2(%)	P_h	OR(95%CI)	P_{OR}	I^2(%)	P_h
Total	5(2234/2380)	1.14(0.89–1.46)	0.306	39.9	0.155	1.11(0.97–1.27)	0.128	0.0	0.424	1.14(0.89–1.47)	0.295	41.6	0.144	1.10(0.94–1.28)	0.224	0.0	0.623	1.30(1.00–1.69)	0.053	77.1	0.002
All in HWE	3(1221/1245)	1.11(0.60–2.05)	0.740	63.3	0.065	1.19(0.97–1.46)	0.090	20.3	0.285	1.15(0.62–2.12)	0.658	64.6	0.059	1.19(0.97–1.47)	0.096	0.0	0.517	1.46(0.90–2.36)	0.124	84.3	0.002
Not in HWE	2(1013/1135)	1.14(0.87–1.50)	0.331	18.2	0.269	1.05(0.87–1.26)	0.606	0.0	0.460	1.14(0.87–1.50)	0.343	16.6	0.274	1.00(0.81–1.25)	0.974	0.0	0.929	1.07(0.93–1.24)	0.346	35.6	0.213

P_{OR}, P values for pooled OR from Z-test. P_h, P values for heterogeneity from Q test. I^2, the percentage of variability in OR attributable to heterogeneity. Random-effects model was used when P value for heterogeneity test <0.05; otherwise, fixed-model was used.

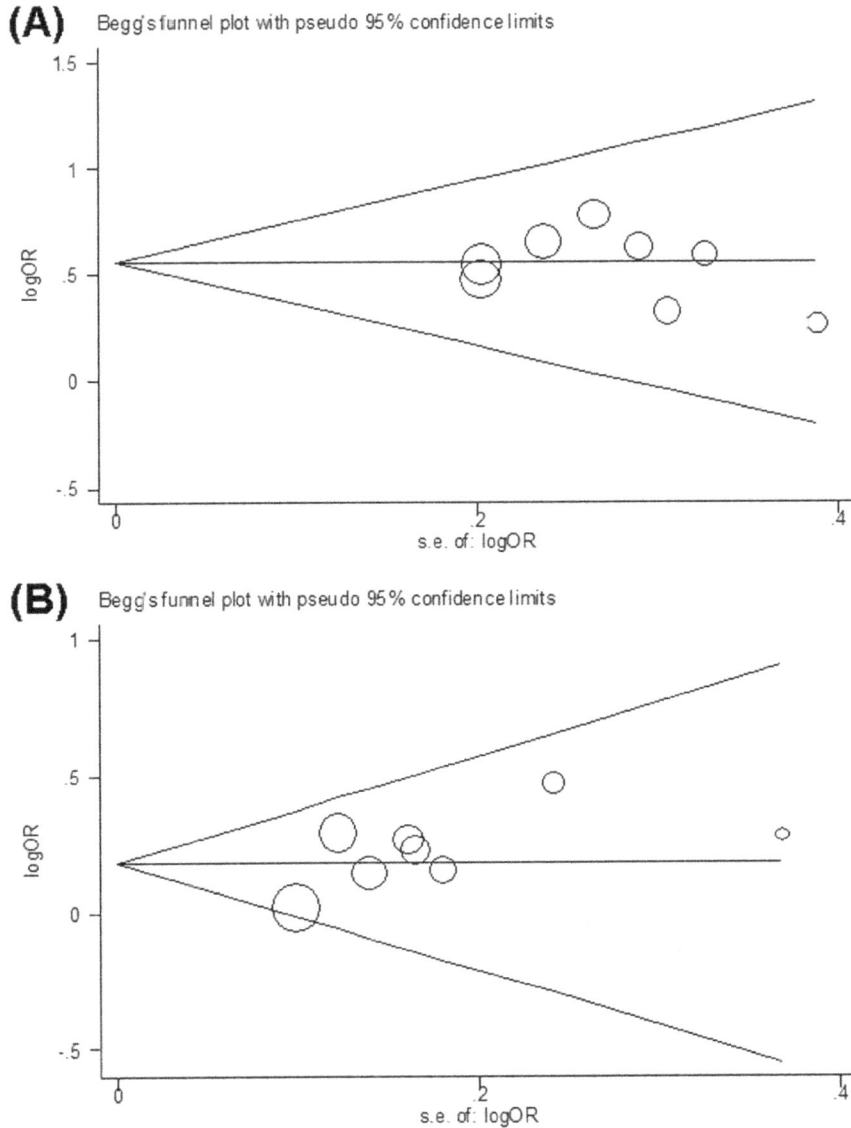

Figure 4. Begg's funnel plots of Arg399Gln polymorphism and glioma risk for publication bias test. Each point represents a separate study for the indicated association. Log (OR), natural logarithm of OR. Horizontal line, mean effect size. (A) Gln/Gln vs. Arg/Arg. (B) Arg/Gln vs. Arg/Arg.

all previous studies [28,37,39,40]. For example, Xu et al. [28] suggested that the Arg280His polymorphism was unlikely to be associated with the risk of glioma.

It is generally agreed that departures from HWE in controls may be due to genotyping error, chance, nonrandom mating, genetic drifting, population stratification, and selection bias. Although there were 3, 2 and 5 studies that deviated from HWE for the Arg399Gln, Arg280His, and Arg194Trp polymorphisms, respectively, the studies that appeared to deviate from HWE should not be excluded mechanically in the meta-analysis unless there are other convincing grounds for doubting the quality of the study [55]. Also, there is no consensus on what to do with studies that are not in HWE in the meta-analysis of genetic association studies. Some authors suggest performing sensitivity analyses, pooling both with and without the studies that appear not to be in HWE and assessing whether studies classified as not being in

HWE provide a different estimate of the genetic effect [56,57]. Furthermore, Mao et al. [58] emphasized that authors of gene-disease association meta-analyses may need to pay more attention to HWE issues, and sensitivity analyses including and excluding the HWE-violating studies may need to be routinely performed in meta-analyses of genetic association studies. In this study we performed sensitivity analyses by excluding the HWE-violating studies to check the robustness of our conclusions, and the corresponding pooled ORs were not materially altered. In addition, we comprehensively assessed the publication bias using several means including the Begg's and Egger's tests as well as funnel plot tests, indicating no publication bias for all these three genetic polymorphisms. In view of this, we are strongly convinced that the methods are appropriate and well described and the results or data of our meta-analysis, in essence, are sound and reliable.

Additionally, there is still a lack of uniform and standardized quality score methods for evaluating case-control gene association studies although it is crucial for a meta-analysis to assess the quality of the individual included studies. Here we used a self-made rating scale for study quality assessment, which was modified based on two previously published meta-analyses [29,30]. The quality score assessment results showed that almost all of individual studies were high quality except for the study by Liu *et al.* [41], indicating that the quality of the included studies was generally high, which lends support to our conclusions. However, considering that high-quality studies may offer quite different outcomes from that of low-quality studies [59], we recommend that researchers carry out study quality assessment and stratification analysis based on the quality appraisal scores when performing the quantitative synthesis of the genetic polymorphism association studies.

When interpreting the results of the current study, some limitations should be addressed. First, lacking the original data for the included studies limited our further evaluation of the association between glioma risk and other risk factors, such as age, gender, smoking status, alcohol consumption and other variables, which might have caused a serious confounding bias. Second, we did not estimate the potential interactions among gene–gene, gene–environment, or even between various polymorphic loci of the same gene, which may alter the risk of cancer. Although the analysis of haplotypes can increase the power to detect disease associations, our study was limited to analyzing a single SNP site owing to only one study [37] focused on determining the XRCC1 haplotype. Third, selection bias should be considered because the controls from the primary literatures were all hospital-based which may not be very representative of the general population. Finally, some inevitable publication bias might exist in the results because only published studies were retrieved although the funnel plot and Egger's test indicated no remarkable publication bias.

In summary, this meta-analysis provides evidence that both the Arg399Gln and Arg194Trp polymorphisms may contribute to genetic susceptibility to glioma risk in the Chinese population, whereas Arg280His polymorphism may have no impact. Nevertheless, large-scale, well-designed and population-based studies are needed to investigate the combined effects of these variants within XRCC1 gene or other BER genes in the Chinese population, which may eventually lead to better comprehensive understanding of their possible roles in gliomagenesis.

Supporting Information

Table S1   Scale for Quality Assessment.

Table S2   Quality score assessment results.

Checklist S1   Prisma 2009 Checklist for this meta-analysis.

Author Contributions

Conceived and designed the experiments: JYZ. Performed the experiments: LWH RS LJ. Analyzed the data: LWH RS LJ. Contributed reagents/materials/analysis tools: LWH RS LJ. Wrote the paper: LWH RS LJ. Revised manuscript: JYZ YZ WLM.

References

1. Goodenberger ML, Jenkins RB (2012) Genetics of adult glioma. Cancer genetics 205: 613–621.
2. Ricard D, Idbaih A, Ducray F, Lahutte M, Hoang-Xuan K, et al. (2012) Primary brain tumours in adults. Lancet 379: 1984–1996.
3. Ostrom QT, Barnholtz-Sloan JS (2011) Current state of our knowledge on brain tumor epidemiology. Current neurology and neuroscience reports 11: 329–335.
4. Schwartzbaum JA, Fisher JL, Aldape KD, Wrensch M (2006) Epidemiology and molecular pathology of glioma. Nature clinical practice Neurology 2: 494–503; quiz 491 p following 516.
5. Gu J, Liu Y, Kyritsis AP, Bondy ML (2009) Molecular epidemiology of primary brain tumors. Neurotherapeutics: the journal of the American Society for Experimental NeuroTherapeutics 6: 427–435.
6. Shete S, Hosking FJ, Robertson LB, Dobbins SE, Sanson M, et al. (2009) Genome-wide association study identifies five susceptibility loci for glioma. Nature genetics 41: 899–904.
7. Wood RD, Mitchell M, Sgouros J, Lindahl T (2001) Human DNA repair genes. Science (New York, NY) 291: 1284–1289.
8. Yu Z, Chen J, Ford BN, Brackley ME, Glickman BW (1999) Human DNA repair systems: an overview. Environmental and molecular mutagenesis 33: 3–20.
9. Caldecott KW, Tucker JD, Stanker LH, Thompson LH (1995) Characterization of the XRCC1-DNA ligase III complex in vitro and its absence from mutant hamster cells. Nucleic acids research 23: 4836–4843.
10. Campalans A, Marsin S, Nakabeppu Y, O'Connor T R, Boiteux S, et al. (2005) XRCC1 interactions with multiple DNA glycosylases: a model for its recruitment to base excision repair. DNA repair 4: 826–835.
11. Siciliano MJ, Carrano AV, Thompson LH (1986) Assignment of a human DNA-repair gene associated with sister-chromatid exchange to chromosome 19. Mutation research 174: 303–308.
12. Almeida KH, Sobol RW (2007) A unified view of base excision repair: lesion-dependent protein complexes regulated by post-translational modification. DNA repair 6: 695–711.
13. Shen MR, Jones IM, Mohrenweiser H (1998) Nonconservative amino acid substitution variants exist at polymorphic frequency in DNA repair genes in healthy humans. Cancer research 58: 604–608.
14. Hamajima N, Takezaki T, Tajima K (2002) Allele Frequencies of 25 Polymorphisms Pertaining to Cancer Risk for Japanese, Koreans and Chinese. Asian Pacific journal of cancer prevention: APJCP 3: 197–206.
15. Moullan N, Cox DG, Angele S, Romestaing P, Gerard JP, et al. (2003) Polymorphisms in the DNA repair gene XRCC1, breast cancer risk, and response to radiotherapy. Cancer epidemiology, biomarkers & prevention: a -

publication of the American Association for Cancer Research, cosponsored by the American Society of Preventive Oncology 12: 1168–1174.
16. Bethke L, Webb E, Murray A, Schoemaker M, Johansen C, et al. (2008) Comprehensive analysis of the role of DNA repair gene polymorphisms on risk of glioma. Human molecular genetics 17: 800–805.
17. Cengiz SL, Acar H, Inan Z, Yavuz S, Baysefer A (2008) Deoxy-ribonucleic acid repair genes XRCC1 and XPD polymorphisms and brain tumor risk. Neurosciences (Riyadh, Saudi Arabia) 13: 227–232.
18. Felini MJ, Olshan AF, Schroeder JC, North KE, Carozza SE, et al. (2007) DNA repair polymorphisms XRCC1 and MGMT and risk of adult gliomas. Neuroepidemiology 29: 55–58.
19. Karahalil B, Bohr VA, Wilson DM, 3rd (2012) Impact of DNA polymorphisms in key DNA base excision repair proteins on cancer risk. Human & experimental toxicology 31: 981–1005.
20. Kiuru A, Lindholm C, Heinavaara S, Ilus T, Jokinen P, et al. (2008) XRCC1 and XRCC3 variants and risk of glioma and meningioma. Journal of neuro-oncology 88: 135–142.
21. Liu Y, Scheurer ME, El-Zein R, Cao Y, Do KA, et al. (2009) Association and interactions between DNA repair gene polymorphisms and adult glioma. Cancer epidemiology, biomarkers & prevention: a publication of the American Association for Cancer Research, cosponsored by the American Society of Preventive Oncology 18: 204–214.
22. Rajaraman P, Hutchinson A, Wichner S, Black PM, Fine HA, et al. (2010) DNA repair gene polymorphisms and risk of adult meningioma, glioma, and acoustic neuroma. Neuro-oncology 12: 37–48.
23. Rodriguez-Hernandez I, Perdomo S, Santos-Briz A, Garcia JL, Gomez-Moreta JA, et al. (2013) Analysis of DNA repair gene polymorphisms in glioblastoma. Gene.
24. Wang LE, Bondy ML, Shen H, El-Zein R, Aldape K, et al. (2004) Polymorphisms of DNA repair genes and risk of glioma. Cancer research 64: 5560–5563.
25. Yosunkaya E, Kucukyuruk B, Onaran I, Gurel CB, Uzan M, et al. (2010) Glioma risk associates with polymorphisms of DNA repair genes, XRCC1 and PARP1. British journal of neurosurgery 24: 561–565.
26. Luo KQ, Mu SQ, Wu ZX, Shi YN, Peng JC (2013) Polymorphisms in DNA repair genes and risk of glioma and meningioma. Asian Pacific journal of cancer prevention: APJCP 14: 449–452.
27. Pan WR, Li G, Guan JH (2013) Polymorphisms in DNA repair genes and susceptibility to glioma in a chinese population. International journal of molecular sciences 14: 3314–3324.

28. Xu G, Wang M, Xie W, Bai X (2013) Three polymorphisms of DNA repair gene XRCC1 and the risk of glioma: a case-control study in northwest China. Tumour biology: the journal of the International Society for Oncodevelopmental Biology and Medicine.

29. Gao LB, Pan XM, Li LJ, Liang WB, Bai P, et al. (2011) Null genotypes of GSTM1 and GSTT1 contribute to risk of cervical neoplasia: an evidence-based meta-analysis. PloS one 6: e20157.

30. Yang X, Long S, Deng J, Deng T, Gong Z, et al. (2013) Glutathione S-transferase polymorphisms (GSTM1, GSTT1 and GSTP1) and their susceptibility to renal cell carcinoma: an evidence-based meta-analysis. PloS one 8: e63827.

31. Thakkinstian A, McElduff P, D'Este C, Duffy D, Attia J (2005) A method for meta-analysis of molecular association studies. Stat Med 24: 1291–1306.

32. Cochran W (1954) The combination of estimates from different experiments. Biometrics 10: 101–129.

33. Higgins JP, Thompson SG, Deeks JJ, Altman DG (2003) Measuring inconsistency in meta-analyses. BMJ (Clinical research ed) 327: 557–560.

34. Mantel N, Haenszel W (1959) Statistical aspects of the analysis of data from retrospective studies of disease. Journal of the National Cancer Institute 22: 719–748.

35. DerSimonian R, Laird N (1986) Meta-analysis in clinical trials. Controlled clinical trials 7: 177–188.

36. Egger M, Davey Smith G, Schneider M, Minder C (1997) Bias in meta-analysis detected by a simple, graphical test. BMJ (Clinical research ed) 315: 629–634.

37. Hu XB, Feng Z, Fan YC, Xiong ZY, Huang QW (2011) Polymorphisms in DNA repair gene XRCC1 and increased genetic susceptibility to glioma. Asian Pacific journal of cancer prevention: APJCP 12: 2981–2984.

38. Liu HB, Peng YP, Dou CW, Su XL, Gao NK, et al. (2012) Comprehensive study on associations between nine SNPs and glioma risk. Asian Pacific journal of cancer prevention: APJCP 13: 4905–4908.

39. Wang D, Hu Y, Gong H, Li J, Ren Y, et al. (2012) Genetic polymorphisms in the DNA repair gene XRCC1 and susceptibility to glioma in a Han population in northeastern China: a case-control study. Gene 509: 223–227.

40. Zhou LQ, Ma Z, Shi XF, Yin XL, Huang KX, et al. (2011) Polymorphisms of DNA repair gene XRCC1 and risk of glioma: a case-control study in Southern China. Asian Pacific journal of cancer prevention APJCP 12: 2547–2550.

41. Liu J, Sun H, Huang L, Hu P, Dai X (2011) Relationship between XRRC1 polymorphisms and adult gliomas. Mod Pre Med 38: 3340–3341.

42. Gao K, Mu SQ, Wu ZX (2014) Investigation of the effects of single-nucleotide polymorphisms in DNA repair genes on the risk of glioma. Genet Mol Res 13: 1203–1211.

43. De Bont R, van Larebeke N (2004) Endogenous DNA damage in humans: a review of quantitative data. Mutagenesis 19: 169–185.

44. Monaco R, Rosal R, Dolan MA, Pincus MR, Brandt-Rauf PW (2007) Conformational effects of a common codon 399 polymorphism on the BRCT1 domain of the XRCC1 protein. The protein journal 26: 541–546.

45. Jiang L, Fang X, Bao Y, Zhou JY, Shen XY, et al. (2013) Association between the XRCC1 polymorphisms and glioma risk: a meta-analysis of case-control studies. PloS one 8: e55597.

46. Li M, Zhou Q, Tu C, Jiang Y (2013) A meta-analysis of an association between the XRCC1 polymorphisms and glioma risk. Journal of neuro-oncology 111: 221–228.

47. Martinez R (2012) Beyond Genetics in Glioma Pathways: The Ever-Increasing Crosstalk between Epigenomic and Genomic Events. Journal of signal transduction 2012: 519807.

48. Sun JY, Zhang CY, Zhang ZJ, Dong YF, Zhang AL, et al. (2012) Association between XRCC1 gene polymorphisms and risk of glioma development: a meta-analysis. Asian Pacific journal of cancer prevention: APJCP 13: 4783–4788.

49. Wei X, Chen D, Lv T (2013) A functional polymorphism in XRCC1 is associated with glioma risk: evidence from a meta-analysis. Molecular biology reports 40: 567–572.

50. Yi L, Xiao-Feng H, Yun-Tao L, Hao L, Ye S, et al. (2013) Association between the XRCC1 Arg399Gln Polymorphism and Risk of Cancer: Evidence from 297 Case-Control Studies. PloS one 8: e78071.

51. Zhang H, Liu H, Knauss JL (2013) Associations between three XRCC1 polymorphisms and glioma risk: a meta-analysis. Tumour biology: the journal of the International Society for Oncodevelopmental Biology and Medicine 34: 3003–3013.

52. Zhang L, Wang Y, Qiu Z, Luo J, Zhou Z, et al. (2012) The XRCC1 Arg194Trp polymorphism is not a risk factor for glioma: A meta-analysis involving 1,440 cases and 2,562 controls. Experimental and therapeutic medicine 4: 1057–1062.

53. Zhang L, Wang Y, Qiu Z, Luo J, Zhou Z, et al. (2013) XRCC1 Arg280His polymorphism and glioma risk: A meta-analysis involving 1439 cases and 2564 controls. Pakistan journal of medical sciences 29: 37–42.

54. Zhu W, Yao J, Li Y, Xu B (2013) Assessment of the association between XRCC1 Arg399Gln polymorphism and glioma susceptibility. Tumour biology: the journal of the International Society for Oncodevelopmental Biology and Medicine.

55. Minelli C, Thompson JR, Abrams KR, Thakkinstian A, Attia J (2008) How should we use information about HWE in the meta-analyses of genetic association studies? Int J Epidemiol 37: 136–146.

56. Attia J, Thakkinstian A, D'Este C (2003) Meta-analyses of molecular association studies: methodologic lessons for genetic epidemiology. J Clin Epidemiol 56: 297–303.

57. Salanti G, Amountza G, Ntzani EE, Ioannidis JP (2005) Hardy-Weinberg equilibrium in genetic association studies: an empirical evaluation of reporting, deviations, and power. Eur J Hum Genet 13: 840–848.

58. Mao C, Liao RY, Chen Q (2010) Sensitivity analyses including and excluding the HWE-violating studies are required for meta-analyses of genetic association studies. Breast Cancer Res Treat 121: 245–246.

59. Camargo MC, Mera R, Correa P, Peek RM, Jr., Fontham ET, et al. (2006) Interleukin-1beta and interleukin-1 receptor antagonist gene polymorphisms and gastric cancer: a meta-analysis. Cancer epidemiology, biomarkers & prevention: a publication of the American Association for Cancer Research, cosponsored by the American Society of Preventive Oncology 15: 1674–1687.

18

Repair on the Go: *E. coli* Maintains a High Proliferation Rate while Repairing a Chronic DNA Double-Strand Break

Elise Darmon, John K. Eykelenboom[¤a]**, Manuel A. Lopez-Vernaza**[¤b]**, Martin A. White**[¤c]**, David R. F. Leach***

Institute of Cell Biology, University of Edinburgh, Edinburgh, United Kingdom

Abstract

DNA damage checkpoints exist to promote cell survival and the faithful inheritance of genetic information. It is thought that one function of such checkpoints is to ensure that cell division does not occur before DNA damage is repaired. However, in unicellular organisms, rapid cell multiplication confers a powerful selective advantage, leading to a dilemma. Is the activation of a DNA damage checkpoint compatible with rapid cell multiplication? By uncoupling the initiation of DNA replication from cell division, the *Escherichia coli* cell cycle offers a solution to this dilemma. Here, we show that a DNA double-strand break, which occurs once per replication cycle, induces the SOS response. This SOS induction is needed for cell survival due to a requirement for an elevated level of expression of the RecA protein. Cell division is delayed, leading to an increase in average cell length but with no detectable consequence on mutagenesis and little effect on growth rate and viability. The increase in cell length caused by chronic DNA double-strand break repair comprises three components: two types of increase in the unit cell size, one independent of SfiA and SlmA, the other dependent of the presence of SfiA and the absence of SlmA, and a filamentation component that is dependent on the presence of either SfiA or SlmA. These results imply that chronic checkpoint induction in *E. coli* is compatible with rapid cell multiplication. Therefore, under conditions of chronic low-level DNA damage, the SOS checkpoint operates seamlessly in a cell cycle where the initiation of DNA replication is uncoupled from cell division.

Editor: Michael Lichten, National Cancer Institute, United States of America

Funding: This work has been funded by grant G0901622 to DL from the Medical Research Council (UK) [http://www.mrc.ac.uk/]. The funders had no role in study design, data collection and analysis, decision to publish, or preparation of the manuscript.

Competing Interests: The authors have declared that no competing interests exist.

* Email: D.Leach@ed.ac.uk

¤a Current address: College of Life Sciences, University of Dundee, Dundee, United Kingdom
¤b Current address: Dept. Crop Science, Oak Park Crops Research Centre, Carlow, Rep of Ireland
¤c Current address: Department of Molecular and Cellular Biology, Harvard University, Cambridge, Massachusetts, United States of America

Introduction

Unrepaired DNA double-strand breaks (DSBs) are a lethal form of damage. In *Escherichia coli*, DNA double-strand break repair (DSBR) is carried out by homologous recombination, a pathway that has been conserved in evolution from bacteria to humans. Recombination mediates repair of a damaged DNA molecule using an undamaged template, which is usually the sister chromosome generated during DNA replication [1]. This reaction is centrally catalyzed by the RecA protein in *E. coli* and by its homologue Rad51 in eukaryotes [2]. DNA damage is also used as a signal to alter a cellular pathway controlling cell division and DNA repair, known as a DNA damage checkpoint. Inhibition of cell division is believed to allow time for DNA repair to occur [3,4]. In *E. coli*, the main DNA damage checkpoint is the SOS response [5]. It is controlled by the same RecA protein that mediates homologous recombination. In the presence of damaged DNA, RecA forms protein filaments on single-stranded DNA, which catalyze auto-cleavage and deactivation of the LexA protein that normally represses genes involved in DNA repair and cell

survival [6,7,8]. Inhibition of cell division during the SOS response is mediated by the SfiA protein (also called SulA) [9,10,11]. SfiA inhibits the assembly of FtsZ, which is a tubulin-like protein essential at the early stage of cell division [12,13,14]. FtsZ polymerizes to form a ring-like structure at mid-cell where it acts as a scaffold for other division proteins. Another system that inhibits cell division is nucleoid occlusion, which is mediated by the SlmA protein that prevents the polymerization of FtsZ filaments into productive FtsZ rings in the presence of DNA [15,16,17].

The counterbalancing priorities of accurate DNA repair and rapid cell multiplication pose a potential dilemma to a unicellular organism. Does it have to sacrifice one in favor of the other? In eukaryotes, a delay in cell cycle progression is observed following induction of a high level of DNA damage [3,4,18,19,20]. Furthermore, in *Saccharomyces cerevisiae*, induction of checkpoint following chronic damage from low levels of UV light can lead to reduced cell viability [21]. In *E. coli*, induction of high levels of DNA damage can result in cell filamentation and death [22,23,24] but experiments using chronic low levels of DNA damage, which may be more frequently encountered under natural environmental conditions, are largely absent from the literature.

Previous work has shown that induction of an I-SceI endonuclease mediated DSB at a single locus in the *E. coli* chromosome can induce the SOS response [25,26,27]. However, that system has certain complexities. First, the I-SceI cleavage site is present on both sister chromosomes, so both chromosomes can be cleaved, which precludes repair. Second, at sites where repair is attempted from an intact sister chromosome, that has by chance escaped cleavage, the products of repair retain the cleavage site and can be re-cleaved. Third, if homologous DNA without the I-SceI recognition site (e.g. on an F′ plasmid) is provided to act as an intact non-sister DNA template, repair from this template will drive the loss of the I-SceI recognition site from the chromosome. These features of chromosome cleavage by I-SceI limit the applicability of this system for the study of chronic DNA breaks. Naturally, DSB repair by homologous recombination is often expected to occur following the formation of a DNA DSB on one chromosome in the presence of an intact sister chromosome. Therefore, the study of chronic DSBR at a single chromosomal location requires cleavage of only one sister chromosome and repair that does not eliminate the source of breakage. These conditions are satisfied by the system used in this study. A 246 bp interrupted palindrome has been introduced in the *E. coli* chromosome [28]. During each DNA replication cycle, this sequence can form a hairpin structure on the lagging-strand template. This structure is cleaved by the SbcCD hairpin endonuclease, leaving a two-ended DSB that is repaired by homologous recombination using the replicated leading strand as a template. In this experimental system, repair does not eliminate the palindrome [28,29,30], allowing a chronic breakage reaction to be established and studied in growing cells.

The present work investigates the consequences of a single chronic DNA DSB in the *E. coli* chromosome. Under these conditions, increased expression of RecA following SOS checkpoint induction is shown to be essential for cell survival. Strikingly, cells subjected to this DNA DSB are longer but their cell growth and viability are nearly unaffected. The roles of SfiA and SlmA proteins in the elongation of cells subjected to a chronic DSB were studied.

Materials and Methods

Strains and plasmids

A list of strains can be found in Table S1 in File S1. *E. coli* strains used were derivatives of BW27784 to allow a homogeneous expression from P_{BAD}, when using the P_{BAD}-*sbcDC* fusion (used for Figure 1), or otherwise were derivatives of MG1655 (please note that this MG1655 also has an *fnr-267* mutation) [31]. Mutations were introduced by P1 transduction or plasmid-mediated gene replacement [28]. Lists of plasmids and oligonucleotides can be found in Tables S2 and S3 in File S1 respectively, and the description of plasmid constructions are in Supplementary material.

Growth of strains

For induction or repression of *sbcDC* expression, strains containing a P_{BAD}-*sbcDC* fusion were grown in LB medium supplemented with 0.2% (w/v) arabinose or 0.5% (w/v) glucose, respectively. To measure the viability of *lexA3* and *lexA*⁺ strains, 10-fold serial dilutions were prepared and 10 µl of these dilutions were spotted onto LB agar plates supplemented with 0.2% arabinose or 0.5% glucose. These experiments were carried out at least three independent times, giving similar results.

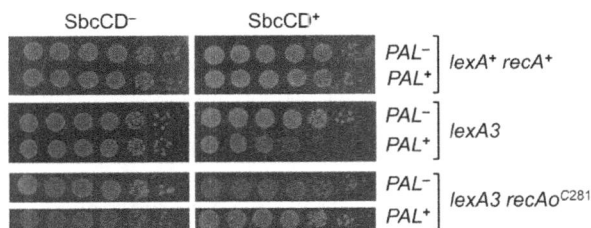

Figure 1. SOS-induced level of RecA is required for viability following DNA cleavage at a palindrome. Effect of SbcCD expression on the viability of *lexA3* and *lexA3 recAo*^C281 mutant strains encoding P_{BAD}-*sbcDC* and containing or not the chromosomal 246 bp interrupted palindrome (*PAL*). Spot tests of ten-fold dilution series were carried out on LB plates complemented with either 0.2% of arabinose (SbcCD⁺) or 0.5% of glucose (SbcCD⁻).

Cell growth measurements

To measure growth levels, *sbcDC*⁻ or Δ*sbcDC* cells containing or not the chromosomal 246 bp interrupted palindrome were grown at 37°C under agitation in LB medium. After an overnight culture, individual strains were diluted and maintained in exponential growth phase (OD_{600nm} <0.5; optical density readings at 600 nm) by appropriate dilution at regular intervals. Growth was monitored by measuring the OD_{600nm} and the number of cells was count by flow cytometry on samples taken every hour from these cultures. Samples were washed three times in sterile filtered PBS and numbers of cells per microliter were counted using an A50 Micro flow cytometer from Apogee Flow Systems. These experiments were carried out at least three independent times and the mean of generation times and numbers of cells were calculated (generation times were calculated using a doubling time program found on http://www.doubling-time com).

Competition experiment

After an overnight culture, individual strains were diluted to an OD_{600nm} of 0.01 in LB medium and grown for 2 hours at 37°C under agitation. Then, *PAL*⁺ and *PAL*⁻ strains were mixed in a ratio of 80% of *PAL*⁺ for 20% of *PAL*⁻. In one set of experiments *PAL*⁺ *yfp*⁺ and *PAL*⁻ *yfp*⁻ strains were mixed together and in a second set *PAL*⁺ *yfp*⁻ and *PAL*⁻ *yfp*⁺ strains were mixed. These cell populations were diluted 10 times and grown in LB medium for 20 minutes and then diluted to an OD_{600nm} of 0.01. For the next 75 hours, cells were kept in exponential phase during the day (OD_{600nm} <0.5) by regular dilution to an OD_{600nm} of 0.01 in new LB medium and at night were either allowed to grow until stationary phase (ON^stat) or kept at 4°C to stay in exponential phase (ON^4°C). The OD_{600nm} of each culture was measured before and after every dilution and the number of cells per microliter expressing or not YFP was similarly monitored using flow cytometry after two washes in sterile filtered PBS. The cell fluorescence and number were measured using the blue excitation laser (488 nm) and detected on the green channel. PMT voltage parameters used were SALS = 220, LALS = 405, Blue = 495, Green = 500 and Red = 520. Gain value parameters used were 1.0 for SALS, LALS, Blue and Green and 2.0 for Red. An example of flow cytometry results from one of these cultures is shown in Figure S1. The percentage of cells subjected to DSBs (*PAL*⁺) was calculated for each culture and time point. Please note that the *PAL*⁺ cells will be the cell expressing the lowest fluorescence in *PAL*⁺ *yfp*⁻ and the cells expressing the higher fluorescence in the *PAL*⁺ *yfp*⁺ cells. The percentage of cells subjected to DSBs (*PAL*⁺) was calculated as 100 times the number of PAL^+ cells per microliter divided by the sum of PAL^+ and PAL^- cells present per microliter of culture. For each time point, the percentage of cells subjected to DSBs (PAL^+) was calculated before and after dilution of the culture and the mean between these two measurements was used to calculate the percentage of loss per generation of cells subjected to DSBs (PAL^+). The number of generations between two time points was calculated on the assumption that $N(t) = 2^{g(t)}$ where $N(t)$ is the number of cells at time t and $g(t)$ is the number of generations that have elapsed at time t. The percentage of loss per generation of cells subjected to DSBs (PAL^+) was the difference of percentage of cells subjected to DSBs (PAL^+) between two time points divided by the number of generations between these two time points. In this study, we have assumed that the effect on growth of the presence of the 246 bp palindrome in the *lacZ* gene was independent from the effect on growth of the presence of the *yfp* gene into the *intC* gene. The results presented are the mean of three independent experiments.

Rate of mutagenesis

The rate of mutation to rifampicin-resistance was measured by fluctuation analysis on 24 colonies for each *sbcDC*+ or Δ*sbcDC* strains containing or not the chromosomal 246 bp interrupted palindrome [32]. After growth overnight of each colony at 37°C under agitation in liquid LB medium, appropriate dilutions of cells were plated onto LB agar plates or LB plates containing 100 µg/ml of rifampicin. Colony forming units were counted the next day. Bars presented in the graph show 95% confidence intervals. This experiment was carried out five independent times, giving similar results.

SOS induction levels

SOS levels in cells containing the pGB150 plasmid (encoding a P_{sfiA}-*gfp* fusion) were measured by microscopy. After an overnight culture, *sbcDC*+ or Δ*sbcDC* cells containing or not the chromosomal 246 bp interrupted palindrome were diluted into fresh LB medium to an OD_{600nm} of 0.02 and grown for 80 minutes at 37°C under agitation (until an OD_{600nm} around 0.2). Cultures were then diluted ten times and grown again for 40 minutes until an OD_{600nm} around 0.1. Microscopy was performed to determinate the average Gray value of a line of pixels in 350 cells per strain (the mean of three lines of pixels taken at different places in the background was subtracted from each cell measurement in each picture). The data presented here are the mean of four independent experiments.

Cell length measurements

Cell length in LB medium was measured by microscopy of early exponential phase *sbcDC*+ or Δ*sbcDC* strains containing or not the chromosomal 246 bp interrupted palindrome. After an overnight culture, cells were diluted to an OD_{600nm} of 0.02 and grown for 80 minutes at 37°C under agitation (until an OD_{600nm} around 0.2). Cultures were then diluted ten times and grown again to an OD_{600nm} around 0.1. Data presented are the mean of four independent experiments investigating 350 cells each.

Microscopy

10 µl of exponential phase cells were mounted on a bed of 1% agarose–H$_2$O for viewing under the microscope. Images were acquired at a resolution of 0.1 µm per pixel using a Zeiss Axiovert 200 fluorescence microscope equipped with a Photometrics Evolve™ 512 EMCCD camera. Image acquisition and analyzes were carried out using the MetaMorph program (Molecular

Devices). For each field of view, a single picture of the sharpest plane was taken and analyzed.

Results

SOS-induced level of RecA is required for the repair of a single DSB per replication cycle

The SOS response requirement for *E. coli* cell viability following the induction of a DSB by SbcCD at the site of a chromosomal 246 bp interrupted DNA palindrome was investigated. For this purpose, the *lexA3* mutation was introduced into strains expressing SbcCD under the control of an arabinose-inducible promoter (P_{BAD}-*sbcDC*) in the presence or absence of the 246 bp interrupted palindrome at the chromosomal *lacZ* locus. The *lexA3* mutant gene encodes an uncleavable LexA protein that prevents the induction of the genes under the control of the SOS system [33]. As seen in Figure 1, the *lexA3* mutation conferred a viability decrease to cells subjected to a chronic DSB (SbcCD$^+$ PAL^+). This result indicates that SOS induction is necessary for the survival of cells enduring a single DSB per replication cycle. Since the RecA protein, that is over-expressed during SOS induction [34,35], is also essential for cell viability following SbcCD cleavage of the palindrome [28], we investigated whether cells subjected to this chronic DSB might need an elevated level of this protein. To determine whether an induced level of RecA protein was required for cell survival, the *recAo*^{C281} mutation was introduced into the *lexA3* mutants [36]. In a *recAo*^{C281} mutant, the LexA protein cannot bind the *recA* promoter, allowing a constitutively high level of RecA expression even in the absence of SOS induction. Notably, the *recAo*^{C281} mutation completely rescued the low-viability phenotype of the *lexA3* mutant strain carrying the palindrome and expressing SbcCD (Figure 1). This finding demonstrates that an increased level of RecA expression is the only SOS-induced characteristic needed for viability of *E. coli* cells subjected to a chronic DSB using this system.

A single repaired DSB per replication cycle induces the SOS response

The observation that an SOS induced level of RecA protein was required for cell survival implied the induction of the SOS response in populations of cells undergoing this chronic break. To measure the induction of the SOS system in individual cells, the fluorescence level was investigated by microscopy in *sbcDC*+ and Δ*sbcDC* cells containing or not the 246 bp interrupted palindrome and carrying a plasmid containing the *gfp* gene under the control of the SOS-inducible *sfiA* promoter (P_{sfiA}-*gfp*) (Figure 2A). The fluorescence level profiles were similar for palindrome-free *sbcDC*+ and Δ*sbcDC* cells and for Δ*sbcDC* cells carrying the 246 bp palindrome. However, the fluorescence level increased dramatically in *sbcDC*+ cells containing the 246 bp palindrome. Therefore, induction of a single targeted DSB per replication cycle significantly activates the SOS response.

Rapid growth, good viability and low mutagenesis are maintained in populations of cells undergoing chronic DSBR once per replication cycle

To investigate whether this level of chronic DSBR and induction of the SOS checkpoint lead to reduced growth and cell viability, cultures of *E. coli* cells were studied in the presence and absence of a chronic DSB. As shown in Figure 3 and Table 1, no differences were observed between growth rates or viabilities of *sbcDC*+ and Δ*sbcDC* strains containing or not the palindrome over a period of 7 hours (corresponding to 24 generations). This result

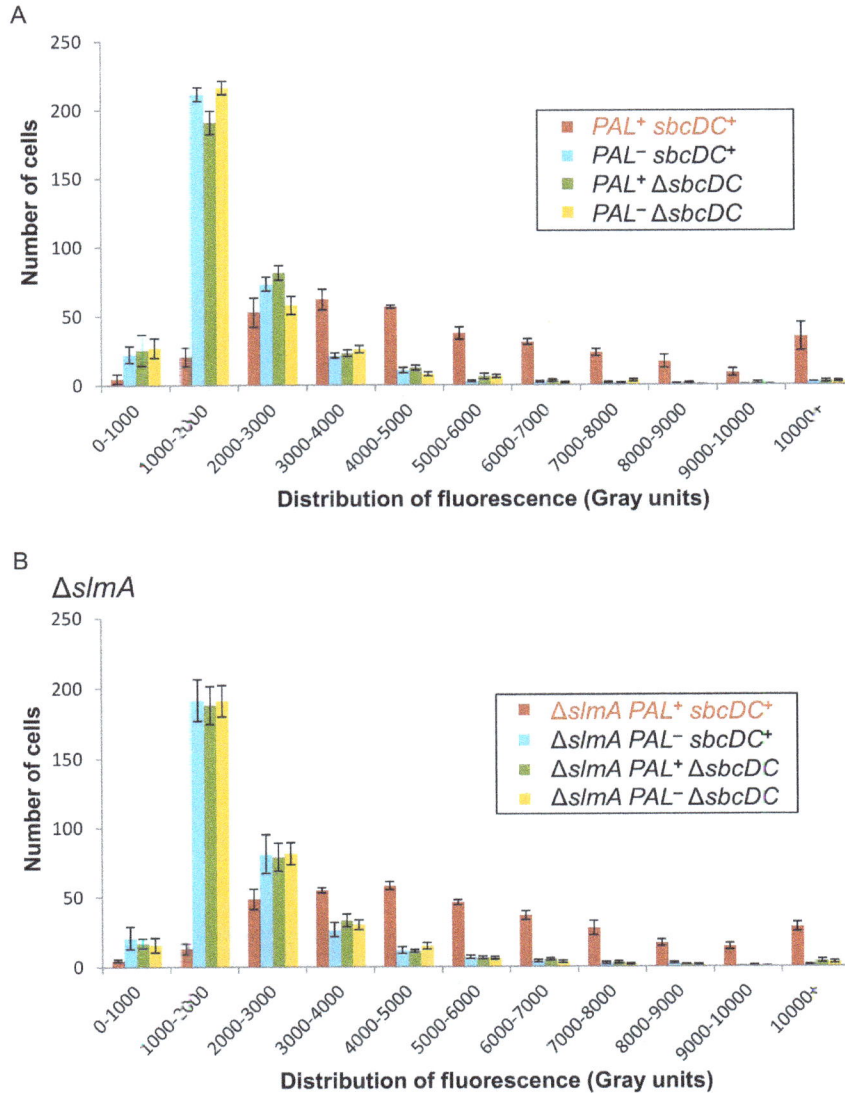

Figure 2. Cleavage of the 246 bp palindrome by SbcCD induces the SOS response. Fluorescence distribution profiles of average Gray value in pixels of populations of $sbcDC^+$ or $\Delta sbcDC$ cells containing or not the chromosomal 246 bp interrupted palindrome (PAL) and carrying a plasmid encoding a P_{sfiA}-gfp fusion (pGB150). Error bars show the standard error of the mean of 4 independent experiments investigating 350 cells each. (A) In a wild-type background. (B) In a $\Delta slmA$ background.

was confirmed by the observation that there was no detectable difference in colony size between any of the studied strains (Figure S2A). These experiments indicated that chronic DSBR must have little impact on cell growth or viability. However, a small growth disadvantage of cells undergoing DSBR (less than approximately 2% per generation) would not be detected in these experiments. Therefore, competition experiments were performed in which $sbcDC^+$ PAL^+ cells were mixed with $sbcDC^+$ PAL^- cells and the relative proportions of the two cell types were evaluated over a longer period of cell growth (75 hours). The two populations of cells were differentially marked with a yfp gene (in both combinations of marking, to account for any effect of the yfp gene on cell viability) and cell numbers were counted by flow cytometry. As can be seen in Figure 4, cells undergoing chronic DSBR had a growth disadvantage of 0.6% per generation.

Induction of the SOS response has the potential to increase mutagenesis due to the activation of one or both of the error-prone

polymerases (PolIV and PolV) [37,38,39,40,41]. $rpoB$ was used as a target gene to determine whether the induction of the SOS system in response to a single DSB per replication cycle leads to an increase in the level of mutagenesis. $rpoB$ mutants were selected by their ability to grow in the presence of rifampicin and their rate of formation was determined by fluctuation analysis (Figure 5) [32]. No increase in mutation rate was observed in the strain undergoing chronic DSBR, indicating that chronic induction of the SOS response in strains containing the 246 bp palindrome and expressing SbcCD does not induce PolIV- or PolV-mediated mutagenesis.

A single repaired DSB per replication cycle causes inhibition of cell division

To determine whether a single DSB per replication cycle inhibits cell division, the length of $sbcDC^+$ and $\Delta sbcDC$ cells

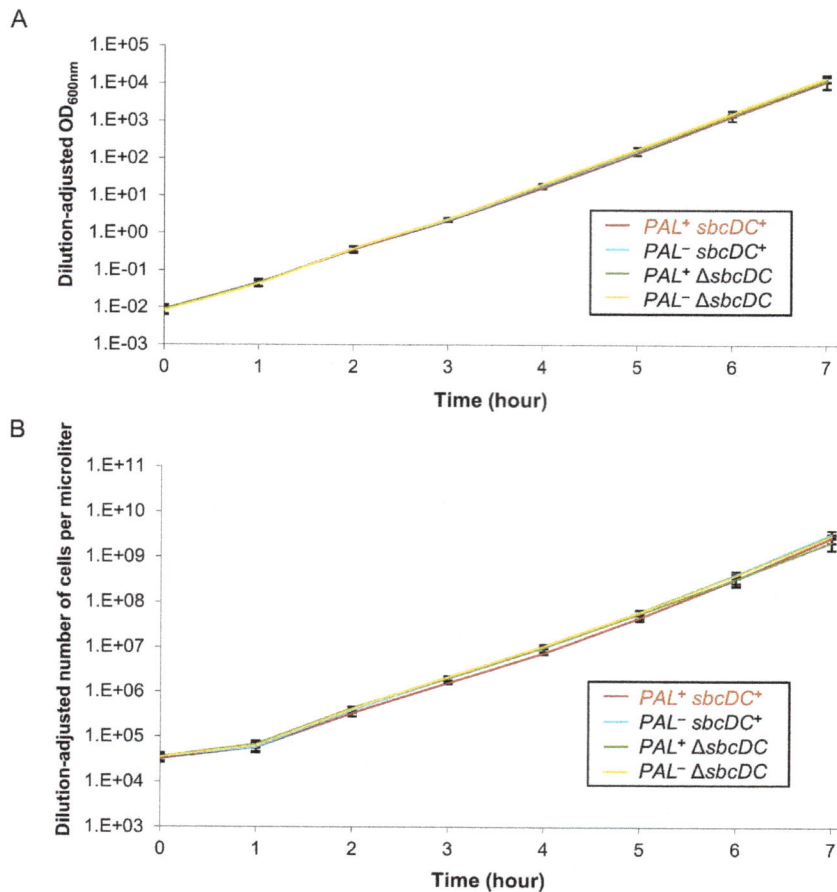

Figure 3. Cleavage of a palindrome by SbcCD has no detectable impact on cell growth. Graphs showing the growth level of *sbcDC*[+] and Δ*sbcDC E. coli* strains containing or not the chromosomal 246 bp interrupted palindrome (*PAL*). Error bars show the standard error of the mean of 3 independent experiments. (A) Dilution-adjusted optical density at 600 nm of cultures kept in exponential phase. (B) Dilution-adjusted average number of cells per microliter of cultures kept in exponential phase as counted by flow cytometry.

containing or not the palindrome was measured. The mean length of *sbcDC*[+] cells containing the palindrome was almost 34% longer than that of cells lacking SbcCD and/or the palindrome (Table 2). The distribution of cell lengths was significantly different in the strain subjected to a chronic DSB (*PAL*[+] *sbcDC*[+]; Figure 6A; Tables 3, 4 and 5). The change in length distribution caused by chronic DSBR was characterized by two principal features, a decrease in the number of small cells (<4 µm in length; Table 3) and an increase in filamentation (defined here as cells longer than 8 µm; Table 4). About 17% of *sbcDC*[+] cells containing the palindrome were longer than 8 µm whereas only 4% of cells that were not subject to a chronic DSB reached that length. In addition, time-lapse microscopy was used to observe live filamentation of *sbcDC*[+] cells containing the palindrome (Videos S1, S2, S3 and S4 in Supplementary data).

Inhibition of cell division can be controlled by the SOS-induced cell division inhibitor SfiA [9,11] or by nucleoid occlusion in which SlmA plays an important role [17,42]. The potential role of SfiA in the elongation of cells subjected to a chronic DSB was investigated. Cell growth and cell length of *sbcDC*[+] and Δ*sbcDC* strains containing or not the palindrome were similar in presence or absence of SfiA (Tables 1 and 2; Figures 6B and S2B), suggesting that other pathways contribute to cell elongation in cells subjected to a chronic DSB. The potential role of SlmA in the

elongation of cells subjected to a chronic DSB was also investigated. There was no significant difference in the growth of Δ*slmA sbcDC*[+] and Δ*slmA* Δ*sbcDC* strains containing or not the palindrome (Table 1 and Figure S2C). Surprisingly, the distribution of length of Δ*slmA* cells subjected to a chronic DSB showed that the whole population of cells was significantly longer in the absence of SlmA (Tables 2, 3, 4, 5 and Figure 6C), indicating that there is an increase in the unit size of these cells. This result suggests that the absence of SlmA induced a nucleoid-occlusion independent pathway that inhibits cell division. Importantly, the levels of the SOS response in Δ*slmA* cells subjected or not to a chronic DSB were similar to those in a wild-type background (Figure 2), demonstrating that this increase in cell size does not originate from a more elevated SOS response in cells subjected to a chronic DSB in the absence of SlmA. To determine whether the action of SfiA and SlmA were both responsible for cell elongation caused by a chronic DSB, cell growth and cell length were studied in Δ*sfiA* Δ*slmA* double mutants. The growth rate of Δ*sfiA* Δ*slmA* strains was unaffected when subjected to a chronic DSB (Table 1 and Figure S2D). However, the cell length of two subpopulations was significantly affected by the deletion of the *sfiA* gene in a Δ*slmA* strain subjected to a chronic DSB (Tables 2, 3, 4, 5 and Figure 6D). Firstly, the number of cells under 4 µm increased back to a similar number as in the *slmA*[+] strains subjected to a chronic

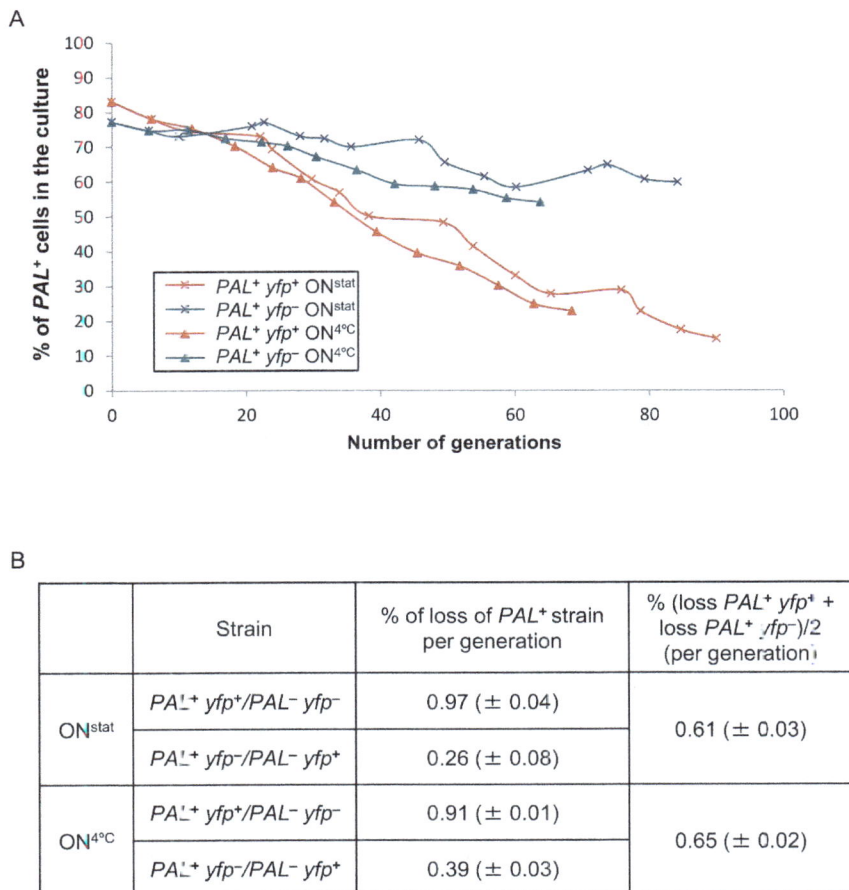

Figure 4. Effect of the cleavage of a palindrome by SbcCD quantified by competition experiments. Competition experiments were carried out between $PAL^+ yfp^+$ and $PAL^- yfp^-$ strains on one hand and $PAL^+ yfp^-$ and $PAL^- yfp^+$ strains on the other hand. Cells were either allowed to reach stationary phase at night time (ON^{stat}; grown for more than 80 generations) or constantly kept in exponential phase ($ON^{4°C}$; grown for more than 60 generations). (A) Example of a graph showing the percentage of cells containing the chromosomal 246 bp interrupted palindrome (PAL) in function of the number of generations of co-culture with a strain that does not contain the palindrome. These results are from the second replicate of the competition experiments. (B) Table presenting the average percentage of loss per generation of strains containing the chromosomal 246 bp interrupted palindrome (PAL) during these competition experiments. Errors indicated between brackets are the standard error of the mean of 3 independent experiments.

DSB (around 31% of the cells in $slmA^+$ and $\Delta sfiA \Delta slmA$ backgrounds compared to 23% in the $\Delta slmA$ background; Figure 6D and Table 3). Secondly, the number of very long cells (more than 15 μm) dropped in the $\Delta sfiA \Delta slmA$ strain subjected to a chronic DSB (around 1.1% of the cells compared to 3–5.6% in the other backgrounds subjected to a chronic DSB and 0.1–0.6% in cells not subjected to a chronic DSB; Figure 6D and Table 5).

These results indicate that the two pathways performed by SfiA and SlmA are together responsible for the majority of the very long cells (cells over 15 μm in length) observed in presence of a chronic DSB. In addition, the increase in cell size observed in the whole population in a $\Delta slmA$ strain subjected to a chronic DSB requires the presence of SfiA but is not due to an increase of the SOS response.

Table 1. E. coli generation time (minutes).

Background	$PAL^+ sbcDC^+$	$PAL^- sbcDC^+$	$PAL^+ \Delta sbcDC$	$PAL^- \Delta sbcDC$
Wild-type	19.7 (±1.2)	19.6 (±0.8)	19.5 (±0.3)	19.4 (±0.4)
$\Delta sfiA$	21.2 (±0.9)	20.7 (±1.1)	21 (±0.4)	21.4 (±0.7)
$\Delta slmA$	18.9 (±0.3)	16.5 (±1)	17.4 (±0.5)	17.5 (±0.9)
$\Delta sfiA \Delta slmA$	18 (±0.5)	17.2 (±0.9)	18.4 (±0.46)	18 (±0.4)

Errors indicated between brackets are the standard error of the mean of 3 independent experiments. No statistically significant differences (p-value <0.05) have been found between strains from the same background using an ANOVA two-factor with replication test (DSBs compared to no DSBs).

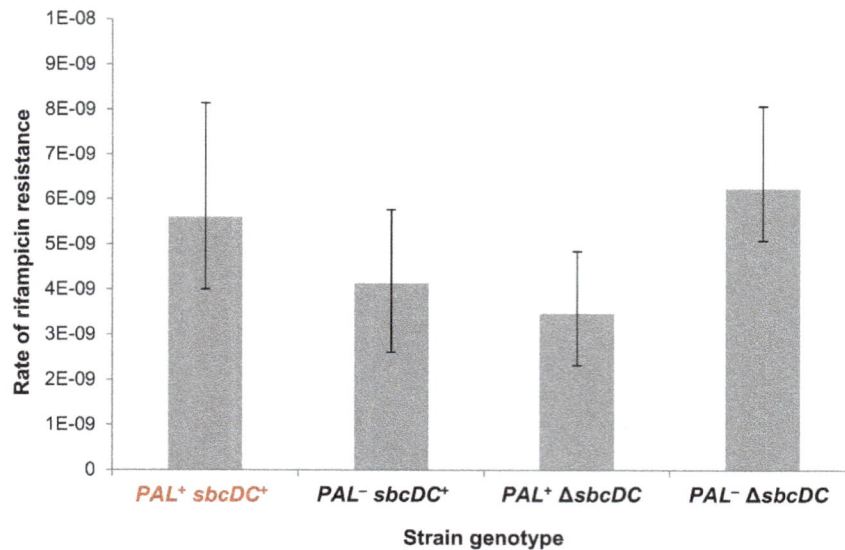

Figure 5. SOS induction following the cleavage of a palindrome by SbcCD does not induce mutagenesis. Fluctuation analysis measuring the rate of mutagenesis (mutation to rifampicin resistance cells) in *sbcDC*+ and Δ*sbcDC E. coli* strains containing or not the chromosomal 246 bp interrupted palindrome (*PAL*). Error bars show the 95% confidence intervals.

It is clear that DSB induction causes three separable effects on cell size. First, there is a reduction of the number of small cells that occurs irrespectively of inactivation of SfiA and SlmA. Second, there is a further reduction of the number of small cells in presence of SfiA but absence of SlmA. Third, there is an increase in very long cells that occurs in the presence of either SfiA or SlmA and is only significantly reduced in the double mutant.

Discussion

This study demonstrates that a single, efficiently repaired, DSB per chromosome per replication cycle is sufficient to induce the SOS response of *E. coli* and that this induction is required for cell viability. The only requirement for the SOS response in the survival of cells following this level of chronic DNA damage is the induced expression of RecA protein. It is possible that the need for an elevated level of RecA protein reflects the repetitive nature of the damage induced since a naïve cell encountering a DSB will not have an induced level of RecA protein and normally survives the damage. The fact that the population of *E. coli* cells subjected to this level of DSB induces the SOS response is consistent with the observation that the level of spontaneous DSBR in cells that are not inducing the SOS response at the population level is lower than one break per replication cycle. Previous estimates are that spontaneous DSBR occurs at a frequency of less than 1% per generation, as measured by SOS induction [25], and that replication restart requiring DnaC (which includes DSBR events) occurs in 18% of replication cycles [43].

We show that chronic DSBR results in an increase in cell size consistent with delayed cell division. It has been proposed that, following DNA damage, inhibition of cell division allows time for successful repair to occur before cell division can proceed [9]. Our data on cell size argue that there are three separable effects of chronic DSB that are differentially affected by the SOS-induced cell division inhibition system mediated by SfiA and nucleoid occlusion mediated by SlmA. First, there is a decrease in the number of small cells (<4 μm in length) that is indicative of a larger size of the unit cell and is independent of SfiA and SlmA.

Second, in the absence of SlmA and presence of SfiA, this decrease in the number of small cells is accentuated. Third, there is a DSB-induced large increase in length that is only significantly reduced in the absence of both cell division inhibition systems mediated by SfiA and SlmA. Recently, the existence of an SOS- and SlmA-independent pathway blocking cell division was revealed by Cambridge and collaborators [44]. Whether or not this is the same system as that causing an increase in the unit cell size observed here remains to be determined.

Importantly, despite the requirement for SOS induction in cell survival and the activation of the checkpoint by this level of DNA damage resulting in a delay in cell division, cells maintain 99.4% growth rate and viability accompanied by no increase in mutagenesis. The prokaryotic cell cycle has partially unlinked its DNA replication and cell division cycles by uncoupling the initiation of DNA replication from cell division while retaining the link between termination of DNA replication and cell division [45,46,47]. In this way, rounds of DNA replication can overlap in situations where the DNA replication cycle takes longer than the cell division cycle. The observation of a cell loss of 0.6% per generation subjected to a chronic DSBR has four implications. First, the period between rounds of initiation of DNA replication in cells undergoing chronic DSBR must be at least 99.4% of that in control cells. A greater difference in this period would result in a corresponding difference in the number of genomes produced that would over the generations affect the number of viable cells. Second, cells increase in mass at approximately the same rate irrespective of chronic DSBR. Therefore, there is no change in metabolism that is sufficient to substantially alter the accumulation of cell mass. Third, at least 99.4% of chromosomes are eventually distributed appropriately to daughter cells even if this may be delayed in some cells that are experiencing a delay in cell division. And fourth, the vast majority of cells in which cell division has been inhibited are fully viable. That all these implications are satisfied in cells that have chronically induced an essential DNA damage checkpoint reveals the seamless operation of the SOS system when cells are experiencing a low level of chronic damage. The present study confirms that *E. coli* has evolved a cell cycle

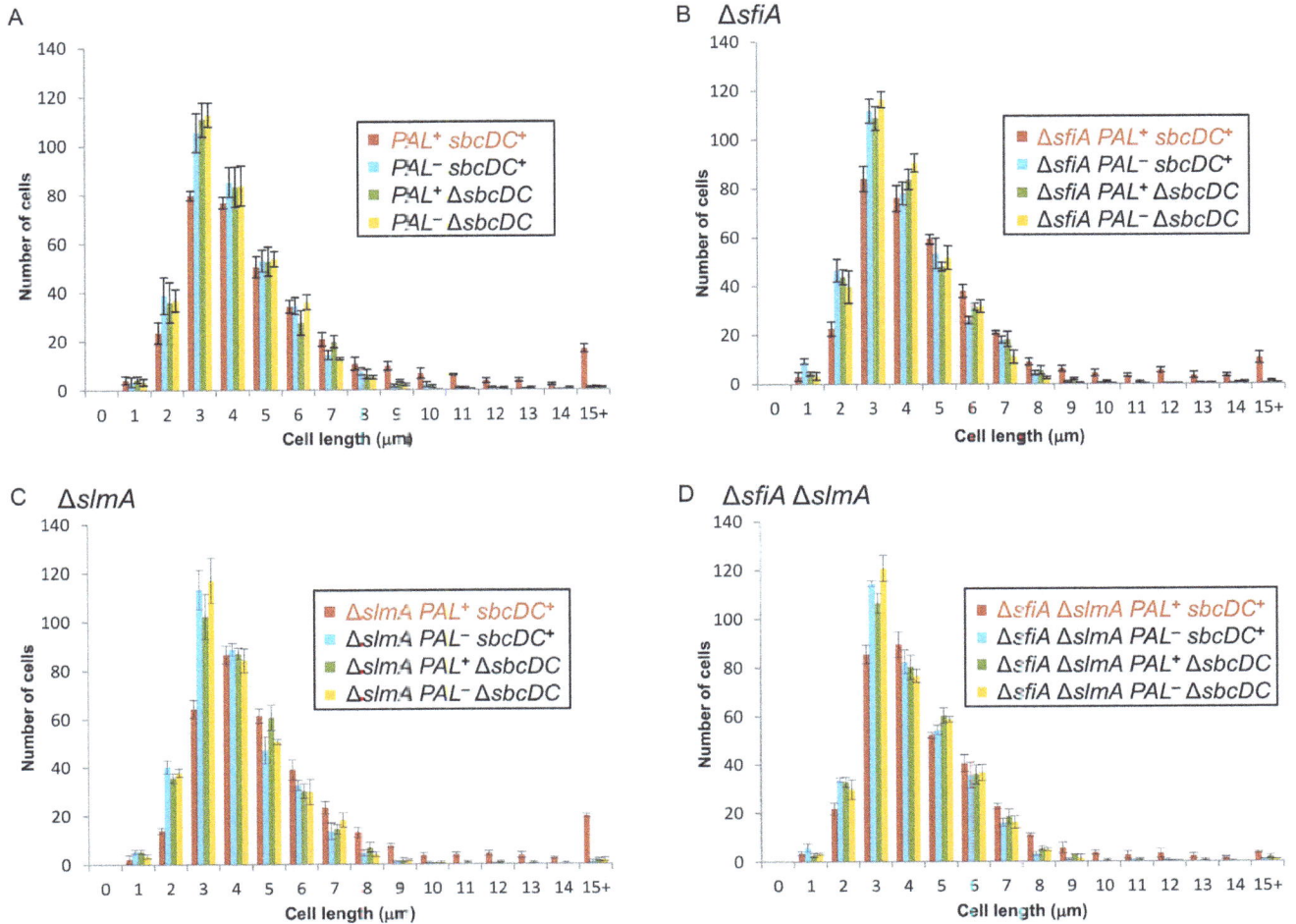

Figure 6. Role of SfiA and SlmA in the delay of cell division following a chronic DSB. Graphs displaying the cell length distribution in micrometers of *sbcDC*[+] and Δ*sbcDC E. coli* cells containing or not the chromosomal 246 bp interrupted palindrome (*PAL*). Error bars show the standard error of the mean of 4 independent experiments investigating 350 cells each. (A) In a wild-type background. (B) In a Δ*sfiA* background. (C) In a Δ*slmA* background. (D) In a Δ*sfiA* Δ*slmA* background.

where it can reconcile the imperative for rapid cell multiplication with the operation of a checkpoint designed to ensure repair of DNA damage prior to cell division. The partially unlinked nature of the DNA replication and cell division cycles implies that *E. coli* can delay cell division in response to chronic DSBR without substantially affecting the time interval between initiations of DNA

replication and can manage the consequences of segregating its chromosomes whatever extra time may be required to undertake DNA repair.

In a wider context, it is interesting to compare the checkpoint strategies adopted under similar situations by eukaryotic cells, in which the DNA replication cycle is more closely tied to the cell

Table 2. Average *E. coli* cell length (micrometers).

Background	PAL[+] sbcDC[+]	PAL[−] sbcDC[+]	PAL[+] ΔsbcDC	PAL[−] ΔsbcDC	% DSB[+]/DSB[−]
Wild-type	6.2 (±0.1) *	4.7 (±0.2)	4.7 (±0.1)	4.6 (±0.1)	133.8%
ΔsfiA	5.8 (±0.2) *	4.4 (±0.1)	4.6 (±0.1)	4.4 (±0.1)	129.7%
ΔslmA	6.5 (±0.1) *#	4.5 (±0.1)	4.7 (±0.1)	4.6 (±0.1)	140.6%
ΔsfiA ΔslmA	5.4 (±0.1) *#†	4.6 (±0.1)	4.8 (±0.1)	4.6 (±0.1)	115.1%

Errors indicated between brackets are the standard error of the mean of 4 independent experiments investigating 350 cells each.
* Statistically significantly different from the other strains in the same background using an ANOVA two-factor with replication test (DSBs compared to no DSBs; p-value <0.05).
# Statistically significantly different from the wild-type version of this strain using an unpaired t-test (p-value <0.05).
† Statistically significantly different from the Δ*slmA sfiA*[+] version of this strain using an unpaired t-test (p-value <0.05).

Table 3. Percentage of *E. coli* cells shorter than 4 μm (%).

Background	PAL⁺ sbcDC⁺	PAL⁻ sbcDC⁺	PAL⁺ ΔsbcDC	PAL⁻ ΔsbcDC	% DSB⁺/DSB⁻
Wild-type	30.7 (±1.2)	42.2 (±4.3)	43.2 (±4.1)	43.7 (±2.5)	71.3
ΔsfiA	31.3 (±2.7)	47.9 (±1.3)	44.8 (±2.2)	45.6 (±2)	67.9
ΔslmA	23 (±1.5)	45.4 (±2.8)	40.9 (±2.7)	45.2 (±2.2)	52.5
ΔsfiA ΔslmA	31.6 (±1)	44 (±0.5)	40.5 (±1)	43.9 (±2.4)	73.8

Errors indicated between brackets are the standard error of the mean of 4 independent experiments.

Table 4. Percentage of *E. coli* cells longer than 8 μm (%).

Background	PAL⁺ sbcDC⁺	PAL⁻ sbcDC⁺	PAL⁺ ΔsbcDC	PAL⁻ ΔsbcDC	% DSB⁺/DSB⁻
Wild-type	17.2 (±1.2)	4.4 (±0.9)	4.4 (±0.6)	3.1 (±0.5)	433.2
ΔsfiA	13.2 (±1.2)	2 (±0.4)	3.4 (±0.7)	1.6 (±0.2)	566.5
ΔslmA	16.9 (±1)	2.5 (±0.6)	4.1 (±0.8)	2.5 (±0.7)	557.7
ΔsfiA ΔslmA	9.8 (±1.6)	2.1 (±0.5)	3.9 (±0.3)	2.4 (±0.5)	350

Errors indicated between brackets are the standard error of the mean of 4 independent experiments.

Table 5. Percentage of *E. coli* cells longer than 15 μm (%).

Background	PAL⁺ sbcDC⁺	PAL⁻ sbcDC⁺	PAL⁺ ΔsbcDC	PAL⁻ ΔsbcDC	% DSB⁺/DSB⁻
Wild-type	4.8 (±0.5)	0.3 (±0.1)	0.4 (±0.1)	0.3 (±0.1)	1454
ΔsfiA	3 (±0.7)	0.1 (±0.1)	0.4 (±0.1)	0.1 (±0.1)	1500
ΔslmA	5.6 (±0.2)	0.3 (±0.2)	0.5 (±0.1)	0.5 (±0.2)	1302
ΔsfiA ΔslmA	1.1 (±0.1)	0.3 (±0.2)	0.6 (±0.3)	0.3 (±0.2)	275

Errors indicated between brackets are the standard error of the mean of 4 independent experiments.

division cycle. There, replication generally takes up a less significant period within the cell cycle and accommodation to chronic checkpoint induction may be possible via the alternative strategy of altering the lengths of G1, S and G2 phases of the cell cycle, while dividing at a higher cell mass. It is also possible for some DNA damage to be carried over from one cell cycle to another [48,49,50]. However, it has been shown that activation of the DNA damage checkpoint can be detrimental to *S. cerevisiae* survival in the presence of continuous low levels of DNA damage by UV irradiation [21]. By contrast, in the same organism, checkpoint function is required for optimal growth and colony formation following chronic checkpoint induction caused by humanized telomeres [51]. Overexpression of Rad24 induces checkpoint activation in *S. pombe*, increases cell size and reduces growth rate [52,53] but the reduction in growth rate may not simply be due to checkpoint activation. To our knowledge, the possibility that eukaryotic cells might be able to delay cell division by chronic checkpoint activation and yet retain growth and viability associated with normal growth conditions remains open. Clearly, this would not be desirable in many cells of multicellular eukaryotes where rapid multiplication would be of no selective

advantage and might be associated with pathogenic consequences (e.g. cancer).

Supporting Information

Figure S1 Example of flow cytometry results from a competition experiment. Results from flow cytometry analyses of the third replicate of the competition experiment between a *PAL⁺ yfp⁻* strain and a *PAL⁻ yfp⁺* strain after 23.5 hours of growth (these cells were allowed to reach stationary phase at night time). (A) Visualisation and selection of cells in function of light scatter angles. The flow cytometer counted and displayed 500,000 particles. A heat map indicated the population density of these particles. Cells were selected (here 466,255 cells were encircled in region of interest 1). (B) Visualisation and selection of cells in function of their green fluorescence. *PAL⁺ yfp⁻* cells were encircled in region of interest 2 whereas *PAL⁻ yfp⁺* cells were encircled in region of interest 7. (C) Number of cells in function of fluorescence when gated by region of interest 1. The cells selected in region of interest 1 in panel A were separated here in function of their fluorescence so that it was possible to evaluate the number of *PAL⁺ yfp⁻* cells indicated in region of interest 5 and *PAL⁻ yfp⁺*

cells indicated in region of interest 6. (D) Number of PAL^+ yfp^- cells in the population. The cells selected in region of interest 2 in panel B were separated in function of their fluorescence so that it was possible to calculate the number of PAL^+ yfp^- cells indicated in region of interest 4. (E) Number of PAL^- yfp^+ cells in the population. The cells selected in region of interest 7 in panel B were separated in function of their fluorescence so that it was possible to calculate the number of PAL^- yfp^+ cells indicated in region of interest 3. Characteristics of regions of interest are indicated under each panel; the numbers of cells per microliter of culture (Evt/µl) were used for subsequent data analyses. (TIF)

Figure S2 ***E. coli* viability is not significantly affected by a chronic DSB.** Viability of $sbcDC^+$ and $\Delta sbcDC$ E. coli strains containing or not the chromosomal 246 bp interrupted palindrome (*PAL*). Spot tests of ten-fold dilution series were carried out on LB plates. (A) Wild-type background strain. (B) $\Delta sfiA$ background strain. (C) $\Delta slmA$ background strain. (D) $\Delta sfiA$ $\Delta slmA$ background strain.

File S1 Main supporting information file. This file includes additional materials and methods (strains and plasmids, spot test, time-lapse microscopy), additional results (time-lapse microscopy), Table S1 (E. coli strains), Table S2 (plasmids), Table S3 (oligonucleotides) and additional references.

Video S1   **PAL+ SbcCD+.**

Video S2   **PAL− SbcCD+.**

Video S3   **PAL+ SbcCD−.**

Video S4   **PAL− SbcCD−.**

Acknowledgments

We would like to thanks Dr Garry W. Blakely for the pGB150 plasmid, Dr Haomin Huang and Dr Millicent Masters for the pMH9 (pHM) plasmid, Dr Rosalind J Allen and Dr Lucas Black for the RJA002 strain, Lisa Iurchenko for the DL5402 and DL5403 strains, Julie Blyth for the pDL1573 plasmid and preliminary experiments, Rebekah Tillotson for preliminary experiments and Charlie Cockram for helping with statistical analyses.

Author Contributions

Conceived and designed the experiments ED JKE MALV MAW DRFL. Performed the experiments: ED JKE MALV MAW DRFL. Analyzed the data: ED JKE MALV MAW DRFL. Contributed reagents/materials/analysis tools: ED JKE MALV MAW DRFL. Wrote the paper: ED JKE MALV MAW DRFL.

References

1. Kuzminov A (1999) Recombinational repair of DNA damage in *Escherichia coli* and bacteriophage lambda. Microbiol Mol Biol Rev 63: 751–813, table of contents.
2. Cromie GA, Connelly JC, Leach DR (2001) Recombination at double-strand breaks and DNA ends: conserved mechanisms from phage to humans. Mol Cell 8: 1163–1174.
3. Harper JW, Elledge SJ (2007) The DNA damage response: ten years after. Mol Cell 28: 739–745.
4. Harrison JC, Haber JE (2006) Surviving the breakup: the DNA damage checkpoint. Annu Rev Genet 40: 209–235
5. Walker GC, Smith BT, Sutton MT (2000) The SOS response of DNA damage. In: Stork G, Hengge-Aronis R, editors. Bacteria Stress Responses. Washington D.C.: American Society of Microbiology. pp.131–144.
6. Brent R, Ptashne M (1981) Mechanism of action of the *lexA* gene product. Proc Natl Acad Sci U S A 78: 4204–4208.
7. Little JW (1984) Autodigestion of *lexA* and phage lambda repressors. Proc Natl Acad Sci U S A 81: 1375–1379.
8. Little JW, Mount DW, Yanisch-Perron CR (1981) Purified *lexA* protein is a repressor of the *recA* and *lexA* genes. Proc Natl Acad Sci U S A 78: 4199–4203.
9. Huisman O, D'Ari R (1981) An inducible DNA replication-cell division coupling mechanism in E. coli. Nature 290: 797–799.
10. Bi E, Lutkenhaus J (1993) Cell division inhibitors SulA and MinCD prevent formation of the FtsZ ring. J Bacteriol 175: 1118–1125.
11. Chen Y, Milam SL, Erickson HP (2012) SulA inhibits assembly of FtsZ by a simple sequestration mechanism. Biochemistry 51: 3100–3109.
12. Rico AI, Krupka M, Vicente M (2013) In the beginning, *Escherichia coli* assembled the proto-ring: an initial phase of division. J Biol Chem 288: 20830–20836.
13. Egan AJ, Vollmer W (2013) The physiology of bacterial cell division. Ann N Y Acad Sci 1277: 8–28.
14. Natale P, Pazos M, Vicente M (2013) The *Escherichia coli* divisome: born to divide. Environ Microbiol 15: 3169–3182.
15. Bernhardt TG, de Boer PA (2005) SlmA, a nucleoid-associated, FtsZ binding protein required for blocking septal ring assembly over Chromosomes in E. coli. Mol Cell 18: 555–564.
16. Cho H, McManus HR, Dove SL, Bernhardt TG (2011) Nucleoid occlusion factor SlmA is a DNA-activated FtsZ polymerization antagonist. Proc Natl Acad Sci U S A 108: 3773–3778.
17. Tonthat NK, Milam SL, Chinnam N, Whitfil T, Margolin W, et al. (2013) SlmA forms a higher-order structure on DNA that inhibits cytokinetic Z-ring formation over the nucleoid. Proc Natl Acad Sci U S A 110: 10586–10591.
18. Lee SE, Moore JK, Holmes A, Umezu K, Kolodner RD, et al. (1998) Saccharomyces Ku70, mre11/rad50 and RPA proteins regulate adaptation to G2/M arrest after DNA damage. Cell 94: 399–409.
19. Weinert TA, Hartwell LH (1988) The RAD9 gene controls the cell cycle response to DNA damage in *Saccharomyces cerevisiae*. Science 241: 317–322.
20. Siede W, Friedberg AS, Friedberg EC (1993) RAD9-dependent G1 arrest defines a second checkpoint for damaged DNA in the cell cycle of *Saccharomyces cerevisiae*. Proc Natl Acad Sci U S A 90: 7985–7989.
21. Hishida T, Kubota Y, Carr AM, Iwasaki H (2009) RAD6-RAD18-RAD5-pathway-dependent tolerance to chronic low-dose ultraviolet light. Nature 457: 612–615.
22. Keller KL, Overbeck-Carrick TL, Beck DJ (2001) Survival and induction of SOS in *Escherichia coli* treated with cisplatin, UV-irradiation, or mitomycin C are dependent on the function of the RecBC and RecFOR pathways of homologous recombination. Mutat Res 486: 21–29.
23. Whitby MC, Lloyd RG (1995) Altered SOS induction associated with mutations in *recF*, *recO* and *recR*. Mol Gen Genet 246: 174–179.
24. Rudolph CJ, Upton AL, Lloyd RG (2007) Replication fork stalling and cell cycle arrest in UV-irradiated *Escherichia coli*. Genes Dev 21: 668–681.
25. Pennington JM, Rosenberg SM (2007) Spontaneous DNA breakage in single living *Escherichia coli* cells. Nat Genet 39: 797–802.
26. Vlasic I, Ivancic-Bace I, Imesek M, Mihaljevic B, Brcic-Kostic K (2008) RecJ nuclease is required for SOS induction after introduction of a double-strand break in a RecA loading deficient *recB* mutant of *Escherichia coli*. Biochimie 90: 1347–1355.
27. Meddows TR, Savory AP, Lloyd RG (2004) RecG helicase promotes DNA double-strand break repair. Mol Microbiol 52: 119–132.
28. Eykelenboom JK, Blackwood JK, Okely E, Leach DR (2008) SbcCD causes a double-strand break at a DNA palindrome in the *Escherichia coli* chromosome. Mol Cell 29: 644–651.
29. Cromie GA, Millar CB, Schmidt KH, Leach DR (2000) Palindromes as substrates for multiple pathways of recombination in *Escherichia coli*. Genetics 154: 513–522.
30. Leach DR, Okely EA, Pinder DJ (1997) Repair by recombination of DNA containing a palindromic sequence. Mol Microbiol 26: 597–606.
31. Soupene E, van Heeswijk WC, Plumbridge J, Stewart V, Bertenthal D, et al. (2003) Physiological studies of *Escherichia coli* strain MG1655: growth defects and apparent cross-regulation of gene expression. J Bacteriol 185: 5611–5626.
32. Spell RM, Jinks-Robertson S (2004) Determination of mitotic recombination rates by fluctuation analysis in *Saccharomyces cerevisiae*. Methods Mol Biol 262: 3–12.
33. Little JW, Edmiston SH, Pacelli LZ, Mount DW (1980) Cleavage of the *Escherichia coli lexA* protein by the *recA* protease. Proc Natl Acad Sci U S A 77: 3225–3229.
34. Courcelle J, Khodursky A, Peter B, Brown PO, Hanawalt PC (2001) Comparative gene expression profiles following UV exposure in wild-type and SOS-deficient *Escherichia coli*. Genetics 158: 41–64.

35. Kenyon CJ, Walker GC (1980) DNA-damaging agents stimulate gene expression at specific loci in *Escherichia coli*. Proc Natl Acad Sci U S A 77: 2819–2823.

36. Thoms B, Wackernagel W (1998) Interaction of RecBCD enzyme with DNA at double-strand breaks produced in UV-irradiated *Escherichia coli*: requirement for DNA end processing. J Bacteriol 180: 5639–5645.

37. Delmas S, Matic I (2006) Interplay between replication and recombination in *Escherichia coli*: impact of the alternative DNA polymerases. Proc Natl Acad Sci U S A 103: 4564–4569.

38. Pham P, Rangarajan S, Woodgate R, Goodman MF (2001) Roles of DNA polymerases V and II in SOS-induced error-prone and error-free repair in *Escherichia coli*. Proc Natl Acad Sci U S A 98: 8350–8354.

39. Wagner J, Gruz P, Kim SR, Yamada M, Matsui K, et al. (1999) The *dinB* gene encodes a novel *E. coli* DNA polymerase, DNA pol IV, involved in mutagenesis. Mol Cell 4: 281–286.

40. Kobayashi S, Valentine MR, Pham P, O'Donnell M, Goodman MF (2002) Fidelity of *Escherichia coli* DNA polymerase IV. Preferential generation of small deletion mutations by dNTP-stabilized misalignment. J Biol Chem 277: 34198–34207.

41. Tang M, Pham P, Shen X, Taylor JS, O'Donnell M, et al. (2000) Roles of *E. coli* DNA polymerases IV and V in lesion-targeted and untargeted SOS mutagenesis. Nature 404: 1014–1018.

42. Wu LJ, Errington J (2012) Nucleoid occlusion and bacterial cell division. Nat Rev Microbiol 10: 8–12.

43. Maisnier-Patin S, Nordström K, Dasgupta S (2001) Replication arrests during a single round of replication of the *Escherichia coli* chromosome in the absence of DnaC activity. Mol Microbiol 42: 1371–1382.

44. Cambridge J, Blinkova A, Magnan D, Bates D, Walker JR (2014) A replication-inhibited unsegregated nucleoid at mid-cell blocks Z-ring formation and cell division independently of SOS and the SlmA nucleoid occlusion protein in *Escherichia coli*. J Bacteriol 196: 36–49.

45. Cooper S, Helmstetter CE (1968) Chromosome replication and the division cycle of *Escherichia coli* B/r. J Mol Biol 31: 519–540.

46. Haeusser DP, Levin PA (2008) The great divide: coordinating cell cycle events during bacterial growth and division. Curr Opin Microbiol 11: 94–99.

47. Zaritsky A, Wang P, Vischer NO (2011) Instructive simulation of the bacterial cell division cycle. Microbiology 157: 1876–1885.

48. Weinert T (2007) Cell biology. What a cell should know (but may not). Science 315: 1374–1375.

49. Lukas C, Savic V, Bekker-Jensen S, Doil C, Neumann B, et al. (2011) 53BP1 nuclear bodies form around DNA lesions generated by mitotic transmission of chromosomes under replication stress. Nat Cell Biol 13: 243–253.

50. Mankouri HW, Huttner D, Hickson ID (2013) How unfinished business from S-phase affects mitosis and beyond. EMBO J 32: 2661–2671.

51. di Domenico EG, Auriche C, Viscardi V, Longhese MP, Gilson E, et al. (2009) The Mec1p and Tel1p checkpoint kinases allow humanized yeast to tolerate chronic telomere dysfunctions by suppressing telomere fusions. DNA Repair (Amst) 8: 209–218.

52. Ford JC, al-Khodairy F, Fotou E, Sheldrick KS, Griffiths DJ, et al. (1994) 14-3-3 protein homologs required for the DNA damage checkpoint in fission yeast. Science 265: 533–535.

53. Lee M (2008) Overexpression of human Raf-1 enhances radiosensitivity in fission yeast, *Schizosaccharomyces pombe*. Cell Biochem Funct 26: 125–131.

19

Potentially Functional SNPs (pfSNPs) as Novel Genomic Predictors of 5-FU Response in Metastatic Colorectal Cancer Patients

Jingbo Wang[1,9], Xu Wang[2,9], Mingjue Zhao[4], Su Pin Choo[3], Sin Jen Ong[3], Simon Y. K. Ong[3], Samuel S. Chong[4], Yik Ying Teo[2]*, Caroline G. L. Lee[1,5,6]*

1 Department of Biochemistry, Yong Loo Lin School of Medicine, National University of Singapore, Singapore, Singapore, 2 Saw Swee Hock School of Public Health, National University of Singapore, Singapore, Singapore, 3 Division of Medical Oncology, National Cancer Centre, Singapore, Singapore, 4 Department of Paediatrics, Yong Loo Lin School of Medicine, National University of Singapore, Singapore, Singapore, 5 Division of Medical Sciences, National Cancer Centre, Singapore, Singapore, 6 Duke-NUS Graduate Medical School, Singapore, Singapore

Abstract

5-Fluorouracil (5-FU) and its pro-drug Capecitabine have been widely used in treating colorectal cancer. However, not all patients will respond to the drug, hence there is a need to develop reliable early predictive biomarkers for 5-FU response. Here, we report a novel potentially functional Single Nucleotide Polymorphism (pfSNP) approach to identify SNPs that may serve as predictive biomarkers of response to 5-FU in Chinese metastatic colorectal cancer (CRC) patients. 1547 pfSNPs and one variable number tandem repeat (VNTR) in 139 genes in 5-FU drug (both PK and PD pathway) and colorectal cancer disease pathways were examined in 2 groups of CRC patients. Shrinkage of liver metastasis measured by RECIST criteria was used as the clinical end point. Four non-responder-specific pfSNPs were found to account for 37.5% of all non-responders ($P < 0.0003$). Five additional pfSNPs were identified from a multivariate model (AUC under ROC = 0.875) that was applied for all other pfSNPs, excluding the non-responder-specific pfSNPs. These pfSNPs, which can differentiate the other non-responders from responders, mainly reside in tumor suppressor genes or genes implicated in colorectal cancer risk. Hence, a total of 9 novel SNPs with potential functional significance may be able to distinguish non-responders from responders to 5-FU. These pfSNPs may be useful biomarkers for predicting response to 5-FU.

Editor: Anthony W. I. Lo, Queen Mary Hospital, Hong Kong

Funding: This work was supported by a grant (SERC 112 148 0008) from Singapore BioMedical Research Council - Science and Engineering Research Council (BMRC-SERC) to A/Professors Caroline Lee, Simon Ong, Yik Ying Teo and Samuel Chong. The funders had no role in study design, data collection and analysis, decision to publish, or preparation of the manuscript.

Competing Interests: The authors have declared that no competing interests exist.

* Email: bchleec@nus.edu.sg (CGLL); yik_ying_teo@nuhs.edu.sg (YYT)

9 These authors contributed equally to this work.

Introduction

Every year, more than one million individuals worldwide will develop colorectal cancer [1], accounting for 10% of the global cancer burden. Colorectal cancer (CRC) is the most frequently diagnosed cancer in Singapore (7,909 new cases between 2005–2009) [2]. More than half of CRC patients develop metastatic disease (stage 4) either at diagnosis or at relapse following initial curative intent therapy. This translates to a substantial proportion of patients who may need treatment for the metastasis or relapse of colorectal cancer.

5-fluorouracil (5-FU) and its pro-drug, Capecitabine, are widely used in treating CRC. It has been proposed that there are two distinct modes of action for 5-FU. First, it acts as anti-metabolite whereby its active form, FdUMP, produced by Thymidine Phosphorylase (TYMP), inhibits Thymidylate Synthase (TYMS). Second, it can induce cell death, whereby incorporation of its active products FUTP and FdUTP into RNA and DNA,

respectively, leads to subsequent cell apoptosis [3]. Uridine Monophosphate Synthetase (UMPS, also known as OPRT) is responsible for converting 5-FU to FUMP, which is the first step of producing FUTP and FdUTP. However, the two pathways may overlap, because the intermediate product in the "cell toxicity" pathway, FUDP, may also be converted to FdUDP and subsequently FdUMP and participate in the "anti-metabolite" pathway. 5-FU is catabolized into the inactive form of DHFU by Dihydropyrimidine Dehydrogenase (DPYD), and DPYD is the rate-limiting enzyme in degrading 5-FU.

At present, there are no reliable tests for early prediction of response to 5-FU. Developing a reliable early predictive biomarker of response to common chemotherapy, like 5-FU, in metastatic colorectal cancer has the potential to lead to appropriate tailoring of treatment for individual patients and help move us closer to a truly personalized care. Overall economic cost benefits are realized in both predicted responders and non-responders. Responders get appropriate treatment with confidence of anticipated response.

Predicted non-responders to conventional treatment avoid wasted expense of 3 cycles of futile treatment, unnecessary toxicities that themselves require remedies and time loss in terms of futile treatment and loss of a window of opportunity for effective treatment. These patients may be selected as candidates for novel therapies and combination chemotherapy.

Thus far, only variants in the "5-FU PD" genes were reported to be significantly associated with 5-FU efficacy measured by tumour shrinkage in some studies [4–7]. Unfortunately, replication of such reported association between "5-FU PD" gene variants and tumour shrinkage remains challenging [4,6,8–13], suggesting the possible presence of other loci in determining 5-FU efficacy.

It was interesting to note that the variants in the "5-FU PK" genes were mainly investigated for their association with 5-FU toxicity, not efficacy [14–17], despite the expression levels of these genes having been previously associated with 5-FU efficacy [18]. Limited efforts [8,19] attempted to explore the possible association for efficacy, but failed.

Furthermore, most studies on response to 5-FU treatment focused primarily on SNPs in a few candidate genes. Only one study examined 21 variants primarily in coding region of 11 genes involved in metabolism/action of 5-FU and other related pharmacological pathways [19]. However, this study still does not comprehensively interrogate all possible variants that may be involved in 5-FU response.

Another limitation of current studies is that only univariate analyses have, thus far, been employed and this may not have sufficient power for detection of association of drug response with less common/rare SNPs with small sample size. Multivariate model was successfully employed to estimate the appropriate dose of warfarin based on clinical and genetic data [20].

Hence, in this study, we employ a novel approach interrogating potentially functional SNPs (pfSNPs) in relevant drug and disease pathway to identify association with drug response. 1,547 potentially functional SNPs+1 VNTR (Variable Number Tandem Repeat) from 139 genes in the drug (both PK and PD pathway) and disease pathways were examined. Potentially functional SNPs were identified using the pfSNP Web Resource (http://pfs.nus.edu.sg/) [21] which included SNPs that were previously reported to be functional or associated with disease/drug response; SNPs that were inferred to be potentially functional from genetic approaches as well as those predicted to be potentially functional from sequence motifs.

As the number of samples was limited, a two-step study design was employed. In the first stage, we examined 62 patients who were only on Capecitabine, a pro-drug of 5-FU, to identify interesting SNPs that are marginally associated with drug response as measured by tumor shrinkage. These SNPs were then examined in another group of 27 patients who were treated with 5-FU and oxaliplatin. Combined Multivariate and Collapsing (CMC) analysis was employed to evaluate the less common (≤5%), non-responder-specific pfSNPs for their association with 5-FU drug response while a logistic regression based multivariate model using stepwise Akaike Information Criterion (stepAIC) procedure was used to interrogate the other pfSNPs for their association with 5-FU drug response in patients that do not carry the non-responder-specific pfSNPs.

Materials and Methods

Patient samples and clinical parameters

The shrinkage of liver metastatic CRC tumour was used as the clinical endpoint for measuring treatment efficacy. Response Evaluation Criteria In Solid Tumours (RECIST) [22] is used to determine tumour response. In the patients recruited, there was no patient belonging to the 'Complete Response' category. Patients with 'Partial Response' were deemed as 'Responders' and patients with 'Progressive Disease' or 'Stable Disease' were classified as 'Non-Responders' in the association analysis.

A total of 89 unrelated Chinese metastatic CRC patients were recruited. All patients had liver metastasis and were given neo-adjuvant chemotherapy prior to operation for the liver lesion. **Table 1** shows the characteristics of the patients in each study.

In group 1, 62 unrelated Stage IV CRC Chinese patients were recruited. These patients were treated with only Capecitabine and they have never been previously exposed to this drug. Of these 62 patients, 13 had partial response, 31 had stable disease, and 18 had progressive disease. Hence, the response rate of this group of patients is only ~21%, which is typical for single-agent treatment [23]. ~79% of the patients were male, and the median age of the cohort was 60 years.

In group 2, 27 unrelated Chinese liver metastatic CRC patients who were treated with 5-FU (a few had Capecitabine) alone (a few) or with oxaliplatin regime (most) as their neo-adjuvant chemotherapy were examined. Some of these patients had also been previously exposed to these drugs. Of these 27 patients, 12 had partial response, seven had stable disease, and eight had progressive disease. Hence, the response rate was ~45%, which is typical for patients undergoing 2-drug combination therapy [24]. Two-thirds of these patients are males, and had a median age of 62 years.

Ethics statement

This study has been approved by Singhealth Centralized Institutional Review Board (CIRB) (Reference No: NC05–22 and 2005/421/B).

Selection of potentially functional SNPs (pfSNPs) for association study

The pfSNP resource (http://pfs.nus.edu.sg/) [21] was employed to identify SNPs in genes associated with 5-FU/Capecitabine, oxaliplatin as well as colorectal cancer. Approximately 2800 pfSNPs in 214 genes were found to be associated with keywords including "fluorouracil", "5-fluorouracil", "capecitabine", "platinum", "oxaliplatin" as well as "colorectal cancer". As only 1,536 SNPs can be genotyped within a single customized GoldenGate Genotyping Array (Illumina, Inc), the following criteria were employed to select a subset of these 2800 pfSNPs: all SNPs within the promoter, coding, 5'/3' un-translated regions which has a GoldenGate Score (GGS: measure of assay quality by their platform) of greater than 0.5 were selected. For the introns, pfSNP with a GGS>0.7 were selected and monomorphic ones reported in HapMap CHB population were excluded, except for those previously reported as functional. For any adjacent SNPs that may interfere with each other in the assay, we selected the SNP according to the following order: "Previously reported → Non-Synonymous → Synonymous → UTR → Intron". A list of all of the SNPs included on the GoldenGate array is available as **Table S1**.

Among the markers that were unsuitable to be genotyped by GoldenGate assay, 14 important markers in 5-FU response prediction were selected to be genotyped by other methods (listed in **Table S2**). The 14 markers include the previously well studied VNTR with embedded SNP [25] as well as the 6bps 3' UTR indel in the TYMS gene because GoldenGate technology could only genotype SNPs. Other markers are SNPs with low GoldenGate scores in the TYMS, TYMP and DPYD genes. A customized Sequenom's MassARRAY panel was used to genotype 11 of the

Table 1. The demographic characteristics of the patients recruited for each study.

	Group 1	Group 2
Number of Patients	62	27
Ages (Median)	36–78 (60)	42–86 (62)
Males (Females)	49(13)	18(9)
Prior Drug Exposure		
5-FU alone	0	2
Capecitabine alone	0	3
5-FU + oxaliplatin	0	2
Capecitabine + oxaliplatin	0	0
5-FU + Radio Therapy	0	2
Drugs Treated		
5-FU alone	0	2
Capecitabine alone	62	1
5-FU + oxaliplatin	0	15
Capecitabine + oxaliplatin	0	8
5-FU + Irinotecan	0	1
Response		
Partial response	13	12
Stable disease	31	7
Progressive disease	18	8

14 markers and 1 SNP was genotyped by ABI TaqMan. In addition, we developed a novel method to genotype the VNTR (rs2853542) and embedded SNP (rs34743033) in the TYMS gene. This VNTR can have either 2 or 3 repeats, and the SNP can occur in both the second and third repeat [26]. We developed a robust method using Sanger Sequencing for this purpose. A fragment of 486 bp was amplified using the primers (F- CTGCTGGCTTA-GAGAAGGCG and R- AGCGGAGGATGTGTTGGATC) and the amplicon was sequenced in both directions using the forward and reverse primers. Different genotypes would yield distinct patterns on the forward and reverse sequencing reads (As shown in **Figure S1**), allowing the genotype to be easily deduced.

In summary, there were 1,536 markers (Listed in **Table S1**) genotyped with a single customized Illumina GoldenGate SNP genotyping array, 11 (Listed in **Table S2**) by Sequenom's MassARRAY, 1 (rs11479) by ABI TaqMan and the VNTR (rs2853542), with the embedded SNP (rs34743033) was genotyped using Sanger Sequencing.

The distribution of the SNPs and genes selected in the three categories (CRC, Fluorouracil and Platinum related) is depicted in **Figure S2**. More than half of the SNPs (863) are from fluorouracil-related genes and 702 SNPs are from platinum-related genes. A considerable portion of the SNPs (656) are from CRC-related genes, although 40% (32 out of 80) of these genes and 88% (579 out of 656) of the SNPs are related to fluorouracil and/or platinum as well.

The numbers of SNPs in each gene region and function category covered in this study are shown in **Figure S3**. Each of the four gene regions, namely promoter, coding, intron and 3' UTR, are adequately covered in general. For promoter and 3'UTR, most of the SNPs genotyped are those that change TF binding sites. In the coding region, SNPs that change ESE/ESS sites are the most abundant, and non-synonymous SNPs that cause deleterious effects are the second most abundant. The intron

region SNPs are enriched with those with a signature of recent positive selection.

The distribution of SNP minor allele frequency for the intronic versus non-intronic region is shown in **Table S3**. For coding, 3'UTR, and promoter regions, a number of SNPs not previously genotyped by HapMap has been genotyped in this study. As the study aims to also explore rare variants, a number of SNPs reported by HapMap to be monomorphic was also genotyped. For the intron region, since most of the SNPs are those with a signature of recent positive selection, they have MAF more than 5%. We did not genotype many monomorphic ones within introns.

Single marker association analysis

Hardy-Weinberg equilibrium and minor allele frequency were analysed using the Microsoft Excel-based SNP Statistics Calculator developed in-house. Single marker association analysis was performed using PLINK [27]. The P-value was calculated by the permutation-based method, and the Odds Ratio (OR) and corresponding 95% confidence interval were determined using regular allele-based association analyses, because the permutation-based method does not provide such information. The genotype of the VNTR (rs2853542) and embedded SNP (rs34743033) in the TYMS gene is re-coded as a bi-allelic SNP comprising the high-expression allele and the low-expression allele according to Kawakami et al [26].

Combined Multivariate and Collapsing (CMC) analyses for non-responder-specific SNPs

Combined Multivariate and Collapsing (CMC) method was first proposed as a method for analysing rare SNPs [28]. CMC utilizes Hotelling's T^2 test to analyse more than 2 groups of collapsed variants. When only 2 groups of such variants are analysed, Fisher's exact test can be used. In this study, we used the Fisher's

Table 2. List of SNPs showing P<0.05 in Group 1 ranked by P value.

SN	Gene	mRNA Location	AA Change	rs No.	Function Summary	P	Allele Count			OR 95 CI	
							NR (98)	Rsp (26)	OR		
1	ATP7A	E23/3UTR/T1960C	-	rs1062472	RPS	0.003	22	14	4.03	1.55	9.29
2	RRM1	5UR//A-2723G	-	rs3750996	TF	0.004	30	1	11.36	1.46	86.66
3	DLG5	E/23/G4442T	P1481Q	rs2289310	Reported, Non-Syn, ProteinDomain, Del AA, ESE/ESS	0.005	15	11	4.06	1.53	10.13
4	RRM1	5UR//T-265G	-	rs1735068	TF	0.010	19	12	3.56	1.26	7.70
5	RRM1	5UR//A-4023G	-	rs3794050	TF	0.012	20	12	3.34	1.26	7.70
6	RRM1	5UR//T-659C	-	rs1662162	TF	0.012	20	12	3.34	1.20	7.24
7	UMPS	5UR//T-1256A	-	rs12492095	TF	0.013	11	9	4.19	1.45	10.88
8	UMPS	E/3/G638C	-	rs1801019	Reported, Non-Syn, ESE/ESS	0.013	11	9	4.19	1.45	10.88
9	APC	I/2/C-230A	-	rs2464805	RPS, ISRE	0.018	6	6	4.60	1.40	16.42
10	SMARCA2	I/28/G-8275T||I/29/G2824T	-|-	rs7048976	RPS	0.021	39	4	3.64	1.09	10.62
11	RRM1	5UR//G-2528A	-	rs1561876	TF	0.023	21	12	3.14	1.20	7.24
12	RRM1	E/19/G2232A	A744A	rs1042858	ESE/ESS	0.023	21	12	3.14	1.14	6.83
13	RRM1	E19/3UTR/C316A	-	rs1042927	miRNA	0.023	21	12	3.14	1.14	6.83
14	WDR7	I/13/A323G	-	rs11664579	Reported	0.024	10	8	3.91	1.30	10.42
15	TFRC	E/4/C424T	S142G	rs3817672	Reported, Non-Syn, ProteinDomain	0.025	14	9	3.18	1.24	8.91
16	ATP7A	E/10/G2299C	V767L	rs2227291	Non-Syn, ProteinDomain, Del AA, ESE/ESS	0.025	22	12	2.96	1.14	6.83
17	ATP7A	I/12/C-882A	-	rs17113617	RPS	0.025	22	12	2.96	1.14	6.83
18	ABCC4	3DR/A75075G|E31/3UTR/A879G	-|-	rs1059751	Reported	0.025	38	17	2.98	1.19	7.20
19	ABCC4	3DR/A74234C|E31/3UTR/A38C	-|-	rs3742106	miRNA	0.029	40	17	2.74	1.10	6.63
20	ABCC4	3DR/T74507C|E31/3UTR/T311C	-|-	rs4148551	Reported	0.029	40	17	2.74	1.10	6.63
21	APC	E/16/T5465A	V1822D	rs459552	Reported, Non-Syn, ProteinDomain, ESE/ESS	0.033	5	5	4.43	1.23	17.40
22	APC	I/6/T-3774C	-	rs2431238	RPS	0.033	5	5	4.43	1.23	17.40
23	CDC2	5UR//C-3953T||I/1/C263T	-|-	rs2448341	TF, ISRE	0.039	42	5	3.15	1.07	8.76
24	RRM1	5UR//C-3890T	-	rs7934581	TF	0.043	13	8	2.91	0.95	6.98
25	ERCC6	I/6/T871G	-	rs4253101	RPS	0.045	50	7	2.83	1.14	7.59
26	SLCO6A1	I/10/A-2493G	-	rs1562961	RPS	0.046	38	16	2.53	1.02	6.01
27	SLCO6A1	I/11/C702T	-	rs10062613	RPS	0.046	38	16	2.53	1.02	6.01

Table 2. Cont.

SN	Gene	mRNA Location	AA Change	rs No.	Function Summary	P	Allele Count		OR	OR 95 CI	
							NR (98)	Rsp (26)			
28	SLCO6A1	I/12/A7020C	–	rs6873738	RPS	0.046	38	16	2.53	1.02	6.01
29	SLCO6A1	I/12/G-738T	–	rs6877722	RPS	0.046	38	16	2.53	1.02	6.01
30	SLCO6A1	I/12/T517C	–	rs1901512	RPS	0.046	38	16	2.53	1.02	6.01
31	SLCO6A1	I/3/T142C	–	rs10041525	RPS, ISRE	0.046	38	16	2.53	1.02	6.01
32	SLCO6A1	I/3/T220C	–	rs10041507	RPS, ISRE	0.046	38	16	2.53	1.02	6.01
33	SLCO6A1	I/4/A-9G	–	rs11746217	RPS, ISRE	0.046	38	16	2.53	1.02	6.01
34	SLCO6A1	I/6/A4781G	–	rs1452057	RPS	0.046	38	16	2.53	1.02	6.01
35	SLCO6A1	I/9/G1986T	–	rs1901521	RPS	0.046	38	16	2.53	1.02	6.01
36	SLCO6A1	I/9/T50A6G	–	rs1901522	RPS	0.046	38	16	2.53	1.02	6.01

Abbreviations: Reported: previously reported in the literature to be associated with disease/function; ESE/ESS: change Exon splice enhancer/silencer; NMD: mRNA nonsense mediated decay; Non-sym: non-synonymous SNP; ProteinDomain: residing in important protein domains; miRNA: change miRNA binding site; RPS: show signature of recent positive selection; TF: change transcription factor binding site; ISRE: change intron splice regulatory element.

exact test to evaluate if the collapsed minor allele of non-responder specific SNPs which are less common (≤5% minor allele frequency) would be a good indicator of responsiveness to 5-FU.

Logistic regression based multivariate model using Akaike Information Criterior (stepAIC) procedure to predict drug response in patients who do not have non-responder-specific SNPs

Patients, who do not have any of the non-responder specific SNPs, were divided into 2 groups. Data from the first group comprising 80% of the patients was used to train a logistic regression based multivariate model by using the Akaike's Information Criterion (AIC) in a stepwise algorithm (using R package "stepAIC") while the data from the other 20% of patients were used to validate the model. The selected model was evaluated by the Area Under the Curve (AUC) of the Receiver Operating Characteristic (ROC) curves. The optimal cut-off point for the logistic regression was chosen where the maximum sum of sensitivity and specificity is obtained [29,30].

Results and Discussion

A high concordance ($R^2 = 0.9494$) was observed between allele frequencies of SNPs in our study and those from the CHB (Chinese in Beijing) population in HapMap (Release 27) (**Figure S4**) affirming the quality of our genotyping. A large proportion of the SNPs examined in this study were either monomorphic (36%) or had a high minor allele frequency (MAF≥0.1, 46%) (**Figure S5**). Seventy-two and 66 SNPs in Groups 1 and 2, respectively, were found to significantly deviate from Hardy-Weinberg Equilibrium and were excluded from further analysis.

Genotype was successfully (97–100%) assigned in 9 out of 11 SNPs genotyped using the Sequenom's MassARRAY. Sanger sequencing successfully assigned genotype of the 2 SNPs to all the samples while TaqMan assay successfully assigned genotypes to 96% of the samples. All the SNPs successfully genotyped by these methods were found to be in Hardy-Weinberg equilibrium.

Single SNP association analysis identified three non-responder specific SNPs in the UMPS gene that may represent potential predictive biomarker for non-response to 5-FU

As the number of samples in this study was small, a cross validation approach was employed where the samples were segregated into 2 distinct groups for discovery and validation to enhance the robustness of our findings.

A total of 36 SNPs in 12 genes were found to be associated with drug response before multiple test correction in Group 1 patients (**Table 2**). As the sample size was small (n = 62), none of these markers were statistically significant after Bonferroni correction.

Nonetheless, there were 68 low frequency pfSNPs in Group 1 that were uniquely found only in non-responders (non-responder-specific pfSNP). To evaluate if any of these non-responder-specific pfSNPs may represent potential predictive biomarker for non-response to 5-FU, we examined a second group of 27 patients. Of these 68 non-responder specific pfSNPs, 24 remained non-responder-specific even in Group 2 and these are presented in **Table 3**. However, only 3 of the non-responder-specific SNPs in the Uridine Monophosphate Synthetase (UMPS) gene, namely rs2291078 (E/4/T1050A C350*), rs3772809 (E/6/A1336G H446Y) and rs3772810 (E6/3UTR/A28G) (**Table 2,** SNPs 42–44) (**Table 3**, SNPs 1–3) were found to be statistically significant (p = 0.036 before multiple test correction) in Group 2. When the 2

Table 3. List of SNPs with non-responder specific allele in both groups.

SN	Gene	mRNA Location	AA Change	rs No.	MAF HapMap	MAF This study	Function Summary	Group 1 P	Group 1 NR (98)	Group 1 Rsp (26)	Group 2 P	Group 2 NR (30)	Group 2 Rsp (24)	Combined P	Combined NR (128)	Combined Rsp (50)
1	UMPS	E/4/T1050A	C350*	rs2291078	-	7.3%	NMD, Non-Syn, ProteinDomain, ESE/ESS	0.140	8	0	0.036	5	0	0.032	13	0
2	UMPS	E/6/A1336G	H446Y	rs3772809	5.4%	7.3%	Non-Syn, ProteinDomain, ESE/ESS	0.140	8	0	0.036	5	0	0.032	13	0
3	UMPS	E6/3UTR/A28G	-	rs3772810	5.4%	7.3%	miRNA, TF	0.140	8	0	0.036	5	0	0.032	13	0
4	TK1	5UR//G-1181A	-	rs8071253	-	3.4%	TF	0.250	5	0	0.367	1	0	0.119	6	0
5	DPYD	I/3/A22444C	-	rs10493895	1.8%	2.8%	Reported	0.305	4	0	0.367	1	0	0.156	5	0
6	DPYD	I/3/A39932G	-	rs10747486	1.9%	2.8%	RPS	0.305	4	0	0.367	1	0	0.156	5	0
7	DPYD	I/3/C30060T	-	rs1931063	2.2%	2.8%	RPS	0.305	4	0	0.367	1	0	0.156	5	0
8	DPYD	I/3/G-27495C	-	rs4537601	1.8%	2.8%	RPS	0.305	4	0	0.367	1	0	0.156	5	0
9	DPYD	I/3/G29092A	-	rs1333717	1.8%	2.8%	RPS	0.305	4	0	0.367	1	0	0.156	5	0
10	WDR7	I/1/A35G	-	rs501415	2.3%	2.8%	TF, ISRE	0.305	4	0	0.367	1	0	0.156	5	0
11	DPYD	I/4/A5229G	-	rs6683957	0.7%	2.2%	RPS	0.376	3	0	0.367	1	0	0.206	4	0
12	DPYD	I/4/G3787C	-	rs4970728	2.2%	2.2%	RPS	0.376	3	0	0.367	1	0	0.206	4	0
13	REV3L	E/26/C8285T	R2762Q	rs3218592	2.9%	2.2%	Non-Syn, ProteinDomain, DelAA, ESE/ESS	0.376	3	0	0.367	1	0	0.206	4	0
14	WDR7	E27/3UTR/C112T|E28/3UTR/C112T	-|-	rs3745032	-	2.2%	TF	0.376	3	0	0.367	1	0	0.206	4	0
15	WDR7	E27/3UTR/C2176G|E28/3UTR/C2176G	-|-	rs3745030	3.3%	2.2%	TF	0.376	3	0	0.367	1	0	0.206	4	0
16	WDR7	I/14/T9751A	-	rs11876256	2.2%	2.2%	RPS	0.376	3	0	0.367	1	0	0.206	4	0
17	WDR7	I/19/T-30795A|I/20/T-30795A	-|-	rs2576415	2.2%	2.8%	RPS	0.376	3	0	0.197	2	0	0.156	5	0
18	WDR7	I/12/C-2229T	-	rs11877604	2.2%	1.7%	RPS	0.467	2	0	0.367	1	0	0.271	3	0
19	SMARCD1	E/4/A423G	V141V	rs2307083	0.0%	1.1%	CodonDiff, TF	0.612	1	0	0.367	1	0	0.374	2	0
20	UPB1	5UR//G-96A	-	rs2232861	-	1.1%	TF	0.612	1	0	0.367	1	0	0.374	2	0
21	WDR7	I/18/A-2783C|I/19/A-2783C	-|-	rs9946253	0.4%	1.1%	Reported	0.612	1	0	0.367	1	0	0.374	2	0
22	WDR7	I/20/A20363G|I/21/A20363G	-	rs2083020	0.4%	1.1%	Reported	0.612	1	0	0.367	1	0	0.374	2	0
23	WDR7	I/21/A532G|I/22/A532G	-|-	rs8094838	0.4%	1.1%	Reported	0.612	1	0	0.367	1	0	0.374	2	0
24	WDR7	I/21/T-2912G|I/22/T-2912G	-|-	rs6566846	0.0%	1.1%	Reported, RPS	0.612	1	0	0.367	1	0	0.374	2	0

Abbreviations: Reported: previously reported in the literature to be associated with disease/function; ESE/ESS: change Exon splice enhancer/silencer; NMD: mRNA nonsense mediated decay; Non-syn: non-synonymous SNP; ProteinDomain: residing in important protein domains; miRNA: change miRNA binding site; RPS: show signature of recent positive selection; TF: change transcription factor binding site; ISRE: change intron splice regulatory element; DelAA: Deleterious amino acid change; CodonDiff: High codon usage difference.

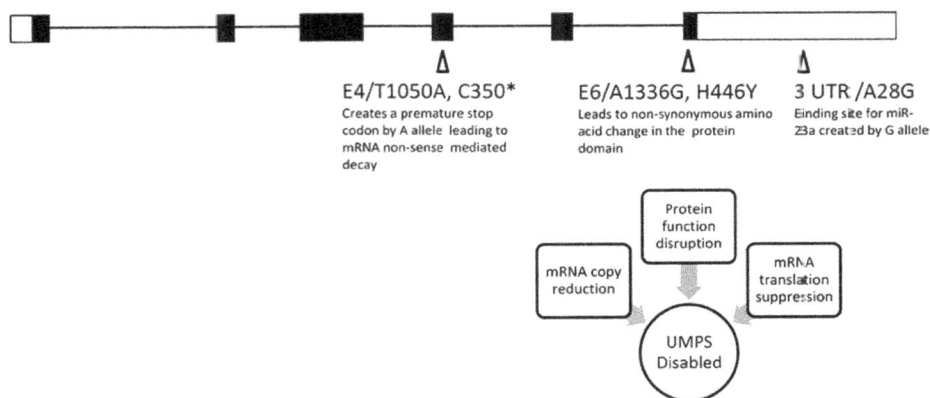

E4/T1050A, C350*
Creates a premature stop codon by A allele leading to mRNA non-sense mediated decay

E6/A1336G, H446Y
Leads to non-synonymous amino acid change in the protein domain

3 UTR /A28G
Binding site for miR-23a created by G allele

Protein function disruption

mRNA copy reduction

mRNA translation suppression

UMPS Disabled

Figure 1. The molecular functions of the three SNPs in UMPS gene with minor allele uniquely found in non-responders are all linked to disabling UMPS.

groups of patients were combined and analysed, these 3 SNPs remained statistically significant (p = 0.032 before multiple test correction). The observation that out of a total of 89 patients in the combined group, no responders were found to carry this allele suggests that this allele may be a "causal" allele for determining the response to 5-FU. The non-statistical significant data obtained (after multiple test correction) suggests that this may not be the only "causal" alleles for 5-FU response and there are likely other alleles that also play a role in 5-FU response suggesting "locus heterogeneity" of response to 5-FU.

The UMPS gene is important in determining 5-FU response, as it converts 5-FU into its active metabolite, FUMP, which can participate in both the cell toxicity pathway as well as in the "anti-metabolite" pathway. In the cell toxicity pathway, FUMP can be further converted into FUTP and FdUTP which is then incorporated into RNA and DNA respectively. In the "anti-metabolite" pathway, FUMP can be converted into FdUMP and inhibits TYMS.

These 3 alleles in the UMPS gene are in perfect linkage disequilibrium (LD) and hence will occur together all the time. The predicted molecular functions of the three alleles unique to the non-responders are all associated with the disruption of the UMPS gene function and support their unique presence in the non-responders (**Figure 1**).

The A allele of rs2291078 (UMPS E/4/T1050A C350*) was predicted to create a stop codon in exon 4 of the UMPS mRNA. UMPS mRNA containing this stop codon may be quickly degraded since stop codon appearing more than 50 bps from the last exon-exon junction would induce non-sense mediated decay of mRNA [31]. Therefore, patients carrying this A allele may have lower UMPS mRNA and protein abundance.

The co-occurrence of 3'UTR pfSNP rs3772810 (UMPS E6/3UTR/A28G) with this pfSNP rs2291078 suggests that the expression of this gene may be further attenuated. The G allele of the 3'UTR SNP rs3772810 (UMPS E6/3UTR/A28G) is predicted to create binding sites for miRNA 23a, 23b and 130a*. The miRNA 23a is shown to be up-regulated under hypoxic condition commonly found in tumors [32]. Notably, a recent publication reported that miRNA 23a is up-regulated in metastatic colorectal cancer [33] suggesting that patients with the G allele may be non-responsive to 5-FU since miRNA 23a may suppress the expression of UMPS mRNA containing the G allele.

Also co-occurring with these 2 pfSNPs, is the non-synonymous pfSNP rs3772809 (UMPS E/6/A1336G H446Y) which have the

potential to alter the function of the UMPS gene. Hence, these 3 co-occurring pfSNPs, which accounted for 17.2% of all the non-responders have the potential to be the causal variants affecting the function of UMPS and thus response to 5-FU although further experiments are required to validate the potential functionality of these pfSNPs.

Combined Multivariate and Collapsing (CMC) analyses revealed that a minimum of four non-responder specific pfSNPs that are not in linkage equilibrium can significantly distinguish non-responders from responders

We proceeded to determine if combination of non-responder specific pfSNPs (**Table 3**) can account for a greater percentage of 5-FU non-responders than the abovementioned 3 non-responder specific UMPS pfSNPs in perfect LD that show statistical significance (before multiple test corrections). Since the 3 non-responder specific UMPS pfSNPs are in perfect LD, only one was selected for further analyses. We then identify the minimum number of additional non-responder specific pfSNPs from **Table 3** that can account for the maximum percentage of 5-FU non-responders and employed Combined Multivariate and Collapsing (CMC) analyses [23] to determine its statistical significance.

Notably, three other non-responder specific pfSNPs together with any one of the UMPS non-responder specific pfSNPs were found to account for 37.5% of all non-responders from the 2 groups of patients (**Table 4**). CMC analyses revealed statistical significance (P = 0.0003) of these 4 non-responder specific pfSNPs (3 non UMPS plus any one of the 3 UMPS pfSNPs) suggesting significant association of these pfSNPs with non-responsiveness.

SNP rs3218592 causes a non-conservative amino acid change in the REV3L gene which encodes the catalytic subunit of DNA Polymerase Zeta. DNA Polymerase Zeta was reported to be significantly down regulated in human colorectal cancer [34] and was suggested to be a tumour suppressor [35]. The T allele of the rs3218592 (E/26/C8285T, R2762Q) which is uniquely found in non-responder in our study is predicted to be damaging to the protein function by both Polyphen [36] and SIFT [37]. We thus hypothesize that the patients carrying this deleterious allele would have more aggressive disease and hence are more likely to be non-responsive to treatment.

pfSNP (rs8071253) resides in the promoter region of TK1 and is predicted to create a xenobiotic-stress activated TGA1a transcription binding site.

Table 4. The list of less-common SNPs with non-responder specific allele and their predicted molecular functions.

S.N	rsNo	Gene Name	mRNA Location	AA Change	Non-responder Specific Allele and Frequency (HapMap/This Study)	Allele Count		P	Potential Molecular Function
						NR	Rsp		
1	rs3772810	UMPS	E6/3UTR/A28G	–	G (5.4%/7.3%)	13	0	0.02	Creates miR23a binding site
2	rs3218592	REV3L	E/26/C8285T	R2762Q	T (1.8%/2.2%)	4	0	0.45	Predicted deleterious by Polyphen and SIFT
3	rs8071253	TK1	5UR//G-1181A	–	A (Unknown/3.4%)	6	0	0.26	Creates TGA1a binding site
4	rs501415	WDR7	I/1/A35G	–	G (2.3%/2.8%)	5	0	0.41	Disrupts a binding site of RUNX1 and possbily RUNX3 (Since all RUNX family proteins are sharing same motif)

The third SNP (rs501415) resides within the first intron of WDR7 and is predicted to disrupt AML1 (RUNX) transcription factor bind site. Since the entire RUNX family share the same binding site (TGt/cGGT) [19], we postulate that this SNP may also affect the binding of RUNX3. RUNX3 had been hailed as a tumour suppressor gene and reduced expression of RUNX3 has been previously associated with poorer survival in colorectal cancer patients [38]. Nonetheless, the role of WDR7 in 5-FU resistance remained unclear. It was reported to be associated with 5-FU by PharmGKB [39] but the publication [39] was recently retracted [40].

The logistic regression-based multivariate model identified an additional 5 pfSNPs which are not non-responder-specific that may distinguish responders from non-responders

In addition to the non-responder specific pfSNPs that are associated with patients who do not respond to 5-FU, we proceeded to identify additional pfSNPs that may be associated with 5-FU drug response by training a logistic regression-based multivariate model with the stepAIC method using data from the other pfSNPs. The multivariate model identified 5 additional pfSNPs, namely, rs2289310 (DLG5, E/23/G4442T, P1481Q), rs1047840 (EXO1, E/12/G1765A, E589K), rs17431184 (PTEN, I/7/T-400C), rs2236722 (CYP19A1, E/2/A115G, W39R) and rs17160359 (ABCB1, 5UR//G-4254T) (**Table 5**) that may distinguish responders from non-responders. The AUC (Area Under Curve) for ROC (Receiver Operating Characteristic) curve of these 5 SNPs is 0.875 (**Figure 2**). A predicted value of 0.794 was identified as the optimal cut-off point to predict drug response, with sensitivity of 62.5% and specificity of 100%. With this threshold, the logistic-based multivariate model can correctly identify 39.1% (25/64) of non-responders. Together with the 37.5% of non-responders predicted by the non-responder-specific SNPs, a total of 76.6% (49/64) of non-responders can be correctly identified by both models.

It is noteworthy that the SNPs in the multivariate model are primarily localized within tumor suppressor gene (PTEN) or in genes which are mainly associated with colorectal cancer (DLG5, EXO1, CYP19A1 and ABCB1) (**Table 5**). Notably, one of the non-responder-specific SNP (rs3218592, REV3L E/26/C8285T, R2762Q) (**Table 4**) residing in the gene, Rev3L, has also been implicated to be a tumor suppressor gene [41].

The PTEN (phosphatase and tensin homolog) gene is a well-known tumor suppressor gene that was recently reported to control DNA repair and sensitivity to genotoxic stress [42]. The higher frequency of the C allele in the responders (26% in the responders vs. 12% in the non-responders) suggests that patients with this allele may exhibit lower tolerance to genotoxic stress caused by DNA damaging agents like 5-FU.

The DLG5 (Disks large homolog 5) gene encodes a member of the membrane-associated guanylate kinase (MAGUK) family of scaffolding proteins which is involved in maintaining the epithelial integrity [43]. The T allele of rs2289310 (DLG5, E/23/G4442T, P1481Q) causes a non-conserved amino acid change in the vicinity of one of the PDZ domains in this gene (aa 1391–1472; Prosite score 13.531). This variant was postulated to impair the scaffolding functions of DLG5 [44] and enhance the tight junction-mediated gut permeability [45]. This polymorphism has also been associated with increased risk of Inflammatory Bowel Disease [45] which may lead to increased risk for colorectal cancer [46]. Since enhanced gut permeability was reported to lead to higher 5-FU absorption in rats [47], we hypothesize that the T allele would lead

Table 5. The list of common SNPs included into the multi-variate model and their predicted molecular functions.

S.N	rsNo	Gene Name	mRNA Location	AA Change	Allele	Allele Count (Frequency) NR (128)	Allele Count (Frequency) Rsp (50)	Potential Molecular Function	Discussion
1	rs2289310	DLG5	E/23/G4442T	P1481Q	T	22 (17%)	17 (34%)	Causes a non-conserved AA change in PDZ-like domain. The PDZ-like domain is important in cell-junction according to SuperFamily database.	DLG5 is involved in maintaining the epithelial integrity. The T allele causes a non-conserved AA change in the PDZ-like domain which is important in cell-junction. The T allele has been associated with increased risk for Inflammatory Bowel Disease (IBD) and Crohn Disease (CD). The authors suggest it may have a role in altering tight-junction mediated permeability. It has been shown that enhanced intestinal permeability would increase 5-FU absorption. Therefore, patients with T allele may have higher 5-FU bioavailability and more likely to respond.
2	rs1047840	EXO1	E/12/G1765A E/13/G1765A	E589K E589K	A	20 (16%)	15 (30%)	Causes a non-conserved AA change in the Exonuclease domain.	EXO1 is a gene controlling DNA repair (OMIM 606063). The A allele causes a non-conserved AA change in the exo-nuclease domain. The A allele has been associated with higher colorectal cancer risk in a UK population. We hypothesize that the increased risk is due to the reduced DNA repairing function of EXO1 caused by the A allele. Therefore, patients having A allele may be more responsive to DNA damaging agents like 5-FU.
3	rs17431184	PTEN	I/7/T-400C	–	C	15 (12%)	13 (26%)	Creates intronic splicing regulatory elements and under recent positive selection	PTEN is a well-known tumor suppressor and part of the apoptosis signalling pathway. The C allele is under recent positive selection. Therefore, patients having this allele may have stronger PTEN activity and respond better to 5-FU.
4	rs2236722	CYP19A1	E/2/A115G E/3/A115G	W39R W39R	G	16 (13%)	1 (2%)	Causes a non-conserved AA change in the CYP_P450 family domain. Predicted to be deleterious by Polyphen. Also alters exonic splicing element.	A number of SNPs in the CYP19A1 gene have been associated with colorectal cancer risk. In the particular paper, this SNP has not been tested in this study because the study was conducted in an US white population and the SNP is likely to be mono morphic according to HapMap. The G allele is detrimental to the protein function therefore patients having the G allele should have lower oestrogen level. This may translates to a higher colorectal cancer risk and more progressive disease therefore less responsive to 5-FU.
5	rs17160359	ABCB1	5UR/G-4254T	–	T	3 (2.3%)	5 (10%)	Creates binding site for HMGA1.	ABCB1 does not transport 5-FU but a few SNPs in it are implicated in CRC risk. The T allele creates a binding site of HMGA1 which is upregulated in various cancers.

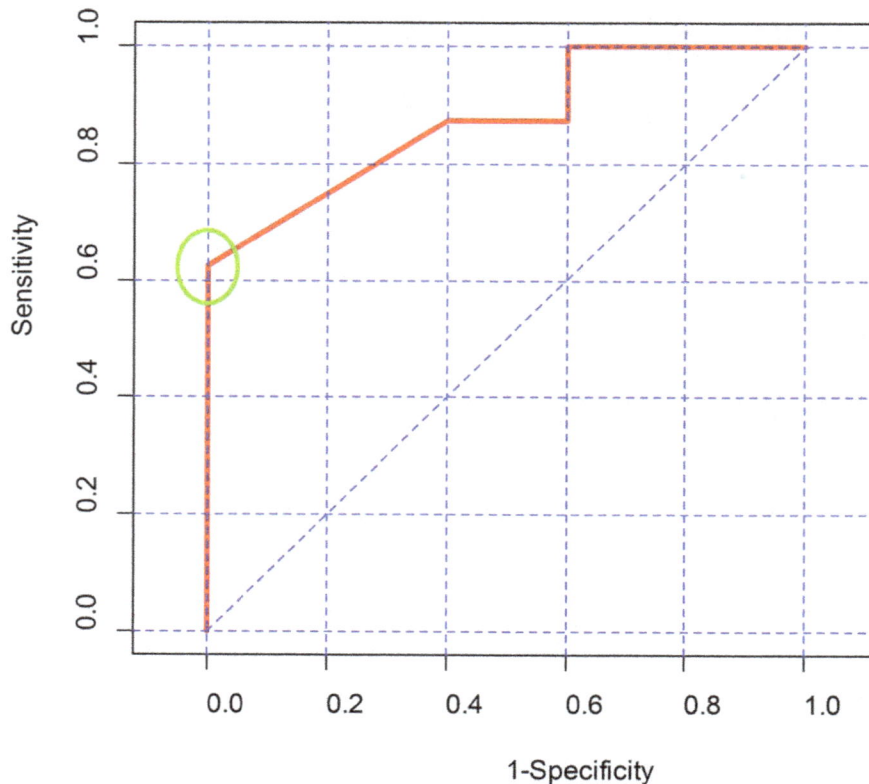

Figure 2. The ROC curve for the logistic regression based multivariate model trained to differentiate non-responders who do not have the non-responder. The AUC of the ROC curve is 0.875. The point of maximum sum of sensitivity and specificity is highlighted by the green circle on the ROC curve. The corresponding sensitivity and specificity is 62.5% and 100% respectively.

to better drug absorption and thus better response. Consistent with our hypothesis, more responders have the T allele (MAF of 34% in responder vs 17% in non-responder) in this study.

The EXO1 (exonuclease 1) gene has been implicated to play roles in DNA replication, recombination, repair, telomere integrity [48] as well as damage signalling decisions [49]. The A allele of rs1047840 (EXO1, E/12/G1765A or E/13/G1765A, E589K) causes a non-conserved amino acid change and is predicted to reside within a region that is highly conserved amongst the XP-G/ RAD2 DNA Repair Endonuclease Family (HMMPanther PTHR11081). In the Kin-cohort analyses, the A allele has been associated with higher risk of colorectal cancer in a UK population [50]. This SNP has also been associated with higher risk for various other cancers in the Chinese population [51–57]. We hypothesize that the increased cancer risk associated with this SNP could be due to less efficient repair of DNA damage in individuals carrying the A-allele. As the metabolites of 5-FU gets incorporated into DNA damaging the host DNA, the inefficient repair mechanisms of individuals carrying the A-allele of this SNP may result in greater cell death hence enhancing the effectiveness of 5-FU treatment. This is consistent with our observations that greater percentage of responders carries the A-allele of this SNP compared to non-responders (30% versus 16%).

CYP19A1 (cytochrome P450, family 19, subfamily A, polypeptide 1) or Aromatase is a member of the cytochrome P450 superfamily of enzymes and plays an important role in the metabolism of oestrogens. Oestrogen has been associated with lower risk of colorectal cancer [58–60]. Although several SNPs in the CYP19A1 gene had been reported to be associated with risk for colorectal cancer in a Caucasian population [61], SNP rs2236722 (E/2/A115G or E/3/A115G, W39R) was not examined in that study as it is monomorphic in HapMap CEU population. Nonetheless, this SNP (rs2236722), which occurs at a frequency of 3.3% in HapMap CHB population and 9.5% in our study, causes a non-conserved amino acid change from hydrophobic tryptophan to charged arginine in the CYP_P450 family domain and is predicted by Polyphen [36] to be a deleterious alteration. Hence, it is possible that this deleterious change in CYP19A1 may lead to lower oestrogen levels leading to higher colorectal cancer risk. We thus hypothesize that patients with the minor G-allele may have more progressive disease and hence are less responsive to 5-FU treatment.

The final gene implicated by the multivariate model to be associated with 5-FU response is the ABCB1 (ATP-Binding Cassette, Sub-Family B (MDR/TAP), Member 1) or the MDR1 (multidrug resistance protein 1). Although 5-FU is not a substrate of MDR1 protein, there's some, albeit controversial evidence that SNPs within the ABCB1 gene, may be associated with CRC risk [62,63]. Nonetheless, the SNP rs17160359 (ABCB1, 5UR/G-4254T) which is implicated in the multivariate model to be associated with drug response in CRC patient, resides in the promoter region and the T allele of the SNP creates a binding site of a transcription factor called HMGA1 which is expressed at very low level in adult human tissues but highly expressed in various tumours [64].

In summary, three perfect LD, non-responder-specific pfSNPs within the UMPS gene which plays a role in 5-FU metabolism together with 3 other non-responder-specific pfSNPs and 5 other pfSNPs in genes that may play roles in modulating tumor risks may collaborate to influence the patient's response of CRC drugs. This study thus provides one of the building blocks for subsequent meta-analysis in larger cohort of patients.

Supporting Information

Figure S1   The different sequencing patterns generated by the different genotype of the VNTR and embedded SNP in the TYMS gene promoter region.

Figure S2   The gene and pathway distribution of pfSNPs chosen for genotyping.

Figure S3   The number of SNPs selected for genotyping in each gene region and function category.

Figure S4   Comparing HapMap CHB reported allele frequency (Release 27) and allele frequency observed in this study.

Figure S5   The MAF distribution of GoldenGate genotyped SNPs.

Table S1   The list of all the SNPs included on the GoldenGate array.

Table S2   The 14 markers not suitable to be genotyped by GoldenGate array and genotyped by other methods.

Table S3   The MAF for SNPs selected for genotyping in each region based on HapMap R27 CHB.

Acknowledgments

We thank Mah Way-Champ and Teo Wei Bing for their assistance in the project.

Author Contributions

Conceived and designed the experiments: JW SSC YYT CGLL. Performed the experiments: JW MZ. Analyzed the data: JW XW YYT. Contributed reagents/materials/analysis tools: SPC SJO SYKO SSC YYT CGLL. Contributed to the writing of the manuscript: JW SSC YYT CGLL.

References

1. Cunningham D, Atkin W, Lenz HJ, Lynch HT, Minsky B, et al. (2010) Colorectal cancer. Lancet 375: 1030–1047.
2. SC R (2011) Singapore Cancer Registry Interim Annual Registry Report. Trends in Cancer Incidence in Singapore 2005–2009.
3. Sobrero AF, Aschele C, Bertino JR (1997) Fluorouracil in colorectal cancer–a tale of two drugs: implications for biochemical modulation. Journal of clinical oncology: official journal of the American Society of Clinical Oncology 15: 368–381.
4. Graziano F, Ruzzo A, Loupakis F, Santini D, Catalano V, et al. (2008) Liver-only metastatic colorectal cancer patients and thymidylate synthase polymorphisms for predicting response to 5-fluorouracil-based chemotherapy. British journal of cancer 99: 716–721.
5. Salgado J, Zabalegui N, Gil C, Monreal I, Rodriguez J, et al. (2007) Polymorphisms in the thymidylate synthase and dihydropyrimidine dehydrogenase genes predict response and toxicity to capecitabine-raltitrexed in colorectal cancer. Oncology reports 17: 325–328.
6. Etienne MC, Formento JL, Chazal M, Francoual M, Magne N, et al. (2004) Methylenetetrahydrofolate reductase gene polymorphisms and response to fluorouracil-based treatment in advanced colorectal cancer patients. Pharmacogenetics 14: 785–792.
7. Jakobsen A, Nielsen JN, Gyldenkerne N, Lindeberg J (2005) Thymidylate synthase and methylenetetrahydrofolate reductase gene polymorphism in normal tissue as predictors of fluorouracil sensitivity. Journal of clinical oncology: official journal of the American Society of Clinical Oncology 23: 1365–1369.
8. Farina-Sarasqueta A, van Lijnschoten G, Rutten HJ, van den Brule AJ (2010) Value of gene polymorphisms as markers of 5-FU therapy response in stage III colon carcinoma: a pilot study. Cancer Chemother Pharmacol 66: 1167–1171.
9. Tsuji T, Hidaka S, Sawai T, Nakagoe T, Yano H, et al. (2003) Polymorphism in the thymidylate synthase promoter enhancer region is not an efficacious marker for tumor sensitivity to 5-fluorouracil-based oral adjuvant chemotherapy in colorectal cancer. Clinical cancer research: an official journal of the American Association for Cancer Research 9: 3700–3704.
10. Vignoli M, Nobili S, Napoli C, Putignano AL, Morganti M, et al. (2011) Thymidylate synthase expression and genotype have no major impact on the clinical outcome of colorectal cancer patients treated with 5-fluorouracil. Pharmacological research: the official journal of the Italian Pharmacological Society 64: 242–248.
11. Marcuello E, Altes A, Menoyo A, Rio ED, Baiget M (2006) Methylenetetrahydrofolate reductase gene polymorphisms: genomic predictors of clinical response to fluoropyrimidine-based chemotherapy? Cancer chemotherapy and pharmacology 57: 835–840.
12. Ruzzo A, Graziano F, Loupakis F, Rulli E, Canestrari E, et al. (2007) Pharmacogenetic profiling in patients with advanced colorectal cancer treated with first-line FOLFOX-4 chemotherapy. Journal of clinical oncology: official journal of the American Society of Clinical Oncology 25: 1247–1254.
13. Cohen V, Panet-Raymond V, Sabbaghian N, Morin I, Batist G, et al. (2003) Methylenetetrahydrofolate reductase polymorphism in advanced colorectal cancer: a novel genomic predictor of clinical response to fluoropyrimidine-based chemotherapy. Clinical cancer research: an official journal of the American Association for Cancer Research 9: 1611–1615.
14. Ichikawa W, Takahashi T, Suto K, Sasaki Y, Hirayama R (2006) Orotate phosphoribosyltransferase gene polymorphism predicts toxicity in patients treated with bolus 5-fluorouracil regimen. Clinical cancer research: an official journal of the American Association for Cancer Research 12: 3928–3934.
15. Zhang H, Li YM, Jin X (2007) DPYD*5 gene mutation contributes to the reduced DPYD enzyme activity and chemotherapeutic toxicity of 5-FU: results from genotyping study on 75 gastric carcinoma and colon carcinoma patients. Med Oncol 24: 251–258.
16. Gross E, Busse B, Riemenschneider M, Neubauer S, Seck K, et al. (2008) Strong association of a common dihydropyrimidine dehydrogenase gene polymorphism with fluoropyrimidine-related toxicity in cancer patients. PloS one 3: e4003.
17. Schwab M, Zanger UM, Marx C, Schaeffeler E, Klein K, et al. (2008) Role of genetic and nongenetic factors for fluorouracil treatment-related severe toxicity: a prospective clinical trial by the German 5-FU Toxicity Study Group. Journal of clinical oncology: official journal of the American Society of Clinical Oncology 26: 2131–2138.
18. Koopman M, Venderbosch S, Nagtegaal ID, van Krieken JH, Punt CJ (2009) A review on the use of molecular markers of cytotoxic therapy for colorectal cancer, what have we learned? Eur J Cancer 45: 1935–1949.
19. Lund AH, van Lohuizen M (2002) RUNX: a trilogy of cancer genes. Cancer Cell 1: 213–215.
20. Deng T, Zhang Y (2009) 5-Aza-2'-deoxycytidine reactivates expression of RUNX3 by deletion of DNA methyltransferases leading to caspase independent apoptosis in colorectal cancer Lovo cells. Biomedicine & pharmacotherapy = Biomedecine & pharmacotherapie 63: 492–500.
21. Wang J, Ronaghi M, Chong SS, Lee CG (2011) pfSNP: An integrated potentially functional SNP resource that facilitates hypotheses generation through knowledge syntheses. Human Mutation 32: 19–24.
22. Schaib A (2012) RECIST rules. Cancer imaging: the official publication of the International Cancer Imaging Society 12: 345–346.
23. Van Cutsem E, Hoff PM, Harper P, Bukowski RM, Cunningham D, et al. (2004) Oral capecitabine vs intravenous 5-fluorouracil and leucovorin: integrated efficacy data and novel analyses from two large, randomised, phase III trials. British journal of cancer 90: 1190–1197.
24. de Gramont A, Figer A, Seymour M, Homerin M, Hmissi A, et al. (2000) Leucovorin and fluorouracil with or without oxaliplatin as first-line treatment in advanced colorectal cancer. Journal of clinical oncology: official journal of the American Society of Clinical Oncology 18: 2938–2947.
25. Kawakami K, Watanabe G (2003) Identification and functional analysis of single nucleotide polymorphism in the tandem repeat sequence of thymidylate synthase gene. Cancer Res 63: 6004–6007.
26. Kawakami K, Watanabe G (2003) Identification and functional analysis of single nucleotide polymorphism in the tandem repeat sequence of thymidylate synthase gene. Cancer research 63: 6004–6007.

27. Purcell S, Neale B, Todd-Brown K, Thomas L, Ferreira MA, et al. (2007) PLINK: a tool set for whole-genome association and population-based linkage analyses. American journal of human genetics 81: 559–575.

28. Li B, Leal SM (2008) Methods for detecting associations with rare variants for common diseases: application to analysis of sequence data. American journal of human genetics 83: 311–321.

29. Zou KH, O'Malley AJ, Mauri L (2007) Receiver-operating characteristic analysis for evaluating diagnostic tests and predictive models. Circulation 115: 654–657.

30. Patti G, Nusca A, Mangiacapra F, Gatto L, D'Ambrosio A, et al. (2008) Point-of-care measurement of clopidogrel responsiveness predicts clinical outcome in patients undergoing percutaneous coronary intervention results of the ARMYDA-PRO (Antiplatelet therapy for Reduction of MYocardial Damage during Angioplasty-Platelet Reactivity Predicts Outcome) study. Journal of the American College of Cardiology 52: 1128–1133.

31. Nagy E, Maquat LE (1998) A rule for termination-codon position within intron-containing genes: when nonsense affects RNA abundance. Trends in biochemical sciences 23: 198–199.

32. Kulshreshtha R, Ferracin M, Wojcik SE, Garzon R, Alder H, et al. (2007) A microRNA signature of hypoxia. Molecular and cellular biology 27: 1859–1867.

33. Jahid S, Sun J, Edwards RA, Dizon D, Panarelli NC, et al. (2012) miR-23a promotes the transition from indolent to invasive colorectal cancer. Cancer discovery 2: 540–553.

34. Pan Q, Fang Y, Xu Y, Zhang K, Hu X (2005) Down-regulation of DNA polymerases kappa, eta, iota, and zeta in human lung, stomach, and colorectal cancers. Cancer Letters 217: 139–147.

35. Zhang S, Chen H, Zhao X, Cao J, Tong J, et al. (2013) REV3L 3'UTR 460 T> C polymorphism in microRNA target sites contributes to lung cancer susceptibility. Oncogene 32: 242–250.

36. Adzhubei IA, Schmidt S, Peshkin L, Ramensky VE, Gerasimova A, et al. (2010) A method and server for predicting damaging missense mutations. Nature Methods 7: 248–249.

37. Sim NL, Kumar P, Hu J, Henikoff S, Schneider G, et al. (2012) SIFT web server: predicting effects of amino acid substitutions on proteins. Nucleic Acids Research 40: W452–457.

38. Soong R, Shah N, Peh BK, Chong PY, Ng SS, et al. (2009) The expression of RUNX3 in colorectal cancer is associated with disease stage and patient outcome. British Journal of Cancer 100: 676–679.

39. Potti A, Dressman HK, Bild A, Riedel RF, Chan G, et al. (2006) Genomic signatures to guide the use of chemotherapeutics. Nature Medicine 12: 1294–1300.

40. Potti A, Dressman HK, Bild A, Riedel RF, Chan G, et al. (2011) Retraction: Genomic signatures to guide the use of chemotherapeutics. Nature Medicine 17: 135.

41. Brondello JM, Pillaire MJ, Rodriguez C, Gourraud PA, Selves J, et al. (2008) Novel evidences for a tumor suppressor role of Rev3, the catalytic subunit of Pol zeta. Oncogene 27: 6093–6101.

42. Bassi C, Ho J, Srikumar T, Dowling RJ, Gorrini C, et al. (2013) Nuclear PTEN controls DNA repair and sensitivity to genotoxic stress. Science 341: 395–399.

43. Festen EA, Zhernakova A, Wijmenga C, Weersma RK (2008) Association of DLG5 variants with gluten-sensitive enteropathy. Gut 57: 1027–1028.

44. Stoll M, Corneliussen B, Costello CM, Waetzig GH, Mellgard B, et al. (2004) Genetic variation in DLG5 is associated with inflammatory bowel disease. Nature Genetics 36: 476–480.

45. Newman WG, Gu X, Wintle RF, Liu X, van Oene M, et al. (2006) DLG5 variants contribute to Crohn disease risk in a Canadian population. Human Mutation 27: 353–358.

46. Triantafillidis JK, Nasioulas G, Kosmidis PA (2009) Colorectal cancer and inflammatory bowel disease: epidemiology, risk factors, mechanisms of carcinogenesis and prevention strategies. Anticancer Research 29: 2727–2737.

47. Hirata K, Horie T (1999) Changes in intestinal absorption of 5-fluorouracil-treated rats. Pharmacology & Toxicology 85: 33–36.

48. Tran PT, Erdeniz N, Symington LS, Liskay RM (2004) EXO1-A multi-tasking eukaryotic nuclease. DNA Repair 3: 1549–1559.

49. Tomimatsu N, Mukherjee B, Deland K, Kurimasa A, Bolderson E, et al. (2012) Exo1 plays a major role in DNA end resection in humans and influences double-strand break repair and damage signaling decisions. DNA Repair 11: 441–448.

50. Webb EL, Rudd MF, Sellick GS, El Galta R, Bethke L, et al. (2006) Search for low penetrance alleles for colorectal cancer through a scan of 1467 non-synonymous SNPs in 2575 cases and 2707 controls with validation by kin-cohort analysis of 14 704 first-degree relatives. Human Molecular Genetics 15: 3263–3271.

51. Luo X, Hong XS, Xiong XD, Zeng LQ, Lim CE (2012) A single nucleotide polymorphism in EXO1 gene is associated with cervical cancer susceptibility in Chinese patients. International journal of gynecological cancer: official journal of the International Gynecological Cancer Society 22: 220–225.

52. Jin G, Wang H, Hu Z, Liu H, Sun W, et al. (2008) Potentially functional polymorphisms of EXO1 and risk of lung cancer in a Chinese population: A case-control analysis. Lung cancer 60: 340–346.

53. Chang JS, Yeh RF, Wiencke JK, Wiemels JL, Smirnov I, et al. (2008) Pathway analysis of single-nucleotide polymorphisms potentially associated with glioblastoma multiforme susceptibility using random forests. Cancer epidemiology, biomarkers & prevention: a publication of the American Association for Cancer Research, cosponsored by the American Society of Preventive Oncology 17: 1368–1373.

54. Hsu NY, Wang HC, Wang CH, Chiu CF, Tseng HC (2009) Lung cancer susceptibility and genetic polymorphisms of Exo1 gene in Taiwan. Anticancer Research 29: 725–730.

55. Tsai MH, Tseng HC, Liu CS, Chang CL, Tsai CW, et al. (2009) Interaction of Exo1 genotypes and smoking habit in oral cancer in Taiwan. Oral Oncology 45: e90–94.

56. Wang HC, Chiu CF, Tsai RY, Kuo YS, Chen HS, et al. (2009) Association of genetic polymorphisms of EXO1 gene with risk of breast cancer in Taiwan. Anticancer Research 29: 3897–3901.

57. Bau DT, Wang HC, Liu CS, Chang CL, Chiang SY, et al. (2009) Single-nucleotide polymorphism of the Exo1 gene: association with gastric cancer susceptibility and interaction with smoking in Taiwan. The Chinese journal of physiology 52: 411–418.

58. Rennert G, Rennert HS, Pinchev M, Lavie O, Gruber SB (2009) Use of hormone replacement therapy and the risk of colorectal cancer. Journal of clinical oncology: official journal of the American Society of Clinical Oncology 27: 4542–4547.

59. Martinez ME (2001) Hormone replacement therapy and adenoma recurrence: implications for its role in colorectal cancer risk. Journal of the National Cancer Institute 93: 1764–1765.

60. Nanda K, Bastian LA, Hasselblad V, Simel DL (1999) Hormone replacement therapy and the risk of colorectal cancer: a meta-analysis. Obstetrics and gynecology 93: 880–888.

61. Slattery ML, Lundgreen A, Herrick JS, Kadlubar S, Caan BJ, et al. (2011) Variation in the CYP19A1 gene and risk of colon and rectal cancer. Cancer causes & control: CCC 22: 955–963.

62. He T, Mo A, Zhang K, Liu L (2013) ABCB1/MDR1 gene polymorphism and colorectal cancer risk: a meta-analysis of case-control studies. Colorectal disease: the official journal of the Association of Coloproctology of Great Britain and Ireland 15: 12–18.

63. Potocnik U, Glavac D, Dean M (2008) Common germline MDR1/ABCB1 functional polymorphisms and haplotypes modify susceptibility to colorectal cancers with high microsatellite instability. Cancer Genet Cytogenet 183: 28–34.

64. Fusco A, Fedele M (2007) Roles of HMGA proteins in cancer. Nature reviews Cancer 7: 899–910.

Permissions

All chapters in this book were first published in PLOS ONE, by The Public Library of Science; hereby published with permission under the Creative Commons Attribution License or equivalent. Every chapter published in this book has been scrutinized by our experts. Their significance has been extensively debated. The topics covered herein carry significant findings which will fuel the growth of the discipline. They may even be implemented as practical applications or may be referred to as a beginning point for another development.

The contributors of this book come from diverse backgrounds, making this book a truly international effort. This book will bring forth new frontiers with its revolutionizing research information and detailed analysis of the nascent developments around the world.

We would like to thank all the contributing authors for lending their expertise to make the book truly unique. They have played a crucial role in the development of this book. Without their invaluable contributions this book wouldn't have been possible. They have made vital efforts to compile up to date information on the varied aspects of this subject to make this book a valuable addition to the collection of many professionals and students.

This book was conceptualized with the vision of imparting up-to-date information and advanced data in this field. To ensure the same, a matchless editorial board was set up. Every individual on the board went through rigorous rounds of assessment to prove their worth. After which they invested a large part of their time researching and compiling the most relevant data for our readers.

The editorial board has been involved in producing this book since its inception. They have spent rigorous hours researching and exploring the diverse topics which have resulted in the successful publishing of this book. They have passed on their knowledge of decades through this book. To expedite this challenging task, the publisher supported the team at every step. A small team of assistant editors was also appointed to further simplify the editing procedure and attain best results for the readers.

Apart from the editorial board, the designing team has also invested a significant amount of their time in understanding the subject and creating the most relevant covers. They scrutinized every image to scout for the most suitable representation of the subject and create an appropriate cover for the book.

The publishing team has been an ardent support to the editorial, designing and production team. Their endless efforts to recruit the best for this project, has resulted in the accomplishment of this book. They are a veteran in the field of academics and their pool of knowledge is as vast as their experience in printing. Their expertise and guidance has proved useful at every step. Their uncompromising quality standards have made this book an exceptional effort. Their encouragement from time to time has been an inspiration for everyone.

The publisher and the editorial board hope that this book will prove to be a valuable piece of knowledge for researchers, students, practitioners and scholars across the globe.

List of Contributors

Kwon Joong Yong, Diane E. Milenic, Kwamena E. Baidoo, Martin W. Brechbiel
Radioimmune & Inorganic Chemistry Section, Radiation Oncology Branch, National Cancer Institute, National Institutes of Health, Bethesda, Maryland, United States of America

Long Gu, Shanna Smith, Caroline Li and Linda H. Malkas
Department of Molecular & Cellular Biology, Beckman Research Institute of City of Hope, Duarte, California, United States of America

Robert J. Hickey
Department of Molecular Pharmacology, Beckman Research Institute of City of Hope, Duarte, California, United States of America

Jeremy M. Stark
Department of Radiation Biology, Beckman Research Institute of City of Hope, Duarte, California, United States of America

Gregg B. Fields
Torrey Pines Institute for Molecular Studies, Port St. Lucie, Florida, United States of America

Walter H. Lang and John A. Sandoval
Department of Surgery, St. Jude Children's Research Hospital, Memphis, Tennessee, United States of America

Haina Du, Nannan Guo, Qian Zhang, Yongqian Shu and Lingjun Zhu
Department of Oncology, The First Affiliated Hospital of Nanjing Medical University, Nanjing, China

Bin Shi, Kai Lu and Tao Chen
Department of Gastrointestinal Surgery, The First Affiliated Hospital of Nanjing Medical University, Nanjing, China

Zhipeng Chen
Department of Oncology, The first people's Hospital of Zhangjiagang City, Suzhou, China

Samir Acharya, Zeenia Kaul, April Sandy Gocha, Alaina R. Martinez, Julia Harris, Jeffrey D. Parvin and Joanna Groden
Department of Molecular Virology, Immunology and Medical Genetics, College of Medicine, The Ohio State University, Columbus, Ohio, United States of America

Na Deng
Tumor Etiology and Screening Department of Cancer Institute and General Surgery, the First Affiliated Hospital of China Medical University, and Key Laboratory of Cancer Etiology and Prevention (China Medical University), Liaoning Provincial Education Department, Shenyang, China
Department of Oncology, The Fourth Affiliated Hospital of China Medical University, Liaoning, Shenyang, China

Jing-wei Liu, Li-ping Sun, Qian Xu, Zhi-Peng Duan, Nan-Nan Dong and Yuan Yuan
Tumor Etiology and Screening Department of Cancer Institute and General Surgery, the First Affiliated Hospital of China Medical University, and Key Laboratory of Cancer Etiology and Prevention (China Medical University), Liaoning Provincial Education Department, Shenyang, China

Martyn K. White, Rafal Kaminski, Kamel Khalili and Hassen S. Wollebo
Center for Neurovirology, Department of Neuroscience, Temple University School of Medicine, Philadelphia, Pennsylvania, United States of America

Jinhua Zhou
Department of Obstetrics and Gynecology, Renji Hospital, School of Medicine, Shanghai Jiao Tong University, Shanghai, China
Shanghai Key Laboratory of Gynecologic Oncology, Shanghai, China
Focus Construction Subject of Shanghai Education Department, Shanghai, China
Shanghai Health Bureau Key Disciplines and Specialties Foundation, Shanghai, China
Department of Obstetrics and Gynecology, The First Affiliated Hospital of Soochow University, Suzhou, Jiangsu, China

Yunfei Wang and Wen Di
Department of Obstetrics and Gynecology, Renji Hospital, School of Medicine, Shanghai Jiao Tong University, Shanghai, China
Shanghai Key Laboratory of Gynecologic Oncology, Shanghai, China
Focus Construction Subject of Shanghai Education Department, Shanghai, China
Shanghai Health Bureau Key Disciplines and Specialties Foundation, Shanghai, China

You Wang, Xia Yin, Yifeng He, Lilan Chen, Wenwen Wang and Ting Liu
Department of Obstetrics and Gynecology, Renji Hospital, School of Medicine, Shanghai Jiao Tong University, Shanghai, China
Shanghai Key Laboratory of Gynecologic Oncology, Shanghai, China

Xiaoling Wang, Tammy Chang and Jiing-Kuan Yee
Department of Virology, Beckman Research Institute of City of Hope, Duarte, California, United States of America

Yingjia Wang
Department of Virology, Beckman Research Institute of City of Hope, Duarte, California, United States of America
Bone Marrow Transplantation Center, The First Affiliated Hospital, Zhejiang University, Hangzhou, Zhejiang, China

He Huang
Bone Marrow Transplantation Center, The First Affiliated Hospital, Zhejiang University, Hangzhou, Zhejiang, China

Buyuan Chen and Xinji Chen
Department of Molecular and Cellular Biology, Beckman Research Institute of City of Hope, Duarte, California, United States of America
Department of Hematology, Union Hospital of Fujian Medical University, Fuzhou, Fujian, China

Jianda Hu
Department of Hematology, Union Hospital of Fujian Medical University, Fuzhou, Fujian, China

Ren-Jang Lin
Department of Molecular and Cellular Biology, Beckman Research Institute of City of Hope, Duarte, California, United States of America

Kendric Wang, Alexander W. Wyatt and Anna Lapuk
Vancouver Prostate Centre, Vancouver General Hospital, Vancouver, Canada

Raunak Shrestha
Vancouver Prostate Centre, Vancouver General Hospital, Vancouver, Canada
CIHR/MSHFR Bioinformatics Training Program, University of British Columbia, Vancouver, Canada

Anupama Reddy and Joseph Lehár
Novartis Pharmaceuticals, Oncology Division, Basal, Switzerland

Yuzhou Wang and Colin C. Collins
Vancouver Prostate Centre, Vancouver General Hospital, Vancouver, Canada
Department of Urologic Sciences, the University of British Columbia, Vancouver, Canada

Lalita A. Shevde
University of Alabama at Birmingham, Birmingham, Alabama, United States of America

Erhong Meng, Aparna Mitra, Kaushlendra Tripathi, Michael A. Finan, Jennifer Scalici, Steve McClellan, Luciana Madeira da Silva, Komaraiah Palle and Rodney P. Rocconi
University of South Alabama Mitchell Cancer Institute, Mobile, Alabama, United States of America

Eddie Reed
National Institutes of Health, National Institute on Minority Health and Health Disparities, Bethesda, Maryland, United States of America

Thomas Pavelitz
Department of Immunology, University of Washington, Seattle, Washington, United States of America
Department of Chemistry, University of Washington, Seattle, Washington, United States of America

Lindsay Renfro
Division of Biomedical Statistics and Informatics, Mayo Clinic, Rochester, Minnesota, United States of America
Department of Chemistry, University of Washington, Seattle, Washington, United States of America

Nathan R. Foster
Division of Biomedical Statistics and Informatics, Mayo Clinic, Rochester, Minnesota, United States of America

Amber Caracol
Department of Immunology, University of Washington, Seattle, Washington, United States of America
Molecular and Cellular Biology Graduate Program, University of Washington, Seattle, Washington, United States of America

Piri Welsch
Department of Genome Sciences, University of Washington Medical School, Seattle, Washington, United States of America

Victoria Valinluck Lao
Clinical Research Division, Fred Hutchinson Cancer Research Center, Seattle, Washington, United States of America
Department of Surgery, University of Washington Medical School, Seattle, Washington, United States of America

William B. Grady
Clinical Research Division, Fred Hutchinson Cancer Research Center, Seattle, Washington, United States of America
Department of Medicine, University of Washington Medical School, Seattle, Washington, United States of America

Donna Niedzwiecki
Cancer and Leukemia Group B Statistical Center, Duke University Medical Center, Durham, North Carolina, United States of America

Leonard B. Saltz
Memorial Sloan-Kettering Cancer Center, New York, New York, United States of America

Monica M. Bertagnolli
Dana-Farber Cancer Institute and Brigham and Women's Hospital, Boston, Massachusetts, United States of America

Richard M. Goldberg
The Ohio State University, Columbus, Ohio, United States of America

Peter S. Rabinovitch
Department of Pathology, University of Washington Medical School, Seattle, Washington, United States of America

Mary Emond
Department of Biostatistics, University of Washington, Seattle, Washington, United States of America

Raymond J. Monnat Jr.
Department of Genome Sciences, University of Washington Medical School, Seattle, Washington, United States of America
Department of Pathology, University of Washington Medical School, Seattle, Washington, United States of America

Nancy Maizels
Department of Immunology, University of Washington, Seattle, Washington, United States of America
Molecular and Cellular Biology Graduate Program, University of Washington, Seattle, Washington, United States of America
Department of Pathology, University of Washington Medical School, Seattle, Washington, United States of America
Department of Biochemistry, University of Washington, Seattle, Washington, United States of America

Irfan Khan, Avvaru N. Suhasini, Taraswi Banerjee, Joshua A. Sommers and Robert M. Brosh, Jr.
Laboratory of Molecular Gerontology, National Institute on Aging, National Institutes of Health, NIH Biomedical Research Center, Baltimore, Maryland, United States of America

Daniel L. Kaplan
Department of Biomedical Sciences, Florida State University College of Medicine, Tallahassee, Florida, United States of America

Jochen Kuper and Caroline Kisker
Rudolf Virchow Center for Experimental Biomedicine, Institute for Structural Biology, University of Würzburg, Würzburg, Germany

Jing Yang and Xiangyin Kong
The Key Laboratory of Stem Cell Biology, Institute of Health Sciences, Shanghai Jiao Tong University School of Medicine (SJTUSM) and Shanghai Institutes for Biological Sciences (SIBS), Chinese Academy of Sciences (CAS), Shanghai, People's Republic of China

Lei Chen
College of Information Engineering, Shanghai Maritime University, Shanghai, People's Republic of China

Tao Huang
Department of Genetics and Genomic Sciences, Mount Sinai School of Medicine, New York, New York, United States of America,

Yu-Dong Cai
Institute of Systems Biology, Shanghai University, Shanghai, People's Republic of China

Chaoyang Sun, Na Li, Dong Ding, Danhui Weng, Li Meng, Gang Chen and Ding Ma
Department of Obstetrics and Gynaecology, Tongji Hospital, Tongji Medical College, Huazhong University of Science and Technology, Wuhan, Hubei, China

Zalman Vaksman, Natalie C. Fonville and Hongseok Tae
Virginia Bioinformatics Institute, Virginia Tech, Blacksburg, Virginia, 24061, United States of America

Harold R. Garner
Virginia Bioinformatics Institute, Virginia Tech, Blacksburg, Virginia, 24061, United States of America
Genomeon LLC, Floyd, Virginia, 24091, United States of America

Li-Wen He1,2.,
1 Institute of Genetic Engineering, Southern Medical University, Guangzhou, China
2 Zhujiang Hospital, Southern Medical University, Guangzhou, China

Rong Shi1., Wen-Li Ma1, Jue-Yu Zhou1*
1 Institute of Genetic Engineering, Southern Medical University, Guangzhou, China

Lei Jiang
Department of Neurosurgery, Changzheng Hospital, Second Military Medical University, Shanghai, China

Ye Zeng
Department of Stomatology, Nanfang Hospital, Southern Medical University, Guangzhou, China

Elise Darmon, John K. Eykelenboom, Manuel A. Lopez-Vernaza, Martin A. White and David R. F. Leach
Institute of Cell Biology, University of Edinburgh, Edinburgh, United Kingdom

Jingbo Wang
Department of Biochemistry, Yong Loo Lin School of Medicine, National University of Singapore, Singapore, Singapore

Xu Wang and Yik Ying Teo
Saw Swee Hock School of Public Health, National University of Singapore, Singapore, Singapore

Mingjue Zhao and Samuel S. Chong
Department of Paediatrics, Yong Loo Lin School of Medicine, National University of Singapore, Singapore, Singapore

Su Pin Choo, Sin Jen Ong and Simon Y. K. Ong
Division of Medical Oncology, National Cancer Centre, Singapore, Singapore

Caroline G. L. Lee
Department of Biochemistry, Yong Loo Lin School of Medicine, National University of Singapore, Singapore, Singapore
Division of Medical Sciences, National Cancer Centre, Singapore, Singapore
Duke-NUS Graduate Medical School, Singapore, Singapore

Index

www.ingramcontent.com/pod-product-compliance
Lightning Source LLC
Chambersburg PA
CBHW082050190326
41458CB00010B/3498